"Shattered Nerves"

"Shattered Nerves"

Doctors, Patients, and Depression in Victorian England

JANET OPPENHEIM

New York   Oxford
OXFORD UNIVERSITY PRESS
1991

Oxford University Press

Oxford   New York   Toronto
Delhi   Bombay   Calcutta   Madras   Karachi
Petaling Jaya   Singapore   Hong Kong   Tokyo
Nairobi   Dar es Salaam   Cape Town
Melbourne   Auckland

and associated companies in
Berlin   Ibadan

Published by Oxford University Press, Inc.,
200 Madison Avenue, New York, New York 10016

Oxford is a registered trademark of Oxford University Press

Library of Congress Cataloging-in-Publication Data
Oppenheim, Janet, 1948–
"Shattered nerves" : doctors, patients, and depression
in Victorian England / Janet Oppenheim.
p. cm.   Includes index.
ISBN 0–19–505781–3
1. Depression, Mental—England—History—19th century.
2. Depression, Mental—Patients—England—Biography.
3. Depression, Mental—Treatment—England—History—19th century.   I. Title.
RC537.066   1991   616.85'27'0094209034—dc20   90–39361

1 3 5 7 9 8 6 4 2

Printed in the United States of America
on acid-free paper

To the memory of Stephen Koss

ACKNOWLEDGMENTS

To derive pleasure from writing a book about depression perhaps reveals something unfortunate about my character, but during the near decade that I have spent thinking about the subject, I have received so much generous assistance that the experience proved immensely rewarding.

The American Philosophical Society, the National Endowment for the Humanities, the John Simon Guggenheim Memorial Foundation, and the College of Arts and Sciences Faculty Development Grant, from the American University, Washington, D.C., all provided help of a most concrete sort—the means first to pursue research abroad and then to stay at home writing. The American University allowed me to remain on leave for two consecutive years, for which I am most grateful and without which this manuscript would have taken far longer than a decade to transform itself into a book.

I would like to thank the staff of the Cambridge University Library for unfailingly prompt and courteous help during several months of research in its splendidly accessible collections. Mrs. C. J. Anderson, at the Library, University College London; H. M. Young, at the University of London Library; Richard Palmer, curator of Western Manuscripts, and Lesley Hall, assistant archivist, at the Wellcome Institute for the History of Medicine, London; Geoffrey Davenport, librarian, Royal College of Physicians, London; Vincent Giroud, curator of Modern Books and Manuscripts, at the Beinecke Rare Book and Manuscript Library, Yale University; Hildegard Stephans, at the Library of the American Philosophical Society, Philadelphia; and Thomas A. Horrocks, curator, Historical Collections of the Library, at the College of Physicians of Philadelphia, helped me to find manuscripts and obscure periodicals, or made photocopies for me, in a way that deserves my fullest acknowledgment. They immeasurably facilitated my work. Florence Goff, reference librarian, Bryn Mawr College—the closest library facility when I am working at home—was always ready with assistance.

A topic like depression sparks discussion wherever it goes, and I have been fortunate in the comments and advice elicited in conversation and correspondence with Robert Beisner, Saul Benison, Ronald Berger, William F. Bynum, Geoffrey Cantor, Jane Caplan, LeAnn Davis, John Eyler, Valerie French, Martha Garland, Alan Kraut, W. C. Lubenow, Mark S. Micale, Jane Oppenheimer, Martin Pernick, M. Jeanne Peterson, Dale Smith, F. B. Smith, Richard Soloway, Susan Thomas, Judith Walkowitz, Anthony Wohl, and J. H. Woodward. I am very grateful to them all, and to Lucy McDiarmid, for showing me splendid allusions to the nerves in the work of Jane Austen, D. H. Lawrence, and T. S. Eliot.

Permission to quote from documents in their collections or from copyrighted material is acknowledged with thanks from the following individuals, institutions, and publishers: Dr. Sarah Pearson, for Maria Sharpe's "Autobiographical Notes on 'Men & Women's Club' "; the Beinecke Rare Book and Manuscript Library, Yale University, for letters from Maria La Touche in the George MacDonald Papers; the Syndics of Cambridge University Library, for letters to and from James Crichton-Browne in Charles Darwin's correspondence; the Royal College of Physicians of London, for material in the William Baly Manuscripts; the University of London Library and the Athenaeum, for documents in the Herbert Spencer Papers; the Trustees of the Victoria and Albert Museum, for a letter in Edwin Landseer's correspondence; Clarendon Press of Oxford University Press, for excerpts from Van Akin Burd, ed., *John Ruskin and Rose La Touche: Her Unpublished Diaries of 1861 and 1867* (1979); Random House, Inc., and Century Hutchinson, Ltd., for excerpts from *The Memoirs of John Addington Symonds,* edited by Phyllis Grosskurth, copyright © 1984 by The London Library; the Belknap Press of Harvard University Press and Virago Press Ltd., for excerpts from *The Diary of Beatrice Webb,* Vol. 1: *1873–1892, "Glitter Around and Darkness Within,"* edited by Norman MacKenzie and Jeanne MacKenzie, editorial matter and arrangement © 1982, 1983, 1984 by Norman and Jeanne MacKenzie, and The Diary of Beatrice Webb, The Passfield Papers © 1982, 1983, 1984 by the London School of Economics and Political Science; Viking Penguin, Inc., for an excerpt from *The Daughters of Karl Marx: Family Correspondence 1866–1898,* edited by Olga Meier and translated by Faith Evans (1984).

Ashley Minihan, my daughter, grew up while I was writing this book. Although she could not read when I began the research for it, she was finding wonderful quotations about the nerves in her own reading before I finished it. All the references to Sherlock Holmes are thanks to her. It has been a very great pleasure to have her as a collaborator. As for my husband, J. H. M. Salmon, this book simply owes more to him than I can calculate.

Twenty years ago, when I began my graduate studies at Columbia University, I did not intend to become a Victorianist, but Stephen Koss made the subject irresistible. Some fifteen years or so into my own career as a college teacher, he still seems to me the model of everything a mentor is supposed to be. This book is dedicated to his memory, with gratitude.

Washington, D.C.   J. O.
June 1990

CONTENTS

"Shattered Nerves"

INTRODUCTION

The Enigma of "Nervous Breakdown"

> One night he went to bed late, and found it difficult to sleep; thoughts raced through his brain, scenes and images forming and reforming with inconceivable rapidity; at last he fell asleep, to awake an hour or two later in an intolerable agony of mind. His heart beat thick and fast, and a shapeless horror seemed to envelop him. He struck a light and tried to read, but a ghastly and poisonous fear of he knew not what seemed to clutch at his mind. At last he fell into a broken sleep; but when he rose in the morning, he knew that some mysterious evil had befallen him. . . . For that day and for many days he wrestled with a fierce blackness of depression.[1]

The experience of nervous breakdown, vividly recalled by the writer Arthur Christopher Benson in this passage from *Beside Still Waters,* published in 1907, achieved a significance in Victorian culture that went far beyond the substantial interest bestowed by the medical profession on so perplexing and elusive an illness. The nerves and their disorders were inextricably interwoven with nineteenth-century British assumptions about more than health and illness, or normalcy and deviance; they were interlaced with attitudes toward success and failure, civilization and barbarism, order and chaos, masculinity and femininity. Just as nerves pervaded the physical body, so did they permeate the images with which the Victorians evoked their society. Nerves existed physiologically and metaphorically, conjuring up complicated and sometimes contradictory associations. Occasionally conveying an idea of courage and vigor, they more often stood for fragility and weakness. They suggested sensitivity, sympathy, and, above all, a suffering that frequently defied medical knowledge and curative skill. "You say truly," the author John Addington Symonds wrote to a friend in 1868, "that when people talk of 'Hell' they often mean a state of their nerves. Is there anything after all that is not a mode of the human nervous system—at least to human beings?"[2]

Nervous breakdown, a popular name for incapacitating depression, is not a specific disease that can be traced to a single cause. It is an abstract concept, encompassing many symptoms that vary from one patient to another, with invariably devastating effect. The characteristic sense of overwhelming hopelessness, emptiness, impotence, and uselessness, the incapacity to focus attention or reach decisions, the obsessive thoughts and fears, the diminished self-esteem, the extreme lethargy, and the inability to take interest or pleasure in any aspect of life make existence scarcely tolerable. Insomnia, weight loss, excruciating headaches, and other bodily pains typically exacerbate the patient's suffering. The illness may attack suddenly, overnight, heralded by sleeplessness or nightmares. Symonds's breakdown early in 1863 began with the dream of a helpless old man being clubbed to death. He awoke the next morning "with the certainty that something serious had happened to [his] brain."[3] In other cases, the symptoms encroach gradually on their victims' peace of mind, over a period of weeks or even months. Readers of Victorian diaries, letters, and fiction will recognize the condition, which often relegated once vigorous men and women to an invalid's sofa or sent them on prolonged travels in search of renewed vitality.

This book attempts to ascertain what nervous breakdown meant to the Victorians, both to patients who experienced the baffling disorder and to medical practitioners who tried to treat it. Such a malady, which respected no barriers of class, age, or gender, is particularly informative about the place that medicine assumed in Victorian culture, and, with its ill-defined physiological contours, nervous breakdown serves to underscore the significance of social influences in the perpetual drama enacted between those who dispensed and those who received medical advice. In recent years, historians of medicine have emphasized the extent to which any form of illness is the product of interaction between biological reality and shifting cultural perspectives. Public perceptions of disease are never merely reactions to discoveries of microbes, toxins, or genes; they are molded, too, by systems of values, ethical codes, religious beliefs, and all manner of preconceived opinion. Scientists and medical doctors, belonging integrally to the public thus affected, share many of its biases and expectations. Their pronouncements are not objective, or free of implicit moral judgment, for science and medicine are interpretative endeavors into which the surrounding social context constantly intrudes. The Victorians developed an ambiguous and shifting response to nervous breakdown, the reasons for which this study attempts to explain.

In somatic diseases, an underlying physiological condition exists regardless of the way people apprehend it. Since the second half of the nineteenth century, as information about the human body has increased in depth and detail, as biomedical research has revealed the agents that cause diverse bodily afflictions, and as pharmaceutical companies have devised means to combat some of them, the physiological foundations have assumed greater importance in comprehending physical disorders than the social myths that accumulate around the sickbed. The same cannot be said of psychiatric disorders, in which cultural imperatives still play a paramount defining role in the absence of any sure knowledge of causation. At the end of the twentieth century, neurologists have gained impressive insight into the cerebral basis of mental illness, but Victorian medical practitioners could only hypothesize about the connection between mind and body. As a result, pressures and prejudices that had nothing to do with medical science impinged all the more heavily on interpretations of mental distress. It is one thing, however, to observe that Victorian medical men lacked the instruments to prove the dependence of mind on body, and quite another to assume that mental illness was a figment of their collective imagination. If it is misleading to depict sickness as a medical absolute, untouched by ideology, economics, and social circumstances, it is equally wrong to insist that the cultural construction known as psychiatric illness lacks foundation in real mental pain—in states of confusion, disorientation, wild excitement, or acute misery. The Victorians who endured nervous breakdown were tormented by something amiss within themselves that destroyed, at least for a time, all chance of happiness or serenity. The way they reacted to the experience, and the way people reacted to them, reflected the circumstances of their lives in nineteenth-century England, but the underlying condition of crippling despair has plagued the human race throughout the annals of medicine.

While medical practitioners today address the problems of "depression," their Victorian predecessors employed a more picturesque vocabulary to designate the same ailment. They spoke of shattered nerves or broken health; they conjured up images of nervous collapse, exhaustion, or prostration, and toward the end of the nineteenth century they brandished a new label—neurasthenia. The term *nervous breakdown* was not itself much employed until the late Victorian period; in earlier decades *breakdown* was more commonly used alone, without a modifier. These diagnostic names evoke striking pictures of ravage and destruction, but they raise serious problems for the historian who may easily misinterpret them a century later. Some sad tales of "breakdown" and "broken health" turn out, on close scrutiny, to signify the onset of pulmonary tuberculosis, a bout of rheumatic fever, or the depredations of some other identifiable somatic disease.

Nor is it always possible to ascertain the severity of the depression afflicting men and women in the nineteenth century. Today, psychiatrists call *dysthymia* the chronic, but milder, forms of depression that rarely require hospitalization,[4] but their Victorian forebears frequently made no clear distinction between the lesser and greater, the chronic and acute, varieties. They and their patients used phrases like "nervous exhaustion" and "nervous collapse" loosely, sometimes indicating a condition of dullness, inertia, pessimism, and deep unhappiness that nonetheless permitted the victim to function and, at other times, describing complete paralysis of the will. Manifestations of depression, furthermore, can be thoroughly appropriate responses to tragic events in life, or so utterly out of proportion to their causes as to demand medical attention. "It is not natural to burst into tears because a fly settles on the forehead, as I have known a melancholic man do," a leading Victorian psychiatrist sagely remarked.[5] This study focuses on the graver examples of Victorian depression, but, with the boundaries so difficult to place, less severe cases have unavoidably been caught in its net as well.

So have occasional diagnoses of hysteria and hypochondriasis, two disorders that appeared prominently in Victorian medical parlance and were frequently confounded with shattered nerves. Nineteenth-century medical literature abounded with efforts to delineate the defining characteristics of each of the three maladies, but with little success. All were assumed to have a physiological foundation, but since each featured changes in mood and behavior, medical commentators acknowledged their psychological aspects as well. Victorian interpretations hovered uncertainly between the physical and the mental; doctors were never sure whether to treat these illnesses with medicines aimed at restoring the body or with moral exhortations designed to rally the mind and return the will to its proper function. Hypochondriasis has become hypochondria today, a purely psychological, and relatively harmless, condition of undue anxiety about one's health; hysteria has been subsumed under the capacious category of psychosomatic disorders, although neither psychiatry nor neurology has yet produced a satisfactory explanation of its bizarre symptoms, which imitate those of many organic diseases. Depression, of course, remains in the forefront of medical inquiry.

The boundary dispute with insanity was the one that most urgently challenged Victorian medical men who treated depressed patients. No one expected a distinct line of demarcation, for it was a commonplace of British psychological medicine throughout the period that soundness of mind merged imperceptibly with unsoundness. Lunacy in its most pronounced form was recognizable enough, but borderline mental states posed particular problems. The melancholy that dominated most cases of nervous breakdown was precisely such a condition, and Victorian taxonomies of madness typically stumbled over its classification. Melancholy, not in itself deemed pathological, could become so profoundly disabling that the patient seemed to have lost the capacity to reason—to have fallen into "melancholia," which *was* considered morbid and classified as a distinct form of mental alienation. Mad-doctors in these decades never reached a consensus concerning melancholy/melancholia. One school of thought interpreted melancholia as merely an intensification of "normal grief and low spirits," while another insisted that it was an unnatural reaction, qualitatively different from more moderate forms of sorrow and despondency. Advocates of the second viewpoint emphasized the presence of delusions, and even hallucinations, in melancholia, which indicated, as they argued, its unquestionable kinship with madness. Samuel Johnson was a convenient case from the past for Victorians to ponder: a man hounded by morbid obsessions, he was held to exemplify some intermediate position neither wholly sane nor certifiably insane.[6]

Many Victorians viewed nervous exhaustion in much the same light. Although, in theory, it was not a form of mental illness, but a disorder of the nervous system, most British medical men during the nineteenth century acknowledged extreme difficulty in separating the two kinds of afflictions. "Practically," Daniel Noble, a Manchester doctor, commented in 1853, "it is always difficult to draw the boundary line between what are commonly considered purely Nervous maladies, and diseases of the Mind, on account of the connection subsisting amongst all the nervous centres and the correlated psychical states."[7] That connection occurred, of course, in the brain, whose function as coordinator of the nervous system and organ of the mind made any precise discrimination between mental and nervous illness impossible for Victorians to establish.

Both doctors and patients knew that nervous breakdown did not necessarily undermine the ability to think coherently. Benson, describing a long spell of depression that preyed on him between 1907 and 1909 stressed precisely the clarity of mind that added to his pain: "Neurasthenia, hypochondria, melancholia—hideous names for hideous things—it was these, or one of these. The symptoms a persistent sleeplessness, a perpetual dejection, amounting at times to an intolerable mental anguish. The mind perfectly unclouded and absolutely hopeless." Michael Faraday's Victorian biographer, Henry Bence Jones, likewise insisted that, during the renowned physicist's breakdown in the early 1840s, he wrote letters that were "free from the slightest sign of mental disease." Like Benson and Faraday, the other victims of depression who appear in this book were all fully aware of their plight and, if so inclined, could discuss their condition with great penetration and lucidity. They were, as a psychiatrist who studied their malady commented at the end of the nineteenth century, "perfectly sane persons who are horribly depressed."[8]

Recognizing the disorder and talking or writing about it with memorable vividness did not, however, always preclude some degree of mental derangement. If mental illness, beyond the narrow legal definition of knowing right from wrong, has been traditionally understood as "disturbance of the reason, judgment, or imagination,"[9] nervous breakdown could certainly involve mental illness. Severely depressed patients frequently revealed totally unwarranted fears of financial ruin or the expectation of professional disgrace, which could not be allayed by any reassurance to the contrary. In the early 1860s, John Tulloch, principal of St. Andrews, experienced a nervous breakdown that was much aggravated by the recollection of an erroneous Latin quotation embedded in a speech he had delivered to his fellow Scottish theologians. The glee with which a particular Scottish newspaper seized on the inadequacies of Tulloch's classical training should have hardly sufficed to keep a widely respected religious scholar in numbing despair for nearly a year. Margaret Oliphant, the versatile author who was also his friend and biographer, wisely concluded that the incident had not in itself precipitated Tulloch's illness, but merely aggravated a liability to depression already undermining the tranquillity of his mind. Such an irrational reaction was not actually tantamount to insanity, but Oliphant regarded Tulloch as a man goaded "to the verge of madness," who, for a time, all but crossed that brink.[10] The doctors who attended men like Tulloch fully acknowledged their precarious hold on sanity and worried that, if prolonged, nervous exhaustion could gradually become complete alienation of reason. For the patients themselves, the dread of going mad was not the least of their agonies.

A considerable area of ambiguity between psychological illness and physiological disorder thus deeply perplexed Victorian medical practitioners. They managed to conceal, perhaps even to themselves, the cracks in the theoretical structure of their expertise by employing obscure terminology, which, when adopted in due course by their patients, spread the confusion in ever-expanding circles throughout society. The notion of "partial insanity," for example, attempted to account for individuals who appeared completely irrational in certain aspects of their thought or behavior, but unexceptionally sane in others. The diagnosis of "mental breakdown," paradoxically suggesting the physical destruction of the metaphysical mind, similarly masked profound medical uncertainty. Sometimes the phrase signified an irrevocable descent into madness; sometimes, merely temporary lapses into incoherence or highly eccentric conduct; and at still other times, it seems to have been used interchangeably with "nervous exhaustion" accompanied by slightly disordered thought, which vanished with the patient's recovery. "Those who have not suffered from mental breakdown," Francis Galton, the freelance scientific polymath, wrote in his memoirs, "can hardly realise the incapacity it causes, or, when the worst is past, the closeness of analogy between a sprained brain and a sprained joint."[11] The difficulty of encapsulating his own experience of depression in a brief, vigorous phrase prompted Galton to employ the vocabulary of corporeal injury. It was an effort to give substance to an illness that persistently eluded physiological analysis in the nineteenth century—much as it continues to escape from the historian's confining definitions today.

Of all the labels that Victorian medical men applied to the vast number of indeterminate nervous and mental maladies they examined, the two most frequently invoked were *neurosis* and its synonym, *functional nervous disorder*. In the late twentieth century, the terms *neurosis* and *neurotic* have passed into popular usage to designate purely psychological "hang ups" that clearly pertain to the psychiatrist's domain. Throughout the nineteenth century, however, the concept of neurosis belonged to the emerging fields of psychiatry and neurology alike. The name and the idea were the contributions of William Cullen, a prominent professor of medicine at the University of Edinburgh in the latter half of the eighteenth century. Building on the work of Thomas Willis and Thomas Sydenham, eminent British physicians of the preceding century, Cullen classified diseases in such a way that the neuroses constituted a principal category—one which embraced all disorders presumed to involve the nervous system, but occurring without any evidence whatsoever of structural change, inflammation, or lesion.[12] Cullen's class of neuroses encompassed all the mental illnesses of his day, including such diverse forms of insanity as mania, dementia, and melancholia. It also embraced diseases whose physical causes, unknown at the time, have since been wholly or partially identified, like poliomyelitis, diabetes, and epilepsy. It included, too, the puzzling conditions of hysteria, hypochondriasis, migraine, neuralgia, convulsions, and nervous exhaustion, among others.

By categorizing such disparate ailments as neuroses, or functional nervous disorders, Cullen and his nineteenth-century successors were, in effect, suspending judgment about their origins. They could not be designated structural disorders of the nervous system because their anatomical basis had not been located, but the Victorian medical profession nonetheless anticipated that scientific research would eventually reveal the physical agents responsible for these manifold disturbances. Indeed, by the final quarter of the nineteenth century, the list of neuroses was beginning to shrink in response to discoveries in bacteriology. In 1882, for example, the first edition of the authoritative *Dictionary of Medicine,* edited by Sir Richard Quain, enumerated tetanus among the neuroses. When the second, revised, edition appeared in 1894, that disease had been dropped from the list, for its pathogenic microbe had been isolated in the interim.[13] Right down to World War I, however, nervous breakdown remained firmly ensconced among the functional nervous disorders, along with other unsolved medical mysteries, like hysteria and migraine. It is true that some British medical men by the turn of the century were speculating that disorders still classified as neuroses might prove to have no somatic foundation, and that "the description 'functional' really means 'psychic,' just as 'organic' means 'physical,' "[14] but few were willing to endorse an unequivocally psychological interpretation of maladies long assumed to have their origin in the functions of the nerves. Most of the medical profession preferred to keep their choices open, hoping that some yet unstudied physiological process or some still elusive microorganism would in future bring the neuroses clearly within the company of somatic diseases, which they considered the legitimate realm of medicine. They regarded the division of nervous disorders into structural and functional largely as a provisional expedient, and they valued the latter as a catch-all classification, despite the confession of medical uncertainty implicit in its very name.

The words *nervous* and *nervousness* themselves scarcely concealed broad expanses of medical ignorance, as some doctors were candid enough to admit throughout the Victorian era. "Many diseases," observed Thomas Smethurst, who presided over a hydropathic establishment at Ramsgate in the 1840s, "are denominated nervous, purely nervous, with which the nervous system—the animal functions, namely, the external and internal senses, the involuntary action of the muscles, &c.,—has little to do; but the causes being difficult to define, the general, significant, and yet often unmeaning, term of nervous affection, 'nervous weakness,' is applied." Fifty years later, no less a figure that T. Clifford Allbutt, regius professor of medicine at Cambridge, issued virtually the same criticism when he complained that "the so-called diseases of the nervous system" were "a vast, vague, and most heterogeneous body, two-thirds of which may not primarily consist of diseases of nervous matter at all."[15] In different Victorian hands, nervous clearly meant different things. Its strict usage referred only to the structure and activities of the nerves, but the popular meaning dealt with personality traits and conveyed the idea of edginess, agitation, and irritability. This broader connotation was not intended to deny the likelihood that such instability arose from the nerves, but, as the century drew to a close, the continuing failure to identify the physical bases of numerous neurotic illnesses encouraged the facile equation of nervous with "emotional" or "psychological." By then, Cullen's convenient umbrella category of neuroses was falling apart.

During Victoria's reign, the nascent psychiatric branch of British medicine, specializing in the treatment of mental alienation, had no monopoly on alleviating a malady that was believed to harbor hidden somatic roots. Every variety of medical attendant, from the family doctor to the costly specialist, encountered cases of shattered nerves and offered advice about their cure. Functional nervous disorders did, however, offer particular enticements to the alienists, as Victorian mad-doctors came to be called. Their efforts to expand their practice, from the lunatic asylums where psychiatry was born to the prestigious consulting rooms of fashionable London, depended heavily on their claim to skillful handling of neurotic illness that did not require institutionalization. The professional development and aspirations of British alienists provide a recurrent motif throughout this book, although I do not offer anything like a history of Victorian psychiatry. The prominent part taken by alienists in treating severe depression means that I have been obliged to devote more space to insanity than I intended when initially planning the study. Not only did nervous breakdown sometimes approach madness in the intensity of its disorientation, but many of the consultants who ministered to nervous prostration among the affluent in the second half of the nineteenth century began their careers as medical officers among pauper lunatics in public asylums and derived most of their views on mental illness from that experience.

Considerations of gender and class further complicated the difficulties that Victorian alienists and their medical colleagues faced in diagnosing nervous breakdown. They responded differently to male and female patients with shattered nerves, while the medical theories behind the forms of treatment they applied also varied considerably from men to women. Doctors' opinions altered, too, with the social status of the sufferer. They rarely hesitated to diagnose insanity in a working-class lunatic, but were sensitive to the implications of that label in families with social pretensions and, in order to spare them humiliation, might call "nervous collapse" what were, in fact, the inroads of madness. (The same misleading diagnosis could similarly conceal advanced stages of alcoholism or syphilis.) Whether one diagnosed nervous breakdown or insanity was, obviously, not an abstract academic exercise; the decision profoundly influenced not merely the patient's experience of illness, but likewise his or her standing in the family and in the eyes of the law. There was not, however, any exact alignment of psychiatric diagnoses and social class—madness for the masses and nervous collapse for their social superiors. Victorian medical men, for the most part, acknowledged the presence of severe depression among the working classes and, equally, of insanity among the affluent. The existence of private asylums catering to ladies and gentlemen bears ample testimony to the intrusions of lunacy in distinguished social circles, although the widespread Victorian anxiety about unlaw-ful confinement, in both private and public institutions, suggests that the record of the medical profession was far from flawless when it came to identifying insanity, at whatever level of society.

Nineteenth-century British alienists were as concerned about their own position as they were cognizant of their patients' social rank. Attempts to improve their status, within the medical profession and among the general public, deeply affected their task as diagnosticians and their relationship with the people who sought their help. During the course of the Victorian era, the occupational needs of the psychiatrists themselves inevitably influenced the way they handled cases of neurotic illness. Yet the articulation of attitudes toward nervous breakdown represented a collaboration between medical men and the community at large, which included their patients. Much recent writing on medical history notwithstanding, doctors did not invariably play the role of powerful oppressor, and patients were not always the impotent victims of medical authority. Nervous patients were, in fact, notorious for consulting a string of medical practitioners in search of relief, both from psychological pain and from the physical symptoms accompanying it. Their willingness to discard one doctor in favor of another strongly suggests that these men and women were not cowed by medical autocrats. Relations involving power are rarely unambiguous; Victorian medical men and their patients participated together in delicate, ongoing maneuvers to delimit their own spheres of influence in defining nervous maladies.

The historian who sets out today to investigate nervous breakdown in nineteenth-century England can thus expect to encounter a formidable array of pitfalls. The inexactitude of diagnostic labels, the laxity with which the terminology of nervous-ness was applied to widely disparate physical and mental states, the imposition of social concerns on medical decisions—all obscure the subject and complicate the task. Such obstacles prevent statistical precision in a study like this. Too many uncertainties intrude to make counting heads an exercise that could produce reliable figures, able in turn to yield valid generalizations. Indeed, generalizations are hard to produce where nervous breakdown is concerned, and all the harder when more than a century intervenes between the evidence and its interpreter. Depression is a highly individual form of illness that follows no predictable pattern, as many Victorian medical men realized. "When shall we learn," asked Alfred Schofield, a doctor who wrote numerous books about nervous patients around the turn of the century, "that each case must be separately and intelligently studied on its own merits, for no two are alike?"[16] Psychologists and psychiatrists working in the late twentieth century concur. Stuart Sutherland, professor of experimental psychology at the University of Sussex, who has depicted his own overwhelming depression with extraordinary intensity, persuasively surmises that "the reasons for breaking down are as multifarious as the goals that different people pursue," and that, similarly, "in the individual case one can never be sure of the factors that bring about recovery."[17]

No single all-encompassing theory exists to explain nervous breakdown, now or in the past, for underlying predispositions and previous experiences react with precipitants in ways that are unique to each sufferer. With historical figures, we simply cannot know for certain what combination of physiological and emotional causes subjected them to incapacitating depression, and we confront the unsatisfactory choice of hazarding no guess at all or permitting our imaginations to reconstruct the past, as best we can, on the basis of surviving medical records and personal documents. The first alternative is flat and disappointing; the second is stimulating, but it is also always speculative. In any case, 100 years or more after the events under scrutiny, we are far better served by the flexibility of an empirical approach to the remaining evidence than by a theoretical rigidity that insists on building explanatory models, even where the foundations are too slight to bear the load.

The geographic and chronological limits that I have imposed on this book doubtless appear arbitrary. The British were not the only people to experience nervous breakdown in the nineteenth century, nor were theirs the only doctors who wrestled with the obscurities of neurotic disorders. On the contrary, British medical practitioners paid attention to continental European and American developments in neurology and psychiatry, even if they were selective in the foreign insights they chose to adopt for their own purposes. Many of the medical themes and preoccupations traced in the following chapters were thoroughly international in scope—the reliance on somatic theories of disease, for example, or the obsession with systems of classifying mental and nervous disorders, the passion for cranial measurements, and the fears of racial degeneration linked with nervous instability. Nonetheless I examine the international contributions, particularly French, German, and American, only where they bear directly on British attitudes, and the British medical profession, working under circumstances unlike those across the Channel or the Atlantic, always remains at the center of my study.

Among all the Victorian medical specialities, psychiatry in Great Britain was particularly subject to influences that marked its difference from German and French psychological medicine. The distinction between cerebral and mental diseases, which troubled British psychiatrists, was largely irrelevant in Germany, where a flourishing school of neuropsychiatry developed after the mid-nineteenth century, based more in the research laboratory than the consulting room.[18] Different professional needs likewise colored the growth of French psychiatry, which was molded by the expanding machinery of central bureaucratic government to a far greater degree than was the case in Great Britain. For social and religious reasons, the subsumption of mental functions under the workings of brain tissue was more problematic there than on the continent. While French alienists learned to tailor their spiritualism or materialism to suit the policies of successive regimes, whether republican, royalist, or Bonapartist,[19] British psychiatrists by mid-century consistently worked within a culture virtually defined by the evangelical religious revival. The Anglican Church, furthermore, remained a partner of the state, at least in England and Wales, throughout the nineteenth century. It was no coincidence that British scientists and theologians were, with a few exceptions, more persistent than their continental counterparts in trying to reconcile science and faith, or that British alienists partici-pated in the endeavor. Even in the United States, where the growth of psychiatry and neurology tended to follow the British pattern, both the structure of society and the place of religion in national life varied so significantly from conditions in Great Britain that striking medical dissimilarities emerged between the two English-speaking countries.

The sheer wealth of material available for a British study provides another reason why I have narrowed the field of inquiry to a single national context. A substantial array of Victorian textbooks concentrated on nervous diseases, both structural and functional, while the various medical periodicals that flourished in the nineteenth century publicized nervous and mental ailments in exhaustive detail. Journals and magazines designed for a broader readership often featured articles on the nerves, which editors knew would attract an eager audience. Doctors' memoirs, casebooks, and correspondence not only expressed widely shared medical opinions, but also revealed idiosyncratic attitudes toward nervous patients—rarely mentioned by name, of course. The patients themselves frequently recorded their experience of sickness in diaries, letters, and autobiographies. Many of these personal sources are available in published form; some can be located in manuscript accounts. Victorian biographies similarly abound, for numerous sufferers were prominent members of the profes-sional and intellectual middle classes whose lives were thought worthy of commemo-ration. Revealing autobiographical material for working-class victims of shattered nerves also exists, but is harder to find, as are annals of depression among the Victorian aristocracy. Nervous prostration occurred at both ends of the social scale, but it apparently did not preoccupy lords and laborers to the extent that it dominated middle-class health concerns, for reasons I hope to make clear. Finally, Victorian fiction reveals a splendid procession of nervous "types" who fully deserve the historian's attention.

The scholar who sits down to such a rich feast can, however, only taste certain dishes. I have not been able to read all the Victorian novels, to track down information about every seriously depressed person I met in the medical literature, or consult all the available biographical and autobiographical material. Each of the following chapters might have grown into a book itself had I not curtailed its attempts at expansion. If some points seem slighted, some publications overlooked, or some fascinating case histories ignored, my sins of omission were prompted by the desire to fit all the pieces together inside a single binding and to show how several themes in the medical, social, and cultural history of Victorian England coalesced around the puzzle of nervous breakdown.

To illustrate this merger, I rely heavily on the figure of Sir James Crichton-

Browne. His work forms the subject of Chapter 2, and he makes regular appearances thereafter. With a medical career that stretched from the early 1860s until 1922, he was personally involved in many of the developments that shaped the British psychiatric profession in the late Victorian and Edwardian decades, just as his father, W. A. F. Browne, had been influential among early Victorian alienists. The tension in Crichton-Browne's own life between neurological research and psychiatric consultation reflects the divergence of neurology and psychiatry in Great Britain and illuminates the choices available in this period to a British doctor whose interests focused on nervous disorders. No individual, needless to say, represents the growth of an entire profession in all its aspects, and Crichton-Browne was certainly extreme in some of his views, particularly with regard to racial degeneration and female intellectual inferiority; however, the readiness with which he mixed social pronouncements and medical theories characterized his generation of British psychiatrists, born between 1830 and 1850, who dominate this study. Although the lines of psychiatry's jurisdiction were anything but clear before World War I, its practitioners claimed the right, in the name of national mental health, to inform public opinion on a wide range of social issues. Crichton-Browne's experiences, assertions, and anxieties were typical of a medical speciality that was still finding its voice and seeking to define its purpose.

Like the geographical confines of this study, the chronological restrictions also require explanation. Depression, after all, has long flourished in Great Britain; it stamped the melancholic man of the sixteenth and seventeenth centuries, as well as the much celebrated "hypochondriack" of the eighteenth. As early as the 1660s, the potential connection between moods and nerves found expression in Willis's observation that a study of the nervous system "revealed the true and genuine reasons for very many of the actions and passions that take place in our body, . . . no less than the hidden causes of diseases and symptoms."[20] It is the eighteenth century, however, that can be designated the era *par excellence* of functional nervous afflictions. An extensive literature from those decades attests to the public appetite for information about hysterical and hypochondriacal disorders, melancholy, lowness of spirits, spleen, and vapors. George Cheyne crowded all these terms into the subtitle of his renowned volume of 1733, *The English Malady,* in which he argued that nervous distempers were peculiarly distinctive of his countrymen. Throughout the century, hypochondriasis and melancholy flourished in polite society as signs of their victims' cultivation. With the label nervous increasingly replacing some of the older diagnostic terminology, nervousness became a badge of honor, to be displayed as a mark of superiority together with the delicate sensibility that usually accompanied it. Nervous patients enjoyed a privileged rank among invalids, even if they were also subject to caricature by the caustic and observant wits of the day. By 1765, Robert Whytt, a leading Scottish physician, felt the need to caution that the appellation of nervous had been too freely applied "to many symptoms seemingly different, and very obscure in their nature."[21] Clearly British society and medicine alike were ready for Cullen's classificatory labors. Although he did nothing to clarify the actual nature of functional nervous disorders, Cullen's work authoritatively established neurosis as a significant pathological entity and placed the nervous system at the very center of the somatic processes that determine health and disease.

By the close of the eighteenth century, the paramount importance of the nervous system in medical science was beyond dispute. Well confirmed, too, was the interpretation of nervous disorders along functional lines, an approach that allowed medical men to emphasize the affected nervous activity, whether voluntary or involuntary, motor or sensory, rather than the nervous structure, about which they remained largely ignorant. The nineteenth century inherited these developments, and Victorians continued to maintain that nervous derangements were the characteristic ailments of their day. The claim made in 1838 that nervous "complaints prevail at the present day to an extent unknown at any former period, or in any other nation," sounded suspiciously like Cheyne's assertion, 100 years earlier, that the "atrocious and frightful symptoms" he studied were "scarce known to our ancestors, and never r[ose] to such fatal heights, nor afflict[ed] such numbers in any other known nation."[22] What justification can therefore possibly exist to treat the nervous culture of Victorian England as something different, and separate, from the Georgian variety?

Although cases of profound depression have occurred in all ages of recorded history, different times and places have invested the illness with differing significance. It has confronted various diagnostic fads over the centuries and suffered reinterpretation in the light of successive theories about the design and functions of the human body. It has contended with black bile, animal spirits, and nerve force. It has been celebrated as a mark of personal distinction and feared as proof of social, economic, and physical impotence. Why a particular society embraces a certain form of sickness in a distinctive way depends on virtually every aspect of its culture, and the Victorian fascination with nervous disorders was not merely a continuation of trends going back through the Elizabethan age to ancient medicine and philosophy. Nineteenth-century British attitudes toward nervous breakdown were initially colored by the legacy of the eighteenth century, by the cult of sensibility, and by the literary glorification of the romantic hero, but with the passage of time, the ways in which the Victorians viewed the disorder diverged increasingly from Georgian perceptions.

The change occurred gradually, under the influence of evangelicalism, industrialization, psychiatry, and physiology. The evangelical stress on self-discipline came to pervade Victorian attitudes toward health and, combined with the emphasis on productivity in a rapidly industrializing nation, discredited lethargy and incapacitation. The appearance of a psychiatric branch within the British medical profession during the course of the nineteenth century meant that alleged experts emerged who were keen to define the meaning of depression for the rest of society. Unlike the eighteenth-century assumption that nervous sensibility graced only the affluent and cultured classes, Victorian alienists eventually found nervous exhaustion afflicting all social ranks. Most important of all, Victorian medicine gained an ever more detailed understanding of how the nerves actually worked. It was expanding knowledge of the motor, sensory, and reflex functions of the nervous system, growing certainty of the electrical nature of the nervous impulse, and enlarged insight into the brain's activities through cerebral localization research that distinguished Victorian medical texts on the nerves, especially in the latter part of the era, from similar works in the preceding century. British obsession with the nerves in the nineteenth century was different in kind from the Georgian version primarily because it was substantially more informed about the nervous system itself. This was, of course, more obvious by the end of Victoria's reign than at the beginning. In the 1770s, Cullen had offered conjectures; in 1895, William R. Gowers, a leading neurologist, was dealing with "a matter of fact" when he observed that "diseases of the nervous system . . . are widening out into other provinces in ever-increasing degree. . . . There is no part of medicine in which a so-called 'nerve specialist' must not be at home."[23]

This study begins at the time when eighteenth-century notions began to encounter new discoveries about the nerves and new attitudes toward the social responsibility to be well; it extends until World War I. If the adjective *Victorian* seems unduly stretched to cover the Edwardian decade, the excuse is simply that the important work in British neurology and psychiatry during the early years of the twentieth century followed lines already established before Victoria's death and represented no striking departures from old inquiries. For most of the period surveyed, men and women wrote or spoke freely about their experiences of nervous breakdown, recognizing it as a fairly common disorder probably attributable to an underlying physical condition, and therefore casting little disgrace on the sufferer. This fundamentally open attitude underwent a slow transformation as the somatic basis of nervous collapse became increasingly doubtful to late Victorian and Edwardian opinion. With the widespread discussion of Freudian theories during the war, thanks to the efficacy of psychoanalysis in the treatment of shell shock, the process accelerated. Although Freud's system never dominated British psychiatry, it was sufficiently notorious to dampen the frank discussion of neurotic symptoms, for his association of sexual tension with the anxiety underlying nervous exhaustion scarcely encouraged people to discuss their condition candidly. Doctors, too, were far less forthcoming about neurotic patients once the general public learned to impute dark significance to their distress. The widespread assumption, after the war, that neurotic illnesses were wholly psychological in origin encouraged popular belief that they were, somehow, under the patient's control and therefore a source of discredit to people who allowed diseased thoughts to dominate their lives. I bring this volume to a close just before the age of openness ended, when the preponderant part of medical and public opinion still perceived nervous breakdown as a torture to be endured, not a sin to be concealed.

A new age of openness, spawned in the 1960s, has brought depression once more into the realm of free and frank conversation. Statistics proclaim the staggering incidence of depression throughout western society and raise questions whether the numbers of victims have themselves mushroomed since World War II or merely the number of people willing to seek help for an affliction they had hitherto sought to hide. In such an atmosphere of acceptance, the temptation to exaggerate despondency, or even a mere sense of being "out of sorts," may prove irresistible to some people, just as two centuries ago there were those who found it advantageous to adopt more extravagant forms of nervous sensitivity than the state of their nerve fibers warranted. This book, however, is not about Victorians who faked nervous exhaustion or allowed affectation to embellish a minor condition of unease. The men and women who appear in the following chapters suffered from no readily controllable ailment. For long periods of time, they were incapable of all exertion—wretched figures of inactivity in a culture that exalted initiative and enterprise.

1

Alienists, Neurologists, and Nerve-Doctors

When the neurologist William Gowers referred to the "so-called 'nerve specialist'" in 1895, he had good reason to cast doubt on the validity, and utility, of that title. By the late Victorian period, medical men with strikingly varied backgrounds and areas of specialization claimed authoritative knowledge of the nervous system and its maladies. Many of them might have breezily explained, like Sherlock Holmes's acquaintance, Dr. Percy Trevelyan: "My own hobby has always been nervous disease. I should wish to make it an absolute specialty, but of course a man must take what he can get at first." One astute medical commentator, T. C. Allbutt, scoffingly inquired at the end of the century, "Is not every large city filled with nerve-specialists? . . ."[1] Amid this heterogeneous array of medical expertise, British alienists were hard pressed to make good their assertion of unique insight into nervous afflictions and particular talent in treating them. That the care of functional nervous disorders was, in fact, increasingly falling to psychiatrists by the eve of World War I was less a measure of their success with such problems than a result of the neurologists' bid to handle cases of identifiable somatic origin. The development of psychiatry in the second half of the nineteenth century involved a long and complicated relationship with neurology, which had not entirely disentangled itself even at the end of the war. The psychiatric profession in Great Britain was slow to assume a coherent identity in large part because, for decades, it remained unsure of its goals and functions. Neurotic disorders, including severe depression, raised questions that belonged at the very heart of that uncertainty.

The growth and divergence of psychiatry and neurology were merely one aspect of the transformation of the entire British medical profession during the course of the nineteenth century. By the beginning of Victoria's reign, the old tripartite division among physicians, surgeons, and apothecaries had collapsed in the face of changing social and economic conditions, and in response to expanding medical knowledge. Throughout the eighteenth century, only physicians had enjoyed any social prestige, although medical prints and caricatures suggested a considerable lack of public respect even for them.[2] An infinitesimally small fraction of the total number of medical practitioners, physicians were the unchallenged leaders of Georgian medicine. Maintaining the time-honored distinction between the learned professions on the one hand and mere trade on the other, physicians exclusively pursued the former. In theory, they restricted their work to the diagnosis of internal disorders and the prescription of allegedly curative drugs, neither performing surgery nor compounding medications themselves. Organized in the Royal College of Physicians of

London, a corporation dating back to the early sixteenth century, they claimed to be gentlemen and boasted a classical education to prove it. Although a university medical degree was necessary for becoming a Licentiate of the College, and specifically a degree from Oxford or Cambridge for aspiring to a Fellowship, medical training mattered far less to the Collegians than the ability to move comfortably among the right sort of people. The venerable English universities could provide the proper social background for a future physician, even if the medical education they offered was haphazard during the eighteenth century. The Fellows both governed the College and cast a supervisory eye over the practice of internal medicine, or "physic," across England. Within London, only those men who held the License or the Fellowship of the College could pursue this lofty branch of medicine; outside London, physicians were not compelled to seek association with the College in order to practice, but possession of the Extra-License gave a university-educated provincial physician particular cachet in his community. That only 179 men in England were Fellows, Licentiates, or Extra-Licentiates of the College in 1800 suggests what an elite institution it was.[3] Clearly, it could not pretend to cater to the medical needs of the country, nor was it interested in doing so.

Surgeons and apothecaries met some, but by no means all, of that need. Skilled craftsmen rather than professional gentlemen, British surgeons in the eighteenth century enjoyed no great social status. Their long-standing affiliation with barbers was not broken until 1745, when they departed from the Barber-Surgeons' Company of the City of London to establish their own, separate craft guild. Trained largely through apprenticeship, surgeons had no prescribed requirements to fulfill in order to gain legal qualification to practice. Unlike physicians, they did not read great medical texts of the past; instead they concentrated on acquiring the skill not only to perform operations, but also to set broken bones, pull teeth, draw blood, dress wounds, burns and other skin afflictions, as well as to treat a few internal ailments, such as ulcers. Surgeons' attempts to improve their position in society received a powerful boost in 1800, with the granting of a charter to found the Royal College of Surgeons of London. Although members of the College did not enjoy a monopoly on the practice of surgery, either in the metropolis or throughout the country at large, the very existence of such a body suggested that surgeons had managed to distance themselves from the stigma of manual labor. Their initiative and ambition gave the physicians no little anxiety.

Apothecaries, too, had humble origins to overcome in their struggle for professional recognition during the nineteenth century. They were, in fact, at the bottom of the recognized medical hierarchy. Originally belonging to the Grocers' Company of the City of London, they had branched off in 1617 to form the Society of Apothecaries under royal charter. Confined at first to the preparation and sale of drugs, they were little more than shopkeepers until early in the eighteenth century, when they were legally enabled to prescribe medication as well. Filling physicians' prescriptions remained, however, a principal part of the apothecary's work, and he trained for it, like the surgeon, through a period of apprenticeship. During the Georgian decades, apothecaries—who now combined the two important roles of druggist and medical practitioner—served a valuable function in providing medical care to a larger section of the populace than physicians, catering to a prosperous urban clientele, could ever reach.[4] Nonetheless, only a small proportion of the total British population in the eighteenth century received the attention of qualified medical men. By far the greater number treated themselves with the contents of the domestic medicine cabinet, consulted healers of all varieties, or consumed the old folk remedies of the village wise woman. Thus, even at the end of the eighteenth century, medical care continued to be fragmented among several competing bodies, without unifying purpose or program. Surgeons and apothecaries, 5,000 strong in 1780, increasingly resented the hegemony of the physicians,[5] while London's dominance in medical affairs provoked the resentment of provincial practitioners.

Significant change was, by the turn of the century, already quietly undermining these apparently rigid distinctions within British medicine. Physicians who did not hold a prestigious Fellowship of the Royal College found compensation in the fact that they were much less limited than the Fellows with regard to the kind of medicine they could practice. Few surgeons outside of London could support themselves and a family on surgery alone. Many had to augment their income by encroaching on the apothecaries' territory, which had itself embraced the pharmaceutical treatment of internal disease. The old corporate divisions, in short, were becoming meaningless before the nineteenth century had begun. The next fifty years continued and accelerated a realignment of British medicine into two basic categories—specialists or consultants, on the one hand, and family doctors or general practitioners, on the other. In large part, the second category arose in response to a rapidly increasing demand for comparatively inexpensive health care among the expanding ranks of the middle classes in the wake of the Industrial Revolution. Recognizing that treatment by a bona fide medical practitioner marked one's membership in a socially elevated circle, yet unable to pay the fees demanded by the leading physicians and surgeons, the vast majority of middle-class families during the Victorian decades patronized general practitioners.

The very notion of *general practice* was legitimized in 1815, with the passage of the Apothecaries' Act that permitted the Society of Apothecaries to issue a license to practice medicine throughout England and Wales. As part of the measure, the Society gained the right to set requisite standards of education and proficiency, and to bar anyone who failed to meet those criteria from advertising himself as an apothecary. Surgeons who qualified for the apothecaries' license and apothecaries licensed by the Royal College of Surgeons could thus pursue all branches of medicine—performing operations, delivering babies, treating and prescribing for internal and external ailments, and preparing medications as well. After 1815, surgeon-apothecaries proliferated across the country, although they preferred to settle in spas, resorts, cathedral towns, and the fashionable neighborhoods of big cities, where they might hope to attract a solid middle-class clientele. Some were extremely successful in their attempts, accumulating incomes worthy of the most distinguished consultant, but the majority had to settle for more modest remuneration, while the least fortunate spent their lives eking out a career under difficult conditions of exhausting, often hazardous, work. By the 1820s, when the term *general practitioner* made its appearance, the English language acknowledged the existence of these medical generalists. In the following decade the title became commonplace, as, indeed, was the general practitioner himself, supplying perhaps as much as 90 percent of the qualified medical services in England at the time.

During the same period, a small proportion of surgeons and physicians were forming the ranks of the consultants, the highest paid and socially most distinguished of Victorian doctors. Slowly, throughout the course of the nineteenth century, these men distanced themselves from the old image of the medical gentleman-scholar, applying general theories to various categories of bodily complaints, with only the most cursory, if any, physical examination of the patient. The proliferation of urban hospitals played a significant part in making this vision obsolete, for it was the gradual relocation of medical practice from the bedside to the hospital, and ultimately the hospital laboratory, combined with the development of medical schools attached to the hospitals, that eventually terminated the style of practice once common among Georgian physicians; it had not, however, altogether vanished even in the early twentieth century.

By the start of Victoria's reign, appointment to the staff of a hospital, whether as physician or surgeon, was essential for the young medical practitioner who wanted to attain the highest rung of his profession. The major institutions that provided in-patient care were voluntary hospitals catering to the poor. Although the staff medical men derived little, if any, salary from treating patients, a hospital appointment usually gave its holder the opportunity to teach medical students, who paid to attend lectures and "walk the wards," and who spread their teachers' reputations abroad. Even more important, hospital appointments brought medical practitioners into contact with the affluent, often aristocratic, lay governors of their institutions, whose patronage outside the hospital could launch a lucrative private practice for the fortunate physician or surgeon. After mid-century, the lucky few were especially well placed to develop those specializations that led to national renown in a particular area of medicine, such as cardiac, pulmonary, gastric, or nervous diseases. While it is true that these consultants might serve as general, or family, doctors to their socially prestigious clients, the distinction between consultants and general practitioners was, nonetheless, readily apparent. In a society where people knew their place, the consultants unquestionably lorded it over the general practitioners.[6]

Despite the obvious differences in income and status between the two types of medical practitioner, the tendency of Victorian medicine was toward professional unity. The Medical Act of 1858 took a long step in that direction, with the establishment of an annual medical register of qualified practitioners and the formation of a General Medical Council to watch over medical education, conduct, and licensing throughout the United Kingdom. As licensing bodies, the law recognized nine medical corporations, including the Royal Colleges and the Society of Apothecaries, as well as ten universities in England, Scotland, and Ireland.[7] No hierarchical distinction was made on the medical register among the licentiates of the various corporations, or between them and the holders of university medical degrees. Anyone who had satisfactorily passed the examination of one or more of the licensing bodies was deemed a "qualified medical practitioner" and duly registered. The law did not eliminate competition from quacks and self-proclaimed healers, but it barred them from pretending to be legally qualified, and a subsequent amendment was specifically directed against the unwarranted use of "Dr." by unregistered practitioners. Even among registered medical men, the adoption of that title was, in fact, the subject of considerable controversy after 1858; general practitioners wished to extend its use to all holders of medical licenses and degrees, while the still-powerful Council of the Royal College of Physicians preferred to restrict it to recipients of the M.D. degree. The public did not come to employ *doctor* as a general term for medical practitioner until the late nineteenth century.[8]

The Medical Act of 1858 did not immediately create a cohesive medical profession in place of competing groups and bitter jealousies. General practitioners were not represented on the General Medical Council until 1886, and the medical elites of the Royal Colleges in London tried to preserve their own bastions of power for as long as possible. The experiences of the typical general practitioner continued to be woefully incomparable to those of the typical consultant, who enjoyed all the perquisites of hospital affiliation. The act, however, defined as a legal entity the medical profession, all of whose members—the qualified and registered practitioners—shared equal standing in the eyes of the law. By the end of the century, when apprenticeship as a means of training had all but disappeared, the development of a common pattern of education in medical schools helped to alleviate the sharp internal divisions within the profession. If it is too much to maintain that all reputable British medical men in the Edwardian decade shared an esprit de corps that bound them into a harmonious professional body, it is fair to say that specialists and family doctors in this period held similar convictions about medicine's lofty role in modern society. They perceived themselves as part of a medical alliance facing a common enemy in dirt, disease, and, occasionally, their patients.

In recent sociological discussions about occupational groups, the defining characteristics of a profession are generally held to be a regular, rigorous system of education that imparts specialized knowledge, carefully defined standards of qualification that limit membership, a monopoly on the performance of certain services, and independence from outside control.[9] The continued presence of quacks on the fringes of medical practice certainly undermined the professional exclusivity of Victorian doctors, but the question of autonomy presented equally weighty problems. Although the Medical Act of 1858 granted the right of self-regulation, through the authority of the General Medical Council, it would be misleading to suggest that the British medical profession was ever truly autonomous at any time in the nineteenth century. It could never entirely escape from dependence on patron-patients.

The relationship between patients and medical attendants changed less from the Georgian to the Edwardian periods than is often assumed. The picture of eighteenth-century medical practitioners virtually at the mercy of a few affluent invalids, who controlled the purse strings, the presentation of their own symptoms, and the progress of their own therapy, thanks to the conditions of a buyer's market, has surely been exaggerated. So, too, has the rosy picture of medical hegemony on the eve of World War I, by which time the development of hospital and laboratory medicine, in partnership with authoritative science, had allegedly shifted the focus of medical attention from the patient to the disease and, in the process, given the knowledgeable doctor the upper hand.[10] The development of career opportunities in public health, as local medical officers, state inspectors, and poor law doctors, is thought to have ended the dependence of the medical profession on private patients, while the increasingly prominent role played by medical men in formulating public health legislation is believed to have augmented their professional status, helping them claim a place as valued experts in Victorian society.[11] The sheer expansion of the market for medical care, one would imagine, freed the individual practitioner from the need to be deferential to patients, especially after the restrictions of 1858 eased apparent overcrowding among the ranks of medical men. Indeed, by the 1880s, a noticeable shortage of registered doctors had become the subject of professional comment—a situation that ought to have made patients compete for medical attendants, rather than vice versa.[12]

Just as the Georgian doctor was not so entirely dependent on the whims of his clients, so the late Victorian medical profession was not in quite so advantageous a position as this summary suggests. While conditions for the practice of medicine had unquestionably, and often strikingly, improved since the eighteenth century, "occupational subservience" was not a thing of the past. Whether in salaried government jobs or prestigious hospital positions, both general practitioners and consultants were subject to control by various lay employers, including ministers of state, boards of governors, and local authorities who zealously guarded the expenditure of the rates.[13] At the lowest level of the profession, the general practitioner in a poor community remained precariously balanced on the edge of respectability all his life. He never ceased having to compete with unlicensed rivals who could charge less and promise more. Successful family doctors likewise had to realize that they enjoyed only a marginal status in the community, unsure whether patients considered them gentlemen or not, and far less socially secure than clergymen or even barristers.[14] At the loftiest peak of the medical hierarchy, consultants derived their stature not so much from scientific accomplishments as from the ranks of society occupied by their private patients, and most specialists remained obliged to court these men and women for the preponderant part of their income. If hospital inmates were passive recipients of medical care, there is no compelling evidence to show that private patients had relinquished all authority in the therapeutic relationship. Beyond doubt, doctors no longer had to rely on subjective symptoms for most of their information about the illnesses they treated; late Victorian and Edwardian medical men did, in general, know considerably more about their patients' maladies than the sufferers could claim to know themselves. Advances in the scientific understanding of health and disease, however, were not as instrumental in bolstering the doctor's authority over the patient as, in theory, they should have been. The identification of pathogenic agents occurred, in most cases, long before medicine possessed the means to destroy them, and thus patients were slow to benefit from the new discoveries. Although, by 1914, consumers of medical services could no longer dominate the arrangements existing between doctor and patient, they were by no means reduced to the role of bit players. Their preconceptions and expectations continued to influence the work of the medical profession.

This was the framework within which British psychiatry took shape during the nineteenth century, sharing the weaknesses of the medical profession as a whole, but few of the strengths. Until the 1840s, in fact, mad-doctors were saddled with a number of particularly severe disabilities in their efforts to achieve professional recognition. Of these, the gravest was public uncertainty whether madness was really a medical problem at all, best treated by trained medical practitioners. The very origins of the psychiatric speciality within British medicine could be traced to the eighteenth-century competition between medical men and lay proprietors for control of "the trade in lunacy"—the establishment and management of private madhouses, which could prove profitable enterprises.[15] A number of successful medical practitioners kept madhouses as a sideline, while continuing regularly to see their sane patients. For those who wanted broader opportunities to study lunacy than a small private asylum could afford, a handful of charity hospitals for the insane existed before 1800, including London's ancient Bethlem and recent St. Luke's, founded in 1751. By 1828, nine county asylums had been established to maintain pauper and criminal lunatics at public expense, following enabling legislation in 1808.[16] In both kinds of institutions, however, management committees composed primarily of philanthropists and magistrates challenged the primacy of medical knowledge about madness and kept control over the appointment and salaries of the medical staff. Moreover, although in London commissioners chosen from the Royal College of Physicians had been charged with the licensing and annual inspection of private madhouses since 1774, in the provinces the same duties were vested in magistrates' hands. Lay commissioners joined the physicians in London after 1828.[17]

One reason for medical vulnerability to lay interference in the supervision and treatment of lunatics was the lack of special training available to mad-doctors. The development of systematic medical education in teaching hospitals and universities throughout Great Britain ignored the category of mental illness until the second half of the nineteenth century. Scarcely any part of their training prepared late Georgian or early Victorian medical men for the tasks they faced within the asylum, or allowed them to pose as informed experts in contrast to the lay amateurs who harassed them. The founders of St. Luke's in London, admittedly, had intended the hospital to offer a kind of postgraduate education in insanity to practicing medical men, and William Battie, the hospital's physician, had offered a series of clinical demonstrations to that end for a few years in the 1750s. Cullen, too, had delivered lectures on mental disease and, in the early nineteenth century, so did Alexander Morison, a Scotsman who received the M.D. degree from Edinburgh in 1799. His annual lectures were presented in Edinburgh and London for more than twenty years, beginning in 1823. Although a society doctor, he acquired some direct experience of insanity as a visiting physician to Bethlem, to private madhouses in Surrey, and to the county asylums of Surrey and Middlesex. It was not until 1842, however, that medical students at the London hospitals were able to combine lectures with clinical observations at the Middlesex County Asylum, Hanwell, under the auspices of John Conolly, the resident medical superintendent.[18] The odd course of lectures or demonstrations, available only in London or Edinburgh, clearly could not reach many of the future asylum medical officers of the country. Most of them came to the work either with previous experience at a private madhouse, through family connections in the business, or simply because they were challenged by the puzzles of mental derangement. As the number of public asylums increased, some medical men turned themselves into mad-doctors in order to gain the newly available jobs. John Charles Bucknill, who subsequently became a leading alienist, initially sought the position of medical superintendent to the Devon County Asylum in 1844 when ill health forced him to abandon his surgical career in London and to seek a milder climate.[19]

In the first decades of the nineteenth century, mad-doctors had to contend, too, with the implications of "moral management," the preeminent theme in early Victorian asylum reform. "Theme" is perhaps a misleading term in this context, because no underlying philosophy or uniform system of treatment characterized the approach taken by "moral managers" toward the insane. They were inspired simply by the conviction that brutal coercive measures were not conducive to curing madness, but only reduced human beings to beasts. The humane treatment of lunatics, they argued in language that blended overtones of enlightened rationalism with strains of Christian brotherhood, would help these unfortunates reaffirm their humanity. Where asylum directors subscribed to such beliefs, strait jackets, chains, straw bedding, sparse diet, purgatives, venesection, and freezing showers gave way as fully as possible to organized activities, decent food, proper beds, patience, kindness, and cheerfulness, in the hope of transforming inmates into orderly, cooperative, and once again rational citizens. What was a humanitarian advance, however, at first posed a serious problem for the medical men who hoped to monopolize the care of lunatics. Surely no medical training was necessary to teach the qualities of gentleness and sympathy, and lay attendants, accordingly, might claim as great a likelihood of success with insane patients as medical practitioners could boast. The fact that the first to implement and publicize a systematic policy of *nonrestraint* in England was the Quaker philanthropist and merchant William Tuke, who founded the York Retreat for Quaker lunatics in the 1790s, did nothing to recommend the idea to medical men. Most of them reacted to the notion of moral management with extreme suspicion, if not outright hostility, when it began to circulate in the opening years of the century, stimulated by Philippe Pinel's work in Paris as well as Tuke's in York. They characteristically insisted that medical treatment—drugging and physical intervention such as bleeding and purging—could alone set lunatics on the road to recovery. Yet within a few years, mad-doctors had learned that they could accommodate the various techniques of moral management within their therapeutic arsenal and that it was advantageous for their professional standing to do so. They had even managed to make the case that men with medical training were far better equipped to practice the methods of moral treatment than men without.[20]

The overriding concern of the early nineteenth-century British alienists was to wrest control of the asylum from laymen, and by the 1840s they had made some notable progress in that direction. Indeed, by the 1820s educated opinion was coming to perceive insanity as a disease that demanded expert medical attention, if inmates were to be cured and not merely constrained. The Madhouse Act of 1828 required that every asylum receive weekly visits from a medical practitioner and mandated that asylums housing more than 100 inmates retain the services of a resident medical officer. The act further strengthened the voice of medical men in the diagnosis and treatment of madness by necessitating medical certificates of insanity for the detention of alleged lunatics. During the 1830s and 1840s, resident medical superintendents became standard features of the public mental institutions, as well as the better private ones, and they increasingly exerted primary authority over the daily management of all that occurred within their domain.[21]

The 1840s witnessed several developments that proved highly significant to the growth of psychiatry as an identifiable specialization within British medical practice. Two lunacy acts passed in 1845 extended the network of county and borough asylums for pauper lunatics and created a national Lunacy Commission, on a permanent basis, to inspect all variety of institutions housing the insane across the country. Asylums were henceforth obliged to maintain a medical visitation book and a medical case-book, recording the details of each patient's treatment. Aspects of the 1828 legislation were confirmed to underscore even more vigorously the importance of the medical presence in the asylum. The laws both promised new jobs at the public institutions, now required by Parliament, and reserved them for qualified medical men. At the same time, it opened up possibilities for employment as national lunacy commissioners.[22] In 1841, even before Parliament delivered these gifts, forty-four mad-doctors, working at both public and private asylums, had launched their own organization, the Association of Medical Officers of Hospitals for the Insane, to mark their self-awareness as a distinct group among medical practitioners. At the end of the decade, in 1848, the first British journal devoted solely to psychiatry, *The Journal of Psychological Medicine and Mental Pathology,* was founded by Forbes Benignus Winslow, the owner of two private madhouses at Hammersmith.[23]

Winslow's career suggests the extent to which professional opportunities were expanding for British mad-doctors by the middle decades of the nineteenth century. Trained in London, at University College and the Middlesex Hospital, he was licensed to practice by the Royal College of Surgeons in 1835. His interest in mental illness revealed itself in such publications as *Anatomy of Suicide* (1840), *The Incubation of Insanity* (1845), and his long essay "On Softening of the Brain Arising from Anxiety & Undue Mental Exercise and Resulting in Impairment of Mind," which appeared as a supplement to the second volume of the *Journal of Psychological Medicine and Mental Pathology* in 1849. In addition to his writings, his journal, and his madhouses, Winslow maintained a very public profile as an expert witness at numerous trials, where he helped to establish the insanity plea in criminal cases. To increase his stature among medical colleagues, he took the M.D. degree from Aberdeen in 1849. By the time he published *On Obscure Diseases of the Brain, and Disorders of the Mind,* which went through four editions in the 1860s, he was recognized as one of the leading authorities in psychological medicine, and he cultivated a flourishing consulting practice in mental disease until his death in 1874.[24]

After the 1840s, however, the more typical launching pad for a successful career in psychiatry was not the private madhouse, but the public institution. As the county asylums expanded, both in total number and in individual size, a kind of training course developed, with young alienists filling the jobs of assistant medical officers, working their way up to a medical directorship or superintendency. From there, they might abandon the asylum to become lunacy commissioners, or perhaps cease to be medical bureaucrats altogether, devoting their time to private practice, usually in London. Bucknill's career followed this pattern. After eighteen years as medical superintendent of the Devon County Asylum, during which time he earned the M.D.

degree from London, he left Devon in 1862 to become one of the Lord Chancellor's Visitors in Lunacy, a position he held until 1876. Thereafter he turned his energies from public to private service, and the consulting practice that he launched was remunerative enough to enable him to bequeath £6,000 to University College, London, when he died in 1897.[25]

Although few mad-doctors had equally rewarding experiences, opportunities outside the asylum were indubitably increasing after mid-century. Even lectureships at medical schools, provincial as well as metropolitan, gradually became available in the field of mental illness, and a number of alienists born in the 1840s found themselves teaching their subject by the end of the century. Thomas Smith Clouston, for example, the medical superintendent of the Royal Edinburgh Asylum, Morningside, lectured on mental diseases at the University of Edinburgh; in London, George Savage, the superintendent of Bethlem, delivered lectures on the same subject at Guy's Hospital and was an examiner in mental physiology at the University of London. Lyttleton Stewart Forbes Winslow, a second-generation psychiatrist, inherited his father's private asylums and lectured on insanity at the Charing Cross Hospital.[26]

The most ambitious of late Victorian alienists typically sought, at the earliest possible moment, to translate the expertise acquired within the asylum into assets outside its walls. Henry Maudsley, one of the great success stories of British psychiatry in this period, received the M.D. degree from London in 1857 at twenty-two years of age, briefly held the job of assistant medical officer at the West Riding Lunatic Asylum, Wakefield, and went on to serve as the medical superintendent of the Cheadle Royal Hospital for the Insane, Manchester, from 1859 to 1862. He had no intention, however, of spending his days among lunatic Mancunians, and thereafter moved back to London to pursue a private career. Although he inherited a small private madhouse at Hanwell from John Conolly, his father-in-law, Maudsley's renown scarcely rested on so slight a foundation. From his base as physician to the West London Hospital from 1864 to 1874 and professor of medical jurisprudence at University College, London, during the 1870s, he built up a consulting practice of enviable proportions. The major difference between the two generations of British psychiatry represented by Conolly and Maudsley is precisely that the latter could, under fortunate circumstances, construct "a practice based almost exclusively on the consulting room."[27] Before World War I, Maudsley's gift of £30,000 to build a psychiatric hospital affiliated with the University of London utterly eclipsed Bucknill's earlier bequest.[28]

There is considerable irony to the fact that while Conolly's generation of mad-doctors, reaching adulthood in the 1820s and 1830s, focused their energies on establishing dominance over the public asylums, Maudsley's generation, coming of age in the 1850s and 1860s, could not wait to move beyond the asylum into the far more prestigious and profitable milieu of the affluent nervous patient. For those lucky and energetic enough to make the transition to consulting practice, considerable income came, not just from families with a lunatic to hide discreetly in a private asylum, but from patients whose functional nervous maladies fell short of insanity. The mental symptoms that distinguished these afflictions—often the signs of severe depression—could be portrayed as requiring the attention of a doctor experienced in treating mental illness. As in the past, association with men and women from the elite ranks of society improved the status of the medical attendant in ways that asylum medicine, particularly as practiced in public institutions, could never accomplish. In neurotic disorders, psychiatrists found a means not only of extending their jurisdiction to a broader segment of the health-seeking public, but also of affiliating themselves with patients whose income and social standing helped to obliterate the taint of the asylum. In a sense, they had come full circle from their eighteenth-century predecessors, who had dabbled in the lunacy business while mingling as physicians or surgeons in polite society. By the late nineteenth century, the demand for health services had grown to such an extent that a fairly high degree of medical specialization was financially possible. Now certain psychiatrists could function solely as consultants in cases of mental disorder, whether mild or acute, and they accordingly sought a clientele among the prosperous reaches of society. In the intervening century, however, they had also claimed the lunatic asylum as their own preserve, a source of jobs for the majority of their colleagues and the supposed foundation of their particular insight into mental illness.

The problem was that asylum medicine carried an ill-defined stigma, despite the best efforts of asylum practitioners to elevate their work in the eyes of their fellow medical men. The job of resident superintendent at a county asylum could not compare to an appointment at one of London's well-known hospitals or a professorship of medicine at some distinguished university. The gradual expansion of lectureships in mental disease did not signify widespread acceptance of the subject's importance, and the rest of the medical profession, even in the last quarter of the nineteenth century, was still not much interested in the treatment of insanity, or other aspects of psychological medicine. In 1877, Crichton-Browne told the Select Committee on the Lunacy Law that "almost all" of the medical schools attached to general hospitals offered "a short course" on cerebral disease "in the summer session, either as part of the course of medical jurisprudence, or as a special course"[29]—an unambiguous indication that it was not considered an essential component of medical education in its own right. Down to World War I, no required course of study marked the training of a doctor who wanted to specialize in mental illness. To a significant degree, alienists who remained throughout their careers at a public asylum post, with its poor rate of pay and exposure to the worst elements of society, stood apart from the rest of British medical practice—isolated, figuratively and literally, in the world of their institutions. No matter how much they controlled daily administration or articulated the medical theories governing the treatment of inmates, they were never able to transcend the fact that they were merely "salaried employees" of lay management committees.[30]

For all their greater economic and professional independence, London's consultant alienists themselves struggled to persuade other doctors of psychiatry's high standing within the British medical confraternity. While the rest of the profession was willing to join ranks to restrain laymen from asserting amateur pretensions in the asylum, doctors in different areas of practice were not for the most part convinced that psychiatry was an authentic medical undertaking, constructed on the somatic foundations that supported all of modern medicine. The need to emphasize psychiatry's rightful place among medical pursuits dictated the names that Victorian alienists chose for their work, for their professional organization, and for its publication—titles that also managed to distance psychiatry from its roots in asylum medicine.

By the time that the Association of Medical Officers of Hospitals for the Insane appeared in 1841, the old label *mad-doctor* was falling out of use, to be replaced by phrases like *medical superintendent* or *resident medical officer*. While more dignified than mad-doctor, however, they were nonetheless redolent of the asylum, and from the 1860s *alienist,* a neutral name, was employed to designate a medical practitioner who specialized in treating the insane. It derived from the phrase "alienation of mind," which dated back to the late fifteenth century. In the vocabulary of the mid-nineteenth, the alienist's concern was not simply madness, but the broader range of problems suggested by the terms *mental pathology, medical psychology,* or *mental physiology,* all of which, in turn, engendered synonyms for alienist, and underscored the location of his work in the mainstream of medical inquiry. From mid-century, too, the word *psychiatry* began creeping into British medical parlance from the continent, particularly Germany, where *psychiatrie* flourished. In England, the medical man who practiced psychiatry or *psychiatrics,* as it was occasionally dubbed, was likelier to be called a *psychiater* than a *psychiatrist* until the 1890s. Even *psychiatrician* made an occasional appearance.[31] By the end of the Edwardian period, psychiatry, psychiatric, and psychiatrist were well established in the English language, with reference to the treatment both of insanity and of less severe mental problems; for example, Charles Mercier, an alienist with experience at public and private asylums, assigned disorders of conduct to the "psychiatric physician" in 1911, the same year in which Clouston asserted that "recent ideas would merge psychiatry into general medicine and pathology."[32] From the Greek word *psyche,* meaning breath or life, the name psychiatrist indeed suggested the wide-ranging relevance of that doctor's work for the entire field of medicine. It did not, however, rapidly replace some of the older terms. "Alienists" continued to practice "psychological medicine" well into the 1920s and '30s.

Victorian psychiatrists were not long content with the title of their association. In 1853, they altered it to the lengthier Association of Medical Officers of Asylums and Hospitals for the Insane, an appellation more indicative of the sources of its members' employment. Yet the new name still consigned alienists exclusively to the company of lunatics and was no more satisfactory than the old one at a time when job opportunities were expanding for them outside the asylum. Accordingly, they once again changed the title, this time in 1865, and the Medico-Psychological Association consequently emerged. Its national scope was indicated when the words "of Great Britain and Ireland" were appended in 1887, and by 1891 it boasted 474 members. Not until 1971 did it bow to contemporary usage and become the Royal College of Psychiatrists. Its own publication, commenced in 1853 as the *Asylum Journal,* underwent a similar transformation of name, first to the *Asylum Journal of Mental Science,* and then, in 1858, simply to the *Journal of Mental Science.*[33] It retained that title for over a century until it was rechristened the *British Journal of Psychiatry* in 1963. Clearly, all the nineteenth-century titular alterations were undertaken with one end in view: to make the point that mental illness was not confined to lunatics or asylums, that it belonged among the catalogue of medical disorders, and that, like all medical problems, it was accessible to the methods of scientific inquiry.

What was not at all clear during the second half of the nineteenth century was where psychiatry stopped and neurology began. The study of the anatomy, functions, and diseases of the nervous system had a long history in British medicine. It was, in fact, Thomas Willis who coined the word *neurologie* in the 1660s; during the subsequent century, it assumed its current form and by the 1830s had spawned the term *neurologist* to signify someone who made the nerves his special subject of inquiry.[34]

Several British medical men early in the nineteenth century contributed significantly to this nascent field of physiology. Between 1810 and 1826, Charles Bell, a surgeon who received his medical education at Edinburgh, recast contemporary understanding of the nervous system's structure and operations. In place of the old assumption that the nerves were unitary fibers, he demonstrated that they were actually bundles of filaments, performing different functions, and he proved that spinal nerves contain separate filaments for motion and for sensation, with distinct roots in the spinal cord. The fact that the French physiologist François Magendie was experimenting with nerve root functions in the early 1820s in no way detracts from the originality of Bell's work, which prompted the *Family Oracle of Health* to proclaim, with premature enthusiasm, in 1825: "The vagueness and mystery which have so long hung over the nervous system are fast disappearing, in consequence of the splendid discoveries lately made in physiology; and the disorders depending on the nerves will, ere long, we are persuaded, be looked upon as no less simple than other diseases." The work of Herbert Mayo also contributed to the journal's optimism. Mayo, who attended Bell's lectures at the Great Windmill Street School of Anatomy in London and followed him around the wards of the Middlesex Hospital, had emulated his mentor by discovering the functions of the facial nerves in 1822. In the following decade, the investigations of Marshall Hall, another British doctor educated at Edinburgh, elucidated the reflex function of the spinal cord, while in the 1840s Thomas Laycock proposed the theory of the brain's reflex action.[35]

These discoveries promised in time to illuminate the physiological foundations of convulsions, paralysis, sensory disorders, and other pathological conditions assumed to involve the nervous system. In place of the nebulous theories about nervous action that had been circulating for centuries, or the equally old and even more unsatisfactory notions of demonic possession to explain madness, hysteria, epilepsy, and the like, the new findings offered specific information that could help to link morbid symptoms with structural damage or deformities. The achievements of the early British neurologists confirmed the growing conviction among medical men that a definite somatic etiology was essential for any disease to assume a legitimate place among the concerns of modern medicine.

Bell, Mayo, Hall, and Laycock were not alienists—that is, they did not specialize in treating the insane. They were primarily anatomists or physiologists who focused their attention on the workings of the nervous system. Yet between them and the Victorian psychiatrists existed a considerable area of mutual interest. Hall was not only a neurological pioneer whose studies extended to the treatment of epilepsy; he was also the consulting physician to Moorcroft House, a private asylum near Uxbridge.[36] Laycock, who became professor of the practice of medicine at Edinburgh in 1855, not only investigated the functions of the cerebral hemispheres and sought to apply evolutionary theory to the development of animal and human nervous centers, but he also lectured on "medical psychology" to his students, offering them his own system of classification for mental diseases and defects. He was fascinated by the role of temperament in molding each patient's pattern of health and sickness and, as Clouston noted in 1906, "gave enormous prominence to what he called 'the neurotic temperament.'"[37] From his first book, *A Treatise on the Nervous Diseases of Women; Comprising an Inquiry into the Nature, Causes, and Treatment of Spinal and Hysterical Disorders* (1840), Laycock retained a lifelong interest in the relationship between the nerves and certain psychological phenomena. He scorned to divide nervous illnesses arbitrarily into structural or functional varieties, believing that, whether the morbid manifestation was mental, as in insanity, or physical, as in paralysis, the root of the problem lay in the nerves. He was as much within his proper province when he investigated neuroses, like hysteria, as when he examined the vascular regions of the brain.

To a considerable extent, neurology in Victorian England developed out of psychiatry, or at least out of psychiatry's milieu and clientele. The asylum population afforded rich opportunities to examine the living and to perform autopsies on the dead. In particular, the prevalence of epileptic and paralytic disorders among the insane provided much material for study by the emerging neurological specialists, who were likelier to be visiting observers at the asylum than part of its staff. The tools they used in their inquiries became the common property of neurologists and psychiatrists alike, as the president of the Medico-Psychological Association exulted in 1881. "To-day the student [of medical psychology] has fortunately a very different position from that which fell to his lot forty years ago," Daniel Hack Tuke, a consulting psychiatrist in London, told the audience at the association's annual meeting. "He has at his command means of research then unknown, as the ophthalmoscope and sphygmograph, and all the modern improvements in the microscope and in preparing sections; and can he not experiment on knee jerks, and a host of reflex and electric phenomena never dreamt of by his predecessors?"[38] Few alienists, it is true, made use of the investigative opportunities thus afforded, but Tuke's remarks illustrate their conviction that psychiatry and neurology were merely two aspects of a common enterprise. That undertaking was nothing less than the great Victorian endeavor to understand the enigmatic interaction of mind and body through painstaking scrutiny of the brain and the vast network of nerves branching from it. During the second half of the nineteenth century, while psychiatrists swore allegiance to a physiological psychology, a psychological neurology—or, at least, a neurology sensitive to the psychological dimensions of nervous pathology—came into being.

The "critical and mature neurological profession"[39] that emerged in Great Britain during the final third of the century was, therefore, a profession willing to cooperate closely with psychiatry. When the Neurological Society of London was launched in the mid-1880s, it drew its members from the ranks of both specialities, and a number of its early officers were alienists. George Savage, for example, served as president both of the Medico-Psychological Association and of the Neurological Society. D. H. Tuke, who had been a medical officer at his family's asylum, the York Retreat, before moving to London and becoming president of the Medico-Psychological Association, was also a founding member of the Neurological Society and its treasurer in 1891. The society's announced objects, furthermore, were not just "to promote the advance of Neurology," but also to "facilitate intercourse amongst those who cultivate it, whether from a Psychological, Physiological, Anatomical, or Pathological point of view."[40] The journal *Brain,* which became the official organ of the society, had been founded in 1878 by four men who were its editors for the first few years. Two of them—John Hughlings Jackson and David Ferrier—became world-famous neurologists; the other two—Bucknill and Crichton-Browne—had both served as asylum medical superintendents.

Appearances, admittedly, were misleading. Beneath the superficial compatibility, differences were already emerging, which by the end of the war would drive British psychiatry and neurology apart. Access to and use of laboratory research facilities became a critical point of distinction. Despite his emphatic endorsement of physiological psychology, for example, Maudsley, the alienist, "was always a clinician who had no laboratory experience or any evident taste for experiment."[41] By the end of Victoria's reign, neurological research had outgrown the limited facilities that asylums might afford, and the focus of that research sharply underscored the emphasis on nervous structure that now clearly characterized neurology. The development of staining methods in the 1850s greatly facilitated the microscopic examination of actual nerve cells and tissue, pioneered in Germany and the Austrian Empire during the first half of the century, while throughout Europe efforts to map out the regions of the brain continued with striking success. In the 1860s and 1870s, the Frenchman Paul Broca, the Germans Eduard Hitzig, Gustav Fritsch, and Karl Wernicke, and the British neurologists Ferrier and Jackson demonstrated that localization of function in the cerebral cortex was not a phrenological fantasy, but a physiological fact.[42] Independently of Broca's identification of the cortical regions associated with speech, Jackson studied the relations between brain disease and speech defect, associated certain epileptic symptoms with specifically located cerebral lesions, and convincingly linked particular areas of the brain to certain movements of the limbs. Using electrical excitation of the cerebral hemispheres, Hitzig, Fritsch, and Ferrier were able further to establish the motor and sensory regions of the brain. In Great Britain, the earliest neurologists all had hospital affiliations, many of them with the National Hospital for the Paralysed and Epileptic (NHPE), the first British institution devoted solely to the treatment of nervous diseases, which opened in Queen Square, London, in 1860. A similar establishment, the Hospital for Epilepsy and Paralysis, subsequently known as the Maida Vale Hospital, opened shortly afterwards. It was there that Rickman Godlee performed the first surgical removal of a brain tumor in 1884, while at NHPE Victor Horsley extended neurosurgery to spinal tumors a few years later.[43]

In the late Victorian and Edwardian decades, however, the future divergence of neurology and psychiatry was still concealed under the harmony of purpose that seemed to characterize their relationship. A handful of alienists *were* performing autopsies on pauper lunatics to see what they could find, while neurologists were sympathetic to the peculiar frustrations implicit in psychiatric medicine. Jackson's often quoted remark—"If there be such a thing as disease of the mind, we can do nothing for it"[44]—signified no lack of interest in psychological phenomena, but merely marked his conviction that the medical man had access only to bodily ills, and that these alone could be successfully treated. He was, nonetheless, a member of the Medico-Psychological Association from 1866, and "discussed psychiatric problems on many occasions." When the psychologist James Sully, suffering from insomnia, sought Jackson's advice in 1878, the neurologist sent him off to the Swiss mountains as readily as any consulting psychiatrist would have done.[45] Although late nineteenth-century British neurologists were less likely to treat neurotic patients than were their American counterparts in the heyday of neurasthenic complaints, they by no means left the care of such cases to the alienists alone. Seymour Sharkey, a pathologist whose career involved no exposure to asylum medicine, considered hysteria and neurasthenia to be appropriate topics for his 1904 presidential address to the Neurological Society because, as he explained: "Whilst gross diseases of the nervous system force themselves most upon the attention, and are the cause of a great number of deaths, I do not think I am wrong when I say that the effects of the ill-health, suffering, and incapacity produced by functional diseases are even more serious and far-reaching. . . . The diseases themselves affect every part of the nervous system and involve the whole subject of nerve physiology and pathology. . . ."[46] Henry Head, a neurologist who had already made a significant contribution to the study of nerve division and regeneration, figured alongside the psychiatric specialists who treated Virginia Woolf during her terrible breakdown in 1913–14.[47]

In fact, the more neurology flourished before World War I, the more psychiatry floundered. For a century, British mad-doctors, alienists, and psychiatrists had persistently reiterated their belief that, to understand madness, one needed to study the brain, while to fathom the nature of related disorders, like hysteria, hypochondriasis, and depression, one had to look to the nerves. By the early twentieth century, neurologists had successfully claimed the structure and workings of the nervous system in all its ramifications, from the brain to the toes, as their own field of expertise. Psychiatrists, whether lunacy commissioners, asylum superintendents, or private consultants, generally lacked adequate research facilities and could not compete in this area of medicine. What remained for them were the less tangible problems—psychological, behavioral, and emotional disorders—all rendered suspect to the rest of the medical profession by their highly uncertain etiology. Yet even here, neurologists threatened to pre-empt psychiatrists' patients, for the mental aspects of illness, although not themselves of primary concern to neurology, were, at least in theory, considered manifestations of an underlying somatic condition, and the medical man who specialized in the pathology of the nerves was accordingly as qualified to offer advice as a doctor with expertise in psychological medicine. Before 1914, British alienists never satisfactorily identified the contributions that they were uniquely qualified to make, apart from the purely managerial chores allotted to asylum keepers and inspectors. They could, at best, handle the insane, although neurologists were likelier to discover the causes of insanity. To make matters worse, outside the asylum neurologists were not the only rivals whom psychiatrists faced.

Medical literature and the biographical records of individual patients leave no doubt that Victorian medical attendants without particular experience in treating nervous maladies or mental illness were frequently called on in cases of functional nervous disorder. The justification for this intrusion was simple: the nervous system, medical practitioners concurred, was involved in virtually every sort of sickness. No one would have argued with the assertion, although articulated in the heterodox *Water Cure Journal and Hygienic Magazine,* that "The nervous system is not a thing apart from the vascular system, but both, to constitute health, must go hand in hand. How, then, shall we rigidly confine ourselves to the brain, when perhaps the cause is located in the stomach, the liver, or the uterus?"[48] If a consultant had won his patient's confidence in medical crises not concerned with nerves or brain, there was, consequently, no good reason not to seek his advice when the distressing symptoms of neurotic illness became manifest. Since psychiatrists were associated above all with asylums and outright lunacy, it is no wonder that many families preferred first to seek out a doctor whom they already trusted and whose reputation for good counsel was not linked with the diagnosis of insanity. In many, indeed in most, cases of milder neurotic problems, the patient never saw an alienist at all.

Gynecologists and obstetricians were particularly prominent among the specialists in other branches of Victorian medicine who became known for treating functional nervous disorders. This was an entirely logical development, because nineteenth-century medical wisdom relentlessly stressed the connection between women's reproductive organs and nervous irritation. Gynecologists, however, by no means excluded men from their "nervous" practice. The leading British advocate of the rest cure therapy for neurasthenia and anorexia from the 1880s was William Smoult Playfair, professor of obstetric medicine at King's College, London, and obstetric physician to King's College Hospital.[49] While the vast majority of his patients were women, he was quite sure that the principles of the rest cure were applicable to men in similar conditions of exhaustion and emaciation. Charles Henry Felix Routh, another prominent gynecologist, felt fully qualified to consider the main cause of nervous prostration in men, and in addition to books on such topics as infant feeding and fibrous tumors of the womb, he published *On Overwork and Premature Mental Decay* in 1876. It is difficult to understand just why Principal Tulloch consulted Sir James Simpson, the most famous of Victorian obstetricians, in 1863 and 1869, during his unbearable experiences of depression, self-consciousness, and insomnia, but perhaps he reasoned that Simpson would have garnered broad experience of nervous derangement from his gynecological practice. Presumably the reason why J. A. Symonds sought the help of T. Spencer Wells in 1864 was not the surgeon's mounting fame as an ovariotomist, but his earlier work in ophthalmology, for one of the most agonizing manifestations of Symonds's breakdown the previous year was terrible inflammation of the eyes.[50] It was precisely this kind of physical symptom of emotional disorder that gave doctors something to treat apart from the elusive nerves.

Medical men with particular knowledge about other organs of the body also attracted their share of nervous patients. Sir Richard Quain, one of the pre-eminent consultant physicians in London during the second half of the nineteenth century, with a clientele at once fashionable, artistic, and literary, wrote papers and lectures on various forms of heart disease that made him a recognized expert in that field. Among his patients who suffered from disabling depression at some stage of their lives were Jane Welsh Carlyle and Sir Edwin Landseer, the popular painter. No one doubted the ability of so distinguished and seasoned a physician to offer meaningful help during health crises precipitated by the nerves. Indeed, Crichton-Browne specifically credited Quain with recognizing the connection between increased heart disease and "the hurry and strain of the age," the "nervous agitations" of modern life.[51] Sir Andrew Clark, like Quain at the very peak of the medical profession in the last quarter of the century, made his specialty pulmonary diseases, and yet he also attracted patients with chronic, nonspecific complaints. Tulloch consulted him in 1881, during a recurrence of depression, and two of the greatest Victorian valetudinarians, Charles Darwin and Herbert Spencer, turned to him for help. Spencer's profound depression in the late 1880s was such, however, that even Clark's cheerful reassurance that he had "the heart of a bullock" was unable to persuade the grim philosopher that his end was not, in fact, drawing near. Darwin, who became Clark's patient in 1873, was treated to an example of the doctor's abiding faith in the therapeutic powers of a controlled diet. It was Clark's attention to the smallest detail of regimen that prompted "most of the hypochondriacs of the time," as the *Dictionary of National Biography* noted, to speak "of him as their dearest friend."[52]

Numerous victims of depression and related disorders never visited a consultant of any sort, but remained satisfied with the care afforded by their family doctor, or general practitioner. These medical men formed the first, and often the only, line of defense against the onslaughts of neurotic illness for countless patients. They were, of course, no more trained in medical psychology than a heart or lung specialist, but where nervous irritability and strain were presumed to be involved, rather than obvious mental imbalance, a generalist in somatic medicine ought to have been qualified to give advice—or so Victorians reasoned. "Year by year cases of neurotic illness assume even larger proportions in the work of the general practitioner," commented David Drummond, a Newcastle doctor, in 1906, "and his inability to deal with them successfully is both a disadvantage to himself and the occasion of much avoidable pain, discomfort, and protracted invalidism in his patients." Drummond's point was not simply that family doctors were scarcely qualified to treat functional nervous disorders, but that, since the neuroses figured so prominently in the practice of the largest segment of the medical profession, medical schools were gravely remiss in neglecting to include the subject in their curriculum.[53]

General practitioners tended to know the limits of their expertise. Henry Ross Todd, the Benson family doctor, for example, not only dealt with the black moods of Edward White Benson, archbishop of Canterbury from 1883 to 1896, but also coped with the manifestations of mental illness in his children, up to a point. In 1907, however, when Margaret Benson, the archbishop's daughter, turned violent and needed to be put under restraint, Todd called in George Savage, the alienist. Similarly, there were occasions when the disabling depression of A. C. Benson, the archbishop's son, surpassed Todd's medical capabilities, and he referred the writer to one or another practitioner who claimed to possess particular skill in dealing with such ailments.[54] When patients evinced symptoms of incipient madness, motor disabilities, convulsive disorders, or seemingly incurable depression, general practitioners were glad to turn them over to some sort of "nerve specialist."

This label, as imprecise and unsatisfactory as everything concerned with the nerves in Victorian and Edwardian medicine, covered neurologists, psychiatrists who practiced outside the asylum, and those various other consultants who gained acclaim for their success with neurotic maladies. It also applied to medical practitioners who sought to capitalize specifically on the fashion for neurasthenic debility perceptible in England from the 1880s. Doctors like Alfred Taylor Schofield, for example, or Thomas Stretch Dowse—a truly Dickensian name for a medical man—were known solely, if at all, for their prolific writings on nervous patients and nervous exhaustion. Dowse claimed to be a Fellow of the Royal College of Physicians of Edinburgh and listed among his credentials positions at the North London Hospital for Consumption and Diseases of the Chest, the Central London Sick Asylum, the Charing Cross Hospital (Skin Department), and the West End Hospital for Nervous Diseases, Paralysis and Epilepsy, in Welbeck Street. With whichever aspect of medicine he felt most familiar, he directed his literary skills to a specific clientele of affluent nervous sufferers. Works with such titles as *On Brain and Nerve Exhaustion: "Neuras-thenia"* (1880) and *The Brain and the Nerves: Their Ailments and Their Exhaustion* (1884) unequivocally staked his claim to this profitable medical territory. Schofield, whose M.D. degree came from Brussels, lacked Dowse's variegated career, but had even more volumes to his credit. *Nerves in Disorder: A Plea for Rational Treatment* (1903), *Nerves in Order or the Maintenance of Health* (1905), *The Management of a Nerve Patient* (1906), and *Functional Nerve Diseases* (1908) represent only a sample of his productivity and amply convey the reason why he felt qualified to call himself a "nerve specialist." He had, furthermore, a precise understanding of the province of such a practitioner: whenever his patients showed signs "of delusions, melancholias, etc."—that is, whenever their symptoms became "clearly mental"—they had "cross[ed] the line and become the care of alienists."[55]

Throughout the nineteenth century, British alienists struggled with an insoluble quandary that hampered their professional growth. They resisted the notion that "clearly mental" disorders existed because they wanted the medical legitimacy that came with ministering to bodily afflictions. Yet to insist that mental illness revealed some malfunction of the nervous system brought alienists into competition with virtually every kind of medical practitioner. Even unlicensed healers advertised their own skill in curing disordered nerves. Whoever offered it, the treatment of functional nervous disorders often actually encompassed what we today consider forms of psychiatric therapy, but, before World War I, psychiatrists offered only a small part of that care. Under the circumstances, it is hardly surprising that they faced for-midable obstacles in their attempts to gain professional standing within late Victorian and Edwardian medicine. No systematic, specialized course of education taught a body of information about mental pathology at once respected by and inaccessible to outsiders. Furthermore, while alienists eventually gained a monopoly on the supervi-sion of asylum inmates, the necessary qualifications for this work were never articulated, and its practitioners enjoyed no autonomy from external interference. Apart from the care of lunatics, they had no clear medical jurisdiction, and many of them yearned, above all else, to move away from madness, or at least to make insanity merely one aspect of a broader medical practice that was both financially rewarding and socially respectable.

The attempt to carve out a remunerative and prestigious medical niche for themselves involved nineteenth-century alienists in what might be called elaborate role-playing.

Throughout the Victorian and Edwardian periods, they posed as scientists, single-mindedly pursuing their physiological inquiries, or as moral guides, firmly but sympathetically redirecting their patients' thoughts away from morbid into healthy channels, or, yet again, as social disciplinarians, resolutely advancing against deviancy on all fronts. These parts occupied no tidy sequential time frame, but rather appeared together throughout the decades, although the moral and social functions tended to become more dominant around the turn of the century, as the likelihood of elucidating major aspects of neurotic illness in physical terms decreased. Alienists were not, of course, alone among medical practitioners in adopting these diverse guises, for the questionable social status of the profession in general prompted its members to seek an authoritative posture in whatever form they could maintain—whether knowledgeable expert, spiritual counselor, or policeman on patrol. Psychiatrists, however, were particularly anxious to insist that they were both medically reputable and socially indispensable, because considerable doubts that they were either heavily tarnished their public image.

The alienists' campaign to bolster their medical reputation consisted chiefly of a determined espousal of what they understood to be the scientific approach to psychological medicine. In pledging their fealty to science, they hoped to impress a public ready to venerate scientific achievements, from the disclosure of electromagnetic mysteries to the discovery of a planet or the isolation of a microbe. Although few Victorians had more than a vague notion of the scientific mode of procedure, they increasingly assumed it to be the surest road to progress in modern branches of knowledge. Like the rest of the medical profession, alienists were keen to establish their place among the ranks of physiologists and pathologists who claimed to base the study of the human body, healthy or diseased, on a rigorous scientific foundation. At the same time, as we have seen, they needed to distinguish themselves from the laymen who challenged their hegemony within the asylum, particularly during the first half of the nineteenth century. Accordingly they stressed—no matter how unjustifiably—that the treatment of insanity was an aspect of medical science, dependent on an intimate knowledge of the physical conditions that gave rise to mental illness. Throughout the nineteenth century, the notion of science was inseparable from the notion of corporeality, as far as British alienists were concerned. Psychiatry could assume the status of science only if it embraced a somatic model of mental alienation, tracing the roots of that disorder to some lesion or malfunction of the body. It was the unswerving emphasis on this approach that marked the medically trained alienist, in contrast to the businessman who owned a madhouse, the philanthropist who supervised a charity hospital, or the magistrate who oversaw a public asylum.

Victorian psychiatrists were, however, driven by more than the anticipation of immediate professional victories when they adopted the pose of scientific researcher. Physiology, they sincerely believed, would reveal what philosophy had kept obscure. The close clinical observation of large numbers of cases, and generalizations inductively derived from them, might solve the riddle of functional nervous disorders, while introspective theorizing about the mind could only offer speculation. No doubt the emphasis on "facts," on hard evidence of a quantifiable sort, can be seen as part of a strategy by which alienists, and medical practitioners in general, used the language of science in an attempt to install themselves as authorities on a range of issues affecting national health and public welfare. Such a goal would not be incompatible with the conviction that the collection and analysis of physical data promised to yield hitherto inaccessible information about the workings of the mind.

Medical research "carried out along physical lines with physical apparatus"[56] made important strides during the nineteenth century across a broad range of concerns, from the arrest of puerperal fever to the measurement of blood pressure. The physical lines of inquiry had been narrowing at least since the mid-eighteenth century, as medical theories based on diffuse bodily states gave way to a closer clinical study of specific alterations in specific organs. By the end of Victoria's reign the focal point of medical investigation was no longer the organ, or the tissue, but the individual cell. At the same time, the physical apparatus of medical research, particularly the microscope, developed greater technical sophistication to meet the demands of the new cellular pathology. It is no wonder that alienists wanted to keep in step with these trends. With "the minute structure of the brain"[57] as their particular object of interest, they had every reason to anticipate success from a materialist assault on insanity, in accordance with the dominant principles of physiology.

British psychiatry evinced a somatic bias throughout the nineteenth century. It informed the work of famous alienists, like Maudsley, and of those scarcely known beyond the asylums over which they presided. Repeatedly, in the early decades of the century as in the later ones, these men informed parliamentary committees of inquiry, the readers of the medical press, and the broader public alike that insanity was the tragic result of organic disease.[58] The classification of lunacy among the functional nervous disorders underscored its presumed physiological foundation and justified the use of diverse medicaments in its treatment. As befitted mental pathologists, the most enterprising of the asylum medical officers sought to identify that foundation by a painstaking scrutiny of the brains of deceased inmates. Bucknill was among the first to undertake a "laborious examination of a number of brains of the insane to determine the amount of cerebral atrophy," while others, including Savage at Bethlem, subsequently applied the microscope to cerebral tissue.[59] Alienists could not only assert with pride, "We are physicians—we treat the body," as W. H. O. Sankey, medical superintendent of the women's section of the Middlesex asylum, announced in 1863; they believed that they could profess to be scientists. "It will not be denied," Tuke insisted in 1881, "that at least the foundations of the pathology of insanity have been more securely laid in cerebral physiology during the last forty years," and he looked forward to "the accumulating knowledge of the morbid histology of the brain and cord in the insane." The advent of microbiology in the final quarter of the nineteenth century further expanded the range of choices open to psychiatrists who sought to explain mental illness in physical, and scientifically orthodox, terms. As Clouston observed in 1903, "adverse bacteria" lurking in the body could henceforth be blamed for a wide array of mental diseases.[60]

The medical model of mental illness, by which alienists hoped to elucidate insanity, was equally applicable to lesser forms of functional nervous disorder, including nervous breakdown. Before, during, and after the Victorian decades, medical men who dealt with the symptoms of nervous exhaustion were kept busy articulating physiological theories to account for them. Whether doctors stressed gastric upheavals, spinal irritation, vascular disturbance, blood abnormalities, local inflammation, irritation of the mucous membranes, cerebral cellular alterations, ovario-uterine derangements, or toxic wastes in the body, the purpose was always to associate depressive states with specific organic causes. The *Family Oracle of Health,* for example, serving up its medical wisdom for a general readership in the 1820s, frequently cited the effect of digestive and circulatory problems on the nerves, in order to account for such complaints as low spirits, headaches, faintness, and fretfulness. In 1814, when Benjamin Collins Brodie, just commencing what became an extremely successful surgical career, evinced the classic symptoms of depression, finding exertion difficult and "life altogether wearisome and uncomfortable," he tersely summarized his condition with the words, "I became dyspeptic." Undernourished nerves were, obviously, prone to nervous collapse, but so were nerves assaulted by various other agents of destruction. Early in the twentieth century, Clouston was quick to point out, not only the links between hostile bacteria and insanity, but also the probability that milder "conditions of mental disturbance, . . . such as lethargy, irritability, inability for work, and depression [were] of microbic origin."[61] In the years between Brodie and Clouston, medical speculation flourished about the origins of disorders like these, and alienists were in the thick of the speculative fray. While no uniformity of opinion emerged from the wealth of etiological options, British medical practitioners could concur on one all-inclusive generalization: functional nervous disorders were impossible without some structural or nutritional change in the body.

Victorian alienists believed that physiological explanations were needed to give psychiatry the authority of science in an era when physics, chemistry, geology, biology, and astronomy appeared to be uncovering the secrets of the universe. Yet, at the same time, the determination to take, and hold, a scientific stance created severe difficulties for psychiatrists in the nineteenth and early twentieth centuries. No amount of assertions could transform what they hopefully called "mental physiology" into an exact science. They could never agree on a single classification scheme for the mental diseases they treated. Furthermore, as they readily acknowledged, both the immense variety within that category of illness and the highly individualized nature of functional nervous disorders placed weighty obstacles in the way of formulating general laws, necessary for psychiatry to become a science in more than name alone. The greater the claims made for psychiatric achievements, the less impressive the reality appeared.

Reality impinged particularly in the failure to locate cerebral lesions—tangible evidence of brain disease—commensurate with the degree of mental derangement evident in lunatics. This "inconvenient fact" had disturbed mad-doctors' peace of mind at the very start of the nineteenth century,[62] but they still retained their faith that further investigations would produce the evidence of physical alteration on which their somatic theories of insanity depended. Most British psychiatrists continued to voice the physiological interpretative orthodoxies down to World War I, hoping that the accumulation of autopsy reports and microscopical inquiry would in due course yield the desired results. In the meantime, they could fall back on the notion of invisible functional lesions—and even lesions of the will or of the understanding—to imply a generalized morbid condition of the brain and nervous system that provided an organic foundation for irrational behavior, but defied material analysis.[63] By the final quarter of the century, however, the invocation of lesions yet to be discovered sounded more and more like psychiatrists whistling in the dark. Even Tuke's optimism in 1881 had a forced ring to it, for he had to admit that the attempt to connect particular symptoms of insanity with morbid appearances of the brain after death had not proved successful in the majority of cases.[64] This realization, combined with the disappointingly low proportion of asylum cases that could be considered "cured" by the supposedly skilled medical officers in attendance, raised grave doubts about the applicability of physiological models to psychological problems.[65]

It is ironic that the more Victorian psychiatrists insisted on their status as physiologists, the more they contributed to the dilemma that challenged their professional identity. To boast that mental illness was increasingly recognized "as an integral part of disorders of the nervous system," and to insist that "medical psychology is less and less regarded as a fragment detached from the general domain of medicine,"[66] was to call in question any separate ground for psychiatry to occupy. A claim designed to rank alienists with biological scientists in fact contributed to a situation in which the late nineteenth-century advances in neurophysiology only brought into harsher light the lack of similar accomplishments in the treatment of functional nervous disorders. As the group of nervous maladies still considered functional contracted in the early years of the twentieth century, the practice of the neurologist expanded, while psychiatrists were left to cope with those remaining neuroses that appeared ever less worthy objects of medical attention.

The contempt which much of the British medical profession expressed for psychological disorders bereft of evident somatic foundations proved less devastating to Victorian and Edwardian alienists than might be assumed from their sustained attempt to play the physiologist's part. For all the homage that they paid to the figure of the empirical scientist, they were powerfully drawn to other roles, which offered invaluable alternative sources both of social prestige and of job satisfaction. In particular, they cultivated the image of trusted family friend and counselor, sagacious advisor on a range of intimate problems, moral guide to the mentally distressed as much as doctor to the physically diseased. It was a character that alienists could readily embrace, for it fitted perfectly their awkward situation on the margins of medical practice. If their "real diagnostic and prognostic skills were rudimentary," they had talent aplenty to foster "a therapeutic ambience"—at least for affluent patients under private care—while "their tact in handling the feelings of their clients won the confidence of patients' families."[67] Unlike other medical specialists during the course of the nineteenth century, psychiatrists did not gain substantially more knowledge about their patients' illnesses than the patients themselves. Especially with regard to afflictions such as depression and hysteria, subjective symptoms continued to dominate the doctor–patient relationship, with medical attendants betraying considerable impotence in the face of intractable conditions. Under these circumstances, alienists often found moral suasion a more promising approach to adopt, even if they continued to prescribe medication or other elements of somatic therapy.

Their signal failure to attain any measure of scientific credibility actually redounded to the benefit of Victorian alienists when it came to attracting a desirable group of patients. Indeed, the importance of a wealthy, leisured class of patrons in the eighteenth century continued to influence the style and values of British medicine for much of the nineteenth, and the personal confidant, not the research-oriented doctor, approximated the Georgian ideal of the gentleman-physician. Patients who wanted sympathy from their medical attendants were looking, not for the latest expertise in physiology, but for a shared outlook on life and common cultural assumptions. Victorian society never ceased to honor the landed proprietor above the bourgeois entrepreneur or the learned intellectual; the initiative and ambition that might lure patients to a particular medical man in the United States or post-revolutionary France, and the scientific accomplishments revered in Germany, had to compete in England with a polished, urbane manner that marked a man at ease among society's natural leaders. It mattered that a medical man appear to be a gentleman, able to display the social graces that made one welcome in the homes of gentlemen. Such traits could, of course, coexist with considerable scientific authority, but among a large segment of potential patron-patients the medical skill they sought did not arise from hours in a hospital ward or operating theater. It was a function of individual character, of long experience in treating patients with suavity and tact, of mixing moral values with medicine, and of circulating among refined people.[68]

While other fields of British medicine obviously felt the influence of such attitudes and preferences, psychiatry was particularly responsive because its pretensions to figure as a scientific pursuit were so easily punctured. Alienists found it immensely reassuring to see among the variety of medical men who treated nervous ailments several enjoying great success because they were sociable rather than scientific. Sir Henry Holland, for example, physician to both Queen Victoria and Prince Albert, and recipient of a baronetcy in 1853, was the author of *Chapters on Mental Physiology*, published in the preceding year. A London physician with an annual income of £5,000, he had no particular claims to prominence as a medical psychologist or as any sort of physiologist, but he was "friend and advisor to almost every man of note," including Darwin. The fact that his work was "more fashionable than scientific," as the *Dictionary of National Biography* observed, was no bar at all to fame and fortune.[69] John Marshall, who reached the pinnacle of the surgical profession in the final quarter of the nineteenth century, contributed no significant innovations to the practice of surgery. Nonetheless he was esteemed by his private patients, including Dante Gabriel Rossetti, who "mostly sought out not the surgeon but the wise and tolerant general practitioner."[70] Even Sir Andrew Clark's appeal, the *Lancet* had to concede, had nothing to do with his medical publications or his gifts as "a great clinical teacher." "The public thronged to him . . . because they were quick to detect in him the qualities that, above all others, they valued in their physician. They saw him attentive, eager, sympathetic, and in particular practical." Marshall Hall, by contrast, although a distinguished physiologist, never obtained a London hospital appointment nor earned from his private practice the kind of income that accrued to the most popular consultants. His wife could only conclude that this was due to "the vulgar prejudice that the cultivation of physiology is incompatible with the character of a *practical* physician."[71]

Alienists eager to ascend the social ladder by expanding their practice beyond the asylum into the ranks of the upper middle classes could not fail to understand that this desirable clientele required solace from kindly, mature medical practitioners who shared their patients' tastes. In warning their sane, but troubled, patrons about healthy modes of life, the avoidance of vicious habits, and the cultivation of nervous stability amid the tensions of modern civilization, Victorian psychiatrists did little to enhance their renown as scientists, but identified themselves as men of common sense who could be relied on for sound advice. Such a reputation was, quite literally, worth its weight in gold, or at least pounds sterling. It was patronage by royalty, aristocracy, and fashionable society in the first half of the century that had ensured the successful career of Sir Alexander Morison, knighted in 1838, and of Henry Herbert Southey, a physician who served as metropolitan lunacy commissioner from 1828 to 1845 with virtually no qualifications for the job, except good looks and athletic prowess.[72] The lesson continued to impress alienists after mid-century. Those who aspired to heal the socially prominent tried to imitate their lifestyle, nurturing a passion for sports and joining the right sort of clubs. George Savage, for one, enthusiastic about fishing, fencing, and mountain climbing, was a member of the Athenaeum and boasted a country address—The Island, Hurstbourne Priors—in Hampshire. By the time he was knighted in 1912, he had, needless to say, left his post at Bethlem and had established a lucrative consulting practice in London.[73]

During the Victorian period, alienists rarely received royal honors. Baronetcies and peerages eluded their grasp altogether. The latter, in fact, remained closed to medical men throughout the nineteenth century, with the one exception of Joseph Lister, the founder of antiseptic surgery, who was created a baron in 1897. Forty-seven baronetcies, however, were bestowed on physicians and surgeons, usually in recognition of services to the Queen, her family, or the royal household. Although none of the medical baronets were psychiatrists, several, including Sir Andrew Clark, were well known to have strong interests in mental and related nervous disorders. Sir William Withey Gull received his baronetcy in 1872, the year after he attended the Prince of Wales through a severe bout of typhoid fever, and during the period when he was trying to establish anorexia nervosa as a form of mental illness. Sir Samuel Wilks became a baronet in 1897, the year he was named physician extraordinary to the Queen. Physician at Guy's Hospital for many years, Wilks turned his attention to a variety of medical inquiries, among which diseases of the nervous system figured prominently. His lectures on the subject went through two editions.[74]

With knighthoods, Victorian psychiatrists fared only slightly better. Few were distributed to men whose work was solely, or even closely, bound up with the menacing world of lunatic asylums. A rare exception was Sir William Charles Ellis, the first resident medical superintendent of the West Riding Lunatic Asylum in 1818 and subsequently of the Middlesex County Asylum, who was knighted in 1835.[75] Far more typical was the experience of Bucknill or of Crichton-Browne, knighted respectively in 1894 and 1886. Although both men began their careers as asylum doctors, their recognition came long after they had left that milieu; it was less for their contributions to the study of mental disease than for their services to the state as Lord Chancellor's Visitors in Lunacy. Not until the Edwardian period did psychiatrists' chances for knighthood somewhat improve, with Allbutt, Clouston, and Savage all being so honored between 1907 and 1912. By then, however, Allbutt had ceased his service as a commissioner in lunacy and held the regius professorship of medicine at

Cambridge, while Savage, as we have seen, was well on the road to becoming a country gentleman. Only Clouston's career had stayed close to its foundations in asylum medicine, although his presidency of the Royal College of Physicians, Edinburgh, had added considerable distinction to it.[76]

By the eve of World War I, therefore, the leading British alienists had made some progress toward obscuring the taint of the madhouse, but they had done so only by distancing themselves from the vast majority of their colleagues who remained permanently mired in asylum medicine. The most visible representatives of late Victorian and Edwardian psychiatry achieved their improved social status, furthermore, at the expense of their professional standing, for the image of the gentleman-physician that they embraced had, according to other medical viewpoints, lost most of its luster by the end of the nineteenth century. The rest of the medical profession *was* relying more and more on scientific methods and equipment, but psychiatry derived little practical benefit from them. Although alienists never repudiated the role of physiologist, they purposefully nurtured another persona as well, simultaneously exploring other avenues to advancement. They sought, in fact, to enjoy the best of both worlds: they hoped to gain the eminence that increasingly accompanied scientific research, but, realistically assessing their poor record in that regard, worked to assure their authority as trusted family friends purveying moral lessons essential for happiness and, above all, for health.

Morality was always closely linked with health in Victorian medical theory, and psychiatrists were scarcely alone among doctors in believing that the moral amelioration of the people was a legitimate medical task. Public health officials were particularly keen to underscore the cause-and-effect relationship between depravity and disease.[77] For alienists, the emphasis on morality, whether public or private, had the undoubtedly welcome effect of giving them an important assignment outside the asylum—one that needed no grounding in cerebral physiology, cellular pathology, or microbiology.

Victorian alienists could only work effectively as moral guides if they truly acknowledged the power of moral agents in causing illness. By *moral,* they understood both the synonymous adjective *ethical,* but also the idea of emotional, mental, or nonphysical influences. Thus if they spoke of the moral causes of insanity, they referred to emotional trauma, such as overpowering grief, passion, disappointment, or fright. It seems utterly inconsistent that they should have stressed the organic bases of functional nervous disorders while recognizing that strong emotions could exert a devastating impact on physical health, yet it is historically demonstrable that they did so. Indeed, in 1863, when David Skae, resident physician at the Royal Edinburgh Asylum, proposed that types of insanity be classified according to the bodily diseases from which they arose, he expected his colleagues to protest that "insanity is a mental affection, brought on most frequently by mental or moral causes." Even Maudsley, the arch-somaticist, appreciated the influence of ideas and violent feelings in producing disease.[78] Such beliefs were commonplace throughout Victorian medical literature, which underscored the potency of distressing passions in provoking, not only mental disorientation, but even such tangible evidence of somatic disarray as fever. Especially concerned about the impact of profound emotions on the sensitive tissue of the brain and nerves, alienists could convincingly persuade their patients that healthy attitudes were as necessary for physical well-being as any mixture from the apothecary's shop. The fact that the heyday of psychiatric confidence in the physiological foundations of insanity—until the 1860s or early 1870s—coincided with the attempt to implement a policy of moral management in the asylums illustrates beyond any doubt how thoroughly Victorian alienists mingled the categories of physical and moral, with regard both to the causation and the treatment of functional nervous disorders. There was never a time in the Victorian and Edwardian decades when somaticism alone characterized British psychiatric theory or practice.

Among medical historians, Victorian doctors have suffered a bad reputation for destroying the psychosomatic or, to use current terminology, the holistic thrust of Georgian medicine. Throughout the eighteenth century, and in the early decades of the nineteenth, so the argument goes, mind and body were treated together, "within the context of the total body system." When medical attendants commanded comparatively scant information about the human body, they considered relevant all aspects of a patient's health, emotional as well as somatic, and forced their comprehension of sickness into no artificial, arbitrary categories of mental and physical. By contrast, Victorian medicine, particularly in the latter half of the nineteenth century, is perceived as separatist. Increasingly detailed and accurate knowledge, linked with the emergence of laboratory research in physiology, allowed practitioners to focus exclusively on the organic causes of disease, allegedly minimizing the significance of psychological ones. Medical specialists had no time for, or interest in, the vague etiological role of emotional distress and mental perturbation, which they tended to place outside the domain appropriate to medical science.[79]

If nineteenth-century medicine *was,* very slowly, moving away from a unified vision of mind and body, the therapeutic implications of the drift did not begin to emerge until the end of the Victorian era. Throughout the period, medical men of all varieties continued to address the mind in their attempts to heal the body. By the final quarter of the century, however, such an approach was starting to fall into disrepute, to the regret of those who still judged it an effective form of treatment. Benjamin Ward Richardson, editor of the *Journal of Public Health and Sanitary Review,* found cause to lament in 1883

> . . . how very little the question of the origin of physical diseases from mental shock or influence has been studied. Even physicians have let this question largely stand aside, as if content with the contemplation of the grosser and more material evidences of the origins of disease. To consider how a person should be injured by taking some deleterious substance into his system through his breath, his stomach, his skin, his blood, were a truly scientific and rational pursuit; but to consider what shall enter by the senses or windows of the mind, and so invisibly entering be potent for evil or for good, that were too refined and indefinite a pursuit.[80]

Although some members of the late Victorian medical profession came to take a dim view of what we now recognize as forms of psychotherapy, alienists were not among them, for they could ill afford to scorn a mode of treatment that sometimes proved successful when pharmaceutical means failed. For all his interest in microbes, Clouston nonetheless paid close attention to "the mental hygiene of bodily disease" and fully acknowledged that mental influences could cure numerous conditions of physical sickness, a viewpoint widely shared by his fellow psychiatrists. Moral guidance, in fact, assumed so prominent a place in the Victorian alienist's therapeutic armory that his work has recently been described as, not mental, but "moral physiology."[81]

At the center of this moral physiology was the concept of the will, on which virtually all Victorian and Edwardian attitudes toward adult mental health and illness were constructed. In a healthy condition, the will was credited with exercising a supervisory function over all activities of the mind—ideas, sensory impressions, emotions, desires, imagination—and over the so-called lower impulses, or instincts, of humanity's animal nature as well. The ability to reason, to exercise judgment, to fulfill one's role in life were all contingent on the operations of the will, for if that became inadequate to its directing task, the personality disintegrated. Mental illness, both severe and mild, was the manifestation of just such a catastrophe, resulting from pathological conditions of the brain and nervous system, or, less frequently, of some other organ. The sufferer lost all ability to regulate thought, feeling, or conduct, and the power to govern instinctual drives.[82]

The dominance of will in Victorian psychiatric theory seems to cast a mentalist glow over nineteenth-century British medical psychology. Although associated with the highest nervous centers of the cerebral cortex, presumably in the frontal lobes, the will was generally interpreted as a mental faculty, not reducible to physiological attributes. It was, in fact, often used interchangeably with *mind,* as when a reviewer for the *British and Foreign Medico-Chirurgical Review* in 1856 portrayed the nervous system as "the instrument by which outward realities around us affect the mind; and by which the mind, as force or will, reacts in its turn upon the world without."[83] Although some attempts were made to encapsulate the will within a vaguely somatic description, such as "neural act," for most Victorians and Edwardians who grappled with the subject the will remained utterly distinct from any bodily components. The fact that D. H. Tuke had to include an article on "Disorders of Will" in his highly regarded *Dictionary of Psychological Medicine,* published in 1892, suggests that the topic would not fit under any other category of mental or nervous illness.[84] Maudsley, notoriously impatient with what he considered an "irrational dualism" impeding the establishment of psychology on physiological grounds, nonetheless himself published a book entitled *Body and Will* in 1883.[85] Despite his concerted efforts throughout the volume, he was unable to make the will entirely coterminous with a cluster of nervous centers in the brain. Psychiatrists, in short, encountered great difficulties in trying to explain human behavior without reference to the will as a managerial force, certainly dependent on the nerves to do its bidding, but existing somehow outside and apart from the nervous system.

Reliance on a nonmaterial organizing concept, the will, to make sense of mental activity in all its extraordinary intricacy did not necessarily invalidate Victorian psychiatric commitment to the bodily foundations of mental illness and functional nervous disorders. When alienists described such maladies in terms of the will's failure, they generally perceived that failure as evidence of an underlying physical disturbance—although that, in turn, might have been precipitated by some emotional crisis. "Failure of the will" was a convenient way to indicate the gravity of the medical problem, without being able to pinpoint its material source. If alienists liked to think that the centrality of will in psychiatric theory was entirely compatible with the theory's somatic emphases, however, they did acknowledge that the critically important role they assigned to the will undermined any tendency toward a deterministic view of human nature. The Victorian public did not want to hear that neural impulses or chemical reactions, operating according to predictable laws, could alone explain the complex behavior of individual people, and few psychiatrists, apart from Maudsley, cared to hint that it was so. The will allowed them to hedge on the issue right down to the war, and long after. It remained the pivotal psychiatric concept, the focus of the irresolvable tension between mental and somatic interpretations of neurotic illness that dominated Victorian psychiatry.

All these themes came together in the interpretation of nervous breakdown as an illness that particularly demanded moral counseling for its victims. Medical practitioners outside the confraternity of alienists assumed as wholeheartedly as the psychiatrists themselves that the inability to exercise will was precisely what barred these patients from undertaking any activity, caused their painful indecisiveness, and prolonged their oppressive lethargy. Whatever the specific reason for the will's enfeeblement, its virtual absence wrought havoc with the personality of the sufferer, making impossible all exercise of self-control or intentional effort. A variety of causes, particularly morbid conditions of the nervous system, could "alter and disturb more or less the action of the will," Sir Henry Holland observed at mid-century, "in some cases rendering it feeble and uncertain, in others apparently for a time abolishing it altogether." When that happened, "a man or a woman . . . is said to have broken down," B. W. Richardson commented, "or to have lost self-control, or energy, or heart." "Of all the pains of consciousness the most painful is the sense of the mental self going to pieces," wrote Maudsley, unable to avoid using another abstract mentalist construct—the self—to explain why depression frequently prompted thoughts of suicide.[86] Under such circumstances, the medical attendant's primary duty was to restore the will to its coordinating role, so that the incapacitated person could once again display the characteristics of a healthy, normal, self-disciplined adult. Often enough, the doctor had to reason the patient back to health, as Bucknill explained in memorable terms. "The true mental physician," he told the Association of Medical Officers of Asylums and Hospitals for the Insane in 1860, "transfers for the moment the mind of his patient into himself in order that, in return, he may give back some portion of his own healthful mode of thought to the sufferer."[87] Bucknill's idealized alienist was to take on, if not the sins, at least the diseases of his patients, replacing them with some measure of his own mental balance. There, Bucknill implied, lay the real source of psychiatric authority and power. Clearly, the chances for success in such a delicate maneuver appeared far greater when patients were depressed, rather than insane. Even after hopes for the moral management of lunatics had faded, British alienists continued to address the invalid's own will to recover when serving moral arguments to victims of shattered nerves.

Despite Bucknill's sacramental language, alienists were no more unique among Victorian medical men in offering their patients the services of doctor-cum-father confessor than they were in standing guard over issues of public morality. Darwin recalled about his father, Robert Waring Darwin, a highly successful physician in Shrewsbury during the first half of the nineteenth century, that thanks to his "skill in winning confidence he received many strange confessions of misery and guilt."[88] While confessions of some sort may be implicit in the relationship between patient and doctor, Victorians were even likelier than their Georgian grandparents to unburden emotional woes onto medical shoulders, for the gradual secularization of British society in the nineteenth century meant that some segments of the population found themselves turning less to clergymen and more to doctors in times of stress and unhappiness. "Moral-pastoral" responsibilities were, indeed, an integral part of the job performed by virtually every Victorian medical man. None worked harder at the effort, however, than psychiatrists. Not only did their patients obviously need to control irrational or disturbed conduct, but, without a demonstrable somatic explanation for mental derangement, alienists were most dependent on a moral approach to the disorders they were supposed to know how to cure.[89]

The assumption of moral-pastoral duties by nineteenth-century British doctors did not mean that medical men were actively seeking to replace clergymen in Victorian society or overtly competing with them for the souls and bodies of neurotic, depressed, or insane patients. Occasionally, a case of professional rivalry did occur, such as Wilks reported in his *Lectures on Diseases of the Nervous System*. He told of a young woman, bedridden for several years with "an affection of the hip," who consulted all the leading medical practitioners in London, to no avail. At length, a clergyman was summoned; he prayed over her and had the considerable satisfaction of seeing her arise and walk. The religious press declared a miracle, while the woman's medical consultants dismissed the case as an example of hysteria all along. Wilks told the story, not to scold the priest for interfering, but to criticize his professional colleagues. If they had, from the start, identified the woman's illness as hysterical, he asserted, they were foolish to have dosed her with physic for three years, instead of trying the moral suasion which, he believed, was essential in such instances.[90] Direct confrontations, however, were exceedingly rare. Through a process both subtle and gradual, medical men—and psychiatrists, in particular— came to realize that they were performing roles once assigned to the clergy. As the traditional range of priestly tasks contracted during the nineteenth century, public agencies and private philanthropies undertook many of the welfare responsibilities once performed by religious bodies, while those Victorians who still attended church increasingly looked to their ministers solely for the theological teaching that no other source could provide. Among the many new purveyors of secular morality for young and old, psychiatrists emerged as prominent figures. Leonard Guthrie, a late Victorian and Edwardian doctor who would today be called a child psychiatrist, seemed almost surprised to find that the public had "learnt that morality is largely a question of health and temperament and environment," with the result that "medical men [were] frequently called upon to advise in cases which formerly were dealt with by disciplinarians." "Hence our professional armamentarium," he observed in 1907, "is no longer completed by a set of infallible prescriptions for coughs, worms, stomach ache and fits; we must often be obliged to dispense more platitudes than pills."[91] In fact, moral platitudes had been part of the medical attendant's bag of tricks throughout the nineteenth century.

British psychiatrists, of course, were fully conscious that clergymen, at least Anglican ones, occupied a more securely elevated and authoritative position on the social ladder than medical men could claim, and such considerations could scarcely have failed to increase the attractions that alienists found in the moral-pastoral role. Yet it would be seriously misleading to depict them imitating their French counterparts, who consciously and methodically "sought to establish [their profession] at the expense of the clergy."[92] The strident anticlerical zeal, inherited from the eighteenth century, that particularly colored French science and medicine under the Third Republic had little appeal in Great Britain. Nor did the scientific materialism fashionable in certain German intellectual circles. British psychiatrists, like other British medical men, saw more to gain from an alliance than a power struggle with the clergy. Somatic and spiritual ministers were often allied in the campaigns to eradicate sin and disease that characterized the Victorian approach to environmental reform, particularly in the first half of the nineteenth century;[93] many doctors, furthermore, were as eager as the clergy to avoid the hostile opposition of science and faith in the second half of the century.

For most of Victoria's reign, any British doctor who sought professional advancement, royal honors, or the patronage of society's leaders found formal adherence to the Christian faith essential, but more than pragmatism or ambition underlay the profound concern with which many medical practitioners viewed the materialism implicit in physiological interpretations of mental illness. The warning issued in 1853 by Daniel Noble, who specialized in medical psychology, was repeated with varying degrees of sophistication through the Edwardian era. "There is nothing in the physiological study of the brain and nervous system," he wrote, "which *ought* to suggest the approaches even of materialism. Whilst here below, the actions of the spirit occur through organic intervention. . . . Yet is it no more the case that the material brain is the thinking principle, and the separate parts divisions of the soul, than it is true that the music of the lyre inheres in the instrument, and that the melodies which art can elicit from it, are self-produced by the particular strings."[94] Preservation of spirit or soul mattered more to British psychiatry, and medicine in general, before World War I than its formal adherence to a physiological psychology would lead historians of a later generation to expect.

Victorian medical theorists attempted to accommodate the soul largely by employing the concept of psychophysical parallelism. With such a theory, it was not necessary to consign the mind to the physical properties of the cerebral hemispheres, for psychophysical parallelism assumed that both mind and brain existed, distinct but not separate from one another. Mental and bodily states were two different aspects of the same reality, the theory asserted. They were corresponding conditions within a single context, never directly impinging on each other, as parallel lines do not intersect, but both essential parts of the functioning organism, each responsive to and affecting the other. The beauty of this theory, as historians of psychiatry have been quick to note, is that it allowed all disease and corruption to reside in the physical matter of the brain. The mind could not help but reflect such alteration, but in itself remained untouched, untarnished. "It is now a pretty generally received doctrine," Thomas Stretch Dowse announced in 1880, summarizing at least a half-century of medico-psychological thought, "that there can be no abnormal condition of mind *per se*. It must arise,'' he continued in more up-to-date terms, ''from some molecular derangement of the brain-cells, from poisonous material floating in the blood, or from an altered condition in the arterial current either in quantity or quality.'' Since the immaterial mind generally figured as synonymous with the spirit in Christian writing, protecting the mind from morbidity was, of course, tantamount to preserving the soul from mortality.[95] The concept of psychophysical parallelism at least served as a delaying tactic, postponing through compromise difficult and painful controversies over the place of spirit in the material universe. As a means of bridging the gulf between mind and body, or of actually attempting to explain the impact of each on the other, however, the theory was singularly uninformative.

With psychophysical parallelism, the easy transition from psychological to cosmological concerns is readily apparent.[96] It was impossible to consider the nature of mind and will without implying something about the source of movement and change in the natural world. Laycock understood this and boldly accepted the consequences of his determination to construe the workings of mind as manifestations of physical properties: not only did he deny that humanity was qualitatively different from the rest of the animal kingdom, but he saw no evidence to support the hypothesis of an immaterial, immortal soul or to uphold the independent activity of spirit in the universe. The majority of Victorian alienists, however, sought above all to avoid explicit engagement in these profound considerations and tried to distance such issues from their attempts to reinvigorate the will of depressed and disoriented patients. The will they celebrated was purely individual volition, without which they could neither account for purposeful human conduct nor conceive of meaningful moral choice. Psychiatrists proceeded in the belief that the far vaster theological problem of free will was irrelevant to their inquiries. Whether or not the conscious efforts of men and women were foreordained by an omniscient deity did not preoccupy them, in part because the harsh doctrine of predestination in all its ramifications commanded slight adherence by the nineteenth century, but mainly because they shared the dominant middle-class commitment to the principle of individual freedom—particularly the freedom to choose right over wrong. If they recoiled from the idea that impersonal physical laws controlled human beings who were nothing more than molecules of matter, they were hardly eager to enslave humanity to the unfathomable designs of divine foreknowledge.

For Victorian and Edwardian psychiatrists, a belief in the existence and real efficacy of human will did not, therefore, necessarily imply the existence and predominance of cosmic will, with the unavoidable conclusion that Providence dictated human destiny. They were certainly disingenuous to think they could have mind writ small—and even the possibility of individual immortality—while downplaying the role of Spirit writ large, but they generally acted on that conviction. Alienists, in short, assumed they could espouse physiological psychology selectively, leaving room for personal moral responsibility and taking care to bypass sensitive theological issues.

In the role of moral guide, they worked to fit cultural creeds into a medical framework. Faith in the possibility of self-improvement and applause for individual effort were central to the system of values which the Victorian middle classes had so solidly constructed by the mid-nineteenth century, and which Crichton-Browne's generation of alienists inherited almost as a birthright. Despite the encroachments of the regulatory state, most members of the bourgeoisie hailed voluntarism as the necessary basis for a healthy society, just as their doctors considered the autonomous will requisite for personal well-being. Medical practitioners combined these two strands of thought when they insisted on the individual's duty to choose health. Ultimately, they argued, patients were as morally responsible in the field of medicine as in all other aspects of life. The doctor could advise and exhort, but only the patient could cultivate the self-discipline that alone ensured soundness of mind and body. When alienists built their psychological theories around the potency of the will, they were closely conforming to the ethos of self-help cherished by the clientele they served. Without the concept of will, furthermore, British psychiatrists in the nineteenth century would have lacked moral authority over their patients, for they could have claimed no reason to exercise those pastoral tasks that generously compensated for the vulnerability of their position as medical scientists.

Equally laden with the values of the Victorian middle class was the psychiatric guise of social disciplinarian, a functionary closely related to the moral guardian, but with particular interest in promoting the interpretation of illness as a punishment for sin, or at least for deviation from accepted forms of behavior. This Victorian adaptation of the ancient medical tradition depicting disease as a means of divine retribution for misconduct suggests how limited was the modernity of nineteenth-century medicine. Ironically, while medical men celebrated their distance from old superstitions attributing sickness to diabolic possession or the triumph of witchcraft, they were persistently incorporating a vestige of older attitudes into their own ideology. The conviction that disease could be the penalty exacted for moral trespassing emerged in many forms throughout Victorian medical literature, particularly in psychiatric texts. The argument clearly worked best where no specific external causative agent had been identified, and it was thus most applicable, by the end of the century, to those functional nervous disorders whose origins still remained a mystery. With unimpressive rates of cure both in the asylum and in private practice, psychiatrists naturally welcomed any opportunity to minimize their own shortcomings, but there is no evidence to indicate that they did not also genuinely believe in the theories they articulated.

Not only did contravention of the unwritten code governing society merit punishment in the form of ill health, according to Victorian alienists, but, what was more, the breach of social convention itself might be pronounced equivalent to sickness, as the concept of "moral insanity" implied. This protean disease construct was first proposed in 1835 in James Cowles Prichard's *Treatise on Insanity,* and it remained in intermittent use throughout Victoria's reign. Also renowned as an ethnologist and one of the very few British alienists to enjoy a reputation outside Great Britain in the first half of the nineteenth century, Prichard participated as a founding member of the Association of Medical Officers of Hospitals for the Insane, as a metropolitan lunacy commissioner from 1841 to 1845, and as a national lunacy commissioner from 1845 to 1848.[97] Building on the work of Pinel, the famous French psychiatrist, he became convinced that there existed a kind of insanity that exhibited disordered conduct in the absence of serious, or even noticeable, mental alienation.

Historians of medicine have had no difficulty demonstrating the authority that "moral insanity" gave to psychiatrists who endorsed Prichard's theory. Since he contended that the disease typically manifested itself "in a want of self-government, . . . an unusual expression of strong feelings, in thoughtless and extravagant conduct," all manner of unseemly behavior might be interpreted as proof of moral madness. As late as 1881, Savage made explicit the social concerns implicit in the diagnosis: "The eccentric person who neglects his relationship to his fellow men and to the society and social position into which he was born must be looked upon as morally insane."[98] It was left to the psychiatrists to judge what was appropriate conduct for different groups in the population. Violence and vulgarity, which might scarcely raise an eyebrow when exhibited by a docker, attracted immediate medical concern in a polite drawing room.

The manifold questions raised by the concept of moral insanity, which the legal profession was quick to condemn, affected depressed as well as more overtly unconventional patients. For the most part, men and women suffering from nervous prostration were not likely to find themselves wrongfully confined in asylums, and the flexible category of moral insanity was reserved for those who offended the standards of normal—that is, respectable—behavior established by the Victorian middle class. Yet nervous breakdown certainly violated its stereotype of adult normalcy, and Prichard himself had suggested the connections between nervous collapse and his problematic diagnostic category. Indeed, his initial discussion of moral insanity included among its "most striking" features the following description of what would now be treated as profound depression: "The faculty of reason is not manifestly impaired, but a constant feeling of gloom and sadness clouds all the prospects of life: the individual, though surrounded with all the comforts of existence, and even, exclusively of his disease, suffering under no internal source of disquiet, at peace with himself, with his own conscience, with his God, yet becomes sorrowful and desponding. All things present and future are to his view involved in dreary and hopeless gloom." That such a condition was unnatural was obvious; that it was morally reprehensible was only suggested in 1835. Nearly a half-century later, Savage carefully explained the reasons why Victorian psychiatrists found such behavior, not merely worthy of censure, but fully deserving consideration as a sort of madness. "The patients neglect their business, their duties, and their rights," he complained, "so that they would willingly allow their nearest and formerly dearest relations to suffer in consequence of their laziness; and this they fully appreciate, but fold their hands and do nothing. In some of these cases, technically one may say there is a want of will, a want of power to balance motives. . . . There seems to be a moral languor that prevents them from acting."[99] Although psychiatrists thought that they could readily distinguish the perversity of moral insanity from the exhaustion of shattered nerves, the implications of Prichard's and Savage's remarks are nonetheless obvious. Failure of will was abnormal. Rendering the sufferer useless to society, and perhaps even harmful to his family, it was fit object of the social disciplinarian's concern.[100]

Perhaps the most serious question raised by the diagnosis of moral insanity did not tax Victorian doctors and lawyers at all, but has emerged to challenge historians today. It is the question of social control—a term that, sky-rocketing into fashion during the last twenty-five years, has seemed particularly applicable to the work of psychiatrists. In the wake of Michel Foucault's vastly influential volume, *Madness and Civilization* (1961), nineteenth-century alienists have been pilloried as covert conspirators on behalf of the capitalist system, masquerading as medical experts in order to force the middle-class values of self-control and personal responsibility on unruly, unproductive members of society. While other figures of authority were rendering criminals, vagrants, paupers, and the unemployed socially harmless in prisons and workhouses, alienists were deflecting the potential danger of madness by incarcerating lunatics in asylums, where the so-called moral management of inmates proved as effectively repressive and punitive by its internalization of discipline as were the old physical methods of external restraint. Through their exercise of the power to label people normal or abnormal—a power supposedly resting on their scientific knowledge—Victorian psychiatrists were able to isolate whomever the middle classes deemed dangerous to social stability. Individual families, deriving their authority from the medical certification of insanity, could use the asylum as a convenient way to deal with disruptive members. This scenario of social control, pregnant with ideological significance, has worked its forceful way into a wide variety of studies that examine Victorian psychiatry.[101]

The difficulty is, however, that the social control hypothesis remains more theoretically compelling than factually demonstrable. In recent years, a few scholars of Victorian psychiatry have begun to question its underlying assumptions and, on the basis of detailed local studies, have suggested a far less simplistic historical narrative that refuses to reduce the complexities of history or to portray the nineteenth-century asylums as mere "dumping grounds for social misfits."[102] That mental illness as a medical category reflects shifting social and cultural contexts is beyond dispute; a more open question is whether psychiatric labels were brandished as agents of class oppression in Victorian England. To contend that they were is to assume that alienists were in a position of social dominance, with the authority "to protect and preserve the state of things which [gave] them power."[103] It is also to make definite judgments about the motives, conscious or otherwise, that impelled nineteenth-century alienists in the performance of their duties.

Most attributions of motive in historical analyses are, at best, educated guesses, for historians can rarely know with certainty the intention or inspiration behind human action. In such an instance as this, involving several hundred men, rather than a single individual, the guesses are perhaps less educated than usual. Certain assumptions nonetheless seem justified, in light of the fact that medicine was not a prestigious profession in Victorian England, except for a small number of fortunate practitioners. The vast majority of their colleagues found that the chances of achieving money and power were slight, while the dangers inherent in constant exposure to disease and infection loomed large. For alienists, who practiced the least reputable branch of legitimate medicine, the opportunities for accumulating wealth and social status were slightest of all, as Tuke ruefully acknowledged in 1881. It was the duty of the Medico-Psychological Association to secure adequate remuneration and retirement annuities for asylum superintendents, he argued, even though they "wooed [mental science] for her own sake, knowing full well that . . . she may hold no dowry in hand or pocket."[104] He was talking, of course, of the alienist who served at a public institution, not the owner of a private madhouse. By the second half of the nineteenth century, the former had become more prominent among British psychiatrists than the latter.

If psychiatry was unlikely to lead to power, social prestige, and professional respect, it is reasonable to surmise that less self-regarding motives inspired its practitioners. It is likely that men chose to become alienists, not simply because some poorly paid jobs were available in asylums, but because they were fascinated with the problems posed by mental illness and were eager to alleviate the suffering of its victims. It is clear from their own writings that Victorian alienists were baffled and disconcerted by insanity and other functional nervous disorders, which would not fit neatly into somatic models of illness. They were, furthermore, profoundly dismayed to realize how fragile was the reign of reason over the human personality. Many of them were deeply compassionate men who longed to return their patients to health and happiness. When they strove to restore lunatics to some semblance of self-discipline and, where possible, to the ranks of useful, industrious people by giving them regular work to perform and appealing to their moral nature, it is just as plausible to believe that they acted out of real concern for what they considered the best interests of their patients as to assert that they were prompted by social fears or animosity. While trying to bolster the inmates' capacity for self-control, they may also have encouraged the ability to feel self-respect. If the two kinds of motivation, altruistic and self-serving, came together so closely as to become indistinguishable in the work of asylum doctors, the existence of the second kind does not necessarily invalidate the sincerity of the first. Psychiatrists, like the Victorian middle class in general, predicated their notion of personal happiness on a social setting; thus the alienation from humanity that insanity inflicted seemed to them an appalling fate, and they hoped that their program of moral treatment, in an asylum atmosphere supposedly reminiscent of the home, would help patients to participate once again in social intercourse. It is easy to denounce their pretensions, to underscore the depths of their ignorance, and to argue that their methods amounted to the arbitrary exercise of power over helpless people; it is impossible to contend that their goals can be satisfactorily encompassed within the phrase "class hegemony."

With profoundly depressed patients, alienists were similarly moved by the desire to end their isolation from other human beings and to reestablish them as engaged participants in life. With these men and women, however, the position of the psychiatric attendant was more complicated than with the lunatic poor, for the victim of shattered nerves whom he treated was far likelier to come from the middle, and even the upper, classes than the lower. If social control represents an effort to remold "values and attitudes in an approved framework imposed or provided from above,"[105] alienists treating nervous exhaustion could hardly be accused of practicing social control when the patient often occupied a loftier social position than the doctor. It has been argued that, both in their relentless emphasis on personal responsibility for health and in their glowing descriptions of the moderate habits and useful activity that promoted it, middle-class psychiatrists were not only criticizing the dissolute, shiftless poor, but also implicitly denouncing the mores of the aristocracy and the idle rich.[106] Yet the evidence suggests that, in their eagerness to doctor the elevated segments of society, Victorian and Edwardian psychiatrists kept their criticism of the upper class very muted. In any case, they rarely managed to exercise unchallenged control over the therapeutic relationship when it involved their social equals or superiors. Not only did alienists have to contend with demanding patients, suffering from a mysterious and refractory malady, but they often had to satisfy the patient's family as well. Indeed, it seems likely that in many situations involving affluent invalids the psychiatrist's authority derived more from the fact that relatives had delegated him to deal with a difficult family member than from any power inherent in his own medical position. In other instances, furthermore, the patient might connive at a particular diagnosis, for personal reasons seeking release from responsibilities under the protection of a pathological label. The powers psychiatrists wielded, in short, were often handed to them by their clients.

There remains, however, another aspect to the debate over psychiatric social control, which focuses on theory rather than practice, and which is both more subtle and more compelling than the effort to cast Victorian alienists in an overtly coercive light. Ignoring issues of work discipline and supervision in the asylum, it identifies the concept of will as the element of authority in nineteenth-century psychiatry. Whether will was invoked as the key to that self-control which obviated the need to repress lunatics by force or as the agent which roused the depressive from lethargy, it stood for government, stability, and ordered activity. The contest that pitted the individual's will against the lower anarchic drives of animal nature represented on the personal level the same struggle to assert order over chaos that society at large experienced. The triumph of the patient's will, and the establishment of the proper hierarchy of nervous centers, could be perceived as a blow struck for the forces of social authority in the community and in the nation. Although the connection between the will as a psychiatric construct and respect for law and order as social necessities lies beyond the possibility of definitive proof, it was not coincidental that the psychiatric theory emerged during the same decades—from the late eighteenth to the mid-nineteenth century—in which the rapid growth of cities, mounting political agitation, and social unrest revealed the inadequacy of traditional British agencies of control. The will that made self-restraint possible could prove as valuable in its way as the new London metropolitan police force. Beyond any doubt, alienists actively disseminated the image of humanity directed and tamed by the workings of the will, and implicit in this image was a particular system of values that served the interests of society's rulers.[107]

The Victorian middle classes were unquestionably involved in a widespread and ongoing struggle to achieve a social position commensurate with their economic power, and alienists certainly shared their aspirations, if not their overall financial strength. Unavoidably, psychiatrists sought to protect and advance their own interests, but it is extremely important to realize that they did so from a general position of weakness, not vigor. Throughout the nineteenth century, psychological medicine remained in an inchoate condition, with its practitioners unable to defend their territory against diverse raiders from other branches of the medical profession. In its vulnerable infancy and childhood, psychiatry was even more absorbent of prevailing cultural moods and dictates than is the case today; alienists dared not contest the moral precepts of the social groups who controlled their professional destiny, whether as members of asylum management committees or as private neurotic patients. The interpretation of normalcy and deviance, which Victorian psychiatrists have been accused of imposing on a defenseless public, was, in a very real sense, imposed on them as well. The interaction between medical beliefs and social prejudices is a process of immense intricacy, and it is no exaggeration to say that alienists were caught in the crossfire.

They were not, of course, innocent bystanders. They enthusiastically shared the values they tried to enforce, and, in the process, they tirelessly worked to improve their own social and professional reputations. If their approach to treating mental and nervous illness was shaped by cultural constraints as well as by the limits of medical knowledge, few Victorian or Edwardian psychiatrists questioned those constraints, or even understood their influence on medicine. They never acknowledged, and probably never realized, what seems so obvious today: that layers of cultural presupposition enveloped every case of mental and nervous illness and interfered with the real comprehension of patients' needs.

It should be emphasized, however, that Victorian psychiatrists hoped to save their patients from misery and devastation when they issued warnings against the consequences of what they defined as deviant behavior. Whether the anticipated result was nervous exhaustion or outright madness, the price was one that nobody could afford, and alienists were utterly earnest in their endeavor to lead men and women away from such a tragedy, both for the sake of the individual patient and for the good of society. Alienists were eager to assume the duties of social disciplinarians, not only because these responsibilities placed them among the leaders of society's search for stability, but also because the task seemed intrinsic to their medical role. Unable to cure many of the patients who came under their treatment, alienists could at least take an energetic part in trying to prevent the ravages of madness and nervous debility among the rest of the British population. Their intentions cannot be simply encapsulated in the formulaic notion of social control. As far as we can tell, they tried, at one and the same time, to enhance the psychiatric profession and to fulfill a medical function. As far as they could tell, both tasks demanded that they advertise the virtues of self-restraint and moral sobriety.

2

Sir James Crichton-Browne

No Victorian or Edwardian alienist assumed the scientific and moral responsibilities of his work with greater confidence than did James Crichton-Browne.[1] During the course of his extremely long career, he sampled nearly all of the professional opportunities open to British psychiatry in these decades, serving as resident medical officer at several public asylums, lecturing on mental disease at provincial medical schools, editing journals, inspecting the treatment of lunatics as a government official, and advising private patients as a fashionable psychiatric consultant. Shortly before his death in 1938, at the age of 97, he described himself as "the Doyen of the Medical Psychologists of Great Britain," and so familiar a figure had he become, discoursing on a range of issues affecting public and private health, that the *Times,* in its obituary notice, dubbed him "the orator of the medical profession." Yet, after his death, he was memorialized more because he was an interesting relic from the past than for his contributions to medicine—the *Times,* for example, noting that "he was one of the last, if not the last, to wear a pair of magnificent Victorian whiskers." Other obituaries stressed his gifts as a public speaker, his fluent pen, or the way his enthusiasm and helpful criticism had stimulated the work of others. None, however, could point to "original work of his own" that produced a significant impact on psychiatry. The *Times* observed that his several volumes of memoirs were "pleasant miscellanies, which made excellent bedside books,"[2] hardly distinguished grounds for remembering a man who had served as president both of the Medico-Psychological Association and of the Neurological Society. His was, indeed, a strangely unfulfilled career, for his early success as a physiologist was ultimately eclipsed by his guardianship of the nation's moral welfare.

Crichton-Browne was virtually born into the psychiatric profession. His father, William Alexander Francis Browne, was a leading participant in the growth of nineteenth-century Scottish psychiatry, which developed along the same lines as English medical psychology. Born in Stirling in 1805 and raised there, W. A. F Browne studied medicine at Edinburgh in the early 1820s, where he may well have attended Morison's lectures on mental disorders. Cullen's legacy, too, gave psychological medicine a small, but noteworthy, foundation at Edinburgh, which could have stimulated Browne's interest in the subject. Like his colleague David Skae at the Royal Edinburgh Asylum, Browne became a proficient medical administrator, concerned as much with the practical issues of running a mental institution, whether public or private, as with the theories behind the therapy.

His first experience of asylum medicine came in 1834 when, after a few years in general practice, he was appointed medical superintendent of the Montrose Royal Lunatic Asylum. He must have quickly mastered the requirements of his new job, for he was soon delivering a series of lectures, entitled *What Asylums Were, Are, and Ought to Be,* to the Montrose managers. Published as a book in 1837, these lectures attracted the attention of Elizabeth Crichton, the widow of Dr. James Crichton, a physician who had made a fortune in the service of the East India Company around the turn of the century. On his death, the childless Crichton left an enormous bequest, of approximately £100,000, for charitable purposes, to be administered by his wife. The fruit of this munificence was the Crichton Royal Institution, a lunatic asylum outside Dumfries, designed to implement the most up-to-date practices in the treatment of the insane. Very impressed with Browne's views on asylum government, Mrs. Crichton invited him to serve as the first resident medical officer of her modern facility when it opened in 1839, and he accepted. Browne remained at Crichton Royal until 1857 when, following the passage of a new Scottish Lunacy Act, he left to become senior medical commissioner in lunacy for Scotland. It was the Board of Lunacy Commissioners, created by the legislation, whom Tuke subsequently credited with ameliorating the egregious ''suffering and degraded state'' of pauper lunatics in Scotland. After his retirement from the board in 1870, Browne returned to Dumfries, where increasing blindness limited his activities until his death in 1885. Throughout his life, he took an energetic interest in all concerns of the nascent psychiatric profession, helping to launch the Medico-Psychological Association in 1841, under its first, lengthier name, and serving as its president in 1866.[3]

Browne's approach to mental illness revealed the uneasy coexistence of physiological and psychological interpretations that characterized the work of British psychiatrists throughout the nineteenth century. On the one hand, he espoused the physical model, unequivocally affirming the conviction that somatic conditions— ''morbid changes in our bodies''—gave rise to the symptoms of mental derangement. Medical experience, he explained, taught that ''we cannot reach the mind even when employing purely *psychical* means, when bringing mind to act upon mind, except through material organs.'' It was likely, he surmised, ''that even moral means exercise *their* influence by stimulating or producing changes in organisation.'' On the other hand, it is clear that Browne conceded real potency to moral means, even if their impact could only be perceived somatically. He was far from embracing materialism, and a strong motive for his emphasis on the organic manifestation of insanity was precisely to leave the mind, soul or spirit, free from corruption.[4]

Browne's strong interest in phrenology allowed him delicately to balance his physiological and moral viewpoints. Having become acquainted with the Combe brothers, the leading Scottish advocates of phrenology, while a medical student in Edinburgh, he found in the ideas they espoused a plausible theory to mold his own studies of the mind. Phrenology, it is true, appeared to advocate a strictly organic approach to mental faculties and moral sentiments, dividing the brain into more than thirty separate regions, each responsible for a highly specific intellectual activity, propensity, or emotion, and each occupying a particular place on the surface of the brain's hemispheres. In theory, there was no space for spirit in this assembly of closely-packed cerebral organs; in practice, the materialism implicit in phrenology was strikingly modified by an unavoidable deduction from phrenological principles, for even the strictest disciples agreed that the individual personality emerged from the subtle interaction of all cerebral parts. They could not help but assume the existence of some organizing, nonmaterial agent at work among these organs, guiding them to function as a harmonious whole and thereby producing rational behavior. As the author of a mid-century lecture on *The Senses, the Brain, and the Mind* observed: "A phrenologist may believe in the immateriality of the mind itself, as fully as the most determined spiritualist."[5]

Harmony could not be maintained among the manifold regions of the brain, however, if a single organ, or group of organs, became too dominant. Such a situation, phrenologists argued, quickly led to irrational, disordered conduct—the symptoms of mental illness—although the derangement did not, in fact, pertain to the mind. It reflected instead a somatic dysfunction that obstructed the mind's operations. Believing that each organ of thought and feeling was strong or weak as it was used or neglected, phrenologists hoped to bring order out of chaos by encouraging the exercise of the enfeebled organs and the atrophy, comparatively speaking, of the overpowering ones, until some measure of balance was achieved. Since they perceived mental health as intimately linked with careful training and education, insanity seemed to them both preventible and curable. It is hardly surprising that such leading early Victorian alienists as Browne, Sir William Ellis, and John Conolly were attracted to this school of thought.[6]

Phrenology was not the only source of Browne's optimism, nor the only reason why he considered moral management an effective method of treating the insane. He was also deeply influenced by his experience in Paris, where he studied in the late 1820s and early 1830s, after qualifying as a doctor in 1826. In the 1820s, Paris was the center of training for the ablest of European and American medical students, who found there a group of brilliant pathologists, diagnosticians, and teachers busily expanding the frontiers of medical practice. Among the several fields of medicine flourishing in the French capital during the first half of the nineteenth century not the least was psychiatry, over which Pinel presided until his death in 1826. When Browne arrived a few years later, he took up his studies with Jean Etienne Dominique Esquirol, Pinel's disciple and colleague, from whom the young Scotsman imbibed the hopeful perspective on lunacy that marked late eighteenth- and early nineteenth-century French medical thought.

While making his own highly significant contributions to psychiatry, Esquirol perpetuated the work of his mentor in diverse ways. He continued, of course, to elaborate and publicize the *nonrestraint system* for the insane, which Pinel had done so much to call to international medical attention. He embraced, and further propagated, the methods Pinel had advocated for the exact observation of patients and the maintenance of accurate case records. Eventually, too, he endorsed Pinel's concept of *manie sans délire,* which foreshadowed Prichard's notion of moral insanity. After initial rejection of Pinel's new category of mental illness, Esquirol not only accepted it, but even incorporated it into his own influential diagnostic creation—"monomania," or partial insanity, "a single pathological preoccupation in an otherwise sound mind."[7] The intellectual baggage that Browne took back to Scotland from Paris thus included much that became essential to him when he began his career as an asylum medical superintendent in 1834.

At Montrose from 1834 to 1838, Browne tried to give expression to his faith in moral management. He was not the first British psychiatrist to attempt to govern his asylum with the least possible recourse to coercive restraints. Purposefully following the example of the York Retreat, Ellis had sought partially to implement a system of moral management at the Wakefield asylum when it opened in 1818 and had experimented with agricultural work as a form of occupational therapy for his patients. When he moved to the Middlesex County Asylum (Hanwell) in 1831, he and his wife continued the experiment, offering a range of occupations that combined therapy with a degree of job training for future employment outside the asylum. Browne was, nonetheless, among the earliest pioneers of nonrestraint in British psychiatry, establishing its principles at Montrose before Robert Gardiner Hill did likewise at the Lincoln Asylum in 1838, or John Conolly aroused public interest in moral management at Hanwell between 1839 and 1844.[8] It was Conolly's flair for self-promotion that established nonrestraint as psychiatric orthodoxy by mid-century, but others had laid the foundations for him.

The optimism inherent in the theories of moral management merged with the meliorism implicit in phrenology to give Browne strong grounds for hoping that the right sort of asylum environment could cure the majority of insane patients. In his 1837 lectures he described in great detail the buildings and grounds best suited to achieving these results, and he also emphasized the importance of assigning each inmate some allotted task, whether among the flower beds, in the kitchen, or at the laundry, as an exercise in disciplining the passions and fortifying the will. Compulsion or corporal punishment played no part at all in Browne's scheme, which he was able to realize in large part when he moved to Crichton Royal. The variety of recreational and occupational diversions available there in the name of therapy was, indeed, impressive for the 1830s and 1840s. Patients were encouraged to participate in theatrical productions, for which a small theater was built after Browne arrived. There were lectures, concerts, and dances for them to attend, excursions into the surrounding countryside, and even into Dumfries. In 1844, patients at Crichton Royal produced the first issue of *New Moon,* a monthly publication which they wrote and edited themselves. In the following decade, Browne launched a series of lectures and discussions on mental illness among the patients—prompting a recent commentator to suggest that he was the originator of group therapy.[9]

Browne also understood the critical importance of keeping thorough clinical records. Such attention to detail was an essential part of his skill as a medical administrator, which his Parisian training had doubtless sharpened and which found expression in his annual reports from Crichton Royal. Like virtually all Victorian psychiatrists, he devoted much time and attention to diagnostic categories of mental illness, classifying his patients according to the symptoms they manifested, but he was more innovative in recording accounts of patients' dreams. His general supervision of the asylum also included the nursing staff and attendants, for whom he established a course of lectures on insanity to help them deal with their patients. Clearly he was a man who found deep satisfaction in his work and who believed in what he was doing.[10]

Moral management, in theory, involved a great deal more than institutional ambience; it required the asylum doctor to attempt individual psychotherapy with every one of his patients. Browne did not recoil from that daunting task, as he indicated in his annual report from Crichton Royal in 1844: "Much of what is designated moral treatment consists in the conferences and controversies of the officers with the patients in the attempt to disentangle the intricacies and confusions of thought; to substitute precise for vague conceptions, hopes for fears, reason for impulse, to convince of error." He assumed the responsibility of making "a philosophical analysis of the individual mind, of its history, condition and capabilities, so that the physician may know and be able to act upon and mould the moral nature of each patient committed to his care."[11] Nor did Browne's moral guardianship of inmates apply only to the indubitably insane; perhaps his studies with Esquirol made him particularly sensitive to forms of mental disorder that fell short of outright lunacy, for he apparently excelled at treating the kinds of depression that crippled the will without destroying the reason. In its obituary of his son, the *Times* described Crichton Royal in Browne's day as "almost the only resort to which sufferers from 'nervous breakdown' could retire for seclusion and treatment." Crichton-Browne himself recalled that one of his father's patients at Dumfries was Henry Scott Riddell, the Scottish shepherd-poet and clergyman. When "the cloud descended on him," Crichton-Browne wrote, "profound mental despondency" required that Riddell seek treatment at Crichton Royal. "After a time the cloud lifted and he was restored to health and happiness, ascribing his recovery to my father's skill and personal attention."[12]

It is clear that the dual meaning of *moral* enhanced the import of Browne's work at Montrose and Dumfries. For him, moral management was both a form of treatment aimed at the mind, rather than the body, and an attempt to restore responsible, self-disciplined conduct among asylum inmates. In either case, however, he was convinced that trained medical men were uniquely capable of using the nonrestraint system to benefit patients. It was "the physician" who had to "mould the moral nature of each patient," not the well-meaning, but unskilled layman. Furthermore, Browne neither discarded pharmaceutical medicaments nor minimized the somatic aspects of mental illness, which also underscored the need for medical expertise in treating lunacy. If by 1864, his writing betrayed some disappointment with the results of moral management and an insistence on the need to minister directly to bodily afflictions, he was not executing a dramatic volte-face from the days of heady optimism at Crichton Royal.[13] He had never placed his faith in benevolence alone, but had recognized that more than humanitarian sentiments were needed to cure the cerebral disorder from which insanity arose. As a phrenologist, he could always pay tribute to the infinite complexities of the brain, yet still leave ample room for the mind.

Browne's eldest son was born in Edinburgh on 29 November 1840. With Elizabeth Crichton consenting to serve as godmother, the baby was christened James Crichton Browne. From both parents he inherited a deep pride in Scottish history and culture, as well as something of a microcosmic war of religion. His mother, Magdalene Howden Balfour, was the daughter of a fanatic Presbyterian, while his father's side boasted a tradition of staunch Anglicanism. Crichton-Browne was raised, apparently peacefully, in the latter creed, but the central place of religious faith in his family's background may have played a part in his determination to preserve the role of religion in national life. Scientific distinction also ran in the family, on the Balfour side. James Hutton, the eminent eighteenth-century geologist and propounder of the uniformitarian theory, was a distant relation, while John Hutton Balfour, professor of botany at Glasgow and Edinburgh in the following century, was Crichton-Browne's uncle.[14]

Crichton-Browne grew up at Crichton Royal, where his parents occupied a house on the asylum grounds. He attended Dumfries Academy and, subsequently, Trinity College, Glenalmond. In 1857, the year his father became a commissioner in lunacy for Scotland, he began his medical studies at Edinburgh. This was only the first of a series of developments that marked striking similarities between the father's career and the son's. Through those parallels, and through the ways in which the two careers differed from each other, it is possible to trace changes in the British psychiatric profession during the course of the nineteenth century. As a second-generation Browne to pursue the study of mental illness, the son's medical interests were more focused, at an earlier age, than his father's had been. More job opportunities certainly awaited him as a psychiatrist after he completed his medical training in the 1860s than William Browne had found in the 1830s. Crichton-Browne never had to perform the duties of a general practitioner in order to earn a living; he was a medical specialist from the start of his career.

When Crichton-Browne entered the University of Edinburgh, it was beginning to lose that preeminence as a center of medical studies that it had enjoyed in the previous century. Founded in 1582, the university had no medical faculty until 1726, but prior to that date students could learn from members of the Edinburgh Guild of Surgeons and Barbers the skills of the medical craft. Within a few decades after 1726, Edinburgh had become the focal point for medical studies in Great Britain, drawing future practitioners not only from the British Isles, but from the American colonies as well. The flowering of intellectual activity that gave Georgian Edinburgh its reputation as the "Athens of the North" did not exclude medicine, and well into the nineteenth century medical education in Scotland, particularly at Edinburgh, was significantly superior to anything available in England. Doctors trained in Scotland between 1750 and 1850 occupied positions of prestige and importance in English medicine throughout Victoria's reign, while a number of Edinburgh's medical students, like Morison, Bell, Conolly, and Hall, figured prominently in the early development of British psychiatry and neurology.[15]

Contrary to medical myth, propagated largely by practitioners jealous of the power wielded by Oxford and Cambridge graduates through the Royal College of Physicians in London, the quality of medical education was improving in England, at least at Oxford, during the second half of the eighteenth century. It is true that medical students at Oxford had to receive part of their clinical training either at Edinburgh or at one of the great London teaching hospitals, but the Oxford medical curriculum was not as abysmally insufficient as its critics pretended. At Cambridge, medical education began to show a marked improvement in the first half of the nineteenth century. What neither English university could offer between 1750 and 1850, however, was the systematic instruction available at Edinburgh, the "well planned and co-ordinated" lectures that covered "some basic science as well as the essential medical subjects such as anatomy, materia medica, and physics," the "organised clinical teaching, and a lengthy final examination at the end of three years."[16] There remained, furthermore, even in the nineteenth century, a lingering Scottish bias toward a broad philosophical foundation for university studies, in contrast to the narrower training offered to Oxford and Cambridge medical students during the early Victorian period. Forbes Winslow regretted that "mental philosophy" formed no part of English medical education in the 1840s and that "the study of psychology has been . . . only preserved in Scotland, as affording to the philosophical classes abstract subjects for disputation. . . ."[17] The Scottish "philosophical classes"— that is, those for whom university education was considered appropriate—included a far greater segment of the population than was the case in England.

If the glory days of Edinburgh medicine were over by the mid-nineteenth century, the university did not cease to produce distinguished medical graduates. Its decline can be attributed, not to a fall in the caliber of student whom the medical faculty attracted, but to the kind of medical training it provided. As modern medicine became more inextricably linked with biological research, a medical faculty that did not emphasize work of this nature was bound to fall from the highest rank of institutions. Already in the first half of the nineteenth century, Edinburgh's clinicians had suffered eclipse at the hands of Parisian pathologists, with their penchant for performing autopsies; in the second half, Edinburgh and Paris were both outdistanced by German medicine, which, finally shaking off the influence of romantic natural philosophy, led the way in developing research facilities where laboratory investigations flourished. From the 1860s, European and American medical students who wanted a place in the vanguard of their profession found essential a year or two of study in Germany. Even within Great Britain, Edinburgh's dominance faded during Victoria's reign, as medical education in England—at Oxford, Cambridge, the University of London, and at the new medical schools and universities in the provinces—gradually came to duplicate what Scotland could provide.

By any standards, the men under whom Crichton-Browne studied at Edinburgh between 1857 and 1861 were, nevertheless, a distinguished group. Joseph Lister, although not yet a professor in the faculty of medicine, was assistant surgeon to the Edinburgh Royal Infirmary, where Crichton-Browne was briefly his pupil. At the time, an even more eminent teacher was James Syme, Lister's father-in-law, professor of clinical surgery and one of the most celebrated surgeons of his day. Crichton-Browne studied, too, with Robert Christison, the renowned toxicologist, and Lyon Playfair, professor of chemistry, who combined the public advocacy of science with his chemical discoveries and was later raised to the peerage. John Goodsir, professor of anatomy and prolific author of scientific papers, also taught Crichton-Browne.[18] The teacher who influenced him the most, however, was Thomas Laycock, professor of the practice of medicine, whose groundbreaking inquiries in cerebral physiology merged with an interest in medical psychology and the less tangible aspects of mental activity in a way that impressed future psychiatrists and neurologists alike. (Both T. S. Clouston and David Ferrier, for example, were among his students.) Crichton-Browne found Laycock simply "the most original and inspiring" of all the medical professors he encountered at Edinburgh.[19]

Laycock, no doubt, only confirmed Crichton-Browne's already resolute intention to make mental illness his particular field of inquiry. His thesis, part of the requirement for the M.D. degree that he earned in 1862, investigated the vexed question of hallucinations, and he had claimed considerable knowledge in the area of medical psychology even before then. The forum for his early presentation of psychiatric opinions was the Royal Medical Society, an association founded in the 1730s to give medical students at Edinburgh an opportunity for frequent discussion of the subjects they were in the process of mastering. The Society elected four presidents annually from among its student members, and in the nineteenth century, James Simpson, Marshall Hall, John Conolly, and William Browne were among the future distinguished doctors who served in that capacity. In 1861, Crichton-Browne assumed the particularly prestigious role of senior president and gave, as his inaugural address, a paper on no less a subject than "The History and Progress of Psychological Medicine." The talk was noteworthy for the young author's remarkably self-confident and authoritative voice, but the address itself had nothing particularly novel to impart. Inevitably claiming the status of skilled expert, the speaker emphasized that psychological medicine was taking its place as "a great and distinct department of the science of medicine," demanding from its practitioners "special tastes and special studies." The influence of William Browne was evident throughout. His son lavished praise on those doctors, from Pinel onwards, who had fought against the "cruelty, barbarity, and injustice" formerly meted out to lunatics, and he coyly referred to a Scottish "labourer in the cause of humanity, of whom it becomes not me to speak." Together, he maintained, physiology and phrenology had substantially helped to elucidate mental disease, and with a solid "physico-psychical basis," he concluded, "psychology cannot fail to advance."[20]

Crichton-Browne had already read a more original paper to the Royal Medical Society in December 1859. While only in his third year of medical studies, he had articulated views on the "Psychical Diseases of Early Life" that became central themes in his mature psychiatric work. Warning that the infant nervous system was extremely susceptible to external stimuli, he urged his audience to discourage all signs of precocity in children, for such early development invariably signaled "a morbid psychical condition." Above all, he exhorted his colleagues to remain constantly alert to the slightest hints of future mental illness or nervous instability, and in a rousing peroration the nineteen-year-old authority asserted: "We believe that states and communities will become great, and good, and healthy, and civilized, in proportion as they attend to early training."[21] Even before he had finished his medical schooling, Crichton-Browne had fully embraced the roles of physiologist, moralist, and social disciplinarian.

Having qualified as a licentiate of the Royal College of Surgeons, Edinburgh, in 1861 and having earned the M.D. degree with honors one year later, Crichton-Browne again followed his father's example and went to Paris to complete his medical education. He wrote very little about his experience in France, which evidently extended from 1862 to 1863, except to note that he came down with a mild case of smallpox while observing at La Charité Hospital.[22] Had he finished his training in Scotland a few years later, he might have decided to make Germany his destination rather than France. As it was, his choice of Paris influenced the rest of his career, for clinical observation in hospital or asylum wards and the performance of autopsies, on the French model, became Crichton-Browne's basic approach to psychological medicine. By the early 1860s, the atmosphere for psychiatric studies in Paris had changed dramatically since William Browne's visit some thirty years before. Esquirol had died in 1840, and the therapeutic optimism that accompanied faith in the efficacy of moral management no longer colored French psychiatric theory. The rise of hereditarianism in psychological medicine allowed far less reason to hope that mental disorders could be helped by moral suasion and environmental reforms. Pathological inheritance became a leading subject of psychiatric inquiry, with the threat of mental degeneracy raising the terrible possibilities of racial decline. The crushing pessimism of degeneration theory clashed harshly with the rosier beliefs that Crichton-Browne had inherited from his father, and for the rest of his life, in his writings for professional colleagues and for the general public, he sought to steer a course between the two perspectives.[23]

On his return from France, Crichton-Browne held a series of brief appointments that functioned, in effect, as his psychiatric apprenticeship. His first assignment, as assistant physician to the Derby County Asylum, under the superintendency of John Hitchman, actually seems to have occurred before he left for Paris, because an article published in the October 1862 issue of the *Journal of Mental Science* describes him as already holding the Derby position. Between 1863 and 1865, he served as assistant medical officer at the Devon and Warwick county asylums, and finally in 1865—the year he married Emily Halliday, the daughter of a Cheshire surgeon—he obtained a medical superintendency of his own, at the Newcastle-upon-Tyne Borough Asylum. At the same time, he was appointed lecturer on mental disease at the Newcastle College of Science. Like Maudsley, Crichton-Browne had attained, in his twenties, the highest appointment his profession could offer. British psychiatry in the mid-Victorian decades was still an open field in which the energetic and industrious could rise rapidly to the top.[24]

The extent of Crichton-Browne's ambition and determination to succeed became obvious when he assumed his next job, as medical director of the West Riding Lunatic Asylum in Wakefield (with the post of lecturer on mental disease to the nearby Leeds School of Medicine). The institution over which he presided from 1866 to 1876 was not only one of the older county asylums, but also one of the biggest. During Crichton-Browne's tenure there, the Wakefield asylum consistently housed some 1,500 patients. No one at the time of its establishment in 1818 had envisioned so sizeable a lunatic population under one roof. Even Colney Hatch, the new asylum for Middlesex that was the largest in England when it opened in 1851, was designed for no more than 1,250 patients—although by the 1870s the number of its inmates had surpassed 2,000. The administrative skills needed by the superintendents of such crowded institutions were considerable, not only to oversee the treatment of lunatics with widely varying needs, but to supervise the supporting staff of assistant physicians and attendants as well. At mid-century, the Wakefield asylum had one attendant to every twenty-two patients, a ratio suggesting nearly seventy attendants on duty.[25]

Crichton-Browne, like his father, was a gifted superintendent who concerned himself with all aspects of running the asylum, from keeping detailed records of his patients to installing a water purification system. Building on Ellis's work at

Wakefield, he encouraged occupational therapy for the inmates, mentioning in his case notes, for example, when a patient performed masonry work or kept himself busy in the tailor shop.[26] Such employment, clearly, was in the tradition of non-restraint that Crichton-Browne had been taught to endorse since childhood, and, indeed, amid all the demands on his time and attention he managed publicly to maintain the note of cheerful confidence characteristic of the previous generation of alienists. In an early quarterly report from Wakefield, he discussed the question of asylum nurses—a problem that had engaged his father's interest—in tones redolent with the optimism of moral management convictions. "How to provide suitable and trustworthy attendants is certainly the great problem of the day in the management of our lunatic asylums," he observed, before proceeding to recommend that female nurses be appointed to serve in male wards. Such an arrangement proved highly advantageous to the patients, he argued, on the basis of experience at Wakefield. Once a woman was introduced among male lunatics, they became "quieter and more orderly." "A singular power of self-control seems to have been awakened in them," he continued, "so that they are enabled to suppress those outbursts of violence, that abusive language, and those offensive habits, to which they used formerly to give way."[27] No moral manager could have asked for anything more.

Public statements of this sort did not, however, reflect Crichton-Browne's private sentiments, for the work of running a huge public asylum was not at all congenial to him. The satisfaction that his father's, and John Conolly's, generation of psychiatrists had derived from the belief that they were effecting a revolution in the care of lunatics and restoring these blighted people to the company of human society eluded the next generation. Overcrowding and inadequate staffing were the realities that confronted asylum superintendents in the second half of the nineteenth century, and no proof of the benefits of moral management helped to lighten their task. On the contrary, alienists and public health offficials faced evidence that pointed exactly in the opposite direction—toward a mounting wave of insanity, undiminished by humanitarian treatment, which threatened to overwhelm the available asylum facilities. The population of lunatics appeared to expand as rapidly as institutions were built to receive them.

Starting in the 1850s, when it was becoming obvious that numerically significant recoveries had not occurred in asylums, and persisting through the Edwardian decade, a debate about the swelling ranks of lunatics raged within the British medical profession. No one doubted that the total number of men and women accommodated in lunatic asylums had substantially increased from the earlier part of the century; the controversy surrounded the possible interpretation of these burgeoning figures. Did they reflect an increase in the actual incidence of madness that exceeded the growth rate of the population in general—a frightening situation with dire implications for the future—or were they merely the result of such nineteenth-century medical developments as a broader definition of insanity, the more extensive institutionalization of lunatics in a greater number of asylums, the longer lifespan of inmates in the new facilities, and other social or environmental causes? Neither side in the debate ever definitively established the validity of its case, but the very nature of the controversy reveals how profoundly misplaced had been the optimism of the early nineteenth-century asylum reformers.[28] Patients may have enjoyed pleasanter surroundings and better treatment under the nonrestraint system, but the influx of lunatics into the asylums destroyed the domestic atmosphere that moral managers had striven to create and placed intolerable strains on the buildings themselves. The great increase in numbers, furthermore, made it impossible to implement that individualized therapy on which theories of moral management were predicated.

By 1867, with nearly 25,000 insane patients held in public asylums and hospitals in England and Wales, asylum superintendents considered more than 20,000 virtually beyond the chances of recovery and less than 2,500 curable.[29] Therapeutic pessimism enveloped British alienists in the second half of the nineteenth century, as their much vaunted medical expertise, on which they had based their claim to monopolize the care of lunatics, failed to achieve the successes they had anticipated. They did not, of course, cease to assert their unique qualifications to minister to the mad, medicinally and morally, but they were themselves struggling against embarrassment and de-moralization. Under the weight of numbers, the nonrestraint system was threatened with reversion to the custodial drudgery that had characterized the treatment of insanity before belief in moral management exerted its appealing influence. A custodian's chores, needless to say, conferred no scientific distinction or social prestige on the men who performed them. In fact, after 1845, the national lunacy commissioners discouraged public asylum superintendents from undertaking re-search projects that might distract them from administrative duties. As the pressure of work mounted, asylum medical directors found themselves increasingly isolated within the confines of their institutions and cut off from the rest of a medical profession that had scant reason to respect the psychiatric speciality. Even oppor-tunities to confer with fellow alienists were few for the overworked administrator, while, at the larger asylums, assistant medical officers distanced him from his patients by undertaking most of the day-to-day work of handling the insane. It is no wonder that Tuke evoked the "strange land of shadows" inhabited by asylum superinten-dents and urged "a very liberal supply of holidays" for them.[30]

Crichton-Browne vented the frustrations he experienced at Wakefield in a series of letters written to Charles Darwin between 1869 and 1873. The celebrated naturalist had initiated the correspondence, using Henry Maudsley as an intermediary, in the hopes that Crichton-Browne could help him with his own research on the facial expressions of insane people. This line of inquiry reflected a Victorian suspicion, presumably confirmed by evolutionary biology, that lunatics, as atavistic creatures in the modern world, provided insights into the primitive origins of humanity. While Darwin incorporated much of Crichton-Browne's material into *The Expression of the Emotions in Man and Animals,* published in 1872, it is significant that he began his investigations while working on *The Descent of Man,* which appeared a year earlier. Crichton-Browne was an amateur photographer who, following the photographic work of Hugh W. Diamond at the Surrey County Asylum in the 1850s, believed that photography could prove extremely helpful, not only in classifying types of insanity, but also in understanding its physical manifestations. With 1,500 patients at his disposal and a lively enthusiasm for photographing them, Crichton-Browne was the perfect psychiatrist for Darwin to approach. The asylum director, highly flattered by Darwin's attention, was more than willing to help in any way he could. Their correspondence has been analyzed for what it reveals about the preconceptions that each man brought to the study of psychiatric photography—the younger seeking to illustrate different categories of insanity, the older examining evidence that the expression of emotions in lunatics ran parallel to similarly uncontrolled expressions in the higher mammals.[31] No one has read the letters as testimony to the miseries of asylum management in the 1860s and 1870s.

Crichton-Browne's first letter to Darwin, dated from Wakefield in June 1869, struck the note that dominated the alienist's subsequent contributions to the correspondence. He was sincerely pleased, he assured Darwin, "to afford any little assistance in [his] power to so distinguished & revered a naturalist," but feared that his "numerous and harassing duties" gave him little time for such "congenial pursuits" as research along the lines of Darwin's inquiry. He lamented "the mass of interesting material which is as it were going to waste . . . in this huge hospital for want of accurate observation & which might be of immense value." "My limited opportunities," he hastened to reassure Darwin, however, "are diligently employed & the fruits of my researches are very much at your service, if you care to avail yourself of them."[32]

The same sense of harassment and tone of self-pity colored Crichton-Browne's letters to Darwin in 1870. For a young doctor anxious to impress a giant among scientists, Crichton-Browne made a poor start. He failed to respond to a letter Darwin wrote him at the end of January 1870; he neglected to thank Darwin when the naturalist sent him a copy of the new edition of *The Origin of Species,* and, worst of all, he lost a book belonging to Darwin—Duchenne's *Mécanisme de la physionomie humaine.* Finally, in March, Crichton-Browne wrote in a burst of self-reproach, making his excuses on the grounds of family sorrows, onerous duties, and his own ill health. In June, Crichton-Browne wrote again, palpably relieved to have found the Duchenne volume lying in a cupboard where a negligent manservant, instructed to post it back to Darwin, had left it. "Enclosed in Duchenne," Crichton-Browne told Darwin, "you will find a few crude notes on expression. I promise more, in a little time, although I fear you will scarcely trust to me after all my carelessness. Bear in mind, in extenuation of my faults that I am one of the hardest worked men in her Majesty's dominions. As a rule I *toil* daily from 8 a.m. to 11 p.m. contending all the while with bad health & great anxiety."[33]

The situation at Wakefield showed no improvement the following year. When Darwin wrote to thank Crichton-Browne for his *"invaluable"* observations "on the expression of the insane," the asylum superintendent was grateful for Darwin's approbation, but confessed that

> I have often been ashamed of the insignificance of the help which I have been able to afford you—and of the inadequacy of my answers to your searching questions. The fact is however that the duties of my position leave me very little time for congenial studies. The exigencies of the public service have already ruined my health, & curtailed my capacities. They now threaten to shorten my life. Pardon so much personal detail and accept my warm thanks for the promise of a copy of your new book [*The Descent of Man*] which will be a genuine solace to me in this house of bondage.[34]

Even in March 1873, when Crichton-Browne wrote, with characteristic tardiness, to thank Darwin for a copy of *The Expression of the Emotions in Man and Animals,* he pleaded delicate health and "the hurry and worry of professional work." Indeed, he confided to Darwin that his work was "more arduous than ever."[35]

It is hard to take seriously the claims of a man who lived to 97 years of age that his health was ruined and his lifespan curtailed by the time he had reached his early thirties. In his letters to Darwin, Crichton-Browne never identified the precise nature of his illness, and one cannot help suspecting that the hard pressed medical director put forward an excuse calculated to arouse sympathy in a notorious valetudinarian. Darwin rose to the bait and expressed sincere concern about the state of his correspondent's health. "I very truly grieve to hear," Darwin wrote in February 1871, "that your continued labours and anxiety have at last injured your health seriously. I know from long-tried experience what misery continued ill-health causes, but my health affects only comfort, and is not otherwise serious, which I fear from what you say is far from your case."[36] Alternatively, Crichton-Browne may have been genuinely ill, with the kind of nonspecific nervous complaint which he soon became a specialist in treating. If so, the years of unremitting, tedious labor in "this house of bondage" at Wakefield provided him with valuable insight into the potential effects on the body of long sustained overwork amid unpleasant surroundings and personal unhappiness. As for Darwin, after much initial enthusiasm over Crichton-Browne's notes and photos, and an assertion that the volume on the expression of emotions "ought to be called by Darwin & Browne," the naturalist came to realize how little information was really imparted by photos of the insane. "I suspect," he informed Crichton-Browne, "that our judgement is in most cases largely influenced by accessory circumstances."[37] That was a point Crichton-Browne would never concede.

Even as he bemoaned his slavery at Wakefield, Crichton-Browne was busy creating more work for himself. It was the kind of work he craved, however, and it brought him considerable professional renown. Having determined that the opportunities presented by a huge public asylum should not be wasted any longer, he decided to transform his institution into a neurological laboratory of sorts—the "first asylum research laboratory in Europe," as he was still proud to boast fifty years later.[38] While at Wakefield, it galled him that public asylums were the objects of "harmless, but vindictive, attacks," on the grounds "that no scientific work is accomplished in them."

> It has been an often repeated accusation that the medical officers of these establishments are so absorbed in general or fiscal management, in farming or in devising ill-judged amusements for their charges, that they have no time nor energy left to devote to professional research. And it has been further asserted that when these medical officers have by any chance ventured to enter the field of original investigation, they have, as a rule, signally failed in achieving any useful result, because they are blinded and misled by an erroneous method and by philosophical phantasms, and are destitute of that strict inductive faculty, which their censors are of course presumed to possess in a pre-eminent degree.[39]

Crichton-Browne keenly felt the disdain of other medical men toward asylum doctors, and he accordingly set out to demonstrate how much asylum practice could, in fact, contribute to the study of the brain and nervous system. At the same time, he aimed to counter the isolation in which he worked by turning the West Riding Lunatic

Asylum into a clearinghouse for the exchange of information about insanity's physiological foundations.

"For a time," the *British Medical Journal* reported after Crichton-Browne's death, "Wakefield Asylum was the centre of neurological interest, and many eminent men congregated there and made their contributions at the monthly medical conversaziones which were organized at that institution by its director" between 1871 and 1875. Through Crichton-Browne's "energy and enthusiasm," the *Times* recorded, the West Riding Lunatic Asylum became "a great training centre for men specializing in mental disease, by whom the influence of its methods was spread all over the country."[40] He established a system of clinical assistantships, which enabled young medical men to study insanity at first hand while residing at Wakefield for three to six months, and he invited more seasoned practitioners to pursue research within his asylum's walls. Sometimes their inquiries centered in the pathological department that Crichton-Browne instituted, where autopsies on pauper lunatics were routinely performed; sometimes they looked to the wards, where inmates provided living material for investigation. T. C. Allbutt, a physician at the Leeds General Infirmary at the time, came to the West Riding Asylum to examine patients with the ophthalmoscope, which he championed as an invaluable diagnostic tool. An outstanding clinician, Allbutt was often frustrated by the suspicious wariness with which his compatriots in medicine tended to greet new technology, and he found the Wakefield doctors, both resident and visiting, a welcome exception. In 1871, he gratefully acknowledged Crichton-Browne's assistance—"especially in the supply and description of pathological specimens"—when he published his study, *On the Use of the Ophthalmoscope in Diseases of the Nervous System and of the Kidneys.* Even as late as 1901, the psychiatrist Charles Mercier effusively dedicated a volume to Crichton-Browne, "to whose persistent stimulation of scientific work English alienism owes, more than to any other influence, its present scientific spirit."[41]

The asylum superintendent had no difficulty supplying pathological specimens for the Wakefield researchers. Ever since the Anatomy Act of 1832, the body of anyone who died in a public institution, if unclaimed by relatives, became available for dissection, and Crichton-Browne was a vigorous advocate of autopsies following all deaths in county asylums. Even where relatives objected, he was skilled in overcoming their protests. (It was not a procedure that he recommended for the deceased inhabitants of private asylums, however, as he hastened to assure the Select Committee on the Operation of the Lunacy Law in 1877.) Nor were Wakefield's inmates allowed to die before they became involuntary volunteers. Allbutt was involved in a series of experiments on the use of electricity in treating the insane, in which he daily administered a continuous current to the heads of patients suffering from acute primary dementia. Other medical investigators tested the effects of drugs, like nitrous oxide, ergot, opium, and amyl nitrite, on various forms of insanity. This work, hailed in the annals of British psychiatry and neurology, bears all too ample testimony to the Victorian equation of poverty and powerlessness. The helpless inmates of the West Riding Asylum were the unacknowledged foundation of Crichton-Browne's subsequent reputation.[42]

The most significant research undertaken at the Wakefield asylum under Crichton-Browne's stimulus was Ferrier's study of cerebral localization. Ferrier, three years younger than Crichton-Browne, was a friend and fellow Scotsman. He had recently begun his long affiliation with King's College, London, and King's College Hospital, where he held posts progressing from demonstrator of physiology to professor of neuropathology. In the pathological department of the West Riding Asylum, which Crichton-Browne placed at his disposal, Ferrier pursued a series of decisive experiments on the electrical excitation of the cerebral cortex, using rabbits, cats, dogs, guinea pigs, fowls, and pigeons to trace the connection between specific parts of the brain and distinct body movements.[43] Crichton-Browne fully appreciated the magnitude of what was happening under his roof. He wrote, for once enthusiastically, to Darwin in April 1873:

> Professor Ferrier of Kings College has just completed an experimental investigation in my pathological laboratory which cannot fail to interest you. . . . By exposing the brains of living animals, under chloroform, and stimulating the cerebral grey matter by an electric current . . . he has discovered that every convolution of the brain is in direct relation with certain groups of muscles, and controls their actions . . . In all different animals analagous [*sic*] convolutions are found to regulate analagous movements. . . . Professor Ferrier's researches . . . will I believe constitute the most important advances yet made in cerebral physiology.

Darwin's reply some months later, after he had read Ferrier's report of his experiments, was flatteringly succinct: "I have been profoundly interested. It seems clear that the physiology of the Brain will soon be largely understood. What a step it is."[44]

In the early 1920s, Bernard Hollander, a doctor who wrote widely on such subjects as brain functions, insanity, phrenology, and hypnosis, asserted that Crichton-Browne's motive for inviting Ferrier to Wakefield was "to confirm—or possibly to contradict—phrenology."[45] There is plenty of evidence that Crichton-Browne harbored a lifelong interest in phrenology, doubtless acquired from his father. He believed that Franz Josef Gall and J. C. Spurzheim, the founders of phrenology, had notable insights into cerebral physiology for which they had never received adequate recognition. In an early paper on homicidal insanity, published in the *Journal of Mental Science* in 1863, Crichton-Browne assumed as a given the existence of "the phrenological organs of destructiveness and combativeness," while a late lecture, "The Story of the Brain," delivered at the University of Edinburgh in 1924, still defended some phrenological wisdom. He always remained convinced that the shape of the skull was indicative of the kind of mind housed inside, and he even surmised that particular cranial contours could be paired with specific professions.[46] He may very well have believed that cerebral localization research verified, if not phrenology's detailed map of the brain, at least its fundamental claim that the brain's many parts perform separate, and diverse, functions. No evidence, however, supports Hollander's contention that phrenology inspired the invitation to Ferrier. In 1873, Crichton-Browne was bent on making his asylum a nationally renowned leader in neurological research, at the forefront of British investigations into cerebral physiology and the pathology of madness, and Ferrier's investigations were clearly part of that endeavor. Crichton-Browne's allegiance to phrenology, in any case, was not swayed by proof or refutation. He clung to old phrenological concepts long after they had been resoundingly discredited, not as an act of excessive filial piety, but because he valued the merger of mind and body that they facilitated.

While stimulating and encouraging the work of other medical men at Wakefield, Crichton-Browne pursued his own projects as well. His study of the effect of cranial injuries on mental disease, for example, cited many of his own patients. He was certain that blows to the head were ''prolific sources of mental derangements,'' and he developed the argument with considerable elaboration in two papers, published in 1871 and 1872. He obviously intended the second of these as a contribution to cerebral localization research, for he contended that the varying effects of cranial injuries depended on which part of the brain received the blow. In another line of inquiry, Crichton-Browne experimented with amyl nitrite on epileptic patients at Wakefield, in the hope that it might avert their fits. At the same time, he carefully scrutinized the autopsy reports on sixty epileptic patients who died at the West Riding Asylum between 1866 and 1873 in an attempt to offer some general observations on ''the coarser and more obvious changes in the appearance and structure of the brain which result from epilepsy.'' He incorporated case studies from Wakefield in papers on acute dementia, chronic mania, and the sensory functions of cerebral nerve ganglia known as the optic thalami.[47]

His most ambitious research project, and the one for which he entertained the greatest hopes, focused on general paralysis of the insane. Identified in the 1820s, this frequent accompaniment of insanity was recognized by the 1870s as a grave indication that the victim's case was incurable. Trembling facial muscles, slurred speech, memory failure, unsteady limbs, together with delusions of grandeur and a wholesale alteration of personality—these were the signs of a rapidly advancing illness that, usually within three years, led to utter incapacitation and death. Psychiatrists were particularly struck by the personality changes that typically revealed a total loss of moral sense in the general paralytic. This could be explained readily enough by the breakdown, through cerebral disease, of the will's inhibitory control, thereby giving free rein to ''instinctive appetites and desires . . . regardless of propriety, and in violation of those habits which education had conferred.''[48] Thus perceived as a degenerative disease that reduced man to his animal nature, general paralysis became linked, in psychiatric interpretation, with vicious habits. In the 1890s, the demonstrated connection with syphilis only confirmed a long-standing medical suspicion that general paralysis was the outward manifestation of sin. Discovery of the syphilis spirochete in 1905 made possible the final identification of general paralysis as the terminal stage of venereal disease.

Prevalent among the inmates of public asylums, this affliction was an obvious subject of inquiry for asylum doctors. Already by 1871, Crichton-Browne had dealt with ''several hundreds of cases'' at Wakefield, five in men to every one in a woman. He believed at the time that the disease did not always have to prove fatal, if ''recognised and attacked at its outset.''[49] The leisure he could devote to investigating general paralysis was, however, severely limited, and by the end of 1873 he had determined to employ bolder measures, as he explained to Darwin:

> Impatient of the slowness of the advance which is made in our knowledge of the Pathology and Treatment of Nervous Diseases, I am about to try a new method of dealing with these subjects. Instead of trusting any longer to independent exertions scattered over a wide area, I propose to test the efficiency of combined effort upon one point. Having selected one well marked variety of mental disease—General

Paralysis— . . . I have induced a number of able and distinguished friends to
undertake its investigation in different aspects. . . . Each investigator will briefly
and clearly set forth the results at which he arrives and the monographs thus produced
will I believe when collected together form a complete natural history of the disease
and greatly elucidate its causes, course and treatment.

His co-workers in this campaign were Ferrier, Hughlings Jackson, Allbutt, and
Thomas Lauder Brunton, the physician who pioneered the use of amyl nitrite in
treating angina pectoris.[50]

By the time Crichton-Browne's own monograph on the subject appeared in 1876,
he had examined "upwards of 1,500 morbid brains" at, or after, autopsies. His
contribution centered on the appearance of the brain after the occurrence of death
from general paralysis, and he claimed originality in finding a consistent pathological
feature common to all his specimens, which previous investigators had overlooked. It
was not microscopical examination of cerebral tissue that had revealed this characteristic, but old-fashioned "hand-and-eye examination of the brain," combined with
a new method of soaking brains in nitric acid, which Crichton-Browne had adopted
for his purposes. The resulting observations led him to insist that, in the great majority
of cases, autopsies on general paralytics revealed adherence of the pia mater—the
delicate inner membrane enveloping the brain—to the gray matter beneath. Although
Crichton-Browne's investigations suggested no means of treating the illness, he did
attempt, in the most up-to-date neurological fashion, to connect "the localisation of
the adhesions" with "the psychical and motor symptoms in general paralysis."
Above all, what his study illuminates is the investigator himself, fully immersed in
the role of objective physiologist. In this extended research project, he assiduously
followed the prescribed inductive method of science, amassing huge quantities of
data from careful observations and drawing the conclusions that they apppeared to
dictate. Crichton-Browne prided himself that he had taken a major step toward "the
strictly scientific knowledge" of general paralysis, whose symptoms had "not yet
been traced out with scientific truth."[51]

Nor did he neglect to guarantee due publicity for the investigations that his asylum
promoted. In 1871, he launched a journal, the *West Riding Lunatic Asylum Medical
Reports,* which was published annually for six years under his editorship. He
persuaded Churchill, the London medical publisher, to bring out the first two volumes
and lined up Smith, Elder for the last four. The entrepreneurial element in Crichton-
Browne's personality emerged clearly and effectively in his management of the
journal, for which he secured a distinguished roster of writers. Ferrier contributed
three articles and Jackson five—most of the latter concerning aspects of epilepsy. In
the fourth volume, William B. Carpenter, the eminent naturalist and physiologist,
offered an appreciation of Ferrier's experiments. Sixty-two of the seventy-nine
papers published in the *Medical Reports* dealt with original research accomplished at
the West Riding Lunatic Asylum. These papers contained a much greater emphasis
on neurological inquiries than could be found at the time in the *Journal of Mental
Science,* and the *Medical Reports* answered a real need that was subsequently met by
Brain. The fact that three of the four founders and first editors of *Brain*—Ferrier,
Jackson, and Crichton-Browne—had only a few years before been collaborating on

the *Medical Reports* indicates how much the earlier, little known journal paved the way for the later, famous one.[52]

To a remarkable degree, Crichton-Browne had succeeded in establishing the West Riding Lunatic Asylum as the place in Great Britain where the most exciting work in neurology and psychiatry was being performed during the early 1870s. By bringing together doctors in both areas of medical inquiry, and, indeed, in pathology, physiology, and pharmacology as well, he had underscored the mutual interdependence of psychological and somatic approaches to mental illness. He had demonstrated that the director of a large public asylum need not be reduced to custodial chores, merely keeping track of hundreds of deranged men and women, but could work in the vanguard of the psychiatric enterprise. Having managed to make his institution "known and respected throughout the scientific world,"[53] however, he became anxious to find a post that would free him from the onerous administrative tasks that devoured his time. He was, accordingly, glad to accept the job of Lord Chancellor's Medical Visitor in Lunacy when it became vacant, with Bucknill's retirement, at the end of 1875. He occupied the position from 1876 until 1922 when, a venerable octogenarian, he at length retired from public service. Ironically, the government inspectorship virtually blocked Crichton-Browne from original research and altered the tenor of his professional life.

It is easy to understand why he welcomed the appointment, offered to him by Baron Cairns, the Tory Lord Chancellor.[54] The chance to follow his father's path yet again, by resigning an asylum directorship to become a government lunacy inspector, may have provided some inducement, but far greater must have been the attraction of London itself. In the late 1870s, the chance to move to the metropolis held abundant promise of success in private consulting practice for an alienist with good social connections. These were virtually assured to Crichton-Browne with the assumption of his new duties, for the Chancery Visitor in Lunacy was responsible for overseeing the treatment of affluent lunatics.

When a person with property valued in excess of £1,000, or with an annual income greater than £50, was considered insane, special legislation governed the procedures both for committal and for institutional supervision. Typically motivated by the fear that the individual in question was squandering family money, relatives or heirs had to petition the Lord Chancellor to hold a commission of inquiry into the case; the Chancery Visitor in Lunacy only became involved if the "accused" were, in fact, judged to be insane. While the lunacy commissioners established in 1845 were charged with inspecting the asylum conditions under which less privileged inmates existed, it was Crichton-Browne's duty to visit only Chancery lunatics, whether lodged in private asylums or attended in private homes. In 1877, there were 1,012 such patients, 676 of them in the former accommodation and 336 in the latter. By law, the Lord Chancellor's Medical Visitor was required to see Chancery lunatics in private asylums at least once a year, while those in a domestic setting, where the chances for abuse were considered greater, received quarterly visits. Although he had no control over the administration of his patients' estates, which passed under Crown protection, the Chancery Visitor made sure that they were maintained in a situation suitable to their wealth. The comforts they enjoyed were certainly very different from the conditions at Wakefield, where the inmates "had to wear the pauper clothing and be treated in all respects as paupers." While Crichton-Browne's new job was a "very laborious one," the number of visits that he actually had to make was considerably reduced by the fact that a single private asylum might house "as many as 40 Chancery patients."[55] Nor did he have to perform the work alone, for at any one time three Lord Chancellor's Visitors in Lunacy divided the responsibilities among themselves. Thus Crichton-Browne was left ample time for private practice.

In his new official capacity, he readily embraced the role of spokesman for his country's psychiatric practitioners. In 1877, in one of his first public appearances, he defended them before the Select Committee on the Operation of the Lunacy Law, insisting that public anxiety over the wrongful confinement of lunatics was grossly distorted. He felt certain that adequate safeguards existed to protect sane men and women from being unjustly admitted to and detained in asylums, or under domestic confinement; he belittled charges that "malice or ill will," on the part of relatives and with the connivance of doctors, might suffice to label a person insane. If mistakes *were* occasionally made—as when delirium was a symptom, not of lunacy, but of some grave somatic disease, like consumption—these cases were released, he assured the committee, as soon as the error became apparent. He even turned such mishaps to advantage, arguing that they proved the need for training in the study of mental disease as a necessary part of all medical education. "I think," he explained, carefully placing psychiatry at the heart of the medical enterprise, that "if they [medical men] had a little knowledge of mental disease they might be able to treat it in its earliest stages, when it falls under the notice of the general practitioner, and prevent it passing on to a more hopeless condition. I think cerebral diseases are so intimately bound up with all other diseases, that it would increase their general efficiency in the practice of their profession to have a knowledge of those diseases." Above all, he put a brave face on conditions at the large public asylums, telling the committee that they were "becoming day by day more like hospitals, and less like mere houses of detention." Although the nonrestraint system had proved sadly inadequate to stem what he himself, in his *Medical Reports,* had called "the great and growing tide of insanity," Crichton-Browne nonetheless insisted to the committee that the advantages of the modern asylum over older institutions arose from "the general humanity and gentleness of the mode of treatment and the scientific knowledge brought to bear on it." "Insanity," he confidently told his questioners, "is an eminently curable disease if taken in time and properly treated."[56] It is no surprise that so staunch a champion of the profession should be chosen president of the Medico-Psychological Association in 1878, thus achieving in his thirties an honor that had eluded his father until William Browne was in his sixties. In 1880, Crichton-Browne served, too, as president of the Psychological Section of the British Medical Association when it held its annual meeting in Cambridge.

As he settled into the public duties that he obviously found congenial, Crichton-Browne's consulting practice likewise began to flourish. Even at Wakefield, he had not considered insanity his sole area of expertise, but had spoken of nervous disorders in general as his "special practice."[57] In London, residing at Cumberland Terrace,

Regents Park—an area readily accessible to a fashionable clientele—he became, in effect, a "nerve specialist." Principal Tulloch, during one of his struggles against depression, consulted Crichton-Browne in 1881, when the theologian's "brain state was indescribable, the darkness at times reaching a horror of madness, in which suicide presented itself as a welcome relief." Managing to resist the temptation, Tulloch traveled from Scotland to consult Andrew Clark and Crichton-Browne. It is a measure of how quickly the latter had made a reputation for himself that he should have been paired with so eminent a physician as Clark, although the fact that the patient and his two doctors were all Scotsmen may have had some bearing on this case. In his diary, Tulloch mentioned Crichton-Browne's "unbounded kindness" and strong interest in his patient's troubles. The alienist was awaiting Tulloch's arrival by train at King's Cross and played the leading part in arranging for Tulloch to reside in Torquay, under the treatment of yet another Scottish doctor, Hamilton Ramsay, who had taken up practice in the English resort. Tulloch's "mental discomfort" gradually lifted at Torquay, and, with Crichton-Browne's permission, he left Ramsay's care after a stay of nearly two months. In early 1886, when he once again fell into "a very miserable state," Tulloch sought the advice of Clark and Crichton-Browne for a second time. Sadly, on this occasion, as his biographer wrote, "it was no longer a hypochondriac overwhelmed with mysterious miseries" who asked for help, but an extremely sick man dying of advanced kidney disease.[58]

Around 1880, Crichton-Browne was consulted on a very different sort of "nerve" case. Charles Eliot, later knighted for his service as a diplomat and subsequently the British ambassador to Japan in the 1920s, suffered a nervous breakdown—to use Crichton-Browne's term—after being tarred and feathered at school. Apparently his success at winning a Balliol scholarship, and his studious habits in general, had aroused the wrath of sixth-form bullies at Cheltenham, who vented their spleen in this particularly humiliating fashion. Eliot's mother brought him to see Crichton-Browne, who urged the young scholar to "throw the Classics aside for a little" and dispatched him on a sea voyage to the West Indies and South America. Eliot returned fully recovered and proceeded to achieve brilliant success at Oxford. Crichton-Browne's advice to another patient, Henry Arthur Jones, was less helpful. The playwright consulted him about recurrent fits of black depression, appalling periods of "stagnation and misery," which Jones feared "would end in a complete mental overthrow." Late Victorian psychiatry had no idea how to respond to what was certainly manic-depression, for Jones's suffering alternated with spells of "great intellectual activity, accompanied by intense nervous energy and excitement and high spirits." Crichton-Browne reassured Jones that his bouts of depression were "mere mental dyspepsia" and left it at that.[59]

Such advice seems a far cry from the kind of inquiry Crichton-Browne had encouraged, and himself undertaken, at Wakefield just a few years earlier. After his move to London, he never again launched any major new research project. It was not just that the demands of his government position left little time for sustained investigations. Far more serious was the lack of material to investigate, for without asylum patients of his own to examine he had no source of data. He never held a hospital appointment in London, furthermore, and was therefore deprived of the opportunities for empirical inquiries that hospital wards provided. In his desire to quit asylum medicine, he created a situation that placed utterly beyond his reach the prestigious neurological contributions he wanted to make.

Crichton-Browne did not abandon his aspirations immediately on entering a new phase of his career, but, for a while, apparently still hoped to figure among the pioneers of cerebral pathology. After he helped to found *Brain* in 1878, he contributed a lengthy original article to the first two volumes. Based on observations and records taken at Wakefield, it revealed his enthusiastic participation in the passion for weighing brains and measuring crania that swept over Europe and the United States in the second half of the nineteenth century, providing much of the alleged evidence in support of racist and sexist "science." Crichton-Browne claimed to have supervised "the weighing of the brains of 1200 insane patients" at the West Riding Lunatic Asylum and to have developed new methods for ascertaining the weight of the brain's various component parts. Although his investigations were cut short by his removal to London, he did provide elaborate tables comparing the weight of eight different cerebral lobes, the cerebellum, and the medulla oblongata in the brains of sixty lunatics. Subsequent contributions to *Brain* were less ambitious, and after the sixth volume, in 1883–84, he contributed no further original articles.[60] He continued, nonetheless, to support the journal in an editorial capacity until 1887, the year after the establishment of the Neurological Society with which it became affiliated. One of the society's first vice-presidents, Crichton-Browne served as president in 1888 and the following year assumed a place on the governing council. He seemed securely ensconced among the leadership of the new society, as appropriate an officer as Jackson, its first president, or Samuel Wilks, its second. His election as a Fellow of the Royal Society in 1883 had only added to his sterling scientific credentials, and he looked to belong squarely in the neuropsychiatric school of medicine—an approach to mental illness fully acceptable to the infant Neurological Society. Yet by 1894, his name had disappeared from the list of that society's members, regular or honorary.[61] He had, in effect, severed his ties with neurology, although he made no public announcement of the divorce.

In the absence of any explanation from Crichton-Browne, one can only speculate about the reasons why he broke off a relationship that he had been cultivating for at least two decades. It is true that, from its very origin, the Neurological Society witnessed an alignment of neurologists and experimental physiologists that eventually made the psychiatric members feel less welcome;[62] Crichton-Browne's presidency, however, and that of George Savage in 1897, suggest that the process had hardly proceeded far enough by the 1890s to drive out an alienist of Crichton-Browne's stature. He may, perhaps, have recognized that there were limits to what he could accomplish with his set of cerebral measurements from Wakefield and that, without further research opportunities, his future contributions to neurology would be negligible, but, surely, it is curious that the realization did not strike him before the 1890s. He had never, in any case, required ample data to support his medical pronouncements. His first papers, written while he was still a student at Edinburgh, rang with conviction, despite their slight evidential basis; thirty years later, it is highly unlikely that he would have perceived the absence of new material as a bar to participation in the work of the Neurological Society. Furthermore, the distinction between medical scientists who theorize from their armchairs and those who perform actual laboratory research, which seems fundamental today, was far less obvious at a time when research laboratories were still a very novel feature of the scientific landscape, at least in Great Britain. Among the affluent clientele he treated as a consulting psychiatrist, Crichton-Browne may have discovered that the guise of experimental neurologist found less favor than that of the cultured gentleman-doctor, able to sympathize with and cure the weaknesses of human nature. Yet membership in the Neurological Society would not have tarnished his image with such patients, so long as he conformed to their expectations and needs in other respects.

The likeliest reason for Crichton-Browne's departure from the Neurological Society centers on his recoil from the implications of materialism that he found in the latest neurological research. Already in his final contribution to *Brain,* a brief commentary in the tenth volume (1887–88), he expressed profound misgivings about the drift of Ferrier's studies. He was uneasy over the reduction of purposeful activity to a matter of sensory and motor responses. "Perception is not the 'be all and end all,'" he remonstrated, "and to relegate our whole thought-material to sensory centres, for that is what it comes to, according to Ferrier's most recent theory—is to degrade a large region of the cerebrum from its high estate, and leave it a mere superfluous intrusion in the brain mass." He refused to accept that a command from brain to muscles was "merely a haphazard motor impulse" and described it instead as "a nice adjustment of means to the end to be attained." He cound not endorse the fragmentation of "the unity of consciousness."[63]

In alluding to the cerebrum's "high estate," Crichton-Browne referred, of course, to the will, believed to reside within its nervous tissue. To deny that volition, or will, played a role distinct from sense perception or motor impulse was implicitly to deny the self-directed autonomy of individual behavior. It was not a vision of human conduct that Crichton-Browne cared to embrace. Throughout his career and regardless of all the current neurological vocabulary that he incorporated into his writing, he clung to the concept of will in order to make sense of rational behavior, just as he pointed to the absence, or incapacitation, of will to explain mental disorder. As late as 1924, he could not resist speculating that "will-power intervenes" in the synapse between afferent and efferent neurons in the brain.[64] By the early 1890s, he had evidently grasped how easily neurological research could lead to conclusions that challenged the notion of will as constructed by Victorian psychiatry. He may have likewise acknowledged that the neurologist's perspective could henceforth prove utterly incompatible with that of moral guardian, a role he adopted with particular fervor after 1876.

It is a measure of how much the British psychiatric profession had expanded its authority outside the asylum by the late Victorian period that, while William Browne had been content to "mould the moral nature" of his patients, his son preached to the nation at large. After he left Wakefield, education and public health became Crichton-Browne's special areas of concern, and subjects of such breadth allowed him manifold opportunities to sermonize. At Leeds in 1889, he told the British Medical Association about "The Hygienic Uses of the Imagination." At Finsbury Town Hall in 1891, his subject was tuberculosis. The Medical Society of London (of which he was the president in 1895) heard his "Oration on Sex in Education" in 1892. He went twice to Manchester in 1902, addressing the jubilee conference of the Manchester and Salford Sanitary Association on "Light and Sanitation" and, a few months later, lecturing on "The Dust Problem" to the Congress of the Sanitary Institute. Numerous other organizations, including the British Nurses' Association, the National Health Society, the Sanitary Inspectors Association, the Preventive Medicine Section of the Royal Institute of Public Health, and the Incorporated Society for the Destruction of Vermin, also engaged his time and his tongue. In his many public speeches, he found it easy to slip from examining specific problems of mental health to discussing the nebulous concept of mental hygiene, and from there to delivering judgments on the even vaguer notion of moral hygiene.[65]

Assorted honors attested to Crichton-Browne's professional reputation. He was knighted in 1886—a mark of distinction that his father had never received—while over the years he collected honorary degrees from the universities of St. Andrews (1879), Aberdeen (1906), and Leeds (1909). (His own university, Edinburgh, held out until 1933, by which time the LL.D. was awarded more for longevity than scientific distinction.) He became a member of the Royal Institution in 1880 and subsequently served as its treasurer for many years. All these signs of recognition came, however, not to a doctor in the thick of clinical work or to a scientist immersed in research, but to a medical dignitary who issued social commentary from the public lectern. Some of the earlier honors, such as the LL.D. from St. Andrews, may have been a belated tribute to his work at the West Riding Lunatic Asylum, but most were bestowed on him as a government official trying to preserve the nation's health against the debilitating and demoralizing forces that he feared were rampant in modern society.

These efforts were inextricably affiliated with Crichton-Browne's repudiation of materialism. It would be easy to portray the social conservatism of his later years, when he was a J.P. for Dumfriesshire and a member of the Conservative and Athenaeum Clubs, as the anxiety of an elderly man faced with bewildering social changes, but that is too simplistic an explanation. The emphasis on moral principles and religious beliefs, the fear of socialism, and the paeans to family life as the bulwark of social order, which are scattered throughout the reminiscences he wrote at the end of his life, found their roots in attitudes articulated in the 1880s and 1890s, when he was just reaching middle age. Some of these views appeared even earlier, during the 1870s. When he was only in his late thirties, for example, he took advantage of his presidential address to the Medico-Psychological Association to proclaim psychiatry's debt to religion. He called for "the spirit of scientific inquiry" to animate the work of asylum doctors, but he admonished his audience that scientific research without religious inspiration could never discover the secret of mental health. "For religion is still in the ascendant," he insisted.

> It is not, as Feuerbach would have us believe, a brain-sickly fancy, but a conquering power, and the abnormality is not in those who yield themselves to its sway, but in those who profess to have shaken it off, and possess themselves in blank apathy or despair.

> . . . It has ever tended to preserve the equilibrium of the nervous system by the relief which it has afforded in the anguish of remorse, by the consolation which it has

supplied under bereavement, and by the support which it has given in suffering and sickness. Who can say from what universal madness it may not have saved our race?

With its "benign effect upon the human mind,"[66] Crichton-Browne considered religion essential for individual mental health and, by extension, no less important for national stability. Godlessness could both unhinge a person's reason and unleash social chaos, as it had in France, he felt certain, on more than one occasion. In his own mind, the two forms of catastrophe were easily conflated.

Thus, even as a young man, he sought to protect the foundations of religious belief from the harsh assaults of materialism. His path had diverged from Maudsley's in the 1860s, he explained after World War I, when Maudsley "abandoned the teleological platform on which we both started and advanced into scientific material-ism and agnosticism."[67] To a significantly greater degree than most of his profes-sional colleagues, Crichton-Browne explicitly accepted, and even publicized, the religious implications of his psychiatric theories. It was in the hopes of finding a scientific basis for the independent existence of mind, and support for a belief in some kind of immortality, that he participated in thought-transference experiments at the Society for Psychical Research in 1883. He was disappointed, however, and disgusted with what seemed to him obvious attempts by charlatans to trick the earnest psychical researchers. Toward the end of his life, he lamented that he could not believe in "telepathy as an established fact," although he had sought after "really trustworthy evidence of its existence" for many years.[68]

Like his father's, Crichton-Browne's somaticism, was, therefore, severely quali-fied and restricted. Although both men embraced the physiological model of mental illness, each firmly believed in the efficacy of mental therapeutics, of appealing to the patient's moral nature, and of trying to arouse his or her will to recover. With regard to insane, rather than merely depressed, patients, the son's optimism in moral management was, admittedly, weaker than the father's. Thanks to advancing knowledge of the brain, furthermore, Crichton-Browne could locate far more precisely the areas where research was likely to discover the physical bases of insanity and other mental disorders. He looked with confidence, he said in 1878, to "the future of localization of cerebral function, of neuro-embryology, of the pathological chemistry of the brain," and to the study "of intracranial condition and changes."[69] For all his anticipation that psychiatrists would someday pinpoint the causative cerebral lesions in all cases of insanity, however, he was no less fascinated by the moral components of mental and nervous afflictions than William Browne had been. Even in his lengthy study of general paralysis, intended as his crowning contribution to neurological research at Wakefield, he stressed the dangerous impact of strong emotions on mental stability, citing anger, "inordinate ambition," "unfettered imagination," "uncontrolled grief," and other forms of worry or intense feeling, as potential precipitants of morbid cerebral states. Indeed, in 1874, J. M. Fothergill, junior physician to the West London Hospital and a frequent contributor to the *West Riding Lunatic Asylum Medical Reports,* quoted Crichton-Browne specifically to buttress his contention that "feverish anxiety, wearing responsibility, or vexing chagrin" could wreak havoc with the nervous system.[70] While Crichton-Browne always looked for the organic causes of mental derangement, he never assumed that mental processes were comprehensible in terms of physical agents alone. He was convinced that other causes, which bore directly on ethical and theological questions of the greatest magnitude, were also profoundly involved.

There are no easy chronological divisions in Crichton-Browne's life. At every phase of his career, his approach to mental and nervous disease was predicated on his belief in the utter interdependence of mind and body, a viewpoint shared by the vast majority of late Victorian psychiatric practitioners, including Allbutt, Clouston, L. S. F. Winslow, Savage, and even Maudsley. What did change were the professional goals Crichton-Browne set for himself and the emphasis he placed on somatic or moral solutions to the medical problems he examined. Until 1876, while he had ready access to an extensive pool of research material, he concentrated on the physiological clues and sought a place among the pioneering neurologists of the day. Thereafter the moral pieces of the puzzle assumed greater significance for him, and he wholeheartedly came to embrace the responsibilities of social watchdog, at the expense of his neuropsychiatric inquiries. Diverse developments simultaneously influenced this major shift in his professional orientation. Certainly the loss of research facilities after leaving Wakefield had a serious impact on Crichton-Browne's career. So did the emergence of such late Victorian movements as mass unionism, feminism, and socialism, which seemed to him to threaten the stability of British society and to demand response from authoritative medical opinion. In the absence of opportunities to demonstrate how the nerves worked, he could at least warn of impending nervous debility on a national scale, if the sources of public and private tranquillity should disintegrate. His attempts to maintain religion as a vital aspect of modern life were, for him, nothing short of a moral necessity, as indeed were his efforts to expose what he considered the absurdity of feminist aspirations. Although he never repudiated the work of his contemporaries in neurophysiology, he eventually acknowledged that it was not supportive of his own psychiatric priorities.

In numerous respects, Crichton-Browne seems a stereotypical figure in that reaction against positivism and materialism which colored late nineteenth-century European culture. Like many scientists in these decades, he was both attracted to the certainty that positivistic methods seemed to promise scientific inquiry and repelled by their theological implications. Yet, to the very end of his life, Crichton-Browne maintained an extraordinary range of interests and a passion for the odd physiological detail that balances the conventional aspects of his thought. There is something endearing, and surprising, about a nonagenarian who could write in 1931, with palpable enthusiasm, to Sir Edward Sharpey-Schafer, the renowned professor of physiology at Edinburgh, requesting an advance copy of his paper comparing the growth rate of finger nails on the right and left hands.[71]

3

Nerve Force and Neurasthenia

In 1837, James Manby Gully, a medical man soon to become the outstanding apologist for hydropathy, or water therapy, in England, asked: "Phenomena which cannot otherwise be accounted for are commonly attributed to nervousness;—but to what is nervousness attributable? The world may rest on Atlas, but on what does Atlas rest?"[1] Throughout the nineteenth century, and even into the twentieth, the answers British medical practitioners marshaled to respond to that query rested in some measure on the concept of nerve force, power, or energy. All malfunctioning of the nervous system was believed to be attributable, in one way or another, to what Victorian doctors dubbed the *vis nervosa*. When nervous breakdown occurred, the absence or scarcity of this precious power was specifically to blame.

The notion of nerve force had a venerable ancestry, extending back to the animal spirits that figured in classical medicine. It was Galen, the renowned Greek physician of the second century A.D., who placed these spirits at the center of all subsequent ideas about the nerves, for he invoked them to explain the transmission of sensory impressions to the brain and of motor impulses to the muscles. Galen himself never offered definitive pronouncements on the nature of the animal spirits, and for centuries contrasting schools of thought debated whether they should be considered a subtle material substance or an immaterial essence. Similarly, while all agreed that the animal spirits were conducted from the brain along the nerves, no unanimity prevailed concerning the structure of the nerves themselves. A dominant opinion depicted them as hollow tubes through which the animal spirits flowed, but alternative speculations portrayed them as solid, porous, or spongy. By the early modern era, the diverse theories drew their inspiration from mechanical models, predicated on concepts of motion and force, which required an indubitably physical substance for their action. The elusive animal spirits gradually yielded in scientific and medical literature to the notion of a nervous fluid that, like flowing water, was capable of generating power. Although "animal spirits" and "nervous fluid" functioned interchangeably for a time, and although the venerable former phrase continued to find employment throughout the eighteenth century, "the hydraulic view of the nerves" that fitted so neatly with other seventeenth-century developments in biology and physics permitted no ambiguity about the liquid state of nerve force.[2]

In fact, however, the idea of a nervous fluid offered no less controversy than earlier explanations of nervous activity based on the animal spirits. Weighty seventeenth-century opinion, including that of Thomas Willis, insisted that the nerves were solid, a condition that went far to explain why no one ever managed to

79

find any liquid circulating through them, even under microscopical examination. While some medical investigators, like the famous Hermann Boerhaave of Leyden, disputed this point of view, others sought ways to work around the problem. Increasingly, during the course of the eighteenth century, the idea of a nervous fluid conveyed the sense, not of an actual liquid, as denoted in the previous century, but of a so-called etherial or imponderable fluid. The age of Enlightenment abounded in such invisible, superfine fluids, which—although lacking measurable properties— were deemed material substances possessing physical extension. Indeed, scientists were glad to invoke them whenever they encountered processes that could not be elucidated in physical terms. Thus, even if an imponderable nervous fluid escaped instruments of investigation, its proponents might still insist that it existed. Nor did they have to locate any channels in the nerves through which it flowed, for a subtle fluid did not behave in so liquid a fashion. For those who remained unpersuaded by any of the possible forms of nervous fluid, various theories depending on the vibration or tension of nerve fibers were available to shed light on the mysterious workings of the nervous system. Still another school of thought attempted to compromise by suggesting that the nervous fluid itself transmitted vibrations across the nerves.

Even as eighteenth-century physiologists argued over the competing fluidist explanations or pondered the possibility of vibratory nervous action, nerve force was beginning to be associated with electricity. The connection originally occurred in the context of fluidist theory, for electricity figured among the eighteenth century's imponderable liquids. When, after experimenting with frogs and electrical currents in the 1790s, Luigi Galvani spoke of ''animal electricity,'' he intended to signify a kind of fluid, unique to animal life, that linked nerves with muscles and caused the latter to contract. At that time, since his was merely one of several conflicting modes of perceiving nervous conduction, it did not immediately carry the day. Early nine- teenth-century medical texts often straddled the theoretical fence, as the authors waited to see how the controversy would resolve itself. In his *Treatise on Nervous Diseases,* published in the early 1820s, John Cooke, for example, a former physician to the London Hospital, merely reviewed all available theories, without committing himself to any particular point of view:

> The nature of the medium through which the mind acts and is acted upon, in sensation and voluntary motion, has . . . been a subject of much speculation. By many, the nerves are supposed to be hollow tubes, through which a subtile fluid passes with inconceivable velocity from the brain to the muscles, for the purpose of voluntary motion; and from the sentient extremities to the brain for sensation: by others, sensation and motion are referred to vibrations in the brain and nerves, . . . and some have considered the nervous power as something analogous to Galvanism, or some other modification of electricity.[3]

By mid-century, the electrical interpretation of nervous energy prevailed. Just as developments in seventeenth-century physics had influenced the way contemporaries visualized the nervous fluid, so nineteenth-century physics helped to mold Victorian conceptions of the nervous impulse. When the riddles of electricity were yielding to scientific probe, and electricity was being harnessed for human purposes, it is scarcely surprising that it appealed to physiologists and medical men, impressed by these recent advances, as the form of energy most applicable to the nerves. Repeated experiments, furthermore, had demonstrated that "when the supply of nervous energy is cut off from the brain to a particular organ, that organ may be enabled to exercise its functions by exposing it to an electric current."[4] It became commonplace to compare the gray matter of the brain, generating nerve force, to a voltaic battery producing electricity, with the nerve fibers taking the part of electric wires, conducting power throughout the body. Indeed, by the 1850s, if medicine wanted to keep nerve force within the realm of scientifically reputable natural agencies, sharply differentiated from the suspect vitalistic notions that still lurked within nineteenth-century physiology, there seemed no viable alternative to electricity. "If Electricity be removed from the question of identity with the nervous power," Sir Henry Holland justly remarked, "none other of the known physical forces can for a moment be admitted into the hypothesis."[5] During the second half of the century, further research—by Ferrier and the German physiologist Emil Du Bois-Reymond, among others—eliminated any need for considering alternatives. Although definitive proof that the nerve impulse consists of an electric current was not forthcoming until the 1930s, by the end of Victoria's reign the ancient enigma surrounding the nature of nerve force appeared to have been resolved once and for all.

Whatever physical properties Victorian and Edwardian medical men assigned to nerve force, they all concurred in warning that every person possessed only limited amounts. Heedless overexertion, whether mental or physical, could drain an individual's supply, leaving an exhausted nervous system incapable of all endeavor. Failure of nervous power meant utter incapacitation. Just as the manifestations of an epileptic seizure, the characteristic features of mania, or the agonies of migraine might be explained in terms of excessive accumulation and discharge of nervous energy, so the symptoms of melancholia, depression, and nervous breakdown could be ascribed to depletion of the same force. Whether, as in the past, one thought of a nervous fluid that could run dry, or, as in the mid- and late nineteenth century, of "a faradic battery which had been in use for several hours without intermission,"[6] the end result, conceptually speaking, was identical. Holland vividly described that conclusion in his portrayal of several patients suffering from deficiency of nervous power: "In the most remarkable of these cases, (where the symptoms, coming gradually upon a youthful and vigorous frame of body, lasted for several months) all the voluntary movements of walking, speaking, eating, &c., were in a sort of abeyance—the mind inert, as if unable to force itself into any effort of thought or feeling—the circulation exceedingly feeble—and great torpor of all the natural functions." These bodily symptoms, Holland insisted, were "unconnected with any aberration of mind" or "any obvious bodily disorder," except the inadequacy of nerve force itself.[7] Such inadequacy provided the somatic basis for the psychological failure of will in victims of nervous prostration.

Nor was it necessary to exhaust the body's whole supply of nerve force before nervous collapse ensued. It sufficed to overwork only part of the body, for the interdependence of the entire nervous network meant that depletion anywhere drained away the nerve force needed for other physical functions. Thus overworking the brain, for example, could damage digestion or hinder reproduction. In 1867, Sir James Clark, a society physician with connections at Court, warned Florence Nightingale not to overtax her brain, lest it demand "more than its own natural share of the nervous energy of the system." Since she had already been bedridden for years, however, it is difficult to guess what further debility Clark feared for her.[8]

Medical exhortations to conserve nerve force, constantly reiterated in books and articles, made the public fully familiar with its finite nature. Restricted supplies of nervous power became an easy means of explaining the lethargy of depression without having to examine the emotional aspects of the condition. A. C. Benson's characterization of Hugh, the autobiographical figure whose musings comprise *Beside Still Waters,* relied heavily on the idea of a man who had to husband his nervous energy with care. Herbert Spencer, incapable of prolonged mental effort for nearly the last fifty years of his life, yearned in vain for "a full flow of nervous energy . . . sufficient to *simultaneously* supply all the numerous structures called into action" by the "highest intellectual co-ordinations." The limits of one's nerve force could, equally, provide a convenient excuse not to perform unwelcome tasks. Beatrice Webb, who was compelled to cut a certain figure in society before her marriage, but who anxiously sought to preserve time for her social and economic research, "tried to explain . . . [her] doctrine of nervous energy, that you were only gifted with a certain quantity, and that if it were spent in detail it could not be reserved for large undertakings."[9]

Victorians were scarcely the first to argue that the amount of nerve force in the body affected health and disease. It was an old belief, applicable whether the valuable substance appeared in liquid, etherial, vibratory, or electrical terms and whether the disorder under consideration was centered in the bowel or in the brain. When Schofield, as late as 1905, stressed the links between "breakdowns of nerve-force" and disease—organic as well as functional—he was perpetuating a venerable pathological tradition.[10] Like the earlier versions of this explanatory theory, the nineteenth century's contribution incorporated the latest findings from both physiology and physics, or, to give the specific Victorian sources, from neurology and thermodynamics. Medical men drew on the reflex function of the nervous system, increasingly central to neurophysiology from the 1830s, when they insisted that the exhaustion of nerve force in any single part of the body could produce ramifications harmful to the whole.[11] They turned to the second law of thermodynamics when they wanted to preach the dangers implicit in reckless consumption of nerve force.

The second law of thermodynamics, articulated at mid-century, posited a gradually decreasing amount of energy available in the universe. For obvious, dismaying reasons, this postulate made a powerful impression on the educated public, and its echoes reverberated in areas of endeavor far removed from mechanics and calorimetry. In medicine, it made itself heard in such assertions as Maudsley's claim that "the energy of a human body [is] a definite and not inexhaustible quantity."[12] To argue that the nervous energy in a living organism can be exhausted, however, is not necessarily equivalent to maintaining that it can never be replenished, and it was precisely on this point that doctors who treated cases of nervous breakdown encountered considerable difficulty with the second law of thermodynamics.

Some medical men, it is true, cautioned that the body could never recover its former vitality once nerve force had been rashly consumed and that permanent invalidism must be the inevitable consequence. Abstract warnings, however, rarely translated themselves into practice when doctors confronted victims of nervous exhaustion. Virtually every therapy designed for them was predicated on an implicit faith in the body's ability to restore supplies of nerve force, if given adequate, restful opportunity. Without some message of hope to impart, medical practitioners would have been unable—as they well knew—to treat patients with shattered nerves. Indeed, on a more routine level, the restoration of nerve force was generally assumed to be one of the principal functions of sleep, so that the normal, healthy individual could awaken with ample supplies for the activities of the day ahead. The image of a recharged battery was more appropriate to existing theories of nerve force than the menace implicit in the second law of thermodynamics, but it was also more mundane. The apparently irrefutable teachings of physics resonated with an authority that many Victorian medical men, particularly alienists and nerve-doctors unsure of their social and professional status, were anxious to assume; by invoking the second law of thermodynamics, they managed, at one and the same time, to proclaim their undeniable affiliation with the physical sciences and to establish their right to exercise an admonitory role in society.

In borrowing scientific concepts and terminology with which, often enough, they were not fully conversant, Victorian medical writers resembled novelists and poets, for whom the ambiguities of metaphor enriched the intersection of science and literature.[13] Such phrases as "nervous prostration" or "nervous exhaustion" were not, of course, intended as figures of speech in medical vocabulary, but expressed the presumably collapsed state of a patient's nerves when wanting sufficient quantities of the dynamic, invigorating nervous energy. "Nervous lethargy" or "nervous debility" similarly designated what medical men assumed to be an actual somatic condition of utter weakness. Despite their conviction that nerve force indubitably existed, however, it is equally true that metaphor permeated all Victorian and Edwardian discussion of the nerves. In a manner both subtle and heavy-handed, metaphors have for centuries molded the way in which scientists, medical men, and the general public think about the human body and its relation to the social "organism" or body politic.[14] Certain diseases, like consumption in the nineteenth century and cancer in the twentieth, have in themselves become master metaphors for their times. Where aspects of organic processes are particularly enigmatic and the impact of disease especially frightening, metaphor is all the likelier to slip into the discussion, both at the level of scientific debate and in popular pronouncements. Like analogies and similes, metaphors can bridge the gaps in knowledge, creating an illusion of theoretical completeness. Much that Victorian physiology adapted from physics—all its talk of force, energy, and currents—was employed metaphorically before electricity provided a solid foundation for the application of such vocabulary to the nervous system.

Indeed, no area of nineteenth-century physiology tempted the use of metaphor more persistently than the nerves. Not only was language hopelessly vague with regard to their functions, but they were at the very center of "those mysterious relations of mental and bodily life which form at once the foundation and the crucial problems of all physiology."[15] That mystery had to be resolved before physiologists and medical practitioners could gain a firm grasp of their subject, and right down to World War I, metaphor remained a requisite aid to resolution. Many who employed imagery by way of explanation never appear to have realized that they were dependent on mere literary expressions. For them, turns of phrase gave real meaning to nervous disorders. A few, nonetheless, acknowledged the unstable foundation of their theories, for lack of any more substantial basis. Thomas Dixon Savill, physician to the West End Hospital for Diseases of the Nervous System, insisted, for example, that the study of functional nervous disorders—"the most difficult domain of medical science"—could only be satisfactorily illuminated "by the method of analogy."[16] If even today, with our sophisticated knowledge of the nervous system, medical writers must resort to computer analogies when depicting the brain at work, how much more essential were similes and metaphors a century ago. Victorian and Edwardian medical men relied on them, sometimes unwittingly, sometimes purposefully, to create a context for the nerves in Victorian culture. Figures of speech helped them elucidate nervous illness to their patients and to society at large.

Metaphors of the nerves proliferated in rich variety. In addition to the earlier comparisons with flowing water and the later ones with electrical currents or discharges, medical writers worked with a large selection of mechanical images. Allbutt dusted off the old body-machine trope when he wrote in 1884: "We must have stored-up force, partly for greater occasions, partly to secure the equable running of our machinery. A neurotic person is an engine with a light fly-wheel and a small furnace, whose work, therefore, is fitful and unsteady." Crichton-Browne described infinitely complex and delicate nerves as "readily thrown out of gear," while a hydropathist remarked that, in an overworked brain, "the nervous centres . . . had lost their spring of recoil."[17] Others drew on musical associations, depicting nerves strung to the tightest pitch and wondering if an exhausted nervous system could ever be restored to harmony with the rest of the body. Still others found that the intricate network of nerves most closely resembled fine cloth, spoke of mental and nervous fiber, and warned that the endless repetition of hard, grinding, joyless work could destroy the fabric of the brain.

By far the dominant metaphor employed with regard to the nerves was economic. As the term *animal economy* implied the entire range of physiological functions, so Victorians and Edwardians viewed the nervous system in terms of a nervous economy. Nerve force was a form of precious capital that could be spent wisely, husbanded for future investment, or squandered recklessly to the point of bankruptcy. "Taxing nervous resources," "accumulating funds of nerve force," "wasting nervous reserves"—these and countless similar expressions recur throughout nineteenth-century medical literature. J. M. Fothergill marshaled every single one of them in a list of precepts for the maintenance of health, published in 1874, of which the final six were the following:

8. Man has a reserve of force: like the balance of a prudent firm at its bankers.
9. If this is too far drawn upon, a sudden demand becomes a very serious matter.
10. Unfortunately a man cannot estimate his physiological capital so exactly as he can his financial reserve.
11. Stimulants, though a great means, are not absolutely essential to attain physiological bankruptcy.
12. "Living fast" means living beyond the physiological income, and induces early exhaustion of the force capital.
13. Loans of force may be repaid by economy—by quietude and sleep.

Even in more personal texts, the same imagery often informed perceptions of the nerves. J. A. Symonds recalled in his memoirs that his father, a distinguished physician in Bristol, had advised him: "You have one of those constitutions with just enough nervous strength for the common requirements of life. You cannot draw upon the fund of energy without imperilling your health." Sometime later, Symonds's prolonged literary endeavors fulfilled his father's prophecy. "The tax upon my nervous strength," he conceded, "during four years of intense and feverish industry exhausted my constitution."[18]

The prevalence of financial vocabulary in disquisitions on the nervous system reveals the reasons for the profoundly significant place that the nerves occupied in Victorian and Edwardian culture. It was not merely that they figured, obscurely or prominently, in a bewildering diversity of diseases. It was that they were inextricably intertwined with ideas of wealth and power. Wealth gave its possessor public potency; nerve force was essential for personal potency. Absence of nerve force, like poverty, rendered its victim impotent. Just as the careful financier knew when to invest and when to save, the prudent individual knew when to expend nerve force to achieve personal goals and when to protect his resources. The two notions of public and private efficacy became inseparable, for the impoverishment of nerve force, by debilitating a man, could render him incapable of economic activity—could literally make him poor. Alfred Schofield made the connection explicit when he commented in 1903, "Money now is almost exclusively made at the expense of the wear-and-tear of nerve, as contrasted with muscle tissue; and it is a matter of ever-increasing economical importance to keep the money-making machine, the brain and the mind, at the highest productive pitch—in short, in a state of perfect health."[19] At a time when economic productivity was presumed to be an individual's duty, and bankruptcy the ultimate social sin, the possibility of physiological bankruptcy, or nervous breakdown, posed a particularly devastating threat. Although composed at the start of the nineteenth century, Wordsworth's famous lines,

> The world is too much with us; late and soon,
> Getting and spending, we lay waste our powers: . . .

remained fraught with many levels of meaning for Victorian and Edwardian readers.

British medical men paraded images that made sense in the world's leading capitalist country, and their metaphors of economic potency endorsed the bourgeois standards of success. This observation lends itself readily to ideological fanfare: it is certainly possible to portray these depictions of nervous energy as "symbolic systems whose political function is to reinforce social relations necessary to the capitalist mode of production."[20] Yet, in so doing, we may seriously distort the historical context in which these symbols functioned. What seem obvious agents of class dominance today may not have been intended as such ham-fisted devices in the past. The economic metaphors associated with theories of the nerves were not, in fact, perfectly tailored to a capitalist system, for they could not accommodate profits. No one ever argued that prudent preservation and expenditure of nerve force could augment an individual's reserves beyond a fixed amount, whereas the dreams of Victorian capitalists harbored hopes of expansion. In some respects, economic metaphors for the functioning of the nervous system harked back to an older notion of wealth, more aristocratic than bourgeois, as an inherited resource to be guarded rather than risked. In adapting concepts from the world of finance to the working of the nerves, medical writers adhered no more rigorously to a single mode of perception, or to one exclusive set of principles, than they did when trespassing on the domain of physics. Their goal was to help the public, and themselves, understand the cause and consequence of nervous afflictions by employing ideas and language that were readily accessible to their audience. If the imagery they invoked championed the middle-class values of thrift and self-restraint, their concern was surely less to buttress a particular mode of production than to inculcate the mode of living that they recognized as the only certain path to sustained health.

Victorian and Edwardian theorizing about the nervous system depended heavily on metaphor to span the gulf between the somatic functions of the nerves and their psychological, or emotional, manifestations. In addition to the paramount monetary metaphor, which concealed what the medical profession did not understand about the actual accumulation and expenditure of nerve force, minor metaphorical wordplay helped substantially to smooth the wrinkles in medical knowledge. Every term used to describe and explain the operations of the nervous system—tension, sympathy, excitability, irritability, sensibility, and depression—at once denoted a bodily state and connoted an emotional one. Signifying a somatic condition, each word also carried a heavy psychological cargo, and the line separating the two was virtually invisible. The very word *nerve* designated both a specific part of the body and a quality of character, as in the phrase "his nerve failed him." The readers of Fothergill's book of medical advice in the 1870s would have been familiar with the pervasive interplay of physical and mental implicit in his assertion that "there is an emotional sensitiveness which reveals the irritability of the exhausted nerve cen-tres. . . . The mind is as sensitive as is the skin after a blister: the slightest touch produces pain."[21] That interplay was, in fact, essential to much nineteenth-century medical explanation of the body's activities.

Where nervous breakdown was concerned, clearly the most important *double entendre* lurked in the concept of "depression." In general terms, *depression* means a state of lowered activity, as with the decreased expenditure of money in an economic depression, or the lowering of atmospheric pressure in a meteorological depression. To Victorian and Edwardian medical men, it indicated, first and foremost, a lowering of nervous energy, a drop in the quantity of available nerve force, just as neurophysiologists today understand it to imply "any decrease in the electrophysiological activity of a cell or an organ."[22] Among the numerous maladies "attributable to a depressed nervous condition," according to nineteenth-century medical wisdom, were "headache, backache, neuralgia, dyspeptic troubles, muscu-lar weakness, insomnia, chronic gout,"[23] and even graver afflictions, such as tuberculosis. The causes of decreased nerve force were equally varied. Infectious fevers, like influenza, might be the culprit, or excessive bleeding, as the opponents of venesection averred; all manner of overwork could be involved, or mental strain through prolonged anxiety, fear, grief, and disappointment.

These agents—particularly the so-called depressing emotions—not only lowered their victim's physical power, but also cast a somber shadow over the patient's mental state, thereby creating another context for the idea of "depression." With "general depression of nervous activity," William Thorburn, president of the Neurological Section of the Royal Society of Medicine, observed in 1913, "mental processes are in abeyance," along with somatic functions.[24] Although they could only speculate about the exact relationship between brain and mind, medical practitioners before World War I knew that whatever affected the nervous tissue of the one must have a striking impact on the other. Employing the term depression loosely, they easily, and perhaps unwittingly, slipped from discussions of material processes into commentaries on woeful personalities and gloomy frames of mind. It was the commingling of the two meanings, somatic and psychological, that made depression such an evocative term in Victorian and Edwardian medicine. "Low" or "sinking spirits," expressions often used interchangeably with depression, likewise resonated with double import, referring both to animal spirits in a torpid state and to the resulting melancholic cast of mind. Although Victorian medical theorists rarely intruded the animal spirits into formal physiological writing, the ancient concept lingered on in various turns of phrase, including the common one, "depression of spirits," in which both the nouns held physiological and emotional significance.

The elusive—almost slippery—quality of Victorian writing on nervous breakdown arises from the constant movement between one layer of meaning and another in the vocabulary employed. Used in conjunction with "nervous," "breakdown" itself contained implicit metaphors that endowed the neurotic concept with augmented potency, and not a little ambiguity. At its basic level, it indicated a failure of force, or inadequate supplies of nervous energy, much as we talk today of a "breakdown in communications" to describe a failure in the transmission of information. At a more complex level, it involved ideas of descent (ultimately into madness), of a decline in health, of downward movement, not merely to a lower level of vitality, but to the very loss of selfhood. That last threat emerged more explicitly in yet another layer of interpretation, for *breakdown* also means, as it meant to the Victorians, fragmentation into small pieces—the same image at work in "shattered nerves." Nervous breakdown, at its most terrible, signified the complete destruction of the personality. It was a situation in which the will, through deprivation of nerve force, was somehow deprived of the means to exert its controlling power, and the conscious sense of one's own identity vanished.

In its efforts to understand nervous breakdown, the British medical profession in the nineteenth century sought to associate it with some comprehensive medical ideology that offered illuminating interpretative principles. The ancient humoral pathology, challenged since the seventeenth century, was largely discredited by the nineteenth, but doctors and physiologists had no equally satisfactory organizing concept to embrace until the germ theory of disease emerged after 1850. Gradually gaining adherents and credibility, it offered an overarching explanation for the mass of new information about the human body that medicine had been accumulating for decades. The germ theory, however, was not particularly applicable to the enigmatic symptoms of nervous collapse. While these might be caused by a fever attributable to microbic origin, far more frequently the manifestations of breakdown bore no evidence whatsoever of fever or inflammation. Even during the second half of the nineteenth century, nerve-doctors, alienists, and family practitioners accordingly struggled to articulate a general medical theory to encompass, and make sense of, neurotic disorders. Their efforts focused on the notion of a nervous temperament, in which nerve force and its expendability figured prominently.

The very concept of a nervous temperament was itself a relic from the past, which suggested how long humoral theory lingered on in medical consciousness, particularly influencing the infant disciplines of neurology and psychiatry. From Hippocratic medicine in the fifth and fourth centuries B.C., through Galenic revisions centuries later, early modern medicine inherited the conviction that four basic body fluids, or humors, affiliated with the four basic elements—air, fire, water, and earth—held the key to health and illness. When the humors were in a state of balance throughout the body, health prevailed; when out of balance, disease resulted. Blood, phlegm, yellow bile, and black bile were not only linked with the four elements, and with the four fundamental qualities of matter—heat, cold, moisture, and dryness— but also with four temperaments, or types of personality. If blood predominated among the bodily humors, a person's temperament was said to be sanguineous; if phlegm, phlegmatic. Abundance of yellow bile produced a bilious or choleric temperament, while too much black bile caused a melancholic one. Certain diseases, furthermore, were believed to be associated with the particular temperaments.

Although the humoral theory of disease did not survive intact into the nineteenth century, the doctrine of temperaments did; Victorian medical men for the most part remained convinced that each kind of personality, recognizable by its physical appearance, was especially prone to specific morbid afflictions. What is more, the temperaments they considered in their diagnoses had expanded in number to include the nervous, or neurotic, for Cullen had considered that the nervous power modified temperament. From there it was only a short step to the assertion by James Gregory, Cullen's associate at Edinburgh, that a distinct neurotic temperament existed, as highly responsive to changing levels of nerve force in the body as the other temperaments were to their own affiliated fluids.

Thus the pathological theory based on ideas of balance and imbalance survived to influence Victorian attitudes to nervous ailments, even after the bacteriological approach to disease came to dominate other branches of medicine. The older temperaments continued to receive mention in medical texts, but the neurotic one attracted the lion's share of attention, as befitted an era that acknowledged the involvement of the nervous system in widely diverse disorders. It was the nervous, not the melancholic, temperament that medical practitioners expected to encounter in patients experiencing depression. In the 1890s, Tuke's *Dictionary of Psychological Medicine* eliminated the melancholic as a separate category of temperament altogether and dealt with it merely as "a mixture of the bilious and the nervous."[25]

The concept of nervous temperament was constructed from the ideas of sensibility to external stimuli, excitability, irritability, and exhaustibility that lumbered metaphorically through the pages of medical literature about the nerves. Crichton-Browne defined "an intensely nervous temperament" in terms of "an exquisite susceptibility, an incompetency to sustain the trials of life, and a liability to mental derangement." Patrick Nicol, a Bradford physician who trained under Crichton-Browne at Wakefield, found that people of neurotic temperament were "agitated and fretted by every little cross that happens, and over-excited by every pleasure."

Clouston described them as "very often irritable," while a contributor to Tuke's *Dictionary* observed them to be "very susceptible to sensations. They seem to be particularly liable to insanity, . . . and to diseases of the nervous system." On a similar note, Herbert Mayo had observed earlier in the century that the nervous temperament has a "tendency . . . to exhaust itself, and to use its resources with waste of nervous power."[26] In Victorian medical parlance, such vulnerability to nervous ailments and exhaustion was labeled a nervous diathesis, or constitutional predisposition to disorders of the nerves. It featured, in most cases, either insufficient generation of nerve force or its too ready consumption. Sir Andrew Clark, listing the symptoms of "mere and sheer nervousness"—as he called the nervous temperament—began with "a too rapid production and expenditure, together with an irregular distribution, of nerve force."[27]

Although the "nervous temperament," as with everything else relating to the nerves, implied a mental attitude as well as a bodily condition, nineteenth-century medical men welcomed the idea of an inherent tendency to neurotic illness as an explanation in physiological terms. Like the doctrine of humors in its day, the theory of a nervous temperament was presumed to have a physical foundation that enhanced its credibility. Not only was the nervous temperament associated with the somatic substance called nerve force, but it also appeared closely tied to the biological processes of heredity.

Victorian and Edwardian assumptions about the nervous temperament in fact depended heavily on heredity. If someone possessed an inadequate capacity to produce nerve force or to regulate its use, chances were strong that the unfortunate person had ancestors to thank for the condition. Early in the twentieth century, Schofield expounded the current orthodoxy among alienists and neurologists when he insisted that an array of functional nervous disorders—including asthma, hysteria, neurasthenia, insanity, and migraine—were "all strongly hereditary," while, in the same decade, J. J. Graham Brown, an assistant physician at the Royal Infirmary of Edinburgh, explained the situation more technically when he observed that a patient suffering from nervous exhaustion had "been born with a nervous system composed of neurones [nerve cells], many of which are defective in vitality, in resisting power, and in potentiality of repair."[28] This was merely sophisticated language for an old idea. Since at least the late eighteenth century, the medical profession had recognized that mental and nervous disorders were subject to hereditary influences, and the concept of a specifically nervous temperament provided a vehicle for the transmission of this inherited vulnerability.

Although nineteenth-century medical practitioners remained as ignorant about the actual workings of heredity as their eighteenth-century predecessors, the Victorians were familiar with the notion that they could blame their forebears for the temperament they carried through life. Many of their autobiographies traced with painstaking thoroughness the character of parents and grandparents, in a belief that the exercise furnished much insight into the author's own personality. Men and women troubled by nervous maladies were obviously intrigued by the question of a nervous inheritance. Symonds was convinced that his mother had "transmitted a neurotic temperament" to him; he also noted that the family of his maternal grandmother was "tainted . . . with extreme nervous excitability, eccentricity, even madness,"

while his paternal grandfather was "depressed by a melancholy temperament."
Spencer, a victim of recurrent invalidism after his nervous breakdown in the summer
of 1855, was at pains in his autobiography to show that both his father and a paternal
uncle had suffered similarly devastating collapses. Although he attributed their
prostration to overwork and mental strain, the implications were clear: he had
inherited the "extreme nervous irritability" that made his father's family prone to
nervous exhaustion. For her part, Beatrice Webb traced her own tendency to
depression—what she called her *Weltschmerz,* or, alternatively, her "suicidal constitution"—to her mother's relatives. Benson, whose father's "melancholy moods
. . . were many," had good reason to write that "heredity, temperament, environment" severely curtailed a person's set of choices in life.[29]

A nervous inheritance was not always viewed as wholly disadvantageous.
Symonds certainly believed that his literary accomplishments would have been
impossible without that "high degree of nervous sensibility" that also made his life a
torment. Leonard Guthrie, the specialist in childhood nervous disorders, insisted in
1907 that there was nothing innately morbid about a child who inherited a neurotic
temperament, "unless fostered and indulged beyond measure." He even argued that
"a certain proportion of the neurotic temperament is the spice of life" and that
creative achievement in art, science, and literature required the nervous personality.
Allbutt concurred. Samuel Johnson, Coleridge, Carlyle, and General Gordon, he
pointed out, were "all victims of inherited nervous maladies," and yet, despite their
sufferings, they managed to leave a significant mark on their times.[30] The point that
medical men wanted to underscore was that a nervous temperament did not have to
consign a patient to the invalid's sofa. The individual who accepted his or her
hereditary endowments, for better or worse, could wisely work to maximize strength
and minimize weakness; the person who ignored an inherited predisposition to
nervous illness, however, and who violated the dictates of caution under the
circumstances, could eventually count on succumbing to some form of nervous or
mental affliction, ending, perhaps, in madness. The choice remained with the
individual, as the historian Arnold Toynbee fully acknowledged when, in 1913, he
was contemplating marriage at the age of twenty-four. With his father confined to a
mental hospital, Toynbee was painfully aware how poor a risk he must appear to his
future bride and her family. He consulted a doctor for advice and was somewhat
reassured by medical opinion. "He said I must never overwork, or even do extra
work," Toynbee wrote to a friend, "as my father's case did show I had a tendency to
nerve-exhaustion, though it is not a mechanically hereditary thing: it depends entirely
on myself—on whether I play the fool or not."[31]

The hereditarian emphasis in the theory of nervous temperament allowed alienists
to assume a place among the scientists whose inquiries into the laws of inheritance
made evolutionary biology a subject of public fascination from the mid-nineteenth
century. It seemed to offer, too, another piece in the mind–body puzzle that so
preoccupied Victorian psychiatrists. On the one hand, heredity worked through
undoubtedly physical channels, but, on the other, it did so invisibly. It left no marks
to be exposed at an autopsy—a real advantage to psychiatrists often embarrassed by
their failure to find lesions in the brain tissue of deceased lunatics—and its impact on
character was as obvious as its influence on physical traits. Perhaps most useful of all,

to maintain the central causative role of heredity in typical cases of nervous collapse, or even milder forms of nervous weakness, effectively reduced the attendant doctor's responsibility. He could hardly be blamed for failure to cure a patient whose illness originated at the moment of conception, although the cases that he did treat successfully redounded all the more to his credit.

No one maintained, however, that all cases of shattered nerves could be traced to the *inheritance* of a neurotic temperament. The medical profession unanimously agreed that "a nervous disposition may be . . . acquired during the life of the individual," without any hereditary liability whatsoever, and doctors offered an impressive list of means by which a man or woman could make so troubling an acquisition. It could ensue "as a sequence of some severe illness, of some grave anxiety, or of some physical or moral shock";[32] it could follow in the wake of persistent mental or physical overwork; it could arise from indulgence in all manner of imprudent habits, not excluding religious enthusiasm and excessive emotionalism. Medical practitioners were fond of reminding their patients that there existed certain laws of health, affecting body and mind alike, which could not be contravened without dire consequences. In effect, these laws reduced themselves to the golden mean, "nothing in excess." Schofield, spelling out for his readers the descending steps to broken health, warned that *"Nervousness* is the general result of overstrain of the nervous temperament," but *"Nervous debility* is a still worse disorder. It is the manifestation of nerve exhaustion rather than irritation, and is . . . the frequent result of excesses of all kinds."[33]

"Excess" was a purposely ambiguous word. It could convey the idea of essentially admirable conduct carried to an extreme, as when young men applied themselves too diligently to their studies, or when businessmen spent too many hours at their offices, neglecting to rest and take exercise. When Victorian and Edwardian medical men preached against excess, however, they frequently had in mind a quite different sort of intemperance. "Luxurious living" was a phrase designed to cover a multitude of sins, including too many late nights and fashionable parties, too frequent attendance at the theater or perusal of racy novels, alcoholism, overeating, drug addiction, and overindulgence in sexual activity. By long overstimulation of the nervous system and failure to replenish nervous energy, all could serve to establish a neurotic temperament, which, if the offender neglected a reform of lifestyle, would lead inexorably to chronic nervous prostration. Charles Kingsley, whose own struggles with disabling depression had exposed him to much medical advice, passed some of it along to his readers at the start of *The Water-Babies,* when he compared "fine gentlemen and ladies" to Tom, the little chimney sweep, who rose at "three o'clock on a midsummer morning" to enjoy "the pleasantest time of all the twenty-four hours." "Why everyone does not get up then, I never could tell," the story's narrator mused, "save that they are all determined to spoil their nerves and their complexions by doing all night what they might just as well do all day. But Tom, instead of going out to dinner at half-past eight at night, and to a ball at ten, and finishing off somewhere between twelve and four, went to bed at seven, . . . and slept like a dead pig. . . ."[34]

Kingsley's genial admonition only implied what Allbutt, and many other physicians, made perfectly explicit. Among the nerve-doctor's best customers, Allbutt scoffed, was the "'City man' . . . [who] poisons nerves and blood with champagne, stodges his stomach with rich food three times a day, feeds his mind with vulgar shows and the 'dreams of avarice,' finds his recreation in Zola and the Society journals, and then tells us, forsooth, that the nineteenth century is too much for his nerves."[35] Patients like that were, beyond any doubt, the agents of their own suffering through their deplorable lack of self-control. Allbutt's remark sharply reveals that, just like the hereditary interpretation of nervous temperament, the theory that disordered nerves could result from irresponsible habits exonerated the medical profession from blame. It shifted the focus of discussion from the doctor's task of curing to the patient's role in provoking illness.

In warning that people could bring all the miseries of a nervous temperament on themselves, alienists were balancing the fatalism inherent in any discussion of heredity with an emphasis on personal responsibility. Their conviction that the bearer of a nervous inheritance, such as Toynbee believed himself to be, could activate his neurotic diathesis, or *not* activate it, struck a sharp blow against hereditary determinism. The possibility of an entirely acquired liability to nervous exhaustion, furthermore, strengthened the message that men and women had to take the initiative to preserve their own health or else, deciding to "play the fool," bear the blame for its ruin. If it seems heartless and tyrannical of doctors to accuse patients of choosing to bring illness on themselves, that particular medical strategy is almost always a reflection, not of expertise, but of ignorance, bewilderment, and helplessness in the face of some unusually baffling form of sickness, like nervous breakdown. The accusation, needless to say, allowed alienists and nerve-doctors to launch a moral crusade on behalf of clean living and common sense. Yet it was also fully in keeping with the all-important Victorian doctrine of self-help and, perhaps most important of all, enabled patients to feel some measure of control over their own afflictions—a sensation whose psychological benefits medicine is rediscovering today.

Until the 1880s, British medical literature on nervous exhaustion, extensive though it was, lacked coherence. Contributions to the subject were scattered among diverse sources, such as doctors' memoirs, studies of mental physiology, texts on the nervous system, speculations about various functional nervous disorders, and even philosophical disquisitions on the nature of life itself. From the 1880s to World War I, however, the new diagnostic category of *neurasthenia* provided the missing focus. Building on the already well established conviction that individual supplies of nerve force were limited and exhaustible, the name neurasthenia seemed to impart not merely enhanced medical legitimacy, but also real distinction, to the sundry symptoms of depression formerly subsumed under the less specific concept of nervous prostration. Medical journals abounded with discussions of the catchy new title, which rapidly caught on among the educated public as well.

Although George Miller Beard's name is commonly linked with the emergence of neurasthenia as a pathological construct, the term had been in use for several decades before he adapted it to his own purposes. Nor was he the only American doctor to realize its potential utility. E. H. Van Deusen, medical superintendent of the Michigan Asylum for the Insane, independently bestowed the same name on diverse manifestations of nervous collapse in 1869, the very year that Beard, a lecturer on nervous diseases at New York University, published his initial article on neurasthenia. The fact that Beard, the New Yorker, interpreted neurasthenia as a disorder precipitated by the fast pace of urban life, while Van Deusen, working in a community of farmers, attributed it to rural isolation, aptly illustrated neurasthenia's immense capacity to be all things to all medical men.[36] Despite its impressive Greek etymology, however, the label meant nothing more arcane than nerve weakness, or debility of the nervous system.

While the international medical community had long been familiar with the idea, and appearance, of nervous debility, no one before Beard had so pertinaciously insisted on its status as a distinct disease, with both a specific etiology and distinguishing symptoms. His was the name that became inextricably associated with neurasthenia because the New York neurologist tirelessly publicized its existence between 1869 and his death in 1883. In this campaign, Beard's greatest difficulty arose in the effort to draw up a definitive list of the physical and mental manifestations of neurasthenia, for he could enumerate more than fifty such signs without exhausting all possibilities. His list included profound anxiety, despair, and fear, various phobias, fretfulness, insomnia and nightmares, indecisiveness and inattention, extreme weakness and fatigue, migraine, dilated pupils, frequent blushing, heart palpitations, cramps, dental decay, indigestion, neuralgia, rapid changes in body temperature, sexual impotence, backache, and the fidgets. Just as psychiatrists today recognize that depression may be expressed through loss of appetite or overeating, sleeplessness or the inability to stop sleeping, so Beard acknowledged apparent contradictions among the symptoms of neurasthenia.[37] The catalogue, it seems, was infinitely expandable, and any symptom, evinced by any patient considered neurasthenic, could be added as occasion demanded.

Where the etiology of neurasthenia was concerned, Beard was able to provide more precise information. He had no doubt that only the nineteenth century could give rise to neurasthenia, for contemporary civilization alone had produced the peculiar combination of causative agents so deleterious to nerve force: rapid transportation and communication, great advance in scientific learning, and the widespread education of women. Taken together, these conditions created an environment in which repose was almost impossible. Men and women, deprived of religious certainty, constantly strove for ever more extensive knowledge of the world—and competed strenuously to derive the greatest advantage from it. Such an atmosphere made exhaustion of nervous energy virtually inevitable. While previous civilizations had, of course, known nervous disorders and fatigue, none had ever experienced the particular condition of nervous prostration that he designated neurasthenia. Of all societies, furthermore, none was so prone to the illness as Beard's own United States, that land of unparalleled social mobility, uniquely dynamic enterpreneurs, and ambitious achievers, where the hurried tempo of life was very nearly a matter of national pride. If the eighteenth had been the century of the English malady, Beard seemed determined to stamp the nineteenth with an American affliction.[38]

Beard's British admirers did not have to cede pride of neurasthenic place to America in order to endorse the rest of his views on nervous debility. By the 1880s, many British doctors found the concept of neurasthenia invaluable and gave it a prominent place in their medical vocabulary. During the preceding decade, Silas

Weir Mitchell, Beard's compatriot and fellow neurologist, had published highly successful works with such irresistible titles as *Wear and Tear, or Hints for the Overworked* (1871), and *Fat and Blood: and How to Make Them* (1877), which helped prepare British audiences for Beard's volumes on neurasthenia, when these began appearing in 1880. Since the theoretical core of Beard's assertions about nervous energy and the pressures of modern life merely confirmed long-standing British medical convictions, Beard's special identification of neurasthenia with his own countrymen—and the assumption of American cultural, or at least technological, superiority that accompanied it—was easy to overlook. Some British commentators, it is true, sincerely hoped that their nation's love of athletic sports would spare its inhabitants the nervous exhaustion so rampant in the United States,[39] but most ignored the neurotic rivalry, confident that British men and women could hold their own neurasthenically against Americans any day.

The issue most vehemently debated in the Anglo-American literature on neurasthenia concerned the disorder's novelty. The concept itself was not entirely new; its origins lay in the work of John Brown, a late eighteenth-century Scottish medical theorist and practitioner, who asserted that all diseases fell into the two categories of *sthenia* and *asthenia*—the first denoting an excess of stimulation, the second signifying an incapacity to react to the same.[40] The more immediate diagnostic precursor was spinal irritation, a label much in vogue between 1830 and 1870. The physiological theory behind this alleged functional nervous disorder derived credibility from the great neurological discoveries of the 1820s and 1830s—the work by Bell and Magendie on the motor and sensory functions of the spinal nerve roots, and Hall's exposition of the spinal cord's reflex function.

The diagnosis of spinal irritation, introduced by a Glasgow physician in 1828, was supposed to explain a variety of local pains and debilitating ailments, including mental depression, by reference to inflammation, or, more vaguely, irritation, at certain strategic points along the spinal cord. These were the vertebrae beneath which were located the ganglia of the sympathetic nervous system bringing sensation to the stomach and the heart, as well as to other organs and tissues. Pain at any of the central spinal locations could be transferred to seemingly disconnected parts of the body, like the viscera, through the sensory apparatus of the nervous system, while lethargy and restlessness alike could be explained by dysfunction of the motor and reflex networks involved. Inevitably, "irregular distribution of the nervous energy" also came to figure in this explanatory theory. Complicated though the theory sounded, it pointed to an easy remedy: locate the specific area of spinal tenderness and counteract any inflammation by means of blisters, leeches, or cupping.[41] Both the diagnosis and the therapy belonged to general medical practice, for neurology scarcely existed in these decades and psychiatry was still largely confined to the asylum, unlike the situation that prevailed by the time neurasthenia commanded medical attention. Equally unlike neurasthenia, the theory of spinal irritation was vulnerable to disproof. It became increasingly difficult to uphold as medicine persistently failed to find physiological evidence that primary inflammation of the spinal cord actually occurred. Although "spinal irritation" occasionally appeared in medical textbooks published during the final quarter of the nineteenth century,[42] its days were clearly numbered.

Neurasthenia undoubtedly carried some heavy debts to the theory of spinal irritation, not least of which concerned its reliance on nervous reflex action. In Beard's explanation of neurasthenia, the individual's limited supply of nerve force merged with the reflex function of the nervous system to offer an all-inclusive explanation for every conceivable neurasthenic symptom. For men and women doomed by inheritance to meager production of nerve force, or for those whose style of life and reckless habits jeopardized otherwise adequate supplies, the smallest additional strain, from business worries, domestic woes, excessive mental labor, or anything else, could become the proverbial straw on the camel's back, pushing the hapless victim into neurasthenic decline. Why intellectual labor taken to extremes should cause heart palpitations, say, or why too frequent sexual activity could give rise to facial neuralgia posed no difficulty for Beard. The brain, the reproductive system, and the digestive organs, he argued, were all centers of the body's nervous reflex action. The draining of nerve force through the overuse of any one of these centers sent fatigue and irritation ricocheting through the body, with physical ramifications in what seemed the most unlikely places. In addition to the echoes from spinal irritation theory, Beard's hypothesis bore a certain resemblance, although he would not have acknowledged it, to the ancient Greek medical notion of *sympathy,* an "occult form of communication, hidden from and below the transactions of consciousness," by which doctors could elucidate, for example, the visceral disturbances so frequently accompanying migraine.[43] Indeed, this "sympathy" among the body's organs was long deemed the preeminent characteristic of nervous disorders. Before the notion of psychosomatic illness gained medical legitimacy, the often bizarre manifestations of what would now be called psychosomatic ailments demanded some such explanation, whether dubbed sympathy or reflex action.

Adaptations from John Brown and from spinal irritation theory aside, the question for late Victorian medicine to resolve was whether neurasthenia had appeared in the unique environment of the nineteenth century, as Beard contended, or whether it was the old condition of shattered nerves merely promenading under a new name. The prevalent position among British doctors repudiated Beard and upheld the latter point of view. A few, admittedly, claimed that British medicine had failed to acknowledge the gravity of "wear-and-tear" disorders until the end of the nineteenth century, or to realize that all the associated symptoms constituted a single, identifiable illness, but most assumed that the medical profession had been treating, and taking seriously, the neurasthenic condition—under whatever title—for decades, if not centuries. Sir Andrew Clark observed that its medley of symptoms had "been more or less fully recognised and described by every competent observer and writer from the days of Cheyne and Whytt until now," while others, more sweepingly, argued for its existence since the dawn of human history. Neurasthenia, Guthrie pointed out, "is not a novelty. . . . Under other names it has always flourished." With greater attention to the details of medical history, Rudolf Arndt, a German contributor to Tuke's *Dictionary of Psychological Medicine,* traced a description of its characteristic features back as far as the sixteenth century. In the same source, W. S. Playfair specifically identified neurasthenia with the standard Victorian concept of nervous collapse. Calling his readers' attention to "that species of general nervous breakdown which constitutes a very real and very important malady," he noted that "by some it is called 'nervous exhaustion,' by others, 'neurasthenia.' "[44]

Nonetheless, British medical practitioners generally welcomed the advent of neurasthenia as a useful addition to medical terminology. They were relieved to be able to describe, in a single word, "a condition of prostration of the whole or some of the nervous centres, . . . in which there is no gross lesion, visible to the eye or by the microscope, of any part of the brain or spinal cord," and proceeding "from excessive functional activity of some part of the nervous system." It facilitated medical discussion to be able to encapsulate in the term "neurasthenic" a patient "whose nervous system, from some cause or other, shock, overwork, mental strain, and so on, actually has broken down, and who has thus become a complete invalid, and is incapable of fulfilling the ordinary duties of life." Even Gowers, who had little use for the neologism, conceded that it was simpler to say neurasthenia than any of the older, wordier ways of expressing nervous debility.[45]

Late Victorian and Edwardian medical men found neurasthenia a convenient term not only because it imposed an artificial coherence on a broad array of disparate symptoms, but also because it bestowed an air of precision on an indeterminate affliction whose amorphous contours had puzzled and embarrassed them for decades. They were glad to take advantage of it, even if it did not help them make real progress toward a deeper comprehension of depression. Indeed, far from solving all problems of neurotic taxonomy, the word neurasthenia merely contributed another pathological label to ponder. Whether or not its promoters recognized the fact, the concept of neurasthenia only further muddied already turbid diagnostic waters.

With its related symptoms encompassing virtually the entire range of physical and mental disturbances, it was more than a little perplexing to differentiate neurasthenia from such tried and true categories of neurotic illness as hypochondriasis and hysteria—other misleadingly simple names for complex conditions. Although Beard was perfectly willing to subsume these maladies under the roomy classification of neurasthenia, some of his British counterparts were not so ready to dispense with trusty diagnostic friends. They conceded the difficulty in distinguishing among the several similar neuroses, but tenaciously continued to try. Even in the twentieth century, texts on neurasthenia almost always included a section in which the disorder's characteristic features, although legion, were shown to vary from those of hysteria and hypochondriasis. T. D. Savill, for example, in his *Clinical Lectures on Neurasthenia,* thoughtfully provided a two-page "Table of Diagnosis" that set forth all the differences separating the three functional nervous disorders.[46] No two medical men, however, would have agreed on every aspect of Savill's chart.

One doctor's hypochondriac or hysteric might easily prove another's neurasthenic, and the vast quantity of printer's ink devoted to attempts at differentiation could not provide satisfactory marks of distinction. A telling sentence in Seymour Sharkey's presidential address to the Neurological Society in 1904 reveals the extent of the problem. Acknowledging that neurasthenia resembled hysteria, he insisted nonetheless that they were strikingly dissimilar with respect to certain significant characteristics. "As we are in ignorance as to the actual pathology of either one or the other condition," he added, almost wistfully, "it is very difficult to describe what those characters are."[47] Others observed that neurasthenia, whether chronic or acute, could merge with more severe forms of nervous and mental illness, including suicidal melancholia. Although the British medical consensus was that neurasthenia did not usually end in madness, late Victorian and Edwardian alienists nonetheless perceived neurasthenia "to be common as a kind of connecting link between health and insanity."[48] Under the circumstances, it is hardly surprising that few members of the British medical profession in these years could say for certain whether neurasthenia was a unique condition whose symptoms formed a regular pathological pattern with a consistent etiology or whether it was merely a cluster of accidentally associated disorders with different causative agents varying from victim to victim.

It seems clear, thanks to the wisdom of hindsight, that the concept of neurasthenia offered no substantial improvement, apart from brevity of nomenclature, over the older vocabulary of shattered nerves and nervous prostration. Yet for a while it dominated the important field of medicine claimed by both psychiatry and neurology in the late nineteenth and early twentieth centuries. Perhaps some reason for its popularity, among doctors and patients alike, can be found in its very location at the center of that disputed territory. In a period when the physiological nature of the so-called functional nervous disorders began to be questioned, and the suspicion arose that neurotic patients were feigning illness, neurasthenia, as depicted by Beard and his followers, seemed to reaffirm the somatic basis of nervous breakdown. In their emphasis on nerve force and the workings of the nervous system, they kept alive a mode of explanation that accepted the symptoms of depression as manifestations of a real, physical disease, thereby validating both the doctor's ministrations and the patient's suffering. The former could dispense, and the latter receive, what was "an essentially psychological therapy under a somatic label."[49] It is no wonder that neurasthenia flourished internationally for a season, almost as much a topic of discussion and controversy in France and Germany as in Great Britain and the United States.

The allegedly corporeal etiology of the disorder was nowhere more evident than in the highly specific category of traumatic neurasthenia, which surfaced wherever the general neurasthenic diagnosis found an appreciative reception. When late Victorian and Edwardian medical practitioners spoke of trauma, they generally meant a physical shock to the system rather than a psychological blow. Traumatic neurasthenia was particularly associated with railway accidents and, as such, was a later version of "railway spine," which had figured in the mid-Victorian transatlantic literature on functional nervous disorders, typically in conjunction with the theory of spinal irritation. Since organic lesions of the spine had proved so elusive in cases of presumed spinal irritation, advocates of traumatic neurasthenia did not insist on injury to the spinal column as its sole causative agent, but spoke in broader terms. Herbert W. Page, a London surgeon and the leading expert on the subject in Great Britain, explained that the symptoms of neurasthenia, which often appeared in victims of railway collisions, might be traced to the spine, but could be equally attributed "to lowered nerve force, . . . whereby the various functions of the body, be they muscular, mental, or organic, are thrown out of gear, and rendered incapable of perfectly natural and healthy action." He described at great length the patient who, having survived a train crash with no ostensible bodily injury, nonetheless subsequently evinced all the telltale symptoms of "neurasthenia or nerve weakness and exhaustion":

> . . . he breaks down; his head begins to ache, and he has pains and aches in various parts of the body, most probably in his back; he feels weak and faint, and good for nothing. . . . Whenever he attempts to get up he feels so weak and prostrate that absolute quietude and repose are essential for his comfort, his safety, and his early restoration to health. Bodily exertion brings on muscular fatigue, and aching . . . and any mental exertion has a like effect, pain and a sense of oppression in the head, with inability to occupy the mind. . . . He cannot bear noise, and strong light is very distressing to him; he has lost all inclination for food; he cannot sleep at night. . . . He is nervous and emotional, sighs and pants, is depressed and melancholy, and has so lost control over his emotions that he is ready to cry on the least excitement. . . . Such is an imperfect picture, not of any actual case, but of the kinds of symptoms which in varying degrees of severity, and in every possible variety of combination, you will note in these cases of general nervous shock or neurasthenia. . . .[50]

Page was not only knowledgeable about the impact of modern technology on human health; he also fully understood the varied uses to which a medical diagnosis could be applied. Two of his books discussed the "medico-legal aspects" of railway injuries, particularly to the spine. There must have been a deluge of law suits against railway companies in the wake of accidents—many of which Page investigated himself—for Guthrie quipped in 1907 that neurasthenia was not "solely met in victims of railway accidents and in pleaders for compensation."[51] In any case, neurasthenia was a specific diagnosis that lawyers could parade in court, and with the so-called traumatic variety the causative agent could be pinpointed with legal precision. Even where financial gain was not involved, the tendency to fragment the concept of neurasthenia into subspecies had certain advantages. By specifying whether a patient's illness was the spinal, visceral, cardiac, sexual, or cerebral variant of neurasthenia, a medical attendant could not only pass judgment on the patient's lifestyle, but also prescribe the mode of treatment considered most conducive to recovery. While gentle muscular exercise, for example, was judged beneficial in cases identified as brain exhaustion, or "cerebrasthenia," any physical exertion could prove highly detrimental where spinal weakness was primarily involved and where absolute rest was mandated.[52]

Clearly, there is a law of supply and demand as potent in medicine as in more overtly commercial relationships. It works with regard to medication, and it applies with equal rigor to diagnostic labels. Flora Thompson recalled that the inhabitants of her rural hamlet "Lark Rise" enjoyed excellent health in the late Victorian years, largely thanks to "lack of imagination." "Such people at that time," she surmised, "did not look for or expect illness, and there were not as many patent medicine advertisements then as now to teach them to search for symptoms of minor ailments in themselves." When a new curate arrived, with previous training as a medical student, the situation changed dramatically. Glad to make use of his skills, he dispensed advice and medicine freely, only to find that, suddenly, "nearly every one had something the matter with them. 'My pink pills,' 'my little tablets,' 'my mixture,' and 'my lotion' became as common in conversation as potatoes or pig's food." As the

Journal of Psychological Medicine had noted at mid-century, "the vaunting of specifics" only "magnified our imaginary maladies to excess." So, too, the creation of an authoritative-sounding disease, neurasthenia, persuaded many a late Victorian to seek shelter for indefinable symptoms of depression under its august title. It is not at all remarkable that by 1885 medical observers could report that neurasthenia was "becoming more common, . . . occurring alone, or complicating many every day complaints."[53]

Consumers will always emerge to try new goods, and producers will certainly find ways to satisfy their demands. The two processes interact in an endlessly circular way, for which cause and effect are impossible to assign. Whether medical influence precedes public response or public requirements dictate medical reaction is an extraordinarily complicated question. If doctors found themselves diagnosing nervous exhaustion more frequently at the end of the nineteenth century, they may have been prompted to do so by the ease with which they could flourish the new, all-inclusive designation for a very mixed bag of symptoms. We do not know whether British medical men actually saw greater numbers of severely depressed men and women in private consulting rooms and public infirmaries after about 1880, but we may safely guess that many were glad to identify neurasthenia where previously they might have remained in diagnostic doubt. On the other hand, they may well have been under strong pressure from patients to dispense the neurasthenic diagnosis. Once propagated, disease entities assume dimensions that the medical profession cannot always predict or control. Those that take root and thrive most luxuriantly are the ones that best further the confluence of patient's and physician's needs. Neurasthenia performed that function admirably for a time, bringing consumer and producer together in an intricate collaborative effort.

Both parties benefited. While medical practitioners sold the disease concept to a receptive audience, thus creating a market for their wares that was not easily glutted, they were still dealing with the emotional and physical symptoms of depression, which presented a genuine medical problem regardless of label. Whether family practitioners, alienists, neurologists, or consulting specialist physicians, doctors who treated this problem were eager to persuade the public that it was an objective, medically classified disease, rather than a purely subjective illness defined by the patient. They wanted to emphasize, too, that it posed a real and serious threat to health and happiness. The creation of a formal disease entity with a distinguished title seemed, at least temporarily, to solve their difficulties. On the consumer's side of the exchange, the new label was welcome precisely for its novelty. It was not encumbered by centuries of associations, most of them pejorative or confusingly ambiguous. At the very least, it was a medically neutral term; at the most, it functioned as a kind of compliment, since it could be associated with those who showed enterprise and drive, seizing the opportunities offered by the advances of modernity, albeit too zealously. As far as Savill was concerned, "many neurasthenic subjects are persons of very considerable intelligence and brilliancy, who, therefore, take a leading part in society."[54] The diagnosis of neurasthenia carried a certain cachet that could hardly have failed to appeal to many people experiencing the agonies of depression. Like the eighteenth-century cult of sensibility, the late nineteenth-century incidence of neurasthenia was probably augmented by the potent influence of suggestion and imitation, for neurasthenia was widely perceived as a malady that bestowed on its victims special claims to consideration.

Occupying so prominent a place in the late Victorian and Edwardian literature on the nerves, the concept of neurasthenia figured centrally in the tangled mass of conflicting medical attitudes concerning the impact of modern civilization on human health. Beard's exclusive identification of neurasthenia with the nineteenth century, while not persuading the majority of British medical men, nevertheless powerfully supported those who sought to blame the pace of contemporary life for what seemed an ominous increase in the incidence of nervous illness. To point an accusatory finger at the conditions of modernity itself was, of course, yet another way to reduce the burden of accountability borne by the medical profession, and to promote the diagnosis of neurasthenia created, in effect, a self-fulfilling prophecy about the prominence of nervous weakness in highly modernized societies. Far from endorsing any facile assumptions that civilization was set on an inevitably progressive course, the British medical profession in the late nineteenth and early twentieth centuries viewed the future anxiously, with regard to the nation's nervous stability among much else. The vogue for neurasthenia was by no means alone, however, in stimulating medical concern about the nerves. Victorian and Edwardian doctors were building on a long tradition in British medicine when they voiced the conviction that nervous disorders multiplied with the forward march of civilization.

Among the many Augustan and Georgian contributions to the investigations of melancholy as the preeminent trait of the English character, Dr. George Cheyne's became the most celebrated. In his early eighteenth-century study of *The English Malady,* Cheyne agreed with other observers, including Voltaire, that climate bore some share of responsibility for his countrymen's torments. "The moisture of our air, the variableness of our weather, . . . the rankness and fertility of our soil," he contended, all contributed to the national temperament. By themselves, however, these were not sufficient to cause "almost one third" of the affluent people of England to experience nervous complaints. Additionally, Cheyne argued—in language that resounded down the subsequent decades—medical practitioners had to consider the way their patients lived, particularly "the richness and heaviness of our food, the wealth and abundance of the inhabitants, . . . the inactivity and sedentary occupations of the better sort, (among whom this evil mostly rages) and the humour of living in great, populous, and consequently unhealthy towns." In this conjunction of harmful circumstances lay the reason why the nerves of so many English people were "evidently relax'd and broken." Cheyne regretted the prevalence of luxury and excess among "the better sort" of his compatriots, the lack of exercise to balance the consumption of epicurean meals, the time devoted to overstimulating activities, like dancing and gambling, and, in general, life lived in "over-grown cities," especially London, which Cheyne believed to be "the greatest, most capacious, close, and populous city of the *Globe.*" There was no mistaking Cheyne's pride in the accomplishments of Englishmen, but he nevertheless insisted that prosperity and progress, with their attendant opportunities for self-indulgence and artificial excitements of every sort, cost the English dearly in terms of health.[55] It was thanks, in large part, to Cheyne that the meaning of nervous began to undergo a slow transformation, from the denotation of sinewy, strong, and energetic, which the word had carried since the fifteenth century, to the implication of ready excitability and the likelihood of exhaustion, which it bore in the nineteenth, almost to the exclusion of the earlier signification.[56]

When Victorian alienists and nerve-doctors underscored the connections between the advance of civilization and the onslaught of nervous disease, they stressed, not so much the occasions for dissipation in the modern era, as the perpetual hurry that it seemed to demand, the relentless competition for success, and the constant anxiety attendant on both. "Life at high-pressure is the prominent feature of the nineteenth century," Dowse regretted in 1880, "and we cannot be surprised when we find that the so-called nervous diseases and exhaustions . . . are increasing beyond all proportion to the rapid increase of the population." Innumerable voices expressed their agreement, emphasizing, too, that a century of industrial and commercial advance had effected significant changes in what was often called "the spirit of the age." To all appearances, the accumulation of wealth, rather than the pleasurable expenditure of it, had become the paramount social goal, and the damage wrought to the nerves by the struggle to win the economic race became a recurrent lamentation in Victorian and Edwardian medical literature. "For the blind votaries of Mammon," wrote an anonymous reviewer in the *Journal of Psychological Medicine* in 1849, "tranquillity of mind" was impossible and morbid increase of nervous sensitivity assured. "While Mammon thus reigns in every alley, the health of the body is sapped. . . ." Frederick MacCabe, an Irish alienist, explained more soberly that "undue haste to become rich, which is always a characteristic of high states of civilization, begets an amount of anxiety that becomes an important factor in the production of strain."[57] The frantic pace of life devoted to the relentless pursuit and display of affluence, without adequate time for mental repose and physical relaxation, drained nerve force faster than countless men and women could replenish it.

Nor were nervousness and neurasthenia the only means by which the human nervous system registered the buffetings that modernity administered. Grave pathological conditions of the central nervous system, such as hydrocephalus, could likewise be "attributed to modern civilization, which imposes an ever-growing tax upon the brain and its tributaries," as Crichton-Browne, a frequent contributor to this sort of jeremiad, observed in 1884.[58] Most worrisome of all was a presumed connection between the contemporary style of life and the incidence of insanity. Although Georgian medical practitioners had speculated about that connection, it only became a subject of real concern in the subsequent century, when overcrowded lunatic asylums gave plausibility to old fears. All the major Victorian psychiatrists were certain of a cause-and-effect relationship. Bucknill, for one, called madness "the Nemesis of that ill-directed, ill-regulated development that we call civilization," and Maudsley, eschewing oversimplified generalizations about the causes of lunacy, nonetheless ranked the influence of civilization among the most potent. When, in 1857, D. H. Tuke at least bothered to inquire whether civilization favored the generation of mental disease, his answer was predictably affirmative. Although he relied heavily on nothing more substantial than travelers' tales to demonstrate the rarity of madness among such uncivilized peoples as American Indians, East Indians, Arabs, and South Sea Islanders, few professional colleagues or members of the educated public would have questioned the contention that highly developed societies produced far more lunatics than primitive ones.[59]

One of the principal reasons proposed by medical men and social commentators to explain the correlation between civilization and all manner of nervous disability underscored the prominence of urban life in advanced cultures. The confinement of large numbers of people within a limited geographic space struck most Victorians as profoundly unhealthy, a viewpoint inherited from the eighteenth century and fully substantiated by nineteenth-century mortality statistics. Affluent members of society took what measures they could, not only to avoid the miasmal effluvia of refuse heaps and sewers, but also to counteract the effects of "that general indisposition which, from its frequent occurrence from the anxieties and fatigues of professional or commercial life in the great metropolis, may be called Londonism."[60] They regularly withdrew to the countryside, the seaside, and the mountains, or made their permanent homes in safe, suburban communities. The sense of contamination that clung to the city was both physical—for the filth was palpable—and moral. Vice of every variety was assumed to breed in the urban slums, and even among the city's respectable citizens unhealthy states of mind could fester. It was widely believed that suicide intruded more readily in an urban than a rural setting, although statistics, in this instance, did not support contemporary Victorian assumptions.[61]

By drawing attention to the manifold evils of urban life, alienists joined many of their compatriots in fostering a kind of rural nostalgia. This was by no means a uniform motif in nineteenth-century British medical texts. It was equally possible to portray the countryside as abysmally isolated and dull, where sheer boredom and ignorance spawned mental disorders at a faster rate than the frenzied stimuli of city living could achieve. The opposite point of view, however, was more consistent with the major precepts of Victorian psychiatry, and the many medical authorities who worried that nervous debility was an inevitable consequence of urban civilization looked to the countryside to counteract its toxins. When they idealized rural life, with its regular rhythm, physical exercise, and clean air acting as balm to the nerves, they interwove with their medical opinions the strand of romanticism that faulted industrialized society for violating the organic social patterns presumed to have prevailed in the past. Crichton-Browne returned to the country-versus-city theme throughout his writings, always to glorify rural at the expense of urban existence. While still an aspiring neurologist, he phrased the comparison in terms of cerebral physiology, asserting that "in the busy West Riding of Yorkshire, organic diseases of the brain with extreme wasting of the convolutions are of more frequent occurrence than in the purely agricultural county of Somerset. . . ." Once settled in his role as a socially conservative government official, he drew on a different vocabulary to make essentially the same point, arguing that strength, steadiness, and tenacity characterized the rural community, while urban society was "mobile, fickle, of unstable equilibrium," and far more prone to insanity and suicide.[62]

British psychiatrists in the nineteenth and early twentieth centuries, however, had no desire to halt the advance of civilization. Their denigration of city life, and of the industrialization that typified it, had narrow limits that were quickly reached and rarely transgressed. Not only did their profession, after all, like to locate itself among the champions of science, but it had also profited from the modernization of British society. The weakening of traditional patronage systems based on landed wealth, the growth of an extensive middle class able to afford medical services, and the concentration of patients in urban centers—all redounded to psychiatry's long-term benefit.[63] Clearly those who built a flourishing practice as private consultants to the affluent had more at stake than those whose professional lives were spent among pauper lunatics, for men and women who regarded medical attention as a symbol of their own social importance were not likely to welcome a medical denunciation of the very economic system that promised prosperity to patient and doctor alike. The latter, seeking to confirm his own position among the more elevated ranks of bourgeois society, could scarcely reap advantage from criticizing the foundations on which those ranks rested. It was one thing to deplore the harsh, unyielding competition that pitted man against his neighbor, and threatened to shatter the nerves of both; it was quite another to propound a thoroughgoing economic analysis that illuminated the degree to which the prosperity of some depended on the exploitation and suffering of others.

The psychiatric dilemma over the impact of modernization on the health of the British people was by no means irresolvable. One escape route involved the simple denial of modernity's potential harm to human health—or, at least, a refusal to accept the glib assumption that nervous disorders afflicted society more grievously in the nineteenth century than at any previous era in history. By the late Victorian and Edwardian years, in reaction against the fashion for neurasthenia, some authoritative voices cogently supported this refusal.[64] The problem with such an approach, however, was that it left medical men in general, and psychiatrists in particular, highly vulnerable to criticism of their own performance. If the alleged epidemic of nervous and mental maladies plaguing contemporary society did not result from the very nature of modern life itself, it was difficult to present alienists as heroes struggling against tremendous odds rather than incompetents lacking the skill to heal.

Other strategies, accordingly, attracted medical spokesmen who, although sympathetic to the environmental reform movement, nonetheless sought to mediate between criticism and endorsement of prevailing social and economic conditions. One of the most effective devices was to employ evasion instead of confrontation. As has been noted, alienists regularly invoked "the spirit of the age," the pace of contemporary life, the "wear and tear" wrought by modern pressures—all vague phrases that summoned up so vast and amorphous a causative agent that criticism was deflected from specific abuses in the living and working conditions of the masses. Furthermore, by stressing the tension and anxiety that arose from competition and overwork, psychiatrists were able to suggest that middle-class employers and professionals were as much the victims of advanced civilization as were the workers themselves—probably even more so.[65]

Throughout Victoria's reign, psychiatric orthodoxy upheld the view that nervous and mental illness was an individual tragedy, for which neither society nor the medical profession was fundamentally to blame. With contagious diseases, like cholera or typhoid fever, the public dimensions could not, of course, be ignored, but alienists never viewed neurotic ailments in that light. Functional nervous disorders, including neurasthenia, were either inherited or self-induced through harmful habits. In alluding to the role of modernity in provoking nervous disabilities, psychiatric theorists were not altering this basic interpretation. They were merely adding to it another explanatory layer, one which elaborated the specific, contemporary context that furnished the individual with manifold opportunities to deviate from the ways of health. The context was riddled with dangers, some obvious and some subtle, around which doctors had to steer their patients, pointing out the pitfalls and trying to protect them from the worst risks. Beyond that, the patient alone decided whether to stay on the safe path or fall headlong into the morass of sickness.

Just as the debate over neurasthenia sharpened the medical discussion of civilization and its disorders, so did it color the deeper controversy over social class that was implicit in all Victorian texts on the neuroses of modern life. Whether nervousness, in its mild or debilitating aspects, ever troubled the working class was a question on which the British medical profession achieved no unanimity before World War I. To many doctors, it seemed most unlikely that the laboring masses experienced the sort of sensations associated with vulnerability to nervous collapse—"an acuteness of sensibility, a susceptibility of the emotions, an intense activity of the feelings," and a "cultivated condition of the higher sentiments."[66] While no one doubted that the lower echelons of society fell prey to many maladies, nervous delicacy was excluded from the list by those who assumed that poverty meant lack of opportunity to overstimulate the nerves and absence of pressure to excel at one's work. In his *Treatise on Some Nervous Disorders,* published in the 1830s, Edwin Lee, for example, exempted "the barbarian and the labouring man, occupied in his daily routine of mechanical employment," from the "numerous diseases" exacerbated by "a high degree of sensibility."[67] Influential segments of the Victorian middle class never doubted that cloddish brutality, utterly devoid of imagination and intellectual curiosity, defined the lower orders. These were, according to some medical opinion, spared the suffering that people of good quality endured because of their nerves.

In the final decades of the nineteenth century, British medical practitioners who embraced a socially restricted view of nervous collapse found it confirmed by Beard's interpretation of neurasthenia. The incidence of that disorder, Beard argued, occurred almost exclusively among the educated middle and upper classes—the intellectuals, professionals, and businessmen who participated most fully in the stressful tempo and gruelling economic competition of modern urban life. On the other side of the Atlantic, Playfair concurred, dubbing neurasthenia "chiefly a disease of the cultured classes."[68] As with everything else concerning that malady, however, there was no general medical agreement on this point. Doctors who catered to an affluent clientele assumed an elitist attitude, as often from lack of experience as from social snobbery. Doctors who saw working-class patients found evidence of nervous exhaustion among them. By the close of the century, the dominant medical opinion in Great Britain challenged the assumption that only those in the supposed vanguard of civilization experienced shattered nerves.

Well before then, a significant minority of medical practitioners had questioned so superficial a conclusion. As early as 1807, Dr. Thomas Trotter's study of the nervous temperament had encompassed in its broad sweep the manual with the brain worker, and the more thoroughly the medical profession examined the workings of nerve force, the harder it became to exclude the laboring classes from the consequences of its depletion. They, after all, had their exhaustible ration, just like their social betters, and it was impossible to maintain that relentless physical exertion did not drain precious reserves as harmfully as intellectual effort. Indeed, Daniel Noble included "nervous debility" with "stunted growth, osseous deformity, and pulmonary consumption" among "the morbid effects attributed by large numbers to the prevalence of the factory system."[69] Passing easily from denotation to connotation, medical men merged the idea of physical depression or reduction of nervous energy— believed to result from long hours of work without sufficient rest or nourishment— with the concept of mental or emotional depression. In the 1830s, Dr. James Kay, subsequently Sir James Kay-Shuttleworth and a leading spokesman for public health and education, described with real sympathy the artisan who, eking out a miserable existence at home and at work, becomes "debilitated and hypochondriacal." "The strength fails," Kay continued, "all the capacities of physical enjoyment are destroyed, and the paroxysms of corporal suffering are aggravated by the horrors of a disordered imagination, till they lead to gloomy apprehension, to the deepest depression, and almost to despair." Kay saw such wretchedness ending in the gin shop, but magistrates, policemen, and good samaritans throughout the century also found it leading to suicide, among the urban and rural poor alike.[70]

Other doctors, too, sketched the transition from physical to emotional prostration in working-class lives. Contributors to the *West Riding Lunatic Asylum Medical Reports,* who studied asylum patients in the midst of a highly industrialized region, were particularly aware of this pathological sequence. Fothergill pointed to "a large class" of nervous maladies "very commonly met with amidst the sane," which he traced to imperfect nutrition. Headache and neuralgia were common signs, he explained, that excessive demands were being made upon the nervous system, but so, too, was "psychical pain, . . . the sense of misery, of depression, of low spirits." Fothergill, in fact, perceived such complaints as evidence of an exhausted condition far *less* prevalent among the prosperous classes, who enjoyed better food and more physical relaxation, than among the laboring poor. Charles Henry Mayhew, another writer in the *Medical Reports,* could likewise cite cases of severely undernourished workers who became "intensely dejected" and perpetually depressed.[71] At the same time, changing attitudes toward the notion of sensibility, once the presumed monopoly of the refined and educated classes, suggested that it was no longer a mark of superiority, but rather a personal liability.[72] Under the circumstances, the attribution of nervous vulnerability to working-class men and women won easier acceptance from medical spokesmen, for it was less likely to offend their middle- and upper-class patients.

Thus by the time that neurasthenia became the fashionable way to designate a wide range of indefinite neurotic ailments, the majority of British medical men were generally less receptive to Beard's ideas than they would have been a few decades earlier. Playfair's was not the preponderant point of view. More of his professional colleagues accepted the opposite opinion, that "conditions of nervous exhaustion" were "common amongst all classes of society"[73] and that neurasthenia acknowledged neither social nor geographic barriers. "It is not confined to any class or any district," Guthrie floridly proclaimed. "It may be met with in the castle and in the cottage, in the highlands or in city slums." Savill provided specific examples of working-class neurasthenics in his *Clinical Lectures:* a policeman whose "condition of nervousness and inaptitude for work" Savill called "pitiable"; a male cook "subject to attacks of complete helplessness and prostration," and an engine-fitter who likewise suffered from "sensations of bodily illness, depression, helplessness, and weariness," which the author sympathetically recognized as "some of the most miserable feelings that can curse humanity."[74]

In his insistent acknowledgment of neurasthenia's inroads among British workers, Savill not only registered the reality of national mental health problems, but reflected the influence of the great French psychiatrist Jean-Martin Charcot, who was widely quoted across the Channel in the late Victorian and Edwardian period. As was obvious from his preface to a volume by Dr. Fernand Levillain—*La Neurasthénie, Maladie de Beard,* published in Paris in 1891—Charcot disagreed with essential aspects of Beard's interpretation, for the Frenchman was convinced that neurasthenics were not found solely among the "upper classes, enervated by over-civilization, but are to be counted on a large scale amongst the work-a-day classes." As late as 1910, Albutt still quoted Charcot to support his contention that "the neurasthenic neurosis does not belong exclusively to the men of the privileged classes, softened by culture, worn out by abuse of pleasure, of business, or of intellectual toil." In the United States, too, following Beard's death in 1883, "new ideas coming from Europe" played a significant role in extending the neurasthenic diagnosis downward on the social scale.[75]

If they could have understood the vocabulary, many late nineteenth-century British medical men—psychiatric specialists as well as general practitioners—would have endorsed the conclusion, reached by researchers in the 1980s, that "clinically significant depression occurs at about the same rate in blue- and-white collar workers, whites and blacks, the poor and the rich, college graduates and high school dropouts."[76] The Victorian and Edwardian medical profession was neither indifferent nor insensitive to the manifestations of serious depression in humble men and women. Yet the perspective of class background and bias always intervened between middle-class doctors and working-class patients, inevitably casting a very different light on the suffering of the affluent and of the impoverished.

Numerous constraints molded medical attitudes toward working-class neuroses. Many physicians theorized about the nerves of the poor, as has been noted, without ever encountering a patient crushed by poverty. (Allbutt contemptuously dismissed the belief that neurasthenia afflicted brain-workers alone as "the prepossession of consultants occupied with the middle and upper classes of society."[77]) Furthermore, even those medical practitioners who devoted a significant portion of their time to hospital wards, clinics, and infirmaries often struggled fully to comprehend the nature of existence for a vast segment of the British population. Little in their upbringing, education, professional training, and adult social intercourse prepared them to deal with the emotional troubles of patients engaged in a constant fight to avoid starvation. Medical writers willingly acknowledged the strain and hardship of these lives and expressed concern over the devastating combination of poverty and physical fatigue, but many aspects of the working-class lifestyle appalled them. With their concern heavily diluted by horror and disgust, they could scarcely help viewing men and women from the lower classes as people apart.

Medical recognition that the symptoms of nervous prostration in working-class patients were identical to those in socially superior victims was, acccordingly, balanced by the belief that different causes were at work in the two instances. Victorian and Edwardian doctors rarely looked beyond bodily exhaustion to explain the former, while underscoring the moral agents, such as grief, disappointment, anxiety, and all the other variants of mental strain, responsible for draining the nerve force of the elite. The convenient distinction between physical and mental factors long predated the appearance of neurasthenia on the British scene. In the 1830s, J. C. Prichard had incorporated it into his lengthy discussion of hypochondriasis, whose symptoms were, by then, largely indistinguishable from those of nervous collapse. Hypochondriasis, Prichard conceded, was "not in reality confined to the better classes of society, or to persons of cultivated minds, on whom moral causes may be supposed to act with the most extensive influence." He had seen "instances of hypochondriasis . . . among persons of the lower classes," but, he assured his readers, "the causes which actually gave rise to morbid phenomena in their constitutions could scarcely belong to the class of moral agents: they were circumstances which induced disorder in the physical or natural functions."[78] By the end of the nineteenth century, the contrast between moral and physical causes was implicit in most medical attempts to illuminate the ravages of nervous breakdown at diverse levels of society.

The influence of class also asserted itself at the critical moment when a psychiatric diagnosis needed to be made—when the patient's mental state had to be categorized as sane or insane. Since the severest symptoms of nervous breakdown so closely resembled some milder forms of madness, social considerations often played a determining role in the medical choice. With patients from the middle and upper classes, for whom the diagnosis of insanity could gravely affect professional status and the control of property, alienists were generally slower to identify lunacy than in working-class cases, where no such considerations were seen to apply. There were, of course, instances when family members had their own reasons for seeking to render a relative legally impotent, and suicidal tendencies often sufficed to commit even wealthy men and women to asylum care, albeit of a discreet private variety.[79] Where family self-interest was not at stake and suicide posed no threat, however, the emotionally disturbed patient with means could receive treatment at home, or among friends, while the indigent patient with similar problems had no recourse but the public asylum.

A striking case in point centers on the breakdown of Virginia Stephen (later Woolf) in 1904, following her father's death. There is no unanimity of opinion concerning her actual condition during that painful period; her symptoms included anorexia, a suicide attempt, and bizarre hallucinations. The assertion by her nephew, Quentin Bell, that "all that summer she was mad" has provoked charges of an uncritical and irresponsible use of medical vocabulary. Elaine Showalter has cited Stephen's treatment by George Savage as evidence of the tyranny that Edwardian psychiatrists exercised over women—and Stephen did, indeed, dub her doctor "tyrannical" and "shortsighted."[80] What matters here, however, is not that Savage's program for Stephen consigned her to months of boredom in exile from London, but that he treated her as a neurasthenic who needed tranquillity, rest, sleep, and nourishment, not as a lunatic. Her official diagnosis was loss of nerve force, not loss of reason. She was attended by her close friend Violet Dickinson, by her sister Vanessa, and, at the end of her recuperative period, by an aunt in Cambridge. Private nurses were available during the worst of the crisis. With comparably serious symptoms, but without the social position, domestic arrangements, and economic resources of the Stephen family, a working-class patient would have been quickly admitted to a public asylum. Many were, for less serious symptoms.

Nor are medical inconsistencies and shifting diagnostic criteria the only obstacles confronting the historian today who tries to understand nervous breakdown among Victorians and Edwardians of the working class. The meaning that these men and women themselves assigned to depressive illness is far from evident. The problem is only partly one of source materials. Hundreds of working-class autobiographies, both published and unpublished, have survived from the nineteenth and early twentieth centuries, and although the total is nothing like the mass of autobiographical material from the middle and upper classes in the same period, it is enough to provide a reasonably clear idea of working-class health concerns. The difficulty is that the most severely depressed workers, the ones most prostrated with despair, were least likely to take pen in hand—if they could write at all. If one knows life only as a vale of tears in which individual effort is futile, it hardly seems worth noting down the facts of one's misery. Middle-class autobiographers who suffered nervous breakdown some-times chronicled their state of mind in considerable detail because they felt their cases would command general interest, but the sense of self-importance necessary to prompt such revelations was hardly characteristic of workers who had given up hope. Their stories are occasionally told in the reports of public health officials,[81] but, for most, we lack the words they would themselves have used to describe their suffering.

Other working-class men and women, for whom self-help, self-discipline, and personal initiative meant as much as any middle-class sermonizer could have desired, did compose autobiographies that attest to their own sense of self-worth and achievement against staggering odds that often included deep depression. Yet even their voices are somewhat muffled, for they frequently portrayed the experience of nervous breakdown by means of literary conventions adapted from middle-class models, such as the religious conversion literature of earlier centuries. Dramatic breakdowns, as opposed to merely chronic depression, could serve as the focal point of tension in the tale, the experience crucial to turning the narrator's life from sin to faith. Autobiographies in this vein were written for other workers, as exhortation and encouragement.[82] Where working-class autobiographers had a socially more ele-vated audience in mind, the vocabulary they chose to employ in discussing their illness might not necessarily reflect their own reactions, but rather a set of assump-tions about their readers' expectations. Thus Ben Tillett, the late Victorian and Edwardian trade union organizer, spoke of his "state of nervous prostration" that lasted "for many months" after August 1896, when he was briefly incarcerated in a disgustingly dirty Belgian jail for leading a union demonstration in Antwerp. In his autobiography, published in 1931, when he was a venerable Labour politician with years of parliamentary service behind him, he remembered that during his "break-down of health," he "lingered between life and death for many days." For years Tillett had endured virtually constant health problems, in which physical disorders, like asthma and eczema, mixed with overwhelming emotional distress to incapacitate him repeatedly. In the autobiography, his depiction of suffering stressed nervous debility in terms any member of Parliament would have understood.[83]

None of this is to suggest that middle-class autobiographers did not also have their own motives for drawing on the language of shattered nerves when they depicted the saga of their lives. The invocation of symptoms and diagnostic labels pertaining to the nerves was always a complex act in Victorian and Edwardian culture—even as it is today. Patients grasped the social significance of medical phrases as readily as did their doctors, and were quick to borrow them. For a time, no medical term enjoyed greater currency than neurasthenia, but its glory days were comparatively brief. By the end of World War I, it was no longer the preeminent diagnosis for victims of nervous breakdown. While the word continued to appear occasionally in the 1930s, it was already becoming a medical antique in the preceding decade; its uncompromisingly somatic etiology marked its obsolescence at a time when *neurotic* had, at length, come to designate a mental or emotional, rather than a physical, disturbance. Physicians no longer needed nerve force, on which neurasthenia was predicated, in order to explain depression. For the same reasons, but at a slower pace, "nervous breakdown" has passed from medical parlance.

In many respects, the late Victorian champions of neurasthenia as a distinct pathological entity laid the foundations for its demise themselves. Their claims for it were too vast; the novelty and convenience of the label prompted them to apply it too sweepingly, so that it covered everything from extreme fatigue to temporary insanity. Already in 1894, Savage had joked to his audience at the annual meeting of the British Medical Association: "I am inclined to think that if I gave, in brief only, the many symptoms which are attributed to neurasthenia . . . there are very few of my audience who would not be inclined to believe that they have got it themselves." With such disparate symptoms ascribed to neurasthenia, it became increasingly impossible to maintain its existence as a single, identifiable malady. "To make neurasthenia everything is indeed to make it nothing," Allbutt warned in 1910, and, in effect, this is what happened.[84] The bestowal of a fancy name on the manifestations of depression, furthermore, raised expectations that could not be fulfilled. The manifold signs of illness were no more uniformly amenable to explanation or improvement than they had been before neurasthenia joined the international medical lexicon. After the initial excitement over Beard's "discovery" dissipated, the limits of its usefulness were gradually recognized, and doctors and patients were obliged to acknowledge that assigning new labels is not equivalent to devising new cures.

4

Nerve Tonics and Treatments

When alienists and nerve specialists set themselves to cure patients incapacitated by nervous breakdown, the treatments they designed reflected their awareness that mind and body needed to be healed together. Although there existed no single prescription for the care of shattered nerves, virtually all of the therapeutic methods employed during the Victorian and Edwardian decades sought to address both somatic and psychological distress, restoring the depleted supplies of nerve force that precipitated the collapse and calming whatever form of mental strain exacerbated it. Physical intervention and moral guidance were linked in a seemingly infinite variety of combinations, as doctors worked to return each patient to the medical ideal of healthy adulthood, with the will firmly in control of all mental processes.

Throughout Victoria's reign, most medical men relied on drugs during some stage of a nervous patient's treatment. Although typically administered in conjunction with other forms of therapy, like bed rest or residence at the seaside, drugs were the mainstay of the medical attendant's curative arsenal—at least, he liked to think they were curative. Their widespread employment reflected the dominant physiological interpretation of nervous illness, for their impact was understood to work on the physical substance of the body. During the first half of the nineteenth century, doctors routinely prescribed massive drug dosages, an aspect of the "heroic" practice of medicine that also featured the wholesale bleeding and purging of patients to relieve bodily disorders. It was the golden age, too, of patent medicines and "specifics" that claimed to remedy particular diseases, or certain individual symptoms of them. Quack medicines abounded in an era that lacked legislation to control the sale of drugs. Even after the passage of regulatory laws, such as the Arsenic Act of 1851 and the Pharmacy Act of 1868, doctors had no trouble prescribing large quantities of highly dangerous substances, including mercury, strychnine, lead, antimony, and morphine. Much of the Victorian fascination with drugs arose from the striking expansion of the available pharmacopoeia. In the early years of the century, the discoveries of the alkaloids added morphine, strychnine, quinine, codeine, and atropine, among other vegetable extracts, to the pharmacist's stock, while by the Edwardian period the production of synthetic compounds, including aspirin, veronal, and sulphonal, signaled the birth of the modern pharmaceutical industry.[1]

At the start of the nineteenth century, the dispensing of drugs was a far cry from the big business enterprise that it later became. A pharmacist had to know the diverse processes necessary for preparing infusions, decoctions, tinctures, and extracts, all of which Francis Galton learned while a medical student at the Birmingham General

Hospital in 1838. He found the task of making pills "amusing at first," but the complicated steps involved raise questions about the accuracy of dosage achieved. With medical authorities in London, Edinburgh, and Dublin all issuing their own pharmacopoeias, furthermore, no official standards of pharmaceutical measure or medical formulas existed in the United Kingdom until the appearance of a single authority, the *British Pharmacopoeia,* in 1864. By the eve of World War I, patients could receive their medicine in the accurate form of compressed tablets or gelatine capsules, but a century earlier apothecaries typically had to follow elaborate instructions that drew on a range of supplies in their shops. A prescription for "General Debility of the Nervous System, attended with Costiveness, Flatulence, great Dejection of Spirits, &c.," which the *Monthly Gazette of Health* published in 1816, called for sulphate of zinc, extract of gentian, and extract of bitter apple compound, in varying amounts, to be mixed together and divided into twenty pills. Another recipe, suggested by the same journal for the same malady, required compound spirit of ammonia, compound spirit of lavender, tincture of castor, and camphorated julep. The prescription that Charles Dickens wrote for Bob Sawyer, the aspiring young medical man in *The Pickwick Papers,* to give a highly agitated old lady was an apt reflection of practice in the late Georgian years. " 'Nervous,' said Bob Sawyer complacently. 'Camphor-julep and water three times a-day.' "[2] The eminent consulting physicians of London would not, of course, have advocated such homely remedies, but they were typical of the concoctions produced in vast quantities by apothecary-surgeons and general practitioners for all manner of nervous distempers.

At a loftier professional level, and particularly as new, potent drugs were isolated, Victorian medical men plied their patients with nerve tonics containing more than lavender and bitter apples. Their confidence in the beneficent impact of tonics reflected the legacy of eighteenth-century tension pathology, which attributed illness to the inadequate or excessive tone of bodily organs. If lacking the proper degree of firmness, or tone, the organ in question could not perform its natural functions; on the other hand, too much firmness produced tension that was equally inhibiting. The application of nerve tonics also conformed to the prevalent nineteenth-century medical orthodoxy, known as allopathy, which argued that the most effective way to treat a disease was to produce the somatic condition opposite to the pathological state in question. To combat fever, for example, allopathic medicine insisted that it was necessary to cool the patient's body. Where nervous debility was involved, strengtheners or tonics were required to restore firmness to the patient's collapsed nerves and to stimulate the production of nerve force. Throughout the entire Victorian period, most doctors concurred in designating iron, quinine, and strychnine the most effective of all nerve tonics.

Iron had figured among the mineral components of drugs at least since ancient Chinese medical practice, and its widespread use in British medicine dated from the seventeenth century.[3] It was recognized as an invaluable aid in diseases that required fortifying the blood and, by extension, in other forms of weakness as well. Indeed, since much of what passed for nervous exhaustion, particularly in listless, pale adolescent girls and young women, was the manifestation of anemia, iron was precisely the necessary medicament. Crichton-Browne made that connection in his earliest published paper. Noting that "melancholia of a religious cast" was "not unfrequently observed in girls about the age of puberty," he proceeded to explain that "melancholia is generally dependent upon anaemia, or an impoverished condition of the blood, or an imperfect supply of nutrition, and is hence to be treated by generous diet, stimulants, attention to hygiene and iron."[4] Although he later adopted a less restricted view of melancholia's causes, he always ranked iron among the medical man's most valuable aids in the battle against nervous exhaustion, and countless professional colleagues supported him in the conviction. Of course, in cases where depression had no specific physiological foundation, iron was hardly efficacious by itself, except insofar as it improved general bodily health. If, however, patients were cheered by the simple act of taking medicine whose potency they acknowledged—the so-called placebo effect—iron was as good an ingredient as any, and a lot less harmful than most.

Quinine and strychnine were new additions to the Victorian catalogue of drugs believed to counteract nervous weakness, although cinchona, from which quinine is derived, had been known to British medicine since the seventeenth century, often under the name of "Peruvian bark." Quinine quickly became popular among Victorian medical men. In neurotic illnesses, it was credited both with decreasing "the excitability of the nervous system" and with strengthening "the whole system by invigorating the general nerve power."[5] While medical practitioners conceded that strychnine was dangerous to employ, many nonetheless applauded its impact in bracing the nerves. In the 1830s, Marshall Hall was one of the first to apply it, in small doses, "as a spinal tonic," and the practice soon caught on for diverse conditions of nervous debility. Schofield pronounced strychnine "the stand-by as a nerve tonic," prescribing it two or three times a day in cases of depression. Thomas Henry Huxley periodically took strychnine and quinine, whenever he was anxious about his health or suffering from the melancholy that plagued him all his adult life. Whatever the reason for debility or depression, Victorian and Edwardian medical men placed almost unbounded faith in the revitalizing properties of nerve tonics. They were, Allbutt observed in 1895, "sold behind every counter."[6]

Arsenic, too, was readily available to restore vigor to shattered nerves. Although the Arsenic Act restricted its sale after 1851, no medical qualms limited its use as a nerve tonic for decades thereafter. As the principal ingredient of Fowler's Solution, arsenic had become familiar to medical practitioners by the start of the nineteenth century and was added to the London *Pharmacopoeia* in 1809. Recommending it for "the curative treatment of nervous exhaustion" in 1880, Dowse reported that he had sometimes "gradually increased the dose of Fowler's solution of arsenic to ten drops, three or four times a day, and the same with the solution of strychnine, before the patients have found themselves actually benefited." Some medical authorities contended that the generally tonic properties of arsenic made it valuable, too, in the treatment of hysteria and melancholy. Charles Darwin's chronic ill health, which continues successfully to elude attempts at definitive diagnosis, has been blamed on long-term arsenic intoxication, but the evidence shows only that, as a young man, he took small doses of the drug for eczema during a three-year period. There is no reference to arsenic in his correspondence or medical records thereafter, perhaps because he had been warned by his father of its toxicity.[7]

Toxicity was equally threatening in the case of mercury, and the dangers of that substance received more attention in nineteenth-century British medical literature than those of arsenic or strychnine. Nonetheless, mercury, too, had its advocates where nervous maladies were concerned, and, in the form of calomel (mercurous chloride) or the omnipresent "blue pill," it was a staple item in the care of young and old alike. (The fact that calomel was a powerful purgative did not disqualify it for widespread use with ailing children.) Mercury had a venerable history in pharmacology and, since the early sixteenth century, its use in treating syphilis had promoted the drug's fame. In the eighteenth century, it was also widely employed against fevers— administered in enormous doses until the patient salivated. It was precisely this salivation that prompted Benjamin Rush, the internationally famous American physician, to recommend mercury for hypochondriasis in his treatise on diseases of the mind, published in 1812 and often cited in subsequent British psychiatric texts. "Mercury acts in this disease," he commented, both "by abstracting morbid excitement from the brain to the mouth," and "by changing the cause of our patient's complaints, . . . fixing them wholly upon his sore mouth." "It stimulates every part of the body," he concluded, "renders the vessels pervious to their natural juices, conveys morbid action out of the body by the mouth, and thus restores the mind to its native seat in the brain."[8]

For a variety of reasons, Victorian and Edwardian doctors found mercury helpful in their efforts to combat mental and nervous illness. Sir Henry Holland, who endorsed Rush's claim that mercury afforded quick relief for hypochondriasis, assured his readers that, with proper administration, the benefits of the drug far surpassed any risks to the patient. Peter Mere Latham, an eminent London physician with profound confidence in the medical value of mercury, pronounced it effective against chronic inflammation and, accordingly, advised its employment for "numerous mental affections," as well as for disorders of sensation and movement, whenever these were presumed to stem from an inflammatory origin. Clouston went so far as to argue that a good dose of calomel could ward off insanity. It is curious that Thomas Carlyle, whose experiences with medication made him detest most drugs, never protested against mercury. "The only medicine he believed in," according to his friend William Allingham, "was blue-pill."[9]

Opiates, which particularly aroused Carlyle's wrath, were the most ubiquitous drugs in Victorian society, both as the medical practitioner's alleged panacea and as the most popular form of self-medication. Whether as opium, morphine, laudanum, codeine, or in prepared mixtures like Daffy's Elixir, Godfrey's Cordial, and Dover's Powder, the powerful narcotic could be had for the asking. Opium "has the wonderful properties of mitigating pain, inducing sleep, allaying inordinate action, and diminishing morbid irritability," enthused Reece's *Medical Guide* in 1817. It could quiet screaming infants and soothe jarred nerves, a boon to mother and child alike; not surprisingly, Godfrey's Cordial was the leading children's drug throughout the nineteenth century.[10] Until the 1860s, there seems to have been little anxiety about drug addiction as a social problem, but thereafter medical opinion was increasingly alarmed by its incidence at all levels of British society. The drug habit was not only rampant among the poor, who could readily and cheaply purchase laudanum and patent medicines containing opium at a variety of shops; addiction was also spreading insidiously among the affluent, even among royalty. The subcutaneous injection of morphine by hypodermic syringe, which became the common method for taking the opium alkaloid in the 1860s, made it possible to absorb much greater amounts than heretofore, and when injected, rather than taken orally, "a higher proportion of the drug reached the central nervous system."[11] The cost of morphine and syringes, as well as the need to visit a doctor for the initial prescription, meant that this form of the opium habit ravaged a higher level of society than laudanum reached.

Nor were leisured ladies languishing in boredom and feeling poorly the only ones who found life pleasanter on morphine. Middle-class professionals, businessmen, and intellectuals all figured significantly among the ranks of its addicts. Medical men, in fact, saw their own colleagues overusing morphine, not only to alleviate physical discomfort, such as neuralgia, but to fight off the melancholy that often accompanied the burdens of their work. In 1900, Dr. Martin Grant-Smith, for one, died of an overdose of morphine after suffering from prolonged depression. Cases like his, and the general social milieu in which late Victorian and Edwardian doctors watched morphine addiction taking its toll, prompted them to portray the advent of morphinism as yet another disease of modern civilization afflicting those who experienced life's pressures most acutely. A new Pharmacy and Poisons Act in 1908 placed some restrictions on the sale of opium and morphine, but meaningful controls were not enforced until after World War I. Until then, patients retained their prescriptions and could have them refilled as often as they pleased.[12]

Despite growing medical suspicion that opium addiction was a condition more devastating than most of the disorders the drug was supposed to relieve, doctors continued freely to prescribe the various opiates through the Edwardian decade. The versatility of the drugs made them simply too valuable to discard. For nervous disorders alone, their uses were manifold. Opium was, of course, a widely recognized narcotic, as generously and irresponsibly prescribed to calm agitated nerves as tranquillizers are today. Margaret Oliphant gratefully received such medication when she learned, in 1859, that her husband's illness was incurable consumption. "Whether I took myself, or the doctor gave me, a dose of laudanum, I don't remember; but I recollect very well the sudden floating into ease of body and the dazed condition of mind,—a kind of exaltation, as if I were walking upon air, for I could not sleep in the circumstances nor try to sleep." Opiates, however, were also believed to act as stimulants. Gladstone took laudanum in his coffee before orating in the House of Commons, and much medical opinion supported his assumption that the drug was a "pick-me-up."[13] James Simpson prescribed "strong doses of opium" for Tulloch in 1863, when depression had cast him into "a state of darkness" for "nearly five weeks." E. Mazière Courtenay, an assistant medical officer at the Derby County Asylum who had worked with Crichton-Browne at Wakefield, reported that it was specifically opium's action as a stimulant that made it "so useful and so beneficial in melancholia." "What," he asked, "can be more appropriate in this condition of anaemia and exhausted nerve power than a drug producing increased action both of the [blood] vessels and nerves? . . ." He reminded his audience, furthermore, that opium worked first as a stimulant, and then, as it became fully absorbed into the body, as a narcotic and sedative. The twofold impact of opium, Dowse concurred, made it "the chief" of all the drugs used in "the curative treatment of nervous exhaustion":

"it excites and stimulates for a short time the brain-cells, and then leaves them in a state of tranquillity, which is best adapted to their nutrition and repair."[14] Thus medical men could prescribe opiates in cases of nervous collapse in order to rouse the nerves to action, to quell restless fidgets, and, finally, to conquer the insomnia that often proved the most intractable feature of nervous prostration. Many patients likewise became convinced that opiates were capable of such wide-ranging action. It is no wonder that, despite the appearance of newer sedatives in the late nineteenth century, opiates continued to find a place, not only in the doctor's medicine bag, but in the home medicine chest as well.

Tonics, opiates, arsenic, and mercury were by no means the only pharmaceutical resources with which Victorian and Edwardian medical men experimented when confronting nervous breakdown. In the latter half of the nineteenth century and the opening years of the twentieth, their options expanded to include sulphonal, chloral hydrate, barbiturates, the bromides—of potassium and ammonia, in particular—and much else that boasted either stimulant or narcotic effects. Each drug had its supporters and detractors, who praised its efficacy to the skies or denounced it as a deadly poison. Even quinine failed to win universal approbation as a nerve tonic, while the obviously dangerous medicines provoked sustained controversy in the medical press. Articulate medical spokesmen throughout the nineteenth century warned of the hazards associated with specific medications, and even with pharmaceutical therapy in general. As massive drugging failed to promote the anticipated recoveries, it became increasingly evident that highly toxic substances lurked not only in contaminated and adulterated foods, or in the materials of certain occupations, like house-painting; the very medicaments that doctors bestowed on nervous patients in enormous quantities threatened "the ultimate destruction of nervous function" itself.[15]

By the final quarter of the nineteenth century, as more British doctors embraced a "therapeutic nihilism" than placed confidence in the curative potency of drugs, skepticism about the efficacy of pharmaceutical remedies in combating nervous exhaustion became an acceptable medical attitude. If the skeptics continued to administer sedatives and tonics to nerve patients, they did so because they had found no more successful means of treatment. To some practitioners, however, the evidence was all too persuasive that drugs exacerbated nervous conditions, turning temporary discomforts into chronic maladies. In certain instances, they argued, an extremely dangerous substance might actually provoke neurotic disorders where none had existed. In 1885, J. Strahan, a doctor from Belfast, lectured the British Medical Association on "the nerve-prostration due to many such drugs." For his part, Playfair was convinced that addiction to chloral or morphine was the sole cause of functional neurosis in many cases, while H. Bryan Donkin, a doctor with broad interests in mental pathology and nervous illness, considered mercury poisoning a precipitant of hysteria.[16] Clearly, a segment of British medical opinion was ready to argue that, if the era had witnessed a rise in the incidence of nervous disorders, the reason lay, not simply with the frantic pace of modern life, but with the augmented armory of drugs at a doctor's disposal.

Although drugs could bring sleep to an agitated or tormented mind, they could not, as many late Victorian medical men came to realize, address the deeper disturbances that deprived a patient of hope. Charlotte Brontë had told them as much at mid-century. The conditions of her life at the Haworth parsonage, the deaths of her siblings, her understandable obsession with illness, and her loneliness all made the novelist authoritatively familiar with the state of mind she evoked so powerfully in *Villette* (1853). When partially recovered from "a strange fever of the nerves," the novel's heroine is asked by a doctor to describe her symptoms. In the discussion that followed, Brontë used the term "Hypochondria" to signify profound, incapacitating depression:

> "Your nervous system bore a good share of the suffering?"
>
> "I am not quite sure what my nervous system is, but I was dreadfully low-spirited."
>
> "Which disables me from helping you by pill or potion. Medicine can give nobody good spirits. My art halts at the threshold of Hypochondria: she just looks in and sees a chamber of torture, but can neither say nor do much."[17]

It was a confession, needless to say, that came more easily to fictitious than to practicing medical men. While some of the latter in the late Victorian and Edwardian period made no secret of their disenchantment with pills and potions, they continued to hope that other forms of therapy would rescue their patients from depression's chamber of torture.

Endorsing an approach to treatment that still focused on the body's physiological processes, many medical authorities emphasized the therapeutic role of hygiene. To base the pursuit of health on a systematic regimen of diet, rest, exercise, and cleanliness is, of course, a valuable strategy to employ against a variety of disorders, but it made particular sense in the case of nervous illness. Where the causes of distress were often elusive, the therapeutic campaign needed to be all the broader, encompassing virtually every aspect of the patient's life.

Diet was especially significant because medical wisdom claimed that nervous exhaustion was frequently aggravated, if not occasioned, by a delicate stomach or painful indigestion hindering the transmission of nutriments to weakened nerves. Thus Sir Andrew Clark paid very close attention to dietary prescriptions for his nervous patients, and professional colleagues generally shared his confident belief that the stomach offered an important access route to the nerves. Agreeing on that much, however, Victorian and Edwardian medical practitioners concurred on little else concerning the best food for a victim of shattered nerves. During these decades, they recommended a great variety of diets, with few elements in common besides a warning against spicy and highly seasoned fare. One opinion advised total abstinence from tea, coffee, wine, and spirits; another found all four beneficial in moderate amounts. One school of thought rejected red meat as too rich for a faulty digestive system; another pronounced it essential for regaining strength. Still others urged a diet heavy in fats, or protein, or fruit, vegetables, and bread. While vigorously upholding the merits of their preferred system, doctors acknowledged that no general dietary rule was applicable to all nervous patients, whose ailments exhibited strikingly individual traits and whose constitutions, before illness struck, differed as widely. Medical men might claim to base their advice on scientific principles, invoking the laws of chemistry and biology to persuade one patient that farinaceous food was essential and another that animal fat was out of the question, but, with diet as with drugs, they experimented as they went along. The era of ''scientific dietetics'' was hovering on the horizon, but it hardly influenced medical advice to nerve patients before World War I. Pondering the diverse effects that the same food produced on different patients, Dowse conceded in 1884 that ''our knowledge, vast as it may be, and increasing as it undoubtedly is, leaves us in chaos, when upon minute chemical analysis we endeavour to explain the laws of life, of health, of disease, and of death.''[18]

Diet was a uniquely urgent matter in the numerous cases where refusal to eat accompanied nervous breakdown. Sir William Gull, in his pioneering efforts to identify and treat anorexia nervosa, doubted the wisdom of prescribing potent drugs for maladies that were scarcely understood; while he administered tonics to some of the emaciated young women whose families consulted him, he preferred to concentrate on feeding and nursing the patient. In extreme cases of anorexia, he advised some nourishment every two hours, selecting foods that offered fat and protein, like milk, cream, soup, eggs, fish, and chicken. Sometimes simply persuading the patient to eat represented a major aspect of treatment, as Leonard Woolf recalled about his wife's recurrent illnesses:

> . . . one of the most troublesome symptoms of her breakdowns was a refusal to eat. In the worst period of the depressive stage, for weeks almost at every meal one had to sit, often for an hour or more, trying to induce her to eat a few mouthfuls. What made one despair was that by not eating and weakening herself she was doing precisely the thing calculated to prolong the breakdown, for it was only by building up her bodily strength and by resting that she could regain mental equilibrium.[19]

Leonard Woolf's was the conventional medical wisdom that found expression again and again wherever undernourishment endangered recovery from nervous breakdown. In the famous ''rest cure'' devised by Silas Weir Mitchell, it is fair to say that fattening the patient was the paramount goal of therapy.

Young women were not the only patients with eating disorders. Tulloch's inability to take food during his breakdown of 1881 proved, it seems, a transient problem that disappeared with his gradual return to health, but Charles Booth, the shipowner and social investigator, remained indifferent to food long after his serious depression of 1873–74. His family attributed his broken health to ''multifarious activities,'' both for his business ventures and for the philanthropic causes he championed, which left him little time to eat or sleep. A ''distressing form of nervous indigestion'' set in, according to his wife, and he found the least discomfort in abstaining from food altogether. Even in the late 1870s, when he had recovered from the acute stage of depression, Beatrice Potter, a cousin by marriage, was struck by his odd behavior at table. ''One quaint sight stays in my mind,'' she recollected many years later as Beatrice Webb: ''Cousin Charlie sitting through the family meals, 'like patience on a monument smiling at'—other people eating, whilst, as a concession to good manners, he occasionally picked at a potato with his fork or nibbled a dry biscuit.''[20]

With patients like these, nerve specialists and consulting psychiatrists were fully justified in stressing the suggestive links between depression and eating disorders—an association that continues to engage psychiatric attention today. A further aspect of the Victorian determination to connect the digestive and nervous systems made itself obvious in medical anxiety over constipation in cases of nervous exhaustion. Certain that the accumulation of body wastes could hinder the necessary restorative processes, doctors fussed about their patients' bowel movements, freely prescribing laxatives and enemas when required. They believed that they were conscientiously fulfilling their duties as medical attendants when they concentrated on feeding and removing wastes from depressed and debilitated patients, but the invalids themselves rarely saw nourishment and evacuation as their most besetting problems. So long as the medical profession interpreted its responsibility to anorectic patients largely in terms of digestive processes, doctors failed to help disclose and address the reasons why these men and women had to reject food.

The necessity for adequate evacuation, a cardinal principle of Victorian hygiene, mandated all manner of aperients, emetics, diuretics, and various forms of bleeding in the first half of the nineteenth century. Medical opinion at the start of Victoria's reign still subscribed heavily to the theory that most forms of illness could be traced either to general or to local inflammation, alleviation of which was the doctor's first task. Purging, blistering, and bleeding by lancet, leeches, or cupping-glass were all appropriate remedies, and if patients survived the therapy, they were typically kept on a weak liquid diet to prevent recurrence of the inflammation. These were, clearly, depressant forms of treatment, designed to lower body functions; where the malady to be cured already presented depressed characteristics—as in melancholic derangements—one would assume that medical men avoided evacuative measures. Yet the situation was more complicated than logic would suggest. Various affections of the brain and spinal cord were presumed to arise from inflammation: spinal irritation, for example, as well as the affliction known to Victorians as "brain fever," which is now recognized as meningitis. Interpreting the high temperature, painful headache, and delirium of "brain fever" as manifestations of cerebral congestion, doctors were sure that relief could only come by drawing pressure away from the congested area, and thus they speedily applied the standard anti-inflammatory measures. Even milder headaches were assumed to benefit from the application of leeches to the temples or from some well-timed venesection. It is not surprising that Victorian suicides included the tragic stories of men and women whose profound depression or incipient madness was rendered particularly intolerable by disturbing sensations in the head and who sought escape from their suffering by medically endorsed means—the copious flow of blood from a cut throat or a bullet hole in the brain. In the heyday of medical bloodletting, some asylum doctors considered bleeding and purging perfectly legitimate methods of treating insanity.[21]

Even before reliance on depletive medicine declined dramatically in the second half of the nineteenth century, however, a significant body of respected medical opinion had denounced the use of such measures to treat nervous depression. Already in the 1820s, the *Family Oracle of Health* warned its readers that they erred in attributing a sense of heavy lifelessness to "too much blood weighing down their spirits." Bloodletting, the journal insisted, could only aggravate melancholy. Herbert Mayo illustrated the same point in his popular treatise on hygiene, *The*

Philosophy of Living, published in 1837. Describing a female patient, he remarked that "at the age of thirty-five, she gradually fell into depression of spirits, and terrors of she knew not what. . . . When these impressions were not upon her, she was a high-spirited, intelligent woman. The remedies which had been tried were blisters, cupping, and aperient medicine. These means lowered her strength, and increased the depression of her spirits. The treatment which restored her was a nourishing diet and tonics; and of the tonics principally the carbonate of iron, which had the most remarkable effect, . . ."[22] Patients exhausted by emotional stress or mental anxiety, with nerve force barely adequate for the basic functions of life, had to be aroused and strengthened by tonics and stimulants, he asserted, not reduced to total enfeeblement. Drastic depletive therapies, in fact, were never standard procedure in cases of nervous exhaustion. Like the medical attendants at the York Retreat who, early in the century, gave depressed inmates nourishing food instead of trying, as in the past, to purge away the black bile believed to cause their melancholia,[23] the preponderant part of Victorian medical practitioners, both before and after mid-century, sought to invigorate the unfortunate victims of shattered nerves.

By the late Victorian period, a strengthening regime frequently included massage and electrotherapy. Doctors worried about muscular atrophy if a patient needed prolonged bedrest, and they found that they could obtain "the tonic influence of exercise by daily massage and electricity—skilled rubbing and kneading the muscles, and putting them in action by faradaism." Without massage and electricity, Gowers warned in 1888, bedrest would "probably convert the patient into a helpless invalid."[24] Since neither form of therapy required any effort on the exhausted patient's part, the benefits of exercise could thus be obtained without the risk of fatigue. Here was another means of treating the physical aspects of nervous breakdown that did not rely on drugs, and the popularity of massage and elecrotherapy increased as confidence in pharmaceutical cures declined.

Eighteenth-century medicine had pioneered the application of electricity to mental and nervous disorders. In the Georgian asylums, shock therapy was designed largely to subdue unruly lunatics, but also with a faint hope of improving their mental condition. Electricity was occasionally employed "with the object of increasing the total energy and excitability of the body,"[25] when the patient had sunk into a torpid state. By the 1830s, it received considerable attention in the medical literature on functional nervous disorders. Conolly, for example, was not much impressed with its rate of success in cases of hysteria, while James Gully, by contrast, an unyielding opponent of drug therapy, hailed galvanism "as one of the most vehement of known stimulants of the cerebro-spinal system." He used it "in two cases of inveterate neuropathy," with highly gratifying and permanent results. Dickens, always in touch with the state of popular information about science and medicine, knew that electrotherapy was familiar enough to the reading public to enjoy a little fun at its expense in *The Pickwick Papers.* When the same nervous old woman for whom Sawyer prescribed camphor-julep and water proceeded to faint, Sam Weller commented gravely: "Here's a wenerable old lady a lyin' on the carpet waitin' for dissection, or galwinism, or some other rewivin' and scientific inwention."[26]

Both the medical literature on electrotherapy and its actual employment in medical practice expanded significantly in the second half of the nineteenth century.

In part, the increase reflected growing interest in cerebral localization research and augmented knowledge of electricity's effect on nerve tissue. In a more sophisticated version of eighteenth-century asylum procedures, Crichton-Browne conducted or supervised at Wakefield a number of experiments to test the degree to which electrical stimulation of the brain could improve the mental capacities of lunatics. He was pleased to note that faradic stimulus apparently placed certain nerve tissue "in a state of physiological activity. No structural alteration is effected; but a modification of condition and relation is introduced amongst the existing elements, and healthy metamorphoses are favoured. The molecular equilibrium of the parts involved is disturbed and an opportunity is afforded for natural development, or for the revival of impaired function." In large part, too, the popularity of electrotherapy for nervous disorders in these years resulted from the influence that Beard and Weir Mitchell exerted in Great Britain. Beard experimented with electricity in treating his own neurasthenic symptoms in the late 1850s and 1860s, and he became convinced that it was an invaluable aid in replenishing exhausted supplies of nerve force. Thereafter he played a major role in spreading the electrotherapeutic gospel. Weir Mitchell incorporated electricity, as an effective means of exercising muscles, into his system for treating neurasthenics, which was publicized in Great Britain from the 1880s on.[27] In the final decades before World War I, electrotherapy became securely ensconced among the array of therapies regularly employed by alienists and nerve-doctors. After all, with its close similarity to nervous energy, electrical stimulation was the ideal way to boost the body's production of that commodity. Electricity could even temporarily take the place of the missing nerve force itself.

Electrotherapy came in many guises. Some late Victorian and Edwardian doctors found the faradic, or interrupted, current the most beneficial; others praised the galvanic, or continuous, current. On one occasion, they might prescribe "descending spinal galvanism," "general faradisation of the limbs," or "static electricity"; on another, "high frequency currents" to combat sleeplessness, or "electric nerve vibration" to excite the spinal nervous centers. Patients could don galvanic belts or immerse themselves in electrical baths, which have a deadly sound to them today, but which apparently, through careful insulation, did not electrocute the bather and gave "good results" in cases of neurasthenia.[28] Electricity could be applied to virtually any part of the body—head, neck, spine, abdomen, pelvis, and limbs were particular medical favorites. From the 1860s, electrical stimulation figured as a regular part of the physiotherapy offered at the National Hospital for the Paralysed and Epileptic. Whatever form it took, it assumed a central place in the medical campaign to help patients regain their nervous power, for it was, as Schofield observed on more than one occasion, "the most powerful agent that we possess for direct action on the nerves."[29]

Sleep and inactivity were only slightly less direct in their impact on the nerves, and medical men were not behindhand in championing the physical advantages they bestowed on nervous invalids. In the first stage of treating shattered nerves, doctors invariably stressed the necessity for rest. As Ralph Browne, physician to the Chelsea, Brompton, and Belgrave Dispensary, explained in 1894, "*the nervous system when once exhausted is with difficulty re-established*. Drugs seem to have little effect, or are badly tolerated . . . and at the present time *Rest* is the treatment advocated. Rest of *body and mind* while the system is kept in as hygienic a condition as possible during the period of inactivity." Nervous restlessness and agitation often demanded enforced immobility so that an exhausted nervous system could replenish nerve force. Most British medical opinion, however, strongly deprecated prolonged bed rest as severely detrimental to future health. The extended period that Weir Mitchell recommended—sometimes as much as six weeks—attracted few supporters in England. Maurice Craig, a very successful consulting psychiatrist in the Edwardian decade, insisted that "rest in bed will often save the [neurasthenic] patient months of trouble later," but nonetheless limited it to "two or three weeks." William H. B. Stoddart, a medical officer at Bethlem Royal in the same period, advised one month as the maximum length of time for bed rest; anything longer was liable to make a patient "contract the 'bed habit'."[30] All agreed that, at the earliest possible moment, the patient should be moved to the couch, then encouraged to move around for several hours every day, and finally taken for drives to benefit from fresh air and sunshine.

No one in Victorian and Edwardian Britain doubted that fresh air and sunshine were potent curative forces. "The free exposure of the face and general surface to the breeze," Marshall Hall enthused, had an uplifting effect on his spirits. He was certain that "there is no 'pathy' (to use the fashionable phrase), like Aëropathy." Heliotherapy had its equally ardent disciples. Implicit in Victorian paeans to fresh breezes and solar rays was the conviction that these natural aids to health were a precious antidote to precisely those aspects of urban life that fostered neurotic illness, not to mention the poisons inhaled from a polluted urban atmosphere that promoted other kinds of disease. When medical practitioners evoked the pleasures of life in the open air, they were, of course, envisioning a rural environment, whether among the English lakes, the Welsh valleys, the Scottish mountains, or the Irish hills. In the soothing atmosphere of the countryside, they announced, the tensions generated in London and other urban centers vanished. Pure air cleansed soot-choked lungs, and a relaxing style of life catered to nerves on edge. No admirer of modern social customs and pessimistic about the ability of "modern urban populations" to resist disease, Clouston waxed eloquent about the health-giving properties of fresh air: "The winds of heaven not only cure consumption, they strengthen the nerves and promote nutrition at all ages." "Bracing air with sunshine," he proclaimed, was a powerful medicine, thanks in great measure to "the oxygen of the air giving just the right kind of stimulus which the brain needs for its proper mental action. It accentuates all the nutritive processes of the body."[31] Sitting in a garden chair breathing fresh air was the most that some nerve patients could initially manage, but that in itself represented the first step down the road to recovery.

Greater recuperative progress could be anticipated once the patient was ready to undertake light exercise. In endless refrain, Victorian and Edwardian medical texts reiterated the blessings that muscular activity bestowed on nervous men, women, and children. It was a message that was already familiar to the late Georgians, as the heroine of Jane Austen's novel fragment *Sanditon* (1817) illustrated. A picture of health herself, she reprimanded an egregious hypochondriac with the remark: "As far as I can understand what nervous complaints are, I have a great idea of the efficacy of air and exercise for them—daily, regular Exercise. . . ." Just a few years later, the *Lancet* was telling the same tale to its readers, reminding them that "general nervousness,'' hysteria, and hypochondriasis were all best handled by a lifestyle that included mild exercise in the open air. Indeed, many medical practitioners believed that such activity could ward off depression, or at least keep comparatively mild neurotic complaints from developing into major crises of health. It was in the hope of preserving his precarious health—and perhaps even improving it—that Darwin followed medical advice to take up horseback riding in the late 1860s. He thought his health *was* getting better under the equine regime, ''until one day his horse fell and rolled on him, bruising him seriously, and he then gave up riding.'' Fortunately his friend Huxley had better luck with the pursuit of health through outdoor exertions. During the 1850s, when he was suffering from headaches and depression, Huxley found great relief in his work for the Geological Survey, ''which occasionally took him out of London, and the open-air occupation and tramping from place to place did him no little good.'' For many years afterwards, his son reported, ''his favourite mode of recruiting from the results of a spell of overwork was to take a short walking tour with a friend.''[32]

When a patient was recuperating from the most paralyzing degree of depression, medical men were particularly careful in issuing instructions for exercise. They wanted to induce healthy fatigue, the kind that promised a good night's sleep, without need of sedatives or soporifics; they equally wanted to avoid exhaustion, which would jeopardize the invalid's supplies of nerve force, carefully accumulated during sound sleep and periods of inactivity. Generally speaking, Victorian doctors recommended walking, fishing, and horseback riding (for the more fully recovered), with cycling and golf added to the list toward the end of the period, but they tailored their advice to fit the specific requirements and capabilities of each patient. Walking, for example, might mean an hour's gentle stroll along garden paths, a brisk hike across the moors, or mountain-climbing. To read nineteenth- and early twentieth-century health manuals, one would imagine that it scarcely rained in Great Britain, so full of plans for outdoor exercise were their optimistic authors. They only rarely tendered suggestions for comparable indoor activities, such as the use of dumbbells, because patients were supposed to breath fresh air while exercising. Medical spokesmen extolled the remedial powers of gentle exercise at every opportunity, even indulging in counter-factual speculation to prove their point. If only Carlyle had acquired the habit of regular physical exercise, Crichton-Browne was certain that a few rounds of golf each day would have spared his fellow Scotsman much misery.[33]

Fishing proved a special solace to numerous men recovering from nervous collapse, perhaps because it pleasantly challenged the mind while exercising the muscles. When John Bright broke down early in 1856, hounded by vicious publicity concerning his opposition to the Crimean War and depressed about his future in Parliament, the politician found mental effort an agony. Friends were lavish with offers of help and advice—total rest, a temporary but complete withdrawal from politics, change of diet, and, from his close political colleague Richard Cobden, the suggestion that sunshine would do him good. What Bright found the best therapy, however, was proposed by the hydropathic doctor, William McLeod, who urged him to renew his acquaintance with the fisherman's art. From May through July 1856, Bright visited various friends in Scotland and tried his hand at salmon fishing in the Highlands, with ''great enjoyment,'' as he recorded in his diary, ''and with great benefit to my health." According to George Trevelyan's biography, Bright himself insisted that "from this exercise, from spending many hours almost daily on the river's bank, he recovered the health he had lost in the long nights in the House of Commons, and in the fierce political conflicts of the time." When a similar breakdown in 1870 forced Bright to resign as president of the Board of Trade in Gladstone's first ministry, the process of recovery once again included months of fishing in Scottish waters.[34] For Herbert Spencer, fishing was "the nearest thing to a hobby" that the tormented sage ever acquired. He always retained his fondness for the sport, even when his health scarcely allowed him the pleasure of indulging in it. His secretary recalled that "one of the devices employed when his nerves were in a more than usually perturbed state," and outdoor recreation accordingly impossible, "was a sort of fishing rod with a line at the end of it from which some object dangled—a substitute for angling no doubt." Edwin Landseer, one of the most successful painters of the early and mid-Victorian period, thought that fishing helped him to recover strength after he suffered a nervous breakdown in the spring of 1840.[35]

So great was medical confidence in the therapeutic value of outdoor exercise that it was even incorporated into the regime of the most advanced Victorian asylums, including the York Retreat and the West Riding institution under Crichton-Browne. From the early 1840s, William Farr, the justly renowned public health crusader and statistician, promoted outdoor exercise as a means of reducing the incidence of suicide in Great Britain, though with what effect can hardly be determined. In these perhaps overly optimistic assessments of the impact of exercise under the open sky, alienists and sanitarians were inspired by the realization that the nervous system was not the only beneficiary. The muscles grew firmer, while the heart, too, was strengthened by the accelerated flow of blood that exercise occasioned. An efficient, quickened circulation, furthermore, joined with increased perspiration to facilitate the more rapid removal of body wastes. As far back as the seventeenth century, in fact, Sydenham had recommended horseback riding for hysterical patients precisely because it helped cleanse the blood of waste matter.[36]

The medical profession endorsed mild exercise as a means of treating shattered nerves long before the mania for outdoor sports exploded in Great Britain during the second half of the nineteenth century. Certain aspects of the recuperative program nonetheless benefited from the development of new sporting equipment and new fashions in outdoor recreation. The cycling craze of the 1890s, for example, called attention to an excellent and pleasurable form of exercise, which Beatrice Webb, for one, was glad to pursue in her efforts to maintain good health against the background of frequent depression and nervous strain.[37] Medical advice, however, continued to stress the dangers of excessive exercise for nervous patients. Doctors were not interested in developing body power alone, for their goal, throughout the nineteenth century, was to promote a perfect balance of mental and physical strength, which Victorians always celebrated as the ideal of health.

The mind occupied a very prominent place in Victorian and Edwardian medical strategies for rallying exhausted nerves. It was never long eclipsed by disquisitions on adequately oxygenated blood or the efficient removal of body wastes. Nor did any reputable medical practitioner ever deny that health depended as much on peace of mind as plenitude of nerve force. Particularly as faith in drugs declined, doctors more freely conceded the central part played by mental states in determining which patients recovered and which lingered in invalidism. The various kinds of nature-therapy that enlisted medical advocates—whether they championed the therapeutic power of sunshine, fresh air, a particular climate, water, exercise, or a combination of them all—were actually directed toward psychological woes as much as bodily ills. Medical literature did not always publicize that fact, since commitment to a somatic theory of disease kept the emphasis on physiological cause and effect, but doctors never ignored what they considered the mental aspects of recovery from nervous breakdown.

Naturopathy, or the treatment of disease by promoting the body's own natural recuperation, played a significant part in Victorian medicine, despite the diverse forms of heroic intervention that medical theory sanctioned. The ancient concept of the *vis medicatrix naturae*—the healing force inherent in nature—was no less indispensable to nineteenth-century medicine than it had been 200 years earlier, or than it is today. Invoking the *vis medicatrix naturae* was, of course, a way to mask ignorance and impotence behind impressive Latin vocabulary, but it also meant placing trust in an approach to illness that utterly merged the psychological and physiological. Galton, whose long life was punctuated by spells of severe depression, well understood that combination of curative powers. "There is still," he wrote in his memoirs, "much lack of exact knowledge of what Nature can do without assistance from medicine, if aided only by cheering influences, rest, suggestion, and good nursing." Sometimes all a medical attendant could do was place his patient in the environment most conducive to his or her own spontaneous recovery. He might contribute some pharmaceutical additions to nature's brand of healing, but he nevertheless relied heavily on it. As Allbutt observed in the 1890s, his profession still appealed "to the aid of a certain tricky spirit called 'Nature'" to help out our therapeutics."[38]

To determine what environment would stimulate the *vis medicatrix naturae* to work most effectively for an individual patient, doctors considered the necessary emotional atmosphere as well as the most favorable climate, the best possibilities for rest, and the most appropriate facilities for exercise. Since it was a Victorian medical commonplace that stress, overwork, and mental anxiety could exhaust nerve force, it often proved necessary to withdraw a patient from the situation in which tension and worry arose. Hence the reiterated suggestion that change of scene was essential for recovery from nervous collapse. "Change of air—change of scene; those are my prescriptions," advised the young doctor in *Villette*,[39] and his colleagues outside of novels did the same. Complete removal from the conditions under which the patient broke down became the standard initial instruction from both family practitioners and consulting physicians. Sometimes they specified the patient's destination; sometimes the main object was simply to distance the patient from home.

In a culture that glorified domesticity, it is striking to note the Victorian medical acknowledgment that home life could be detrimental to health. Whether discussing hysteria, hypochondriasis, anorexia nervosa, or neurasthenia and other manifestations of exhausted nervous resources, British doctors were remarkably consistent throughout the nineteenth and early twentieth centuries in stressing that absence from home might hold the key to victory over neurotic ailments. As Craig sagely observed in 1905, "many patients recover more rapidly when in the care of strangers, than in their own homes." It was not just a matter of occupying the invalids' attention with novel impressions that left no room for morbid thoughts; it was necessary to separate them from family and friends whose solicitude only intensified their self-absorption. Even in a happy, loving family, relationships could breed strains that hindered a patient's recuperation. When Charles Kingsley's nervous breakdown occurred late in 1848, following a year of intense political excitement and the pressure to complete his social novel *Yeast,* he temporarily retired from his parish of Eversley, Hampshire, and took his family to North Devon. His recovery was adequate enough to enable him to return to Eversley in June, 1849, but within two months he had suffered a relapse. When he set off again for Devonshire, he went alone. Devoted though he was to his wife and children, he sensed that he needed an utter rest from the role of paterfamilias. As he wrote to a friend and fellow Christian Socialist, J. M. Ludlow, from Clovelly: "I am at last enjoying perfect rest. . . . I am as stupid as a porpoise, and I lie in the window, and smoke and watch the glorious cloud-phantasmagoria, infinite in color and form, crawling across the vast bay and deep woods below, and draw little sketches of figures, and do not even dream, much less think." Such freedom was the perfect form of treatment for a man who, at the start of his illness, confessed that his "poor addle brain feels as if someone had stirred it with a spoon," but the therapy was rarely possible in the bosom of one's family.[40]

If patients were unable to look after themselves and needed trained attendants, doctors might be obliged to dispatch them to the home of a medical practitioner who took lodgers, or to one of the rest-homes that began to appear around the turn of the century. Savill spoke for his fellow nerve specialists when he described grave cases of neurasthenia in which

> it is desirable to place the patient in the house of, and under the care of, a medical man, for these cases generally require constant medical supervision. I have seen valuable time lost, and even still more disastrous results ensue, when relatives—who had formed the opinion that "nothing but a thorough rest and change" was needed— have taken the matter entirely into their own hands. In other cases there has been every reason to believe that the daily watchful care of a skilled medical attendant has restored the mind of a case which at one time appeared hopeless.[41]

It is not difficult to detect a branch of the medical profession staking its claim here to a potentially lucrative monopoly on the rest-home business and parading its special expertise to scare off amateurs, but there was also much truth to the insight that family members were often the last people to realize what a nervous patient needed.

A. C. Benson sought refuge in a Mayfair rest-home, under medical supervision, when depression totally overwhelmed him and he felt himself " 'brought face to face with the ultimate and inexorable darkness' " in November 1907. This particular nursing home accepted patients with a variety of ailments—indeed, operations were apparently performed there—but in January 1908, after trying unsuccessfully to live in the outside world for a few weeks, he was placed under more specialized care, at the Hampstead home of one Dr. Caldicott "who boarded a few mental patients." By then, Benson was, if possible, in an even worse state than he had been in the previous

November, and he was kept under closer watch than the Mayfair establishment had thought necessary. One month at Hampstead, combined with doses of the barbiturate veronal, did not lift Benson's spirits.[42] In fact, they did not lift until 1909, apparently obeying their own timetable over which medicine had no control.

Although Victorian and Edwardian medical practitioners agreed that change of scene and removal from home were frequently essential to initiate the recuperative process, there was as much dispute over the best environment for treating neurotic illness as there was over the most appropriate diet. Crichton-Browne particularly favored the Lake Country of Westmoreland and Cumberland as "a restorative sanitorium for shattered nerves." Allbutt, among many others, preferred the "milder upland airs" of Malvern for combating the neuroses, or the "dry sunny slopes" of the Sussex Downs. Graham Brown, an Edinburgh practitioner, argued that neurasthenics did best in mountain climates and put forward the claims of the Scottish highlands.[43] Every resort and spa had promoters who touted its special climatic conditions. Perhaps his book on *The Influence of Climate in the Prevention and Cure of Chronic Disease* (1829) can help to explain why nervous patients sought the advice of Sir James Clark, a doctor with no particular skills as a diagnostician and certainly no claims to expertise about the nervous system. When Kingsley was once again attacked by "severe illness and great physical depression" in 1864, Clark's counsel was the predictable "thorough rest and change of air." So apparently eager was the medical profession to send its nervous patients up and down the British Isles that Thomas Hughes, the author of *Tom Brown's Schooldays* (1857), issued a tongue-in-cheek complaint against railway company directors who set aside "several millions of money, which they continually distribute judiciously amongst the Doctors, stipulating only this one thing, that they shall prescribe change of air to every patient who can pay, or borrow money to pay, a railway fare, and see their prescription carried out. If it be not for this, why is it that none of us can be well at home for a year together?"[44] The reason for what seemed to Hughes so much unnecessary traveling was not, in fact, the quest for perfect air, but the sad situation that many severely depressed men and women found home and health incompatible.

A large proportion of the stream of invalids flowed toward the ocean, to Brighton, Bournemouth, Ramsgate, Margate and other seaside communities. "Nobody could catch cold by the Sea, Nobody wanted appetite by the Sea, Nobody wanted Spirits, Nobody wanted Strength," Jane Austen had rhapsodized satirically. "The Sea air and Sea Bathing together were nearly infallible, one or the other of them being a match for every Disorder, . . . They were healing, softing, relaxing, fortifying and bracing, seemingly just as was wanted, sometimes one, sometimes the other."[45] If medical men later in the nineteenth century were not quite so absurd as this spoof of Georgian marine propaganda suggested, the number of men and women who were sent to the seaside to recuperate from nervous breakdown certainly indicates the degree of faith that many doctors continued to place in ocean breezes and sea baths. The ozone in the coastal atmosphere was itself presumed to have many health-giving properties—an excellent example of the allegedly scientific rationale behind travel therapy for nervous invalids.

A sense of peace and renewal, such as Kingsley found at Clovelly, was the real goal that drove many sufferers to the seacoast. The celebrated surgeon, Sir Benjamin

Collins Brodie, reminisced fondly in his autobiography about a trip to the coast when he was an overworked young medical man in 1814–15, suffering from depression and losing weight:

> I . . . looked so ill that many of my acquaintance believed that I laboured under some serious organic disease. . . . I attribute my illness to unceasing occupation of mind and body for a long period, and partly to having been during ten years in London, never breathing the air of the country for more than two or three days at a time, and even then only on some rare occasions. . . . I continued to suffer—sometimes more, sometimes less—until the following autumn, when I went . . . for a short time to the seaside. It was remarkable how much, and what immediate refreshment this change of air and freedom of labour afforded me. I returned to London quite an altered person. . . .

John Bright derived comfort from sea bathing in the autumn of 1870, and Michael Faraday, too, found some solace by the ocean. In 1839, at the start of his prolonged breakdown, the great physicist followed Peter Mere Latham's orders and went to Brighton in the hopes of curing an almost incessant headache, accompanied by memory loss. He chose "a situation which commanded a view of the sea, . . . where he could sit and gaze and feel the gradual revival of faith that 'Nature never did betray / The heart that loved her.' But very often for some days after his removal to the country he would be unable to do more than sit at a window and look out upon the sea and sky."[46]

The sight of the sea and the feel of its breezes could not always work miracles. Faraday's illness dragged on. The Unitarian minister Lant Carpenter, taken to the coast by his wife and daughter when depression paralyzed him in June 1839, did not improve. "He complained of giddiness, faintness, headache, sleepless nights, and overwhelming misery." Worst of all, for a man of his calling, he felt certain "of being cut off from God by the weight of his sins." Rachel Grant-Smith, understandably distraught following her husband's lethal overdose of morphine, spent a miserable three weeks at St. Anne's-on-Sea in 1900. After Spencer's "nervous system finally gave way" in 1855, he, too, was disappointed in his hopes that sea air would restore him to health. Yet he nonetheless returned to the seaside, to try bathing and yachting the following year, and in 1886, during a particularly extended period of nervous prostration, he moved himself (traveling "in a hammock slung diagonally in an invalid-carriage" of the train) to Brighton, where he lived for more than a year.[47] It was as if this wretched, irascible man, frustrated by medicine's ongoing failure to alleviate his incapacitation, turned instinctively to the ocean, which, even if it could not cure him, was never a source of irritation.

Spencer's extreme precautions to ensure his comfort while traveling suggested some of the hazards facing a nervous patient who sought change of air and scene. The anticipated benefits had to be balanced against the agitation caused by venturing forth, particularly if the purpose of the trip was to visit foreign countries. Medical opinion concerning travel abroad was, in fact, highly ambivalent. Believing fervently in the power of new surroundings to rouse patients from depression and trusting uncritically in climatotherapy, many British doctors dispatched invalids across Europe and North Africa, typically in the company of a friend or medical attendant. If novel sights and situations provided the mental stimulation, or distraction, to drive away melancholy, then foreign travel seemed to promise greater results than familiar British landscapes could produce. The problem was, however, that travel on the continent, or even further afield, was far less likely to provide the calm restfulness that medical theory also deemed essential for recovery from nervous collapse. The physical discomfort and manifold inconveniences of travel, combined with the anxiety that often accompanied sojourns in a foreign land, could readily aggravate a condition of nervous weakness and jeopardize whatever supplies of nerve force a patient could command. Maudsley ridiculed the idea of sending a deeply depressed man to the Swiss mountains, or anywhere else for that matter, "when he was no more competent to take interest in new scenes than a paralyzed man to embrace Venus."[48]

Nonetheless, desperate measures were occasionally advocated in desperate cases. Benson's doctor, Ross Todd, for example, advised the writer to spend Christmas of 1907 in Italy, after it became clear that the Mayfair nursing home had effected no improvement in his state of mind. Todd's hope was that "a complete change of scene could help to recover his zest for living." It did not, and Benson spent Christmas Day at St. Peter's in Rome, wishing to die. In Faraday's case, however, the decision to send a very sick man to Switzerland proved astute. Although the scientist's condition had worsened by the summer of 1841, with headaches, giddiness, and loss of memory plaguing him mercilessly, he and his wife set off for the Alps in late June. The setting obviously suited him. The beauty of the scenery and the sunsets impressed him deeply; he seized the opportunity for long excursions, "walking thirty miles in a day," his wife reported, "and one day he walked forty-five," with no evil consequences. As his fellow physicist John Tyndall remarked: "His nerves had been shattered, but his muscles were strong." Writing letters was still "quite a labour to him" and conversation with fellow guests at the Swiss inn an impossibility, but it is obvious that the trip to Switzerland, far from draining his nerve force, revived his physical stamina.[49] Clearly, where victims of nervous breakdown were concerned, generalizations were no more valid about foreign travel than about any other aspect of treating that baffling disorder. One patient's cure could consign another to permanent invalidism. As a result, Victorian medical men tended to play it safe, waiting until nervous patients had completed a period of rest on the British side of the Channel, before sending them off to distant parts.

One way to achieve the benefits of travel with few of the attendant risks was to prescribe a sea voyage. On board ship, no sightseeing fatigued the passengers and no worries about luggage or accommodations endangered peace of mind. Crichton-Browne contended that the genuine ocean climate (only available at least thirty miles from land) was even more invigorating than the climate of the seacoast. On a long ocean voyage, perhaps to South Africa, the West Indies, or New Zealand, a number of factors worked entirely to the patient's good, including, of course, the long hours spent on deck in the sunshine and fresh air "free from organic and inorganic impurities, . . . but saturated with saline constituents." Whether it was the saline constituents or the passenger's utter sense of irresponsibility for all shipboard decisions that proved most advantageous to severely depressed people, Crichton-Browne and many of his colleagues were quick to send their patients to sea, whenever possible. Young Charles Eliot, Principal Tulloch, and Charles Booth, for example, all improved after voyages to the West Indies, Greece, and Brazil, respectively.

When money was lacking for such expensive therapy, friends could sometimes be found to foot the bill. A wealthy acquaintance financed Lant Carpenter's voyage to the south of France in late 1826 when the minister had succumbed to deadening despair. Ben Tillett was "compelled to undertake a recuperative voyage to Australia" on two occasions—in 1897, after the distressing incident in the Belgian jail, and in 1907, when his fragile health again evidently required rest and sunshine. In the first instance, he dated the beginning of his recovery from the moment his ship approached Africa and he could luxuriate in the warm sunshine of Capetown. On the second occasion, Horatio Bottomley, the shady business entrepreneur, publisher, and Liberal politician, collected money on the trade unionist's behalf. Friends and acquaintances certainly thought they were helping depressed invalids when they underwrote ocean voyages for them, but occasionally their enthusiasm had to be balanced by the reminder that travel at sea did present one outstanding drawback: the melancholic patient might try to commit suicide by jumping overboard. Indeed, Carpenter disappeared mysteriously at sea in the spring of 1840, during yet another attempt to lift his spirits.[50]

Combining all the reputed benefits of sea air, abundant sunshine, and novel surroundings, the shores of the Mediterranean acted as a particular magnet to draw droves of British invalids to their villas and hotels. In Italy, the French Riviera, Algeria, Egypt, Malaga, and even Malta for a prief period, sickly men and women escaped their native fogs for months at a time. The great thing about the Mediterranean, its promoters were quick to point out, was that its climate was varied enough to serve all types of patients: in parts of Italy, the principal effect of the atmosphere was sedative; in areas of the Franco-Italian Riviera, it was mildly tonic; elsewhere still, it was extremely exciting. The more skeptical Victorian medical men became about the effectiveness of drugs, the more they esteemed the chance to obtain the same effects without resorting to the pharmacist at all. Far better to have a patient addicted to life in the mellow Mediterranean than dependent on morphine.[51] In the second half of the nineteenth century, increasing numbers of doctors came to the conclusion that the Mediterranean could do more to revitalize body and mind than all of the British pharmacopoeia put together.

While the majority of patients who sought Mediterranean refuge from the cold and damp of a British winter suffered from pulmonary disease, the opportunity to pursue outdoor recreation all winter long made the Mediterranean region an appropriate destination for victims of diverse afflictions, including nervous exhaustion. At the end of 1856, John Bright's doctors, including Sir James Clark, bundled him off to Algiers, known as the "Torquay of Africa." After a month there, he traveled to southern France and thence to Italy. He did not return to England until June 1857, by which time he was also ready to return to politics. His diaries reveal him taking an active interest in all he did while abroad, but one suspects that the Mediterranean milieu was less directly responsible for his improvement in health than the sheer distance from the House of Commons. In 1878–79, Spencer spent Christmas and the New Year on the Franco-Italian Riviera, having decided the previous summer that his appetite, digestion, capacity to work, and overall health depended on "avoiding the evils which the winter's cold entails." Despite some chill, wet days in southern France, he seemed to enjoy the seven weeks he spent there and the following

November was persuaded to join a party going up the Nile. This venture was not a success. "As may be imagined," he reported in his autobiography, "five nights on board a cramped Nile-steamer left me in a state of exhaustion." With equally mixed results, countless other depressed Victorians sought relief from their troubles on the shores of the Mediterranean. After a nervous breakdown in 1872, James Sully, attempting to launch his career as a freelance writer on philosophical and psychologi- cal subjects, fled London to "the magic coast" of the Riviera. His reminiscences, published nearly fifty years later, bore tribute to "recuperative Italy" and the power of Mediterranean sunshine to soothe the psyche. Sadly, Italy could do nothing for George Lyttelton, the fourth baron, whose family hoped to dispel a particularly disabling bout of melancholy with a trip to Rome in 1876. Like Benson decades later, Lyttelton found the sojourn a form of torture. "The gloom of his great and slowly over-mastering depression of spirit and increasing restlessness made the trip a time of grievous trial." Shortly after returning to England, he committed suicide.[52]

· Some doctors would not have been surprised at the tragic conclusion of Lord Lyttelton's travels, for one school of Victorian medical thought—albeit small— disagreed with the prevailing passion for the south. The therapeutic merits of different regions of continental Europe offered, of course, even more room for controversy than the climatic variations within the British Isles alone, and the "fashionable resorts in the south of Europe" were not universally approved for nervous patients. Dowse, for one, considered them virtually useless in the treatment of both functional and organic nervous disorders. Pronouncing the Mediterranean climate too mild, moist, and relaxing to provide the stimulus necessary for fortifying the nerves, he questioned those who claimed to have found pockets of atmospheric tonic along the Riviera. While few of his colleagues joined him in a blanket condemnation of the south, many shared his enthusiasm for the "invigorating and toning influence of the splendid mountain air" of Switzerland. The Alpine meadows were as crowded with British invalids in the summer months as the Mediterranean shores were in the winter. Like Faraday, a significant number of them were hoping to rally from nervous collapse.[53] Yet medical spokesmen could also be found who denigrated high altitudes for nervous patients and warned of the consequences to be anticipated from exposing them to such an atmosphere.

Notwithstanding medical assertions to the contrary, so long as a depressed person had the physical stamina to travel, the place of destination did not actually matter. When Galton was recovering from the nervous breakdown he suffered while an undergraduate at Cambridge in the early 1840s, he traveled with his sister in Germany and Austria, about which medical texts had no sanatory theories whatsoever. He visited cities like Dresden and Vienna, and journeyed by diligence, which can scarcely have provided a smooth, restful ride. Landseer, likewise in pursuit of restored vitality after his breakdown, also made a tour of the continent that had no reference to recognized health resorts. Starting in Bruges, where the artist found "everything picturesque and paintable," Landseer traveled through Germany to Geneva, then on to Paris before returning home. "I am as well as can be expected after so much travelling," he wrote to his aunt and sister. "My head soon gets out of order when I am obliged to give up doing anything and go to the open air."[54] If the purpose of travel in cases like Galton's and Landseer's was principally to distract the mind from its troubles, such diversion could just as readily occur among art galleries, cathedrals, and concert halls as among the remote grandeur of mountain landscapes.

The reason for travel in most instances involving severely depressed men and women *was* precisely to provide pleasant mental occupation in congenial company, after the laborious work of replenishing nerve force had been accomplished. While fully acknowledging that the mental component of travel therapy possessed great significance, however, most medical practitioners hesitated to reduce the curative value of travel to mere psychological amusement and preferred to enunciate therapeutic hypotheses based on climate and geography. No British doctor before World War I would have spoken to a patient the way D. H. Lawrence's postwar fictional specialist spoke to Connie in *Lady Chatterley's Lover* (1928):

> "No, no! There's nothing organically wrong, but it won't do! . . . Tell Sir Clifford he's got to bring you to town, to take you abroad, and amuse you. You've got to be amused, got to! Your vitality is much too low; no reserves, no reserves. . . . Nothing but nerves; I'd put you right in a month at Cannes or Biarritz. But it mustn't go on, *mustn't.* . . . You're spending your life without renewing it. You've got to be amused, properly, healthily amused. You're spending your vitality without making any. Can't go on, you know. Depression! avoid depression!"[55]

Amusement alone was not an excuse that Victorian society could sanction for leaving home, and medical advisors accordingly phrased their advice to neurotic travelers in terms of altitude, temperature, and light. Fitting perfectly with orthodox beliefs about tonics and sedatives, climatic theories appeared to furnish plausible physical explanations for the influence of travel on nervous patients, and no doubt doctors genuinely subscribed to them. Yet sincere endorsement of climatotherapy never dulled medical awareness that potent psychological processes were also at work whenever invalids left the scene of their suffering.

The combination of mental and somatic symptoms associated with nervous collapse was tailor made for the water cure, a form of nature therapy that flourished in Great Britain during the second half of the nineteenth century. A visit to one of the hydropathic spas that mushroomed in England and Scotland brought the advantages of new surroundings without extensive travel and exposed the patient to a form of treatment that claimed to promote the body's own recuperative powers. That hydropathy was designed to ease the mind while regulating the functions of the body was not the least of its attractions.

As a formal system of medicine, complete with theory and explicitly opposed to drug therapy, the water cure developed in England from the early 1840s. Long before then, however, the British medical profession had realized that water could prove an invaluable natural aid in the cure of disease. Fashionable spas, like Bath, flourished in the eighteenth century, prospering from the affluent invalid's faith in the remedial effects of mineral water, but Georgian doctors equally acknowledged that plain water, too, had healing potency. They particularly emphasized the efficacy of water in treating nervous complaints, a selling point that continued to bolster medical enthusiasm for the water cure during the early decades of the nineteenth century. Without providing any detailed, methodical program of hydropathy, medical practitioners in these years advocated warm or cold baths for hypochondriasis, tepid bathing for nervous indigestion, warm shower baths for general nervousness, cold baths for hysteria, and so forth. In 1824, the *Family Oracle of Health* even went so far as to announce, in a forecast of subsequent hydropathic manifestos, that proper water treatment in cases of nervous illness would "have more effect than any sort of drugs."[56]

Thus the claims of an Austrian farmer, Vincent Priessnitz, to have discovered the therapeutic impact of nature's pure water seem difficult to swallow. What Priessnitz did achieve beyond doubt was the commercialization of the water cure. Around 1830, he established a hydropathic spa at Gräfenberg, Silesia, where diverse water treatments were employed according to Priessnitzian theory, which particularly featured the alternation of cold baths and hot packs to induce evacuation through perspiration. In addition to the water therapy, patients—who typically spent several months at a time with Priessnitz—followed an entire regime of diet, exercise, and hygiene. Here was a way to harness water power that could appeal to British men and women searching seriously, and they hoped scientifically, for health, while growing increasingly suspicious of heavy drugging. When Richard T. Claridge, captain in the Middlesex militia and deputy-lieutenant of the county, informed his compatriots in 1842 that three months at Gräfenberg in the previous year had cured his rheumatism, he struck an immediately sympathetic chord. Claridge's impeccable social standing naturally helped to obtain an attentive audience for his message, but its content was even more to the liking of Victorian invalids.[57] Already one or two hydropathic establishments had opened in England, but after Claridge wrote and lectured on the Gräfenberg system, the vogue for hydropathy was truly launched.

It was a vogue that, inevitably, attracted unscrupulous opportunists and enthusiastic idealists, as well as serious medical practitioners disillusioned with the therapeutic options available to them. Temperance crusaders, too, seized on the water cure as a means to propagate their own gospel of abstinence from alcohol. One such teetotaler, James Ellis, gave up his business as a lace merchant and set off for the continent, to study hydropathic medicine in Germany and Austria. On his return in 1845, "Dr." Ellis became the manager of Sudbrook Park, a fashionable hydro in Richmond.[58] It was easy enough to become expert in the theory and practice of hydropathy, and many a "hydropathic practitioner," not burdened with formal medical education, ran hydros with varying degrees of success. Richard Metcalfe, for example, supervised two establishments in the 1870s: Priessnitz House, near Edgware Road in London, and Gräfenberg House, in the London suburb of New Barnet. Both offered more than thirty variations of water therapy—every conceivable sort of shower and bath, hot and cold dripping sheets, hot fomentation packs for local inflammations, tepid or cold affusions, and much else. Each form of treatment had its price, from six shillings for a private Turkish bath (by appointment only), to one shilling, sixpence for more commonplace ministrations, like the hot and cold spray bath, cool shallow bath, or plunge bath. These fees were additional to the weekly residence charge, which ranged from two pounds, twelve shillings, sixpence to six guineas for a superior bedroom and private sitting room. Clearly, hydropathy meant big business for the likes of Metcalfe, who also made house calls.[59]

The very possibility of house calls, like the location of Priessnitz House in the midst of London, suggests how far the entrepreneurial spirit had seduced Metcalfe away from the pristine principles of hydropathy. Water therapy was initially intended to be pursued as a way of life, in a controlled environment, where fresh, pure water flowed freely and the opportunities for outdoor exercise enhanced the regimen of drinking and bathing in nature's most abundant liquid. The best known of Victorian hydropathic spas, Malvern in Worcestershire and Ben Rhydding in Yorkshire, were situated in a rural setting that underscored the patients' removal from all that was harassing and hurried in their lives. Both hydros, during their most successful periods, were under the direction of medical doctors who had practiced orthodox drug therapy, realized its dangers and limits, and decided instead to assist the *vis medicatrix naturae* through the natural medium of water.

The partnership of James Wilson and James Manby Gully transformed Malvern into a prominent Victorian health resort, and a mecca for nervous patients. Wilson had studied medicine at Trinity College, Dublin, before completing his training in Liverpool, London, and Paris. While practicing in London during the 1830s, he met Gully, who had recently received the M.D. degree from Edinburgh. Gully's mounting dissatisfaction with current medical practices found expression in his 1837 treatise on "neuropathy," where he lambasted "the excessive use of all medicines," and he was ready for conversion to an alternative system of healing. When his friend Wilson returned from an extended continental tour, including a prolonged stay at Gräfenberg, Gully was receptive to his glowing account of the water cure. Wilson established a hydropathic practice at Malvern in June 1842, and Gully joined him a few months later. Although they ran separate hydros, regulated along rather different lines, their combined influence made Malvern the premier hydropathic haven for thirty years, until Wilson's death in 1867 and Gully's retirement late in 1871.[60]

Gully in particular became the champion of hydropathy in England, writing energetically on its behalf and defending the water cure from its many acidulous opponents. In 1847, he even launched *The Water Cure Journal and Hygienic Magazine,* to represent the hydropathic viewpoint in the burgeoning field of medical periodicals. His co-editor in that endeavor was William McLeod, the doctor whose affiliation with the Ben Rhydding hydro made it a close rival to Malvern from the mid-1840s to the mid-1870s. McLeod, like Gully, earned his medical degree from Edinburgh, where he subsequently lectured on physiology and anatomy. A skilled administrator and an innovative physician, McLeod found in hydropathy the opportunity to attack disease from a number of angles simultaneously. At Ben Rhydding, he pioneered the hydropathic use of Turkish baths and introduced a compressed-air chamber, which removed atmospheric moisture, for the particular relief of asthma and bronchitis. For nervous patients, he prescribed gymnastics, since he believed that "well-regulated therapeutic movements" not only stimulated the circulation of the blood and strengthened the muscles, but also "indirectly increased the vigour of the nervous system."[61]

The beauty, and utility, of hydropathy lay in its very flexibility. It was a form of therapy that could be modified in countless different ways, as the patient's own needs and illness dictated. The water cure could be made "antiphlogistic, or depressive of increased action," when the body's vital activity had to be lowered, as with fever or inflammation; "tonic, or restorative," when bodily functions needed arousal, as with debility, dyspepsia, or many nervous complaints; and "alterative," when somatic action had to be regularized, as with constipation.[62] Its supporters were adamant that hydropathy could assist recovery from diametrically contrasting disorders by warming or cooling the body at the appropriate moment, applying or withdrawing friction, stimulating or soothing. Beneath the diversity of treatments, however, hydropathists were guided by a few comparatively simple precepts. They particularly agreed that the water cure's greatest value arose precisely in those "disorders over which it is *allowed* that medicine possesses scarcely any control— . . . in a word, all depraved conditions of the general health, all functional derangement, all deficiencies of action in any one of the vital organs—for which no specific cause can be assigned."[63] Hydropathy, in other words, was the perfect therapy for nervous breakdown.

In seeking a theoretically compelling way to explain the success of their methods in such cases, hydropathic practitioners stressed the inextricable links that bound the nervous system to every bodily tissue. Any disturbance in the body that communicated itself to the nerves through sympathetic action could give rise to functional nervous disorders. According to this interpretation of somatic processes, morbid conditions of the digestive organs were especially liable to set in motion the pathological chain of events leading to nervous collapse, thanks to the impact of visceral irritation on the brain. It was Gully who developed the argument in greatest detail. Insisting that "the essential nature of nervousness is . . . to be found in the morbid irritation of the visceral ganglionic system," Gully asserted in 1846 that "the unceasing stream of sensations from the viscera is ever acting on the mental organ, maintaining it in a state almost of orgasm, or at least of super-vitality, rendering it thereby constantly prone to the exercise of its function, and that function excessive. . . . It is because the brain is kept in a state of vivid perception, by the irritations proceeding from the ganglionic viscera, that all the external senses are so sensitive, and all the internal senses and the thought are so painfully busy."[64] If allowed to continue, such intense sensitivity of nerves throughout the body led inexorably to nervous exhaustion, but hydropathy could alleviate the victim's suffering, even forestalling the worst effects of visceral irritation when administered in time. Over a period of weeks, the application of soothing water to the abdomen and stomach, in the form of baths, damp cloths, wet towels, or dripping sheets, calmed the gastric and intestinal disturbances, halting their vexatious influence on the brain as no pharmaceutical medicine could. Once the irritation had been removed, furthermore, and the patient's nervous system was ready to be reinvigorated, a sagacious alteration of hydropathic treatment—replacing baths with the more stimulating showers, for example—could provide the desired effect.

Although Gully appeared to be propounding a purely physiological theory when he announced that "the brain only feels as the viscera dictate," he also prized hydropathy as a powerful medicine for the mind, as did his fellow hydropathists. If the brain was eased by wrapping the abdomen in wet towels, the relief was as much mental as physical. Thomas Graham, the proprietor of a hydro in Hertford, pronounced "the *hydriatic* system" "highly satisfactory" both in nervous complaints and in mental maladies[65]—the difference, say, between tic douloureux and melancholy—but, in fact, for the majority of his patients, the distinction would have been meaningless. As far as they were concerned, the nerves and the mind suffered together, and the most successful hydropathists were those who paid close attention to the patient's state of mind at all times.

It was not just the water served up in so many ingenious ways, but the entire ambiance of the hydropathic spas that made them sources of comfort to numerous distressed Victorians. The exposure to fresh air and moderate exercise on foot or horseback, the diet of nourishing but easily digestible food, the enforced abstinence from mental exertion, and, not least of all, the cleanliness that followed frequent immersion in water—all contributed to a hygienic regimen that doubtless proved beneficial to a considerable portion of the affluent, predominantly urban clientele that flocked to Malvern and its competitors. To many of the intellectuals and professionals who patronized hydropathic spas, the time devoted merely to feeling well offered a welcome mental balm. In the hydropathic atmosphere, body and mind alike could relish relaxation from the tensions of busy and often sedentary lives, in a manner at once sensually gratifying and socially acceptable. Gully, and other leading hydropathists, were skilled psychotherapists, who listened attentively to patients' problems and responded with highly individualized treatment for each of them. Despite all his talk of visceral irritation, Gully understood the emotional suffering that prompted men and women to seek relief in the water cure. He knew that physical discomfort could arise from painful thoughts, and he tried to create an environment at Malvern where thinking was, for a while, held in abeyance while the patient cultivated a sense of physical well-being. The real strength of hydropathy lay, not in all the theoretical claims made on its behalf, but in just such a sensible approach to psychosomatic illness.[66]

The other enormous advantage of water therapy was, of course, that its patients were spared massive doses of drugs. Although pharmaceutical remedies were not invariably withheld at hydros, hydropathists were unanimous in condemning medical reliance on drugs and particularly the indiscriminate prescriptions that were still common practice in the 1840s. Already in 1837, Gully had written: "I feel convinced that seven-tenths of the nervous cases that are met with in this country are the result of excessive medication, which keeps the internal sensibility in a continued state of exaggeration, exciting morbid sympathies, particularly with the brain, . . ." After a short time in hydropathic practice, he could be more specific. "Courses of mercury, iodine, iron, colchicum, prussic acid, and creosote," he and Wilson reported in 1843, had driven several patients to Malvern in a terrible state, their minds "emasculated, deprived of moral courage and almost of volition, in a state of hebetude, hypochondriacal anxiety, suicidal depression, or excessive irritability." These patients, whose blood was "charged with the accumulated poison of years," sought in hydropathy "alleviation, not so much of their original maladies, as of the morbid condition into which these have been made to merge by the frightful amount of drugging practised on their systems." To hydropathists, it seemed clear that promiscuous drugging induced exactly the symptoms characteristic of nervous exhaustion—"chronical debility, or weakening of the whole system," as the *Water Cure Journal* described them in 1849, adding "chronical langour and great reduction of power" a sentence later.[67] Even if hydropathists were exaggerating to prove a professional point, it was a point well taken, and they kept their patients off most, if not all, forms of medicine that issued from a pharmacist. The fact that the rules of many hydros also stipulated abstinence from alcoholic beverages further assisted patients in an age when medical attendants administered a glass of sherry, port, or stronger spirits as freely as the blue pill, and alcoholism was as much of a menace in polite drawing rooms as in city slums.

A history of Victorian functional nervous disorders could almost be written from the list of patients who tried hydropathic treatment. Some were attracted as a last resort, after all other known medicaments had failed; others were drawn by the engaging, sympathetic personality of the hydropathist, whose approach to nervous illness seemed, in any case, more promising of success than the bewildering views of orthodox medicine. Some went away satisfied, others disappointed. Bulwer-Lytton, Tennyson, G. H. Lewes, George Eliot, Dickens, Macaulay, Huxley, Thomas and Jane Carlyle, Ruskin, Darwin, and Spencer were only a handful of the celebrated intellectuals who turned to the water cure during periods of prolonged ill health and emotional anguish.[68] Tennyson was in his late thirties when thwarted romantic hopes, the death of Arthur Hallam, and mounting financial anxieties had brought him to the brink of nervous breakdown in 1847. He first tried the water cure at Umberslade Hall, a hydro run by Edward Johnson in Warwickshire, and then at Malvern, under Gully's care. Although he claimed that the treatment "half cured, half destroyed" him, the experience must have proved largely positive, because five years later, the nervous crisis surmounted, he returned with his wife to visit Malvern. The Carlyles, perpetual martyrs to insomnia, indigestion, constipation, and their attendant nervous miseries, were persuaded to spend one month at Malvern as Gully's guests in the summer of 1851. Carlyle's reaction to the doctor's hospitality was typical of his jaundiced attitude, after decades of discomfort, to virtually all types of therapy. "Drank a good deal of excellent water there," he recollected, "and for some time after tried compressors, sitting baths, packing, etc., etc. Admired the fine air and country; found by degrees water taken as a medicine to be the most destructive drug I had ever tried, and then paid my tax to contemporary stupor and had done with it." Between 1849 and 1863, Darwin had uneven results from hydropathy, which he tried several times, at Malvern and other hydros. He was initially enthusiastic, pronouncing water treatment to be "a grand discovery" that "absolutely cured" him, but his optimistic assessment gradually changed to disenchantment, as he ceased to derive benefit from it.[69]

Herbert Spencer's experience with hydropathy may help to suggest why invalids who took their recuperation seriously came to lose faith in the medical claims of the water regimen. In 1849, his uncle, Thomas Spencer, whose health had been strained several decades earlier when he overworked himself as a Cambridge undergraduate, went to Umberslade Hall to see if Johnson could cure his bronchitis and chronic debility. The resulting improvement in his uncle's health persuaded Spencer to try Umberslade himself in the summer of 1854. It was a year before he suffered the strange cerebral sensations that he always subsequently described as his "breakdown," but he was experiencing "signs of cardiac enfeeblement" and thought he would test what hydropathy could do for him. Umberslade Hall was situated in a large park, with paths for walking, lakes for boating, and lanes for carriage rides. With these activities, and the frequently recurring baths, he wrote to his mother, time passed quickly, if not very interestingly. Already in 1854, however, Spencer could perceive the process by which hydros came to resemble vacation resorts rather than nursing homes. "Those who took baths presently came to be outnumbered by those who merely utilized the opportunities for amusement," he remembered in his autobiography; "until at length, the hydropathic element becoming comparatively unobtrusive, there have grown up all over the kingdom places in which people assemble to have games and drives and picnics and balls, to flirt and to make matches." None of those pursuits appealing to Spencer, he subsequently employed hydropathic methods—a shower bath or wet pack to induce sleep—in the privacy of his own home. In 1856, after John Bright spent eight weeks at Ben Rhydding, he came away suspecting that his stay there had been "altogether a mistake. The water treatment may or may not have been injurious to me," he wrote, "but the large company there was certainly most unsuitable for me."[70]

One could go on multiplying Victorian hydropathic histories, pointing to Tulloch's stay at Malvern in 1863, to Florence Nightingale's, or to Samuel Greg's, when he broke down following a strike at his Cheshire cotton mill in 1846. One could quote the psychologist and logician Alexander Bain, who found that his constitutional delicacy derived "great benefit from hydropathic treatment."[71] After a while, such exercises would become pointless. For every patient who praised hydropathy with gratitude, another could be found to denigrate its efficacy. By the late 1870s, however, despite the testimony of numerous loyalists, the denigrators were gaining the upper hand. The mainstream of Victorian medical opinion had, needless to say, never endorsed the water cure, identifying it with rampant quackery that jeopardized the medical profession's scientific credibility. In the final quarter of the nineteenth century, even the open-minded were inclined to agree.

Many developments contributed to hydropathy's fall from popularity. It certainly suffered from association with unabashed money-making schemes and the sort of commercial developments that Spencer chronicled. The emergence of private hospitals, or private wings of public hospitals, also undermined the water cure by offering middle-class patients the personal attention they had received at hydros, without the requisite several months of treatment.[72] No matter how attractive the hydropathic alternative to traditional medical practices, furthermore, the accumulating evidence that water by itself could not cure most, or even some, diseases demanded attention in the end. The Victorian public could distinguish between the temporary benefits derived from several weeks of relaxation, on the one hand, and permanent recovery, on the other. In any case, as massive drugging and bloodletting lost favor, the very need for alternative therapies became less urgent. Finally, in the opinion of many respectable clients, hydropathy was fatally compromised in 1876 by Gully's involvement in a much publicized murder case, for it was rumored that the charming elderly doctor was the lover of young Florence Bravo, whose husband died, under mysterious circumstances, of a lethal dose of tartar emetic.[73] Notoriety of that nature did nothing to enhance the reputation of a movement already full of shady characters.

Interestingly enough, the gradual demise of hydropathy as a formal, albeit unorthodox, system of medical practice by no means signaled the disappearance of water from the assortment of therapies employed by nerve-doctors and psychiatrists before World War I. Just as water had played its part in British medicine long before anyone had heard of Priessnitz, so it continued to find medical favor apart from hydropathic spas long after their vogue had passed. The staunchest enemy of hydropathy was still glad to prescribe warm baths for his patients, both in the interests of cleanliness and as an utterly nonaddictive soporific. Even the advocate of a very different approach to neurotic illness, Ernest Jones—Freud's devoted disciple— recommended trying hot baths or wet packs to induce sleep, "before resorting to hypnotic drugs."[74] If Priessnitzian hydropathy was irrelevant, or absurd, to the majority of doctors who treated shattered nerves in the Victorian and Edwardian decades, the kind of water therapy that could be applied in a domestic setting remained valuable to medicine regardless of fashionable fads.

The irony of nature therapy was precisely its status as a fashionable mode of treatment for the affluent invalid. Although abundantly supplied by nature, fresh air, water, sunshine, and variations of climate proved very costly to obtain. Even if he could afford the expense of a country or seaside holiday—just possible if he had rural relatives—it was the exceptional worker indeed who could afford to lose his job by quitting work for several weeks to recover from nervous exhaustion by nature's means. Even staying at home to rest was, for the same reason, impossible for artisans and laborers. Ocean voyages and foreign travel were simply out of the question for them, except in the rare instance of someone like Ben Tillett, who had supporters with money to spare. As James Johnson, for many years editor of the *Medico-Chirurgical Review,* had observed as early as 1827, when recommending travel abroad as a cure for "depression of spirits": "A few hundred pounds would be well expended by many of our rich countrymen, in applying this pleasant remedy to the mind, when soured and unpoised by the struggle after wealth, rank, or power!"[75] What options were available to his countrymen whose minds might be unpoised by the struggle to survive, but who lacked a few hundred pounds to secure the benefits of travel, were not his concern.

Even at the end of the nineteenth century, when numerous British medical men acknowledged the incidence of nervous breakdown and neurasthenic ailments among the working class, the modes of treatment they suggested had no relevance to the lives of the poor. The diet that Dowse prescribed for nervous patients in 1880, for example, definitely required ample means: he suggested choosing among oyster soup, a variety of fresh fish, beef, lamb, turkey, pheasant, partridge, asparagus, other fresh vegetables, and a variety of beverages, such as Chateau Lafitte and Amontillado sherry. Occasionally, the late Victorian medical literature carried a somewhat sheepish acknowledgment, like Allbutt's in 1884, that there existed comparatively few patients for whom doctors could "write the prescription—to take two months' holiday, to withdraw from all toil and care, and to live in good company on refined and delicate food." In general, however, the Victorian and Edwardian psychiatrist or nerve specialist thought in just those terms, designing treatments for prosperous nervous patients who could afford his services and bypassing the impoverished neurasthenics who could not. As the novelist and poet Amy Levy commented in 1888, with reference to the hero of her novel *Reuben Sachs,* a wealthy young Jewish barrister and aspiring politician who suffered a "nervous break-down": "If Reuben had been a poor man the doctors would never have found out that he wanted a sea-voyage at all." Hydropathists, it is true, made an effort to bring the water cure within working-class budgets. The *Water Cure Journal* in 1847 had publicized an attempt to "erect a Working Man's Benevolent Hydropathic Institution," and Ellis, the former lace merchant, actually opened the Free Private Hospital and Hydropathic Sanatorium in Tower St., London Fields, in order to introduce hydropathy among the London poor.[76] These endeavors were largely inspired by the desire to combat working-class alcoholism and dirt, but they encountered formidable obstacles in the length of time required for the successful conclusion of the water cure. The difficulty of obtaining water in working-class homes only increased the irrelevance of hydropathy to their inhabitants.

The choice of therapies available to these men and women was either the asylum, for cases of extreme depression, or drugs for the less disabled. Without being able to effect any significant alteration in working-class diet or hours of labor, medical practitioners who encountered milder cases of nervous exhaustion in infirmaries and out-patient dispensaries almost invariably had recourse to medication. As early as 1843, Daniel Noble warned that the laboring population of Great Britain was not well served by "the present *dispensary* system," which offered "little or no nursing in sickness, but excess of physic." Like their social betters, working-class men and women could be transformed into permanent invalids by drugs prescribed to fortify shattered nerves, but unlike affluent patients, the invalid poor had no range of therapeutic options. In admitting that the prognosis in neurasthenia depended, "more than in most diseases, on the patient's circumstances and surroundings," John Michell Clarke, professor of pathology at University College, Bristol, was merely making explicit in 1905 the social foundations on which the treatment of neuroses had rested throughout the nineteenth century. He was certain that those who could afford to stop working for a while and secure a change of scene for themselves had a far better chance of recovery from neurasthenia than those who could not.[77] Those who could afford the cost of treatment that addressed emotional needs as well as physical symptoms were, in short, likelier to feel better.

Even for middle- and upper-class patients suffering from nervous breakdown, however, the administration of psychotherapy was, at best, a haphazard business in Victorian and Edwardian medicine. Much of the time, psychotherapeutic practices, so basic to recovery as to escape notice, went unheralded. Doctors recognized their value, but generally considered them ancillary to methods of treatment predicated on physiological assumptions. Thus, for example, if bed rest and nourishment were judged particularly necessary to restore nerve force, the medical attendant's psychotherapeutic task simply involved persuading the patient to sleep and eat.

To engage the patient's mind in the curative process was, nonetheless, considered essential, and the effort to do so justified the long hours spent by medical men—particularly alienists and nerve-doctors—pursuing their moral mission. After the 1860s, as more pressing questions concerning the physical foundations of depression arose, British psychiatrists became more self-conscious about their psychotherapeutic methods and perhaps grew more fully aware of their own role as the model of mental health that patients were supposed to emulate. Schofield actually devoted an entire volume to the healing power of the doctor's own personality, in which he set forth the character traits of medical attendants that proved beneficial to their patients: "dignity, simplicity, brevity, decision, interest, sympathy, candour, naturalness, certainty, cheerfulness, hopefulness, good temper, courage, carefulness, patience, and firmness."[78] Nothing in this list comes as a surprise. Sick people want to hear, from someone who seems authoritative and confident, that they will recover; they want to be able to talk about their suffering to someone who will listen empathetically, but who can also put their minds at ease by telling them when their apprehensions are unfounded. These bland generalizations apply to all kinds of medicine and all kinds of illness. Victorian and Edwardian alienists thought they were particularly relevant to treating nervous breakdown, for cheerful demeanor, unfailing optimism, and persuasive firmness ranked as principal elements in the process of reviving the patient's inoperative will.

British psychiatrists simply proceeded on the assumption that the somatic and psychological avenues to treatment could coexist pragmatically, without occasioning ideological consternation. They tended to ignore theoretical puzzles in their daily work and treated patients empirically, according to whatever means seemed effective in each specific case. There was much that made excellent sense in this "therapeutic eclecticism," which allowed medical men to pick and choose among what one historian has called "little more than a highly heterogeneous 'grab-bag' of techniques."[79] Although alienists may have lamented that such trial-and-error methods reflected poorly on psychiatry, they were occasionally able to provide real benefit to their patients precisely through this approach. That they were not entirely helpless in the face of nervous breakdown may be traced to the common sense with which they shelved insoluble medical problems of mind-body interaction and tried virtually any therapy until, if lucky, they hit on one that proved conducive to the patient's recovery.[80]

The fact remains, nonetheless, that this commendable adaptability barely masked profound medical perplexity. Victorian and Edwardian doctors had no idea why some forms of therapy worked well on some depressed patients and had no effect, or a highly detrimental one, on others. Nor could they understand why the same patient responded rapidly to hydropathy, say, on one occasion, and on another grew worse under its regimen. The spontaneous improvement that many depressives experience, and the self-limiting nature of their illness in most cases, may mean that the kind of therapy employed does not make much difference, so long as it does not hinder "the natural processes of recovery from depression."[81] British alienists, consulting physicians, and family doctors before World War I were saying as much, although not quite so explicitly, when they called on the *vis medicatrix naturae*. They expatiated voluminously on the causes and cures of functional nervous disorders, but their fundamental grasp of neurotic illness was not much more penetrating than that of John Stuart Mill, one of their most famous patients, whose "view of the medical art . . . was, that it should restore a shattered frame by something like magic."[82]

5

Manly Nerves

The fact that shattered frames were just as likely to belong to men as to women caused Victorian psychiatrists no little difficulty in an era when the differences between the sexes were being relentlessly emphasized. The stereotypes that emerged are familiar to all readers of Victorian literature, for novels, poems, social criticism, anthropological analyses, medical texts, and a rich variety of commentary, in serious journals and the popular press alike, underscored the outstanding characteristics of each gender. Men appeared as rational and resolute, capable of violence but generally self-restrained, active initiators and purposeful competitors in the public sphere. Women, by contrast, were typically depicted as emotional and intuitive, tender caregivers, soothing sources of sympathy in the domestic sphere, but spectators rather than participants in the world beyond the home. The great problem with nervous breakdown, as medical men fully realized, was that it made a mockery of these very distinctions, reducing its male victims to passivity, removing them from business activities and public affairs, rendering them utterly indecisive. In short, nervous exhaustion brought men perilously close to the feminine condition. Thus the quandary that the disorder presented to Victorian and Edwardian doctors was interpretative as well as therapeutic, and they sought to resolve the difficulties against the background of significant alterations in British ideals of manliness during the course of the nineteenth century. The solution they achieved helped to confirm stereotypes of masculinity from which men crippled by severe depression could have only derived cold comfort.

The medical profession in these decades never attempted to deny the widespread incidence of nervous breakdown among men. It is utterly erroneous to assume that Victorian doctors perceived the male half of the human race as paragons of health and vigor, while assigning all forms of weakness to women. They could not have done so, even had they wanted to, for the evidence exposing male nervous vulnerability was too familiar to the Victorian public for pretense. Prominent cases, such as John Bright's withdrawal from politics in 1856 and 1870, merely confirmed private experience of incapacitated fathers, husbands, sons, brothers, and uncles, abundantly revealed in the pages of diaries, memoirs, and correspondence. Whether it was A. C. Benson recalling the "exaggerated depression of mind" suffered by his father who, as archbishop of Canterbury, was occasionally "forbidden by his doctors to get up, and lay . . . revolving many things and reviewing his own inadequacy, and the consequent downfall of the Church and the wreck of religion, till he was in complete despair," or the chronic depression of men far removed from national responsibilities, like Margaret Oliphant's brother Frank, who lived off her literary labors for six years, few Victorian families that produced literary remains seem not to have harbored a male relative with fragile nerves. Even working-class autobiographies from the nineteenth century frequently featured debilitated and demoralized fathers.[1]

Medical practitioners had long acknowledged a particularly male variety of functional nervous disorder—hypochondriasis. From the seventeenth century, that diagnostic label began replacing melancholy as the generic term for disorders involving low spirits, apprehensiveness, diffuse physical malaise, languor, irritability, and even pain. As humoral pathology, with its explanation of melancholy in terms of black bile, lost credibility, medical theorists had to find a new way to account for the baffling symptoms of depression, and hypochondriasis was gradually pressed into service. The term's origins stretched back to ancient Greek medicine, where *hypochondria* referred to the viscera located below the rib cage, specifically the liver, gall bladder, and spleen. In the seventeenth century, the pathological conditions associated with the disease concept called hypochondriasis were traced, often rather vaguely, to the "hypchondriacal organs," primarily the spleen, just as the seat of hysteria was usually identified with the uterus. Indeed, Sydenham insisted that hypochondriasis and hysteria were twin disorders, respectively the male and female counterpart of each other. Like his contemporary Willis, Sydenham, while not denying the involvement of the spleen, also recognized the role of the nervous system in hypochondriasis, and it was the nervous etiology that eventually predominated. Cullen's late eighteenth-century categorization of hypochondriasis as a neurosis became the orthodox interpretation in the nineteenth. As with all the neurotic disorders, Victorian medicine upheld, for as long as possible, the assertion that hypochondriasis was a genuine somatic disorder, whose specific origins still awaited discovery.

The psychological manifestations of hypochondriasis, however, also received their due medical acknowledgment. D. H. Tuke, quoting Cullen, observed in 1857, for example, that hypochondriacal invalids were "particularly attentive to the state of their own health, to every, the smallest change of feeling in their bodies; and from any unusual feeling, perhaps of the slightest kind, they apprehend great danger, and even death itself." During the second half of the nineteenth century, as confidence in locating the organic cause of hypochondriasis waned and as neurasthenia became the paramount functional nervous disorder, embracing all the physical and mental symptoms once associated with melancholy, hypochondriasis was increasingly confined to the meaning we give *hypochondria* today. As Schofield announced in 1902: "Neurasthenia used to be called hypochondriasis, being of course put down at first to that long-suffering organ the liver. The term 'hypochondria' is now reserved for a fixed delusive idea of some particular disease or local suffering."[2] He was a bit premature in his proclamation; until World War I, hypochondriasis, in its old denotation, continued to make occasional appearances in British medical texts, but it was clearly a relic from the past. For the rest of the twentieth century, the term *hypochondriac* has described someone tortured by irrational worries over health or morbidly obsessed with bodily conditions.

The dual meaning, somatic and psychological, implicit in the label hypochondriasis explains much of the ambiguity that surrounded the use of the term in

Georgian, Victorian, and even Edwardian medical writing. While the presumption of an anatomical foundation constituted the orthodox viewpoint until about the 1860s, and the suspicion of a purely mental derangement took hold thereafter, much blurring of hypochondriacal categories continued throughout the nineteenth century. Thanks to the careful studies of medical historians, we can understand how the various diagnoses of melancholy, hypochondriasis, hysteria, and neurasthenia, as well as the less precise ones of nervousness and nervous temperament, duplicated, amplified, or replaced each other over the centuries. With the wisdom of hindsight, it is easy to see that Victorian medical authorities who tried to draw tidy distinctions among them all were fighting a losing battle. Where hypochondriasis was concerned, their efforts managed largely to create confusion, from which only two points emerge with anything like clarity or consistency. In the first place, medical opinion reflected the old gender identification of hypochondriasis and assigned it primarily to men. While not barring women altogether from experiencing this particular neurotic affliction, virtually all the major nineteenth-century writers on the subject, including Rush, Prichard, Bucknill, and Tuke, and most of the minor ones, too, found it to be more common among men than women. Secondly, medical spokesmen concurred that a particularly devastating effect of hypochondriasis was enfeeblement of the will. Just like the man who suffered from shattered nerves, the hypochondriac appeared a passive, helpless victim, whether of physical dysfunction or of mental torment.[3]

If hypochondriasis was traditionally a man's malady, hysteria was a woman's, but even that most female of functional nervous disorders found its way into the medical scrutiny of masculine neuroses during the Victorian era. As the seat of hypochondriasis had moved from the viscera to the nerves, so the supposed uterine basis of hysteria had undergone a similar migration over the centuries. Once hysteria gained a place among the functional nervous disorders, its exclusive affiliation with women ceased to make medical sense; there was no reason that men, too, might not evince such bizarre hysterical symptoms as sensations of suffocation, temporary aphasia, and partial paralysis. The possibility of hysteria in men became the focus of heated medical controversy by the early nineteenth century, with traditionalists clinging to the uterine hypothesis in the face of an increasingly articulate opposition that marshaled increasingly solid evidence against it. No less an authority than John Conolly supplied vivid descriptions of male hysteria from his own medical practice. One gentleman, he recalled, "on several occasions . . . was suddenly seized with violent sobbing, gasping, . . . attended with a fear of immediate death by suffocation. During these attacks his face was flushed, the carotids pulsated strongly, and the heart was much disturbed. . . ." Other male patients likewise gave way to "fits of sobbing and crying, with palpitation, a weak pulse, a loss of muscular power, great dyspnœa, painful constriction of the chest, and fear of impending death."[4]

In general, however, Victorian medical authors hastened to minimize, rather than dramatize, the incidence of hysteria among their own sex. They did so primarily by stressing its comparative rarity and by linking it with effeminacy. Reporting the infrequent occurrence of male hysteria, Laycock commented in 1840 that the handful of male hysterics he had observed were scarcely robust specimens of manhood. "Of these, two were fat, pale-faced, effeminate-looking men; in the one the affection was attributed to malaria, and he had flabby wasted testicles. . . ." Another was a "pale and delicate'' youth. This approach remained standard for decades. In the 1870s, the gynecologist C. H. F. Routh remarked that, when a "previously strong-minded" man evinced hysterical symptoms, "it would seem as if he became effeminate in many of his mental emotions." One of the most revealing examples of British medical uneasiness over male hysteria appeared in 1885, in the *Medical Times and Gazette*. The author of an article on "The Systematic Treatment of Nerve Prostration," probably W. S. Playfair, recounted the story of a middle-aged gentleman who, for the past twenty years, "had suffered from one or other manifestation of hysteria." Having treated him according to the methods of Weir Mitchell's rest cure, having bossed and badgered him as befitted a patient with no apparent will of his own, the writer was obviously relieved to report that the therapy ended when "he was . . . seriously talked to as a sensible man—not driven like an hysterical girl— and from that moment he threw off his hesitation, and returned to the life of a healthy man. . . ."[5]

In the 1880s and early 1890s, when Charcot published more than fifty case histories of male hysterics—drawn largely from the ranks of sturdy artisans—British nerve specialists found yet another way to distance themselves from what one historian of medicine has aptly seen as the French psychiatrist's remarkable "diagnostic rapprochement between the sexes." It was not necessary to doubt the accuracy of Charcot's findings, for they were safely across the Channel. As Dowse complacently pointed out in 1889: "The Gallic nature seems to be of less enduring stability than that of the Saxon, and is more liable to exhibit exalted hysterical manifestations." More discreetly but for the same purpose, H. B. Donkin explained the discrepancy in the French and British national incidence of male hysteria by reference to "racial and social differences."[6]

By the time that Charcot's research gained currency in England, hysteria's somatic foundations had become as doubtful as those of hypochondriasis. The suspicion of shamming definitely clung to the hysterical neurosis by the final quarter of the nineteenth century, or, rather, the suggestion of malingering that had colored popular views of hysteria for decades began to find expression in medical texts. Here was a major reason for the reluctance of British doctors to tar their male compatriots with the hysterical brush. No such connotations yet clung to neurasthenia, however. The impeccably physiological origins that Beard assigned to his neurotic creation, problematic though they proved to be, made it a far more respectable affliction for British men. The neurasthenic diagnosis, Donkin admitted, was "often applied to cases where hysteria might seem a term of reproach," especially "by those who insist on confounding hysteria with malingering."[7]

In the face of evidence documenting the extent of severe depression among men, British medical practitioners were accordingly willing to concede the depredations of neurasthenia among their sex. They even acknowledged that it broke down the "strong, well-built men" together with "those of more delicate organisation." "We find sufferers amongst the greatest and the least, the noblest and the basest, the strongest and the weakest," Schofield reminded his readers in 1902. Neurasthenia struck, furthermore, in the prime of life, rarely afflicting the very young or the elderly, but characteristically incapacitating victims between the ages of twenty and fifty years. This, of course, was the period of greatest productivity for a man, the time when he was likeliest to exhaust his nerve force in hard professional effort.[8] With the highest nerve centers deprived of adequate energy, the stage was set for an appalling personal tragedy from which some men might never fully recover.

Victorians evaluated that tragedy very differently as their attitudes toward masculinity changed during the nineteenth century. An object of sympathy in the earlier years became a source of embarrassment in the later ones. What was excusable at first became disgraceful in the end. There were, of course, no tidy chronological divisions, and even within any single, brief span of time the term *manly* carried a heavy load of diverse physical and moral connotations, some of them determined by class and education, some by geography. Bourgeois and aristocratic concepts of masculinity intermingled throughout the century, now one dominating, now the other, but neither ever in complete eclipse. Working-class contributions to the national ethos of manliness were slight, but even these were not entirely negligible. Among all the conflicting definitions and nuances, certain trends are distinct enough to justify partitioning the nineteenth century into three periods, each of which witnessed obvious transformations in the prevailing views of manhood.

Ideals of manliness in the first half of the century are the most difficult to characterize in general terms. A complex merger of late Georgian and early Victorian beliefs produced, at one and the same time, a continuation of many late eighteenth-century assumptions and a reaction against them. Cheyne's influence still echoed down the decades in that association of civilization and sensibility which encouraged so much fashionable indisposition in the Georgian years, when men of feeling, easily moved to tears, congratulated themselves on their cultural superiority over more stolid brethren. In 1831, James Johnson, now physician extraordinary to William IV, was virtually paraphrasing Cheyne when he demonstrated English superiority over the French by advertising his countrymen's vulnerability to the "Wear-and-Tear Complaint,"[9] a strange form of chauvinism to which Beard succumbed, on behalf of the United States, later in the century. The cult of sensibility that the Victorians inherited had, however, encountered romanticism on its way into the nineteenth century and was substantially altered in the process. Romanticism incorporated the cult into a philosophy of life and art that transcended the narcissism and presumptuous posturing of Georgian "hypochondriacks," most of whom suffered only superficially and were a breed apart from the genuinely afflicted victims of severe depression. British romanticism, no matter how tame it seems in comparison to continental excesses in the Wertherian mode,[10] nonetheless celebrated the inner man, the creature of feelings and passions whom the Augustans had preferred to keep concealed. The romantic hero was not the frequenter of salons, dazzling all with his ready wit and cynical repartee, nor a man of merely cultivated sensibilities; he was the artist yearning for freedom, love, beauty, and, above all, insight. His inward vision allowed him to penetrate, beneath surfaces, to the heart of things and thereby justified the intense introspection to which he gave free rein. The examination of his own thoughts and feelings no more branded him as useless or effeminate than did the pursuits of philosophers in this period, who relied on introspection as an essential tool for probing the functions of the mind.

Self-analysis of an even more rigorous sort was promoted by the evangelical movement of the late eighteenth and early nineteenth centuries, which deeply influenced, not only English Protestantism, but the moral climate of the whole country throughout Victoria's reign. In the struggle to recognize one's own imperfections and to experience religious rebirth, the evangelical Christian was supposed to endure virtually constant self-scrutiny, not in the spirit of self-absorption, but in a relentless mood of self-criticism. The call to serve mankind, a powerful motive behind much evangelical activity, required self-sacrifice and self-control, the trait which, above all others, came to exemplify mid- and late-Victorian views of manliness. Evangelicalism, with its moral rectitude and emphasis on self-restraint, can readily be portrayed as a reaction against the excesses of romanticism; yet an intense expression of feeling, particularly in a religious context, was by no means distasteful to the evangelical cast of mind, which harbored no love for rationalism. Indeed, the marriage of mind and heart, after a period of somewhat artificial separation, may go far to explain the potency of evangelicalism in nineteenth-century England.

It was a union that characterized attitudes toward manliness until about the 1850s. The combination of "godliness and good learning," inculcated in the public schools, stressed an approach to manhood that accommodated both intellectual rigor and emotional tenderness. The academic attainments prized by the great Anglican schoolmasters and clergymen of the era were nurtured in an atmosphere saturated with profound spiritual commitment to the Christian faith and redolent with extravagant emotionalism. Passionate attachments between boys, and even close relations between masters and students, were condoned as part of the process that molded a mature man from the materials of exuberant youth. The effusive expression of feeling, including the copious flow of tears, was not deemed unmanly, nor was the exchange of embraces between men. For Thomas Arnold, who, as headmaster at Rugby from 1828 to 1842, played a leading role in propagating the early Victorian ideal of Christian manliness, that ideal had nothing to do with physical prowess. It was a quality of maturity, of intense seriousness about moral responsibility, devotion to religious beliefs, and intellectual pursuits. It was a willingness to eschew frivolity and to work for the greater good instead of the selfish goal.[11]

Throughout the first four or five decades of the nineteenth century, this moral definition of manliness had to contend against an older, secular tradition that did not derive its inspiration from schoolroom or pulpit. The Regency sportsman, the military hero, and even the village athlete offered an alternate model of manliness in which physical valor claimed paramount importance. Popular literature stressed the muscular male paragon, whether a superb horseman or a brave soldier, far more than the Christian gentleman. If the moral exemplar was the product of middle-class culture, shaped by evangelicalism, the ideal of physical manliness derived from a rural and upper-class lifestyle, of which the village champion provided a working-class reflection. There was much that was brutal and coarse in the British tradition of muscular manliness at the start of the nineteenth century, but its ethos also embraced concepts of honor and chivalry that eventually facilitated a kind of merger with its apparent antithesis—the sober middle-class husband and father.[12] Although the head of a bourgeois household was not physically active, he was supposed to be economically busy, securing through his own worthy endeavors a comfortable existence for his wife, children, and other dependent relatives. Nor was he allowed to forget his duty to protect the weaker members of society, even as his own affairs flourished. By the fifth decade of the century, with evangelical values gaining converts among the aristocracy and gentry, the moral vision of masculinity came to predominate over the physical. There could be no doubt that manliness was inextricably bound up with Christian earnestness, with dutiful service to God and humanity, as well as to one's own family, and with kindness toward the needy and helpless.[13] It was not a view that sanctioned the cult of sensibility in any of its excesses, but it could treat with respect and pity unfortunate men tormented by depression.

Early Victorian attitudes toward male nervous collapse were not, in fact, strikingly dissimilar to those characteristic of the late Georgian age. In both eras, parodies of extravagantly sensitive men and women showed that public opinion was wise to the hypocrisy that often lurked beneath the veneer of sensibility; in both, the medical profession thus experienced some trouble in countering the popular assumption that hypochondriasis was an imaginary complaint, not a real physical malady. In both, doctors and patients alike recognized that unbridled passions, left to rage within the human heart, could destroy the mind, but counsels of composure and self-discipline nonetheless warmly endorsed the capacity to feel deeply and sincerely. While nerves that reacted too rapidly to stimuli were considered potentially incapacitating, and a man at the mercy of every fleeting sensation was risible, men and women in the late eighteenth and early nineteenth centuries honored susceptibility to tears and the open expression of true emotion. They valued a certain nervousness in their heroes, if nervousness signified a quickness of response to outside impressions and, therefore, an ability to share what others suffered, a delicacy in one's personal relations. They saluted the empathetic man who felt life's buffetings and was matured, but never toughened, by them. A degree of gentleness was permissible in men, as the popularity of Dickens's hero, Nicholas Nickleby, created in the late 1830s, confirms. Indeed, with his combination of resolute action and emotional tenderness, Nickleby is a perfect expression of contemporary, middle-class ideals of manliness. Perhaps the early Victorians had merely adopted sentimentality in place of sensibility, but their moral climate did not force men to suppress feelings. In such an atmosphere, a man who suffered nervous breakdown could expect to receive sympathy, not scorn.[14]

By the middle of the century, such sympathy was qualified by other considerations. The late 1840s until the 1870s formed a transitional phase in British attitudes toward manliness, when the free expression of male emotions and the ready vibration of masculine nerves were neither discredited nor applauded. The label *muscular Christianity,* which has been somewhat misleadingly applied since the 1850s to the ideals of manhood that emerged at this time, suggests an exaltation of brawn over brain that was not at all the intention of Charles Kingsley and Thomas Hughes, the two men most closely associated with the new mentality. Both men took their religion very seriously; the spiritual and ethical import of their work should not be obscured by the praise they heaped on the value of high-spirited, rough-and-tumble games for boys.[15] The influence of their writings nonetheless played a significant part in promoting the importance of physical hardiness in men, regardless of social rank.

While kind-heartedness remained compatible with manliness, bodily vigor was the necessary accompaniment. From mid-century, the manly man—even in middle-class opinion—enjoyed physical, as well as moral, health. After all, when Kingsley, an Anglican clergyman, wrote in 1849 that his goal as a teacher was "to train not scholars, but men; bold, energetic, methodic, liberal-minded, magnanimous," he was extolling a condition of physical vitality as much as a state of mental alertness. Although Kingsley and Hughes still placed the muscles at the service of the mind, a new tone was definitely beginning to color the way in which the Victorian bourgeoisie evaluated masculinity.[16]

Muscular Christianity, in fact, represented the confluence of moral manliness with the emphasis on robust physique that belonged to the tradition of sporting manliness. For all their complacent confidence that they were morally superior to the upper class, members of the middle class at mid-century were still attracted to the lifestyle of their social betters. They were also, however, registering the impact of medical exhortations to seek fresh air and exercise. What is striking about the intensified middle-class respect for physical fitness in these years is precisely the prominent place occupied by the nerves in its articulation: explicitly and implicitly, medical authors, novelists, and social commentators all used the nerves in order to express changing public attitudes toward manliness. Interpreted in a far less complimentary light than before, nervous sensitivity was coming to be viewed as a severe liability in a man.

Maudsley made the case, strongly and nastily, when he published a memoir of his father-in-law, John Conolly, in 1866. Referring to the late psychiatrist's "fine sensibilities," so unfitted to deal with "life's harsh realities," Maudsley mused:

> In some respects, I think, his mind seemed to be of a feminine type; capable of a momentary lively sympathy, which might even express itself in tears, such as enemies, forgetful of his character, might be apt to deem hypocritical; and prone to shrink from the disagreeable occasions of life, if it were possible, rather than encounter them with deliberate foresight and settled resolution. . . . A character most graceful and beautiful in a woman is no gift of fortune to a man having to meet the adverse circumstances and pressing occasions of a tumultuous life.[17]

By the standards of Maudsley's generation, any manifestation of sensibility, acceptable to Conolly's in a restrained form, now bore a damning stigma of effeminacy. To his son-in-law, Conolly's nervous sensitivity and sympathetic nature, which at times made him irresolute, in effect emasculated him.

The same point was illustrated, with chilling effect, by Wilkie Collins in *The Woman in White* (1860). In that most sensational of Victorian sensation novels, Mr. Fairlie is one of the most subtly sinister male characters in nineteenth-century fiction. He is permanently, and mysteriously, an invalid; "the doctors don't know what is the matter with him, and he doesn't know himself what is the matter with him," but all are agreed in blaming the nerves. Throughout the novel, he uses his agonizingly sensitive nerves, which can tolerate only the dimmest light and the softest sounds—as if he suffered from perpetual migraine—to avoid his responsibilities toward his niece Laura, around whom a diabolical plot has been woven by her husband. Collins, himself tortured by pain of a possibly neuralgic nature, deftly played with his readers' stereotypical gender expectations and well understood that a man who constantly flaunted his nerves to evade life's duties would, in their eyes, be no man at all. Fairlie's feet "were effeminately small, and were clad in . . . little womanish bronze-leather slippers." He had "white delicate hands" and "a frail, languidly-fretful, over-refined look." It is hardly necessary for Fairlie, at a later encounter in the novel, to describe himself as "nothing but a bundle of nerves dressed up to look like a man." The reader already knows that he is not a real man.[18] He is frightening specifically because he is so epicene, like a mythical monster belonging to neither gender, and manipulating his sexlessness to further his selfishness. Lacking a woman's caring heart and a man's capacity to act, he languishes in his cocoonlike room, shielded from life. By contrast, Walter Hartright, the appropriately named hero of the novel, overcomes his own nervous sensitivity to rescue Laura and triumph over her enemies. He is an important fictional figure from this transitional period of Victorian manliness. No athlete or muscle-bound adventurer, he is a thoughtful, compassionate man, strengthened through suffering, very much in the mold of David Copperfield, whom Dickens had created in 1849–50. That both characters were artists—Hartright a drawing teacher and Copperfield a writer—further illuminates their ties to an older, almost outdated, romantic heroic model.

In the new model taking shape during the middle decades of Victoria's reign, the equation of nervous sensibility with effeminacy automatically carried with it the hint of disablement. Sensitive nerves no longer implied quickness of mind or acuteness of sympathy, as in the past, but a virtual assurance that the man so cursed would be unable to play his allotted part on the public stage. When Bright had to retire from politics in 1870, following his second nervous breakdown, Walter Bagehot commented in *The Economist:* "We have only to express our regret at his retirement, and to wonder at the strange dispensations of Providence, which mixed a fine, and to some extent incapacitating, thread of nervous delicacy in a mind so healthy, so vigorous, and on most points so emphatically robust." Bagehot was not unsympathetic to Bright's weakness, but he knew that it effectively removed him from the center of Liberal politics. Four years later, J. M. Fothergill offered a medical endorsement of Bagehot's views. "A mind at once powerful and coarse of fibre has a great advantage, as regards sheer endurance, over another mind of finer fabric," he commented. "Here the fineness of the fibre is a simple unmitigated disadvantage. The fine quality of the material . . . is nothing else than a drawback as regards its power of enduring tension. . . . Polish means loss of substance, put it as we may!"[19]

By the final quarter of the nineteenth century, the ambiguities that obscured the mid-Victorian views of manliness had largely dissolved. While even in this late period, attitudes toward masculinity contained inconsistencies, a generally coherent image of the ideal British man had emerged. It appealed to both the middle and upper classes, and perhaps even to the respectable reaches of the working class. It developed hand in glove with the cult of athleticism at the public schools, and subsequently among the British public at large. While public school headmasters might still delight in praising the young Christian gentlemen whom their institutions molded, the reality was far more secular.[20] The boys themselves, seconded by the most vocal part of British national opinion, idolized athletic conquerors. What had begun as an aspect of elitist educational reform in the 1860s—the imposition of compulsory school games—reached far down the social scale by the 1880s and

1890s. The mania for spectator sports and the establishment of local athletic clubs helped enthrone physical grace, courage, pluck, and toughness among the highest qualities of manhood. In the end, sporting manliness, stripped of its Georgian exuberance, had the last word; vestiges of the Christian manly model had been incorporated in a new synthesis, where they were scarcely recognizable.

The manly ideal that flourished in the late Victorian years did not lack its own ethical content, but its moral message had little to do with religion. Whatever lip-service the heroes of the epoch paid to Christianity, it was clear that the fervent belief of Kingsley, Hughes, and many others, that manliness was inconceivable without sincere Christian faith, no longer prevailed. The code of manly honor at the end of the nineteenth century was, to all intents and purposes, pagan. If it echoed evangelical motifs, with its call for self-control and self-sacrifice, it sounded more stoic than spiritual.[21] The specifically Christian virtues of humility, forgiveness, and charity were conspicuously absent. What element of love survived in this virile ethos was not directed toward the opposite sex, but took the form of devotion to comrades—a loyalty derived from schoolboy friendships. Love of country, likewise, figured prominently among the prerequisites for manliness in this era of strident patriotism. Never had serving one's country, dutifully but stylishly, been more ardently esteemed. The militarism pervading masculine values stretched from the public schools, where rifle corps drill was initiated in the late 1850s, to working-class communities, where the Boys' Brigades attempted to inculcate a similar spirit, albeit with only limited success. The Boy Scouts, needless to say, played an Edwardian version of the same tune.[22] In this climate, it is hardly surprising that achievements of the intellect, already struggling in the 1850s and 1860s to hold their own against athletic triumphs, sank all the lower in the public esteem. The mind busily at work, after all, indulged in too much thought, whereas the best sort of men excelled in disciplined action, responding swiftly to danger and obediently to orders.

The resolute, steadfast man of action could depend on his nerves in moments of crisis. It was nervous stability that Dowse, Donkin, and countless other medical men wanted to extol as a national trait at the end of the century, not liability to the "Wear-and-Tear Complaint." Exalted sensibility was merely, as one public health expert remarked in 1883, evidence of disease, an unnatural state similar to hysteria.[23] Men had to restrain their feelings now; "the training of civilised man, especially in this country," Mercier remarked in 1892, was "directed towards the suppression of the display of emotion." Already in the 1870s, a Frenchman, Jules Verne, had slyly caricatured the new trend in British views of manliness, creating in Phileas Fogg an apparent monument to lack of feeling. When Verne called the hero of *Around the World in Eighty Days* "this man of nerve," he was clearly describing nerves of the steely variety.[24] At the end of the century, they were the only kind worth having.

Thus late Victorian and Edwardian men learned from all kinds of sources about the paramount necessity for self-control in every aspect of their character. It is perfectly true that self-discipline was a hallmark of mature masculinity, at least the middle-class variety, throughout the nineteenth century, even before Victoria ascended the throne, but by the end of her reign it exemplified a hard kind of manliness, purged of tender mercies and ready for combat, whether on the playing fields, in commercial enterprise, or on imperial battle grounds. The expansion of the British empire in the same period contributed heavily toward solidifying this concept of masculinity. With territories to govern and defend around the world, and with jealous rival nations eager to find the weak spot in British armor, the country did not need men lacking determination, whose unreliable nerves were likely to exhaust themselves under stress, and whose will could not exert iron rule over potentially devastating emotions. Nor were the qualities of manly vigor and tenacity needed only in soldiers and statesmen, for relentless international competition was as much commercial as military. Finally, the teachings of social Darwinism in these years combined with the older self-help philosophy to offer an urgent warning: only those who made themselves strong for life's struggles would prevail, at home or abroad.[25] Veneration of success, always a dominant motif in Victorian culture, now struck a harsher note, verging on utter intolerance of masculine failure. Men who succumbed to depression, Maudsley noted in the early 1890s, were "sufferers not doers"; each was "conscious the while how weak it seems on his part to give way to womanish wailings and in amaze at the abject wretch which he is."[26]

Here was a secular creed that took a man's public success or failure as an accurate index of his private worth and judged worth in terms of economic value, not moral worthiness. The model of manliness supported by such a creed could not countenance nervous breakdown; it had become a social as well as a personal catastrophe, for a man incapable of action failed both his own dependents and society as a whole. By withdrawing male victims from the public arena and relegating them to invalidism, nervous collapse underscored their lack of purpose, initiative, energy, and will. The depression that prostrated them thus denied their very claim to manhood.

When medical writers analyzed nervous breakdown in men during the final years of the nineteenth century, they focused more and more of their attention on the failure of will, with considerably less interest in the failure of nerve force that allegedly set the terrible process in motion. The man with shattered nerves was not merely pitiable, but also somehow blameworthy, and by the Edwardian period male neurasthenics were becoming almost as suspect as male hysterics. Whereas in the past, medical authorities had interpreted a paralyzed will as the *result* of nervous exhaustion, they now began to suspect that it belonged at the origins of the disaster. In the years preceding World War I, although few British specialists in mental and nervous illness actually imputed moral insanity to depressed men of socially respectable rank, many did suggest some degree of moral weakness in these patients, an insufficient sense of personal responsibility, a penchant for shirking and shamming. The "diminished brain resistiveness" that lay behind a breakdown, Clouston flatly asserted in 1906, was "closely related to will power and moral capacity." Neurasthenia's characteristic "decrease of will-power," another medical commentator had pointed out a few years earlier, was always associated with "feebleness of character."[27] Baffled by the fact that some victims of nervous breakdown apparently resisted recovery, alienists and nerve specialists seized on constitutionally deficient will as the only possible explanation. It was an explanation that cast no credit on the sufferer.

The experience of World War I confirmed the tendency to associate male nervous breakdown with infirmity of moral purpose. While it is true that the massive incidence of shell shock among soldiers forced British psychiatrists to revise their opinions about the rarity of hysterical symptoms in men, the vast majority of the public saw in shell-shocked servicemen cowards who demonstrated their lack of moral fiber by avoiding duty and repudiating patriotism. The Great War may have demonstrated beyond doubt that psychological agents can, by themselves, utterly disrupt the body's functions, but the lesson did nothing to mitigate the certainty that nervous breakdown unmanned men.[28] The legacy of the changing attitudes toward manliness that developed during the nineteenth century, and crystallized in the first two decades of the twentieth, still profoundly informs current thinking about gender. Today, when depression is "estimated to be two or three times more common in women than in men," medical opinion partly explains that statistical difference in terms of masculine reluctance to acknowledge feelings of inadequacy and despair—an unwillingness even to discuss emotions—for fear of appearing weak and effeminate. If one can trust the recent studies that show the discrepancy to be narrowing,[29] it may be that the late twentieth century has rediscovered some value in male sensibility, a quality widely accepted and, within limits, applauded two centuries ago.

Although medical practitioners altered the emphases in their explanations of male nervous weakness in order to keep pace with prevailing public opinion, they were consistent in distinguishing the nervous collapse that befell men from the same disorder in women. The issue, needless to say, became particularly urgent in the second half of the nineteenth century, not only because popular conceptions of masculinity became more relentlessly scornful of male invalidism, but also because the feminist movement in these decades appeared determined to call in question the existing relationship between men and women. Medical wisdom, backed by evolutionary theory,[30] rigorously upheld the physical and mental superiority of the male sex, but unless the much-vaunted masculine strengths could be made to encompass nervous weakness, paradoxical though that reconciliation seemed, the case for male supremacy was very insecure indeed. Even in the first half of the century, however, British doctors made it very clear that male nervous breakdown was substantially different from the female variety.

In general, Victorian medical spokesmen established that difference by proposing an entirely distinct etiology for the masculine and feminine versions of shattered nerves. They contended that the very nature of female physiology, dominated as it was by the reproductive organs, made the exhaustion of nerve force a constant likelihood in women, who could exercise little control over the disaster. Men, by contrast, were architects of their own suffering, for they typically brought on nervous prostration through overwork. Since men had to compete day after day in the market place; since they toiled year in and out on behalf of their families; since they coped with physical strain and intellectual demands that women never faced, it was entirely understandable that excessive exertion occasionally led to the depletion of their nervous resources. Men broke down, according to medical argument, because they simply overdid the striving for achievement that society honored. They needed strong medical admonition to mend their ways, but they did not merit condemnation. There was no reason for men to feel ashamed of breakdown on these terms, and these were the terms that doctors employed for the majority of their male patients, for most of the nineteenth century.

The argument was not original to the Victorian era. A causative distinction between male and female nervous disorders along the lines of business pressures on the one hand and reproductive physiology on the other had been drawn in the eighteenth century;[31] the conviction that men succumbed to nervous collapse because of the strenuous effort to achieve economic success was implicit in many of the Georgian texts that traced the rise of neurotic illness to the advent of modern life, lived at breakneck speed. It was already a familiar medical theme by the 1830s, when Edwin Lee's *Treatise on Some Nervous Disorders* made the point that men became "extremely liable to mental and nervous affections, in consequence of their being more exposed to numerous sources of cerebral excitement in the worry and turmoil of the world."[32] After mid-century, the point was made with particular insistence.

Every kind of late Victorian and Edwardian doctor who treated nervous disorders joined in the act. Routh, a gynecologist, traced to overwork "the general symptoms of exhausted nervous power" in men. Crichton-Browne, an alienist, explained such "gross structural lesions of the nervous system" as inflammation of the brain and cerebral tumors—which he insisted were more common in men than in women—by one simple fact: men participated in "the struggle for life," while women led "comparatively tranquil and sheltered lives." Seymour J. Sharkey, a neurologist, found the incidence of neurasthenia greater among men than women because "the mental and physical strains which men have to bear are greater than those which befall the opposite sex." Even Conan Doyle, erstwhile medical practitioner, reported that Sherlock Holmes's "iron constitution showed some symptoms of giving way in the face of constant hard work of a most exacting kind," and he ordered his detective to "surrender himself to complete rest if he wished to avert an absolute breakdown."[33] By the early twentieth century, this long-sustained attempt to excuse male nervous exhaustion was, admittedly, beginning to wear thin. It could not, as we have seen, prevent family, friends, and even medical attendants from imputing moral inadequacy to men who suffered from crippling depression. For more than a century, however, it had helped to sustain male dignity in the face of humiliating impotence.

Medical practitioners may have been especially keen to promote the overwork hypothesis because large numbers of their professional colleagues suffered from depression, in its mild and severe forms. In 1860, Bucknill took advantage of his presidential address to the Association of Medical Officers of Asylums and Hospitals for the Insane to urge his fellow psychiatrists to preserve their "mental health by frequent periods of relaxation and variety," for he was convinced that prolonged efforts to help their patients seriously jeopardized the alienists' own mental stability. Nor were they alone among doctors in their vulnerability to breakdown. J. Strahan informed the British Medical Association in 1885 that "one in every ten" of the neurasthenic patients in the country was "said to be a medical man." Indeed, the previous year, Dowse had advised neurasthenics to seek treatment from a "physician who has suffered from nervous exhaustion himself," in order to receive the most sympathetic and knowledgeable care. Dowse hinted, not only that he himself had coped with neurasthenia, but that it would not be hard to find numerous other doctors with similar expertise. The spectacle of nineteenth-century medical men struggling against profound melancholy recurs frequently, both in their professional writings and in personal recollections, like the memoir of John Deakin Heaton, a prominent mid-Victorian physician in Leeds whose low spirits partook "of the nature of 'blue devils'." Countless cases of nervous exhaustion, or at least irritability, among Victorian doctors were attributed to the physical demands of an overly active professional life and the unceasing mental alertness demanded of a medical practitioner. The profession was not, apparently, exaggerating the dangers of depression in its ranks, and Martin Grant-Smith's sad death was not an isolated case: statistics from the late nineteenth century revealed doctors to be among the occupational groups most prone to suicide in England and Wales—a situation contemporaries ascribed not just to the ready availability of poisons in their work, but to its ongoing mental strain.[34]

Victorian and Edwardian doctors, however, were not inclined to claim any monopoly on nervous breakdown among men engaged in business and professional pursuits. The arguments that brought mental fatigue and the intense pressures of modern life to bear on medical men weighed just as heavily on lawyers, politicians, financiers, merchants, and other middle-class breadwinners. In 1876, B. W. Richardson, a physician much concerned with public health issues, singled out four groups of men likely to succumb to "diseased conditions originating in excessive nervous activity" and "arising from excessive mental strain." "We find these phenomena," he reported, "mainly . . . (1) in persons engaged in art, science, or literature: (2) in those who are engaged in political life: (3) in those who are occupied in commerce, exchange, and speculation: (4) in the too laborious scholars or students." Frederick MacCabe, who had served as medical superintendent of the Waterford County Asylum, offered a more precise list, focusing on the higher ranks of civil servants, barristers, journalists, and men involved in commercial enterprises as the ones most liable to feel the ill effects of mental strain and overwork. Dowse whittled the categories down to one, suggesting that clergymen "seem to be more prone to these attacks of brain exhaustion than others," although he could not explain exactly why.[35]

The reason medical men focused on the professional and commercial middle classes when considering male nervous exhaustion was twofold. In the first place, such groups formed the majority of male patients who sought psychiatric counsel outside the asylum. Medical familiarity with their cases easily led to the conclusion that the disorder was most prevalent among them. Psychiatrists and nerve specialists consequently never doubted that these were the men most subject to tensions that ended in overwork and nervous collapse. In the second place, middle-class male susceptibility to severe depression seemed to demonstrate with particular decisiveness the close interaction of physical and mental causes in producing illness. Medical writers emphasized that men from the middle strata of society endured more than demanding work that often denied them adequate relaxation and sleep; they were also constantly subjected to an element of worry that made earning a middle-class income uniquely debilitating for a man. Unlike members of the aristocracy and gentry who had an assured position in society, and equally unlike the workers who had no claim to social standing at all, the middle-class husband and father was always negotiating a place for himself and his family on the social ladder. The need to secure a sufficient income, to keep competitors at bay, and to meet financial obligations all pressed the more ponderously on him, adding a weighty load of anxiety to the daily business of managing his affairs. It was precisely the combination of overwork and worry that could prove his downfall, for a carefree man wisely responded to the physical exhaustion that followed long mental exertion by resting. There was, as Graham Brown insisted in 1905, an "automatic arrangement by which the brain of the healthy man, working hard but free from anxiety, limits its labour in time to prevent catastrophe or indeed any noteworthy injury." In the presence of anxiety, however, "the appetite fails" and "sleep becomes broken and fitful." Nervous tissue, already nearly drained of force, could receive neither the nourishment nor the rest necessary to restore its strength.[36]

Brown's explanation for the onset of nervous collapse was essentially the same as James Johnson's for the "Wear-and-Tear Complaint": "over-strenuous labour or exertion of the intellectual faculties, . . . conducted in anxiety of mind."[37] Throughout the more than seventy years that separated the writings of these medical practitioners, doctors featured the pathological partnership of overwork and worry in their warnings to middle-class men. The place of emotional triggers in the medical theory of male nervous breakdown not only bore testimony to the interpenetration of mind and body, but also helped medical commentators understand why a man might flourish under gruelling work at one point in his life, while breaking down under lesser effort at another. The difference clearly lay in the victim's state of mind and feeling on the two occasions.

The emotions that Victorian doctors enumerated as precipitants of male nervous prostration brought no shame on the patient. Among those most often mentioned were feelings of anxiety related to money—the anguish of failed investments and financial reversals, or merely the fear of such calamities, exacerbated by the expectation of losing social status as a result. In a culture that worshipped Mammon, it was perfectly understandable for a man to be highly sensitive to personal economic indexes. The frequency with which medical practitioners linked "embarrassed pecuniary circum- stances" and financial worries to male nervous collapse, or even graver mental illness, amply illustrates the close metaphorical relationship between notions of monetary wealth and nervous resources, as well as the bond between money and manliness, which became increasingly tight during the course of the nineteenth century.[38] Other stock emotions that were recognized as highly hazardous to a man's nervous stability, if combined with overwork, were intense professional or personal disappointment, grief or bereavement, and any form of powerful shock. The demise of a beloved wife, child, or parent not infrequently served as the final blow in a string of stressful circumstances that pushed even restrained, self-disciplined men over the edge of nervous collapse. The extreme sentimentality with which Victorians ap- proached the subject of death, at the end of the nineteenth century as much as at the start, afforded men some leeway for the expression of feeling in this regard, without diminishing their reputation for manliness. Severe trauma was an equally excusable cause of male breakdown. Conan Doyle knew that readers would forgive Sir Henry Baskerville's shattered nerves after the unfortunate baronet was attacked on the moors by a fiendish hound.[39]

The overwork-and-worry theory of male nervous breakdown was both plausible and acceptable, and it is no surprise that it became the standard explanation that Victorian and Edwardian biographers invoked when the subjects of their work suffered from profound depression. Virtually all of Bright's biographers before

World War I dealt with his illness of 1856 in identical terms: it was, they insisted, the result of incessant parliamentary labors made more onerous by his intense unpopularity during the Crimean War. As the most famous of them, G. M. Trevelyan, observed: "Bright used to attribute his illness to the misery which he had endured during the Crimean War. And indeed no reason can be assigned for it, other than overwork and public cares."[40] Readers of an Edwardian biography of Landseer were told that the artist's breakdown in 1840 arose from the pressure of too many canvases to paint, heightened by the strain of trying to cut a fine figure in the elevated social circles that lionized him. In his article on the historian Henry Thomas Buckle for the *Dictionary of National Biography,* Leslie Stephen told how the death of Buckle's mother in 1859 delivered a "shock to delicate nerves, already weakened by overwork, . . . so great that his sister even feared for his brain." Sometimes biographers assumed that overwork alone was the culprit. In his biography of J. S. Mill, published in 1882, Alexander Bain simply refused to accept Mill's own assertion that "spiritual or mental" causes lay behind his "mental crisis of 1826." "There was one thing he never would allow," Bain explained, "which was that work could be pushed to the point of being injurious to either body or mind. That the dejection so feelingly depicted [in Mill's autobiography] was due to physical causes, and that the chief of these causes was over-working the brain, may I think be certified beyond all reasonable doubt." Faraday's nineteenth-century biographers, too, saw nothing but overwork behind the long period of incapacitation that kept the physicist out of his laboratory for much of the time between 1840 and 1844.[41]

The sufferers themselves were often glad to blame overwork for their incapacitation. Sully, for one, was certain that his breakdown occurred when he unduly emphasized "Goethe's well-known maxim of '*Ohne Rast*' [without rest], to the comparative disregard of '*Ohne Hast*' [without haste]." Galton was equally sure that the reason why he "broke down entirely in health" during his third year at Cambridge was that he "had been much too zealous, had worked too irregularly and in too many directions." "A mill seemed to be working inside my head," he recalled. "It was as though I had tried to make a steam-engine perform more work than it was constructed for, by tampering with its safety valve and thereby straining its mechanism." In a curious simile, which featured Galton as both the machine and its operator, he managed to minimize his own responsibility for the misfortune that befell him as a young man. Machines, after all, are not at fault for breaking down. Interestingly enough, Sarah Austin, the wife of the early Victorian jurist John Austin, who was overwhelmed by depression for much of his adult life, described and exonerated her husband in similar terms: he was, she wrote, "an immense, powerful, beautiful machine, without the balance-wheel, which should keep it going constantly, evenly, and justly."[42] For his part, Spencer, who during his worst periods also suffered from "abnormal sensations" in the head, never doubted that he broke down in 1855 because he had ruthlessly overtaxed his brain for some months previously, in the effort to complete his *Principles of Psychology.* Hours of writing every day were interrupted only by hours of pondering the next passages to be written, he reported in his autobiography. "Practically, therefore, the mental strain went on with but little intermission." According to his account, a photo taken of him a few months before his breakdown confirmed, in his "worn anxious look," that "waste was in excess of repair.'' Despite the agony that Spencer endured for much of the rest of his life, he seemed particularly pleased with the cause that he felt sure had prompted his collapse, as if proud to have been beaten down by his own soaring intellectual ambition. A man who sought to reveal and synthesize the underlying principles of biology, psychology, sociology, and ethics was, clearly, tempting fate.[43]

Spencer's pride in his own fall revealed the darker side of the Victorian Gospel of Work, which aroused considerable concern among medical practitioners. For all their glorification of work and their hatred of indolence, British doctors, together with the general middle-class public, harbored deeply ambivalent feelings about the credo of self-help and individualism that they theoretically celebrated. This ambivalence colored their attitudes toward debilitated men as much, in its way, as their shifting views of manliness. On the one hand, their allegiance to the work ethic and their contempt for idleness enabled them to express sincere sympathy for the man brought low by his own strenuous efforts. Yet, on the other, they had grave doubts about the extent to which competition, and the promotion of individual enterprise, should be allowed to run rampant through society. Perhaps more than other members of the great Victorian middle class, medical men fully understood the potentially devastating impact of a system of values that apparently gave free rein to ambition. Throughout the nineteenth century, as we have seen, they regretted the ''intense efforts for success,'' the pursuit of wealth as ''the only end of life,'' which frequently bestowed on the alleged victor ''a weakened mind and diseased body.''[44] In striving to outstrip his rivals, a man could obviously destroy his own health, but more was involved than merely personal defeat. The individual who ruined his nerves in the quest for wealth and advancement was also socially dangerous, as a comparison between nature and civilization suggested.

It was customary among the middle classes in nineteenth-century Britain to hail competition as a progressive agent in modern society, altogether different from the brutal struggle to survive in nature. After all, competition allowed natural abilities to flourish, opening doors that old systems of patronage kept shut. Certainly the triumph of the fittest in professional or business rivalries could have its tragic side, but few members of the Victorian bourgeoisie would have conceded that the losers in human communities suffered the same fate as nature's failures. The medical profession was not alone, however, in wondering whether civilization was merely a thin veneer through which humanity's latent savagery could burst at any moment. Unbridled competition, a too blatant striving for success regardless of human expense, offered a disturbing glimpse of that very brutality, which, in effect, dehumanized the competitor. It was a theme that perturbed novelists and poets, biologists, and contributors to the nascent social sciences as well. The world of Victorian businessmen had too much of the jungle about it for anyone's peace of mind. When medical advisors warned men against the dangers of overwork, they were not only taking precautions for their patients' welfare; they were trying to hold at bay malevolent forces that could tear society apart. Their high praise for business enterprise or professional initiative, for the self-discipline that kept a man at work instead of indulging in frivolous pleasures, was always balanced by a fear of excessive ambition hazardous to one and all. Self-denial, twisted out of shape, could become the promotion of self to monstrous proportions, just as self-help, carried too far, could hurt others badly. Under control,

competition was an impetus to civilization, but unchecked, it could reduce humanity
to its frightful, natural state.

Even the man who exhausted only himself, without destroying others in the
process, was a menace to society. To have drained his nervous energy was to have
made himself incapable of producing any work of value. Middle-class Victorians
came to believe that health was not only a personal necessity for success, but a social
obligation as well, at all levels of society. When, as a member of the Royal
Commission on the Poor Law from 1905 to 1909, Beatrice Webb treated "illness . . . as a public nuisance to be suppressed in the interests of the community,"[45] she had the working classes in mind, but Benson took a more inclusive view.
"Tracing back the constitution of society to its origin, he saw that it was clear that
every one owed a certain duty of work to the community."[46] Much of the misery that
enveloped Benson during his long periods of depression came precisely from his
inability to work, to fulfill his duty to society, try as he might. Besides denying its
victims the pleasures of social intercourse, nervous breakdown was antisocial in
depriving society of its victims' labor, both mental and manual. The antipathy to male
nervous exhaustion that, by the early twentieth century, appeared in hints of moral
irresponsibility and malingering arose from this realization. Even in the mid-
Victorian years, when laissez-faire principles commanded the widest allegiance, the
rampant individualism that undermined a man's health and social utility earned little
approval.

In their sustained deprecation of overwork, nineteenth-century medical practitioners reflected a conflict between personal and communitarian goals, between
autonomy and altruism, that Victorian culture never resolved. In the early phases of
the Industrial Revolution, the British middle classes revered the solitary entrepreneur
and the heroic trail blazer. In the later stages, with many more men jockeying for the
riches proffered by industrialization, the stakes were considerably higher; competition became more destructive, and the Promethean individual had to be restrained.
The man with too strong a will might prove as detrimental to society as the invalid
with none at all. Ironically, in the process of destroying himself through his own
excesses, the former turned into the latter, or so medical wisdom averred.

If Victorians and Edwardians regarded overwork as a potential form of social
misconduct, how much more anxious was their response to various expressions of
male sexuality that were likewise believed to end in nervous exhaustion. Here, too,
the tension between individual needs and social demands provided a paramount
theme in all considerations of the subject. The unrestrained erotic drives of the natural
man posed obvious dangers, not only to social order, but to the personal well-being of
the civilized man who harbored a wild beast within himself. When medical practitioners cited sexual causes of male nervous breakdown—and, needless to say, they
never mentioned patients' names when they did so—they were certainly not excusing
the victims from accountability. Unlike overwork, sexual excess was not an essentially admirable reason for nervous collapse; the age of the hero as rake or lusty
wencher was finished by the mid-nineteenth century. Nonetheless, to argue that too
much sexual activity, even of a deviant sort, explained some cases of male nervous
exhaustion was still to distance male from female weakness, for voracious sexual

appetites were very rarely attributed to middle-class Victorian women. The man who made himself an invalid through sexual excess had himself chosen that mode of self-destruction. He was still an active participant, not a passive victim, in his own downfall.

The history of human sexuality has been a growth field ever since 1976, when Michel Foucault published *La Volonté de savoir,* the first volume of his unfinished *Histoire de la Sexualité.* In the intervening years, historians have analyzed the language of sexuality in different cultures as modes of discourse whose agenda has far less to do with the reproductive organs than with generalized anxieties about class or gender relations and the pace of social or economic change. In responsible hands, this can be an illuminating approach, but it tends to minimize the very significant degree to which the human body *was* the focus of interest when the subject of sexuality was broached. People wanted to know how their reproductive systems worked; amid much ignorance, superstition, and varying amounts of shame, there was also simple curiosity. The Victorians were no different in this respect. Despite the misinformation that medical attendants so copiously served up, they were just as eager as their patients to understand the mysteries of human sexuality. Unquestionably, many of their pronouncements only perpetuated old myths and, to our way of thinking, cruelly exacerbated needless fears. Nor is there any doubt that, when they patrolled the field of sexual behavior, they were striding forth as moral disciplinarians and social watchdogs, not as scientists. Yet it deserves to be emphasized that, beneath the threatening rhetoric, the *specific* goal of Victorian doctors was not social stability, but the happiness of individual men and women, preferably with each other. That social benefits could be expected to accrue from personal ones made the latter all the worthier to pursue.

It is also important to stress that the sexual repression of the Victorian era, to the extent that it did in fact exist, fell heavily on men—that women were certainly not the only ones to suffer the emotional consequences of prevailing sexual attitudes. Where masculine sexual behavior that led to nervous collapse was concerned, more printer's ink was devoted to censuring the practice of masturbation than to any other topic. A significant portion of the British medical profession joined in the international panic over "self-pollution" that gripped Europe and the United States in these decades. While, after mid-century, most of the attention in England focused on the habit among schoolboys, adult males still continued to receive their share of advice and admonition, as they had in the earlier years of Victoria's reign. Until homosexuality became a growing public concern at the end of the nineteenth century, masturbation enjoyed a dubious distinction as the most antisocial and selfish of vices. Not only was it a solitary habit that cut the perpetrator off from society, but it represented nonprocreative lust devoid of any redeeming social purpose. What was worse, it was believed to violate the Old Testament injunction against a man "spilling his seed on the ground," although the Biblical sin in question may actually have been coitus interruptus. The masturbator, in any case, represented the self-centered individualist at his worst, either unwilling or unable to exercise self-control. Few Victorians would have challenged the *Journal of Psychological Medicine and Mental Pathology* when it argued in 1851 that "many men lose their true manly character, by unnatural stimulation of the reproductive organs." Nor was manly character the only loss attributable to habitual masturbation. Far more serious was the eventual cerebral impact of the disgusting practice, Victorian psychiatrists warned. Forbes Winslow was certain that self-abuse could cause softening of the brain and eventual loss of reason. Many of his colleagues concurred; masturbatory insanity enjoyed a respected place in the increasingly elaborate Victorian taxonomy of madness.[47]

The whole array of medical reasons for deploring masturbation found expression in an article that Crichton-Browne contributed to the *West Riding Lunatic Asylum Medical Reports* in 1874. What strikes today's reader as the absurdity of the argument bears testimony to the depth of Victorian feeling against this secret sin. After asserting that acute dementia was, without question, "often brought on by masturbation," Crichton-Browne continued:

> Anaemia, loss of strength, and nervous exhaustion result from it [masturbation], and after these come forgetfulness, heaviness, and listlessness, which grow and grow until fatuity is attained. I have under my care now a young man who, from time to time, deprives himself of "energic reason and a shaping mind" by this abominable and inveterate vice. When he gives way to it he becomes acutely demented; when he abstains from it, or when by medical interference it is rendered impracticable for a time, he rallies quickly, and is sharp and lively, and an expert tailor. The chief tailor can always tell from the way in which he handles his needle and thread if he is conducting himself with propriety or otherwise. When the former, his fingers move nimbly and his eyes are intent on his work; when the latter, he gazes dreamily about him and dwells drawlingly on every stitch.[48]

The indictment was clear: masturbation meant daydreaming and self-absorption; it curtailed and eventually destroyed a man's productivity; it sapped his vitality and at length rendered him idiotic.

It was obvious to Crichton-Browne that masturbation caused nervous prostration. The belief that excessive stimulation of the reproductive organs could tax an individual's supplies of nerve force to the point of breakdown was a familiar concept and helps to explain the zeal with which Crichton-Browne, Maudsley, and numerous other alienists preached against the solitary vice. Virtually all forms of debility, in the broadest meaning of the word, could be elucidated in terms of chronic masturbation. Extreme fatigue, impaired memory, baldness, deafness, blindness, atrophy of the male sexual organs, impotence, consumption, epilepsy, and, of course, lunacy, not to mention nervous irritability, neuropathy, and neurasthenia, were all laid at the door of masturbation by one medical writer or another. That many of these manifestations of weakness were particularly construed as symptoms of excessive involuntary seminal loss—a pathological condition known as spermatorrhea and often traced to self-abuse—was yet another link in the chain inextricably binding the notions of nervous and virile potency together.[49]

The attention which the nineteenth-century British medical profession paid to spermatorrhea has inspired some recent historians to propose the concept of a "spermatic economy," like that of a nervous economy, to connect Victorian sexual anxieties with the bourgeois emphasis on thrift and self-restraint. According to this theory, sexual activity, even marital intercourse, was a source of constant worry to middle-class men, for they equated loss of sperm with loss of power—not just the power to engender offspring, but the power to create wealth, to accomplish their share of money-making. They believed that they had to conserve semen, just as they had to save money, so the argument goes, lest they should find themselves physically and, in due course, financially powerless.[50] One cannot help wondering if economic considerations really did, in fact, flash through the ardent lover's mind; just as medical advice to conserve nerve force was not likely to stop men from overworking, until it was too late, cautionary tales involving seminal loss probably had little significant impact on sexual behavior. Where they *were* influential was doubtless in their ability to induce guilt after the fact, particularly where an "unnatural" act like masturbation was involved. It would have been difficult indeed for a Victorian masturbator to avoid the conclusion that his despicable habit deprived his "body of something vital,"[51] specifically semen, nerve force, and manliness.

Much of the medical profession, throughout the nineteenth century, sought to frighten men away from masturbation by depicting the dreadful consequences of spermatic profligacy and its resulting train of ever more alarming nervous and mental disorders. Quack practitioners, too, enthusiastically spread the alarm, all the while puffing the properties of their own special salves and medicines to restore potency. Some young men were even driven to commit suicide by the combination of guilt and shame at their own enfeebled condition. Whatever the reason for sexual impotence, or for wasting illnesses that had nothing to do with the reproductive organs, Victorians could be readily persuaded that self-abuse was the cause. There are terrible stories of men suffering from serious organic complaints who, full of remorse, claimed responsibility for their plight—a claim that their medical confessors rarely disavowed. Equally unpleasant are the accounts of operations occasionally performed on masturbators, such as removing the prepuce, or the description of devices, like penile rings, employed to obstruct the practice. British medical men, however, did not show the same zeal for these punitive measures as did their American counterparts. Except in asylums, where lunatic masturbators might be surgically restrained, British doctors preferred to curb masturbation, and what they considered the related problem of nocturnal emissions, by moral suasion, or scare tactics, rather than surgery and mechanical equipment. The moral approach, after all, might appeal to the will and end in restoring manly self-control.[52]

Masturbation obviously had its uses for the Victorian medical profession. It provided a convenient causative hypothesis that, like depletion of nerve force in general, distracted attention from the doctor's frequent inability to offer meaningful therapeutic assistance and concentrated instead on the patient's presumably wayward conduct. It may actually have offered some perverse comfort to patients who chose to blame themselves for mysterious, nameless maladies, rather than feel victimized by forces beyond their control. Even false confessions can afford some sort of psychological relief.[53] Yet it is too easy for us today to relegate the Victorian preoccupation with masturbation to a form of gamesmanship, played by doctors and patients alike.

There is no reason to doubt that those medical practitioners who crusaded mercilessly against masturbation were impelled by a genuine belief in its power to work great evil. Since the very start of the eighteenth century, a steadily increasing number of books, pamphlets, and articles had exposed the mental and physical damage supposedly wrought by onanism, as masturbation was generally named.[54] By the mid-Victorian decades, the chorus of panic-mongers had reached a particularly shrill crescendo, in which doctors were joined by a brigade of miscellaneous spokesmen for morality. Just why anxiety about masturbation attained almost obsessional proportions at this time is by no means clear, although the explanation, as usual, lies somewhere in the conjunction of cultural trends with social, demographic, economic, and scientific developments. The rejection of Georgian sensuality, the conflation of moral and physical health, and the emphasis on self-discipline in Victorian definitions of manliness all contributed to the campaign for continence; so, too, did long engagements and marriages delayed for economic reasons, although this practice was not unique to the nineteenth century.[55] Finally, the slowly expanding knowledge of the human nervous and reproductive systems promoted intensified speculation about the influence of sexual behavior on the mind and nerves, not to mention the impact of emotions on the sexual organs. Whatever the precise combination of causes, the Victorian medical campaigners against masturbation prided themselves on protecting society from a potentially lethal habit and on saving individual men from blighted lives. If they caused intense anxiety and mental suffering along the way, the end surely justified the means.

Not all British doctors agreed. Particularly from about the 1870s, despite mounting pressure to combat masturbation in the schools, a number of Victorian and Edwardian medical men opposed the alarmist response to onanism, at least with regard to adult male patients. A significant strain of common sense in British medical opinion rejected extravagant claims about the destructive effects of masturbation, for which no persuasive evidence existed, and refused to acknowledge spermatorrhea as a disease.[56] One of the leading spokesmen for this point of view was Sir James Paget, a prominent London surgeon affiliated with St. Bartholomew's Hospital, who held appointments to the royal family. In 1870, he delivered a clinical lecture on "Sexual Hypochondriasis" in which he sought to bury once and for all some of the more egregious myths about male sexual diseases. Symptoms of fatigue, including "incapacity for mental exercise," "defect of will," and "restlessness at night" were not indications of something seriously wrong with a man's reproductive organs, he insisted, but were problems of nervous origin. He found nothing unusually harmful about masturbation as a form of sexual activity and was particularly reassuring about nocturnal emissions, which he considered perfectly normal. No less a figure in the medical world than Hughlings Jackson likewise denied that masturbation could cause mental illness, while Schofield, the nerve specialist with something to say about everything, considered masturbation "greatly overrated" as an exciting cause of functional nervous disorders.[57] Voices of moderation never attract the audiences that prophets of doom can draw, and it is not surprising that historians have paid far more attention to the second than to the first where Victorian reactions to masturbation are involved. The solitary sin, signifying utter loss of self-control and the defeat of the will by base animal passions, *did* exert a powerful hold on some segments of the Victorian imagination; it was not, however, the only way in which Victorians and Edwardians were capable of thinking about male sexuality.

The same divide in medical opinion regarded other modes of sexual behavior that were believed to drain a man's supplies of semen and nerve force, leaving him a useless, irresolute wretch. Heterosexual relations obviously aroused very different sentiments from those provoked by unproductive and unnatural sexuality. Hatred and fear of masturbation or sodomy did not necessarily, or even customarily, translate itself into disapproval of sexual relations between men and women. Yet even here, even among doctors for whom the idea of human sexuality caused no tremors of alarm, the concept of excess—that omnipresent object of Victorian dread—molded the terms of discussion around the opposite poles of intemperance and moderation.

That sexual overindulgence could exhaust and weaken a man was a medical view dating back at least as far as Hippocrates,[58] and the Victorians wrought no fundamentally new variations on the theme. Fornication, needless to say, was publicly anathematized, but too frequent sexual activity within the bonds of matrimony also provoked medical protests, for not only did it threaten the husband with nervous exhaustion, it likewise represented the collapse of self-control and the triumph of man's animalism over his spiritual nature. Some medical opinion assumed that the male sexual instinct was a force too predatory and uncontrollable to be denied, but most practitioners urged men at least to try self-restraint. Even William Acton, the self-proclaimed expert on male and female sexuality, never quite decided whether the masculine sexual urge was capable of continence or not.[59] Menacing and unstable, it loomed in the Victorian imagination, threatening to destroy the conventions and compromises on which society depended. When medical advisors cautioned that sexual intercourse, too often pursued, could end in functional nervous disorders, they were working to achieve the same control over male sexual aggression as they sought over male economic aggression: to restrain it within bounds, for both public good and private health.

As with masturbation, heterosexual excesses were blamed for the full range of neurotic illness, from mild hypochondriasis to incurable madness. The lack of consensus as to what degree of activity actually constituted excessive venery never stopped a voluble section of Victorian medical opinion from issuing warnings and denunciations. The appearance of neurasthenia on the scene, furthermore, only encouraged medical literature in the admonitory vein. Beard himself identified a particular variant of that disorder as sexual neurasthenia, and a number of British doctors were quick to publicize the connection between sexuality and the new category of neurotic disease. "Neurasthenia may be a sequel of any exhausting disease," wrote James Ross, a Manchester physician, "but it is generally caused by overwork and worry, or by sexual and other excesses." Strahan explained that the morbid fears so familiar to neurasthenics indicated, not just general debility, but "sexual exhaustion. Sexual excess, of whatever kind, nearly invariably produces them in the end, and is their most common cause." Maurice Craig's observations in 1905 may summarize this school of thought in the years before World War I:

> The sexual variety of neurasthenia is perhaps one of the most frequent types. The patient believes himself to be impotent, and not infrequently adds to his mental distress by reading quack literature on the subject. Spermatorrhœa may be a prominent symptom, and the frequency of the emissions may further tend to weaken the patient. Lack of confidence interferes with the due discharge of daily work; the patient becomes introspective, and may, if untreated, develop acute depression with suicidal tendencies.[60]

It was easy for Craig to accuse quacks of irresponsibly frightening impressionable, neurotic men. He did not acknowledge the extent to which legitimate medical authorities, by relentlessly underscoring the dangers of sexual excess, must have magnified the guilt and despair felt by men whose nervous breakdowns featured temporary impotence, even if their private lives had been blameless. Nor did any medical man before World War I concede the strange inconsistency that undermined the cogency of his views about nervous collapse and sexual overindulgence. Implicit in the condemnation of unrestrained venery was middle-class disapprobation of the alleged promiscuity of the lower classes and the sexual profligacy of the upper. Yet there was, in fact, remarkably little medical discussion of nervous exhaustion from sexual causes at either extreme of the social scale.

If some doctors chose to emphasize the dangers of too much sexual stimulation, however, there were others who stressed the hazards of too little. It is simply not true that the Victorians had lost the ability to enjoy sexual intimacies as fully and freely as had their Georgian forebears. A crushing burden of shame and ignorance doubtless marred the happiness of many men and women, as had been the case before the nineteenth century, but the Victorian banishment of sensuality from the public sphere by no means signaled its removal from the private. The historiographical debate on this subject within the past twenty years or so may reveal more about the debaters than about the Victorians, since many of the latter kept silent about the most personal events of their lives.[61] What *does* form part of the historical record is the widely articulated medical opinion that sexual relations were healthy and, indeed, essential for most men. Sexual potency was, implicitly if not explicitly, an essential aspect of all the Victorian and Edwardian definitions of manliness. The ability to create, to be a molding influence in the world, was inextricably connected with the idea of man as the dominant sexual partner. To be a man, virtually by biological definition, was to sire offspring.

There was no question, from the medical viewpoint, that a man's nerves suffered from excessive sexual abstinence. Doctors who wrote on hysteria in men often noted that prolonged chastity or enforced celibacy could give rise to hysterical symptoms, a belief that echoed the classical interpretation of hysteria in women.[62] Writers on neurasthenia proposed a similar argument, citing the unmarried state as a relatively common cause of neurasthenic symptoms and suggesting marriage to cure many a young man's nervous debility. The advice that the prominent surgeon T. Spencer Wells gave the shattered Symonds in 1864—after Acton had cauterized him through the urethra for painfully swollen genitals—must have been heard countless times in consulting rooms around Great Britain. "He impressed upon me," Symonds recollected, "the theory that marriage ought not to be regarded as a matter of idealized passion, but as the sober meeting together of man and woman for mutual needs of sex, for fellow service, and loyal devotion to the duties of social and domestic life in common."[63]

The vast majority of middle-class couples in Victorian and Edwardian Britain would have applauded Wells's vision of domestic happiness within marriage. Sometimes it was placed in a specifically religious context, as when Elizabeth Blackwell, the first woman listed on the British medical register and a self-styled "Christian physiologist," wrote in the 1880s that "there is nothing necessarily evil in physical pleasure. . . . The sexual act is really a divinely created and altogether righteous fulfilment of the conditions of our present life." More frequently, medical authorities left divine approbation out of the discussion and dwelt on the physiological ramifications of sexual gratification, about which they felt more knowledgeable. They all agreed, needless to say, that marriage was the framework in which such pleasure should occur. Wells, it is true, suggested that Symonds take a mistress, if marriage did not suit his plans; the havoc that celibacy was wreaking on the young man's constitution demanded strong and unusual measures, Wells believed. He made it clear, however, that marriage was the preferable course of action, and no reputable medical man recommended the bohemian lifestyle as a matter of policy to sexually frustrated bachelors. Clouston spoke for the entire medical profession when he asserted, without equivocation, in 1906:

> There is only one natural mode of gratifying sexual *nisus* [desire] and reproductive instinct, and only one truly social arrangement—that of marriage—while there are many unnatural methods. Science, sociology, and Christianity are at one in their conclusions and prohibitions. If natural law is not obeyed we have emotional instability, impairment of manliness and of such social virtues as modesty, purity, control of imagination, and true chivalry. It will be observed that I am not now pressing any conventional or moral rules or any social or religious dicta, but the laws of body and mind and purely scientific facts. If those laws are broken we find arrested nervous energy, less capacity for work, tendencies to nervous excitement with frequently arrested growth of the body.[64]

Although other Victorian and Edwardian medical practitioners might have distinguished scientific facts from moral precepts more successfully than Clouston, few would have challenged his paean to the health-giving properties of sexual relations between husband and wife.

The healing powers of marital sexuality were celebrated beyond the consulting room, not just in the ecstatic letters exchanged between Charles Kingsley and Fanny Grenfell, his betrothed, but in more restrained circles, too. Beatrice Webb's family, the Potters, were pillars of upper-middle-class respectability and not known for indulging in overt displays of sensuality; Herbert Spencer was as passionless a man as one can imagine. Yet Richard Potter, Beatrice's father, and Spencer felt no embarrassment in identifying the likeliest cure for the latter's nervous disorders. In the winter of 1856, Spencer wrote to his good friend: "You are doubtless perfectly right in attributing my present state to an exclusively intellectual life; and in prescribing exercise of the affections as the best remedy. No one is more thoroughly convinced than I am that bachelorhood is an unnatural and very injurious state." Some time later, Huxley echoed Potter's advice, recommending that Spencer "should try what he facetiously termed gynœopathy: admitting, however, that the remedy had the serious inconvenience that it could not be left off if it proved unsuitable."[65]

Spencer readily confessed his loneliness, telling Potter that since boyhood, as an only child, he had "been longing to have [his] affections called out." "I have," he confided, "been in the habit of considering myself but half alive; and have often said that I hoped to begin to live some day." His autobiography makes it clear that he was happiest when he felt part of some family circle, and his secretary, Walter Troughton, likewise attested to Spencer's need for companionship of a more than casual nature. It is extremely touching to read about his request to Mrs. William Harrison Cripps (one of the married Potter daughters) "for the loan of two of her family" in the late 1880s and the extreme solicitude he showed to Judy, aged ten, and her brother Standish, aged eight, during the several weeks that their visit lasted. Despite the disapproval of their nurse, he gave them warm underwear, enriched their diet, and substituted hot baths for the cold or tepid ones to which they were accustomed. In his autobiography, however, Spencer did not dwell on the absence of affection in his life—the lack of intimate friendships and familial bonds of love—as a contributing cause of his prolonged illness. When his doctor, W. H. Ransom of Nottingham, urged him "never in future to live alone," Spencer interpreted the advice to mean that his brain needed occasional distractions from unremitting labor in order to forestall another "physiological diasaster."[66] He did not consider that the disaster might have been in some sense psychological and that overwhelming loneliness, personal unhappiness, and a profound feeling of social isolation may have contributed to the insomnia, the inability to concentrate, and even the nameless physical discomforts that ruined much of his life.

It is pointless and presumptuous of us to blame the Victorians for not possessing psychological insights which belong to a post-Freudian era and which may, in fact, themselves be jettisoned by a future generation of psychiatrists. Nor should we forget that Victorian and Edwardian medicine provided a serviceable somatic explanation for male shattered nerves, in the depletion of nervous energy through overwork, indulgence in assorted excesses, or the effects of trauma. With such a theory on hand, the search for any other was largely wasted effort. What persuasive alternative could skeptics have provided, in any case, at a time when purely psychological explanations enjoyed no credibility? Although nineteenth-century medical practitioners conceded the profound impact of mind and body on each other, and specifically underscored the potent role of emotional strain in triggering nervous breakdown, the emotions they routinely identified in this context were not individualized, but rather followed certain conventional lines. It is the formulaic tone of so many nineteenth-century psychiatric analyses that disappoints today's readers, no matter how sincere their effort to accept Victorian psychiatry on its own terms.

The silences of Victorian and Edwardian commentary on male nervous collapse are most deafening to late twentieth-century ears in cases where young men, just embarked on adulthood, were concerned. A significant number of them broke down at this stage in their lives, often at university or just after completing their studies: Benson, Symonds, Galton, Sully, Ruskin, Mill, Joseph Lister, and Arnold Toynbee are among the best known of those who suffered prostrating depression in their early twenties, but there were countless others.[67] William Stainton Moses, for example, who eventually abandoned the Anglican ministry to become a spiritualist medium, experienced a breakdown shortly before his final examinations at Oxford in the early 1860s, so that he had to settle for a pass degree, and Ransom, Spencer's medical advisor in the mid-1850s, was "specially fit" for that task, having celebrated the attainment of highest honors on *his* examinations with a "collapse from which it took a long time to recover."[68] Indeed, while the social response to the breakdown of young men on the threshold of independence altered with the changing cultural attitudes toward manliness, the nervous vulnerability of that age group does not itself seem to have varied much over the decades. Whether one looks at the 1820s, when

Mill's crisis occurred, or at the end of the Edwardian decade, when Toynbee broke down, there are cases of young male adults whose deep depression interrupted progress toward career goals and disappointed parental hopes.

Medical practitioners recognized that the advent of responsible adulthood could be a trying time for young men, especially of the middle classes, as they faced the need to prove themselves professionally and financially. Sir William Gull pointed out in 1874 that he occasionally saw cases of anorexia nervosa in male patients between the ages of sixteen and twenty-three, while in the same year Elizabeth Garrett Anderson, a pioneer among female doctors, observed that many men broke down at university because of the pressure to excel at examinations that determined "pecuniary rewards" and fellowships. These, in turn, could "affect a man's whole after-life." Edwardian medical commentators found young men more predisposed to neurasthenia than older ones, for it was a disease that typically appeared "after the person leaves school and has a certain amount of responsibility."[69] Clearly, the explanation of breakdown implicit in these comments depended on the standard overwork-and-worry hypothesis, with the combination of elements varying only slightly from case to case. The victims themselves, as we have seen, together with their families and friends, generally concurred.

Students of Victorian lives today, however, look for something more. We are interested to note that, contrary to the account in his autobiography that blamed overwork for shattering his nerves before he could even compete, Galton actually broke down *after* taking the Cambridge mathematical examination and failing to achieve the first he so intensely coveted. We remark that Toynbee's collapse in 1910, while an Oxford undergraduate, came shortly after his father had been committed to a mental institution and his mother had decided to break up the family home. Toynbee collapsed on her sofa, as he admitted, "in the extreme edge of hysteria," receiving electrical massage. The treatment "was so potent," he wrote to a friend, "that it fused my nerves." (He was not so ill that he failed to note "what a whole new field of metaphor electricity gives.")[70] Ruskin's parents may have attributed his breakdown in 1840, during his undergraduate years at Oxford, to "the disastrous effect of excessive studying," but current scholarship is more inclined to censure the parents, for their fierce possessiveness and inability to let Ruskin find new objects of affection.[71]

In the late twentieth century, interpreters of the depression suffered by young men in Victorian and Edwardian England tend, in fact, to stress the areas of potential conflict between the son and his parents, particularly his father. Assuming that certain domestic situations created tensions in the nineteenth century, as in the twentieth, they argue that these were particularly explosive within the Victorian middle-class home, where the father's authority rested on a formidable foundation of moral and economic power, and where offspring and parents were not distanced from each other by the child-rearing methods characteristic of upper-class families. Yet if paternal authority was held to be legitimate, so the argument goes, it was all the more galling to a young man eager to find his own voice. Resentment, love, guilt, and fear all seethed together within him, as he contemplated the divergence between his own needs and his father's power. The perception that enormous family aspirations rested on a son's shoulders could, furthermore, create intense bitterness, as well as a crippling terror of disappointing those hopes. The self-reproach and self-hate that any anticipation of failure could induce were as potent as the ambivalent sentiments aroused by the desire to rebel against familial restraints and to escape to a freer environment. The tragedy for many young middle-class men in the nineteenth century was that the only environment holding any promise of such liberation was the sickbed. Nervous breakdown allowed them to opt out of the conflict, enabling them to express dissent from parental goals and values without overt confrontation. By withdrawing from the field of competition, the young invalid gained a kind of power over his father. At the same time, however, shattered nerves terminated incipient rebellion and punished the offender, not only by reducing him to further dependency, but by placing him under the control of yet another authority figure—the medical attendant.[72]

This psychologically plausible, and very neat, scenario provides a framework into which many of the youthful nervous breakdowns mentioned here could fit comfortably. Sully's breakdown in the early 1870s, for example, may well have been related to his departure from paternal goals, and the uneasiness that step aroused in him. Although his father, a devout Baptist businessman, had first intended Sully to join the family firm and then allowed him to study for the Baptist ministry instead, Sully himself had come to realize that his gifts and interests lay in the utterly secular study of the mind. In 1866–67, the completion of his B.A. degree from the University of London, in conjunction with the Baptist College in Regents Park, had already caused "a depressing reaction, and the sense of drifting from ancient moorings," which he attributed to the strain of mental labor and the shaking of his religious faith. By the early 1870s, however, the strains were even more severe. He had determined on a career that he knew distressed his father, and he thus sensed all the greater need to prove himself, with all the greater dread of failure. He had no very ample source of income, although he had recently married; he had definitively severed his ties with past beliefs and associations, and was trying to establish himself among London's intelligentsia. The long period of education behind him was now supposed to bear fruit, and the pressure on Sully was palpable.[73]

A striking case of filial rebellion, wretchedness, and nervous instability appears in the diary of Jeannette Marshall, the daughter of the London surgeon John Marshall, whose career encompassed some of the highest honors the medical profession could offer in the late Victorian period, including the presidencies of the Royal College of Surgeons, the Medico-Chirurgical Society, and the General Medical Council. His son, also named John Marshall, had gone up to Trinity, Cambridge, in the late 1870s, without any clear idea of what he wanted to do in life, but with parental certainty that he would distinguish himself academically, probably winning a Trinity Fellowship. His mood swings, from intense vitality to extreme lethargy, worried his family while he was an undergraduate, and his increasingly hostile behavior finally provoked a confrontation in 1879, after his twenty-first birthday, when he seems to have experienced some sort of personal crisis. As his older sister noted in her diary: "He behaved in a very rude & disrespectful way to M[ama]., & at last was so insulting that she complained to P[apa]., who took him out in the carriage & gave him a good talking to. J. wept & sobbed like an infant of four, said no one liked him, that he wished he was dead, had been miserable for years, & so-forth, going on like one demented. He quite upset both P. and M. by his extraordinary behaviour.'' After his final examination results dashed the family hopes of a Fellowship, the choice of a career became urgent. With his son unable to reach a decision, Marshall, Sr., chose the Bar for him, with predictable results. For several years in the 1880s, the young man antagonized family and friends alike with his wayward conduct, to be treated like a child by parents who had no idea what ailed him. On more than one occasion, the father hinted at a possibility of real mental instability. There was also the hint that he was a homosexual—''as full of vice as he can be'' was how Jeannette described his relations with a series of male flatmates. In 1888, he finally accepted employment in St. Petersburg, as a private secretary, and left for Russia without saying good-bye to his family.[74]

It is not difficult to suggest psychological explanations that make the pieces of a life, like young John Marshall's, come together into a coherent pattern, but the preeminent problem always remains: historians have no assurance that the reasons they offer for past nervous breakdowns are the correct ones. Some Victorian men clearly broke down under stress early in their adult lives, at a time of sexual maturity and continuing economic dependence, but whether their illness was necessarily occasioned by suppressed conflict with parents is impossible to determine beyond doubt. Others, like Faraday and Landseer, suffered from disabling depression in the midst of highly successful careers. In their cases, are we justified in speculating about some inadequately repressed fear of failing to continue their high standards of achievement, of disappointing their admirers, or of being overtaken by rivals? Or can we point to their rejection, through illness, of the Victorian work ethic that hardly let them pause for breath? When the historian John Seeley ''exhausted his nerve power'' in the mid-1860s, after completing *Ecce Homo,* the highly controversial book about the life of Jesus, should we agree with the acquaintance who thought that the sheer act of composition drained his strength, or can we justly surmise that the faith-shattering implications of his own book unnerved him? When the radical politician Sir Charles Dilke fled to Paris in the autumn of 1874 and stayed there in hiding for weeks, communicating with no one and, in his own estimation, virtually mad, was it overwhelming grief over his wife's death in childbirth that drove him to such extravagant conduct, or some exacerbating degree of guilt and remorse?[75] Many psychological interpretations seem persuasive, but none are absolutely demonstrable.

Nor can historians always ascertain at this remove what were the physiological elements—of brain chemistry, perhaps, metabolism, or nutrition—that precipitated a particular crisis at a particular time, and without which the victim might have been able to endure psychological pressure more successfully. One astute psychiatrist, and historian of psychiatry, who possesses scant regard for freewheeling psychiatric theories imposed on the defenseless dead, has suggested that Faraday's puzzling illness in the 1840s may have been the manifestation, not of severe depression, but of ''an episode of brain damage'' late in 1839, specifically ''a transient ischæmic cerebro-vascular attack . . . in which a part of the brain is transiently deprived of its blood supply.'' In 1847, Lister's father was sure that a recent attack of smallpox had combined with ''too close study'' to shatter his son's nerves and drive him temporarily from University College, London. By the eve of World War I, medical men considered it proven that influenza led to depression.[76] Who knows what microbes, eluding any nineteenth-century system of detection, lurked in the bodies of depressed Victorians? Firm in their conviction that nervous breakdown was a functional disorder of physical etiology, which they intended to identify more precisely as soon as they had the means to do so, Victorian medical practitioners minimized the psychological dimensions of nervous collapse, relying on terms like "worries and strains," "financial anxieties," "bereavement and loss" to summarize as much as they considered important of the emotional elements involved. They may have consciously aimed to spare patients and their families much pain by not investigating further, or it may never have occurred to them that further questions needed to be asked. As far as they were concerned, their psychologizing went far enough, and most of the Victorian public heartily agreed.

Some segment of that public, however, remained dissatisfied with the generalizations and pushed against their limits in an effort to explain why specific individuals suffered nervous collapse. This was largely a literary and philosophical challenge to medical authority, never mounted on a large scale, but only surfacing in scattered biographies, memoirs, letters, and even novels. It was mostly, although not exclusively, focused in the late Victorian and Edwardian decades, when the inadequacy of medical theories about the neuroses became increasingly obvious in contrast to advances in other fields of medicine. It was usually more a matter of nuance than assertion, as when Mr. Home (later the Count de Bassompierre) in Brontë's *Villette* broke down after his estranged wife's death, not from grief but from guilt over his treatment of her. Occasionally, however, an author directly confronted the medical clichés about nervous prostration. Margaret Oliphant, who had much experience to draw on within her own family, brought her doubts to bear when she wrote the biography of Tulloch in the late 1880s. Describing his first encounter with crippling depression in 1862–63, she commented:

> I am far from pretending to throw any light upon what that illness was. Principal Tulloch has not been the only sufferer among his contemporaries, and it has been among the finest minds of our age that it has found its victims. By what subtle action of mind on body, or body on mind—those undefinable partners in the unity of human being—it comes about that this mysterious malady should have so much power in our day, is a question too profound to be discussed by the ignorant. For want of a better explanation, it is generally attributed to overwork or overstrain of the intellectual faculties, nervous exhaustion—whatever words it may occur to the medical faculty to connect with processes which they are unable to fathom. Tulloch did not, I am sure, even when under the immediate influence of those who attribute to this cause everything they do not understand, believe that it was overwork. Perhaps further medical investigations may disclose by what miserable accidental jar the fine machinery of being can be put out of trim, and so much suffering be evolved without any apparent or sufficient cause. It rose upon him like a cloud out of a clear sky, no one knowing why or wherefore.[77]

Around the same time that Oliphant's memoir of Tulloch appeared, William Leonard Courtney also questioned the validity of the overwork hypothesis as the primary explanation for male nervous breakdown. In his biography of J. S. Mill, Courtney, an Oxford philosopher and subsequently a prominent journalist, took Bain to task for his simplistic account of Mill's period of depression that began in 1826.

Courtney acknowledged that, during 1825, Mill had engaged in "remarkably laborious industry" for a nineteen year old, editing Bentham's book on evidence, writing numerous articles, engaging in debates, and fulfilling his clerical duties for the East India Company. "Here was a list," Courtney conceded,

> which was enough to tax even so untiring a brain as Mill's. Yet, perhaps, it is a prosaic opinion to attribute the mental crisis, as Dr. Bain does, principally to physical causes and to the overworking of the brain. Mill treats his malady almost entirely on the subjective side, and that he passed through some kind of a spiritual crisis can hardly be doubted by anyone who studies its sequel in the altered tone of his later writings. . . . He had to get himself out of Benthamism; and the process was rendered doubly difficult and painful owing to the respect and admiration he entertained for the Benthamism of his father. When the light of newer thoughts breaks upon cherished opinions, a mental tragedy, which is by no means the less real because it is subdued, makes havoc of a man's peace and self-control.[78]

The loss of childhood faith, whether religious or rationalist, could be a deeply disturbing process, Courtney realized, especially when it involved a filial declaration of independence, even an unspoken one.

It is not surprising that, as a biographer, A. C. Benson was alive to the psychological subtleties that sparked nervous breakdown. In his own case, he implied that a religious crisis, particularly threatening to the son of an Anglican prelate, was at least partly responsible for his "intolerable depression" at Cambridge in 1882. In Ruskin's undergraduate breakdown, Benson—who published a study of the celebrated critic in 1911—found other forms of psychological torture at work. At the age of seventeen, Benson noted, Ruskin had fallen in love with Adèle Domecq, the daughter of his father's Spanish partner in a highly successful wine importing business. With "intense self-consciousness," Ruskin nurtured his one-sided passion until at length, four years later, "the result was a serious breakdown in health with symptoms of consumption." The combination of bitter disappointment in love heightened by morbid self-absorption was potentially devastating, and Benson was certain that the two psychological states had joined forces to shatter Ruskin's nerves, and lungs. There is no suggestion that overwork at university played any part in the tragedy. Even E. T. Cook, Ruskin's far weightier Edwardian biographer, believed that the news of Adèle's marriage to a Frenchman in March 1840 "doubtless was a cause contributory to his breakdown at Oxford."[79]

With biographers like Oliphant, Courtney, and Benson, one glimpses a growing perception that the problems they narrated did not really concern the nerves, or, at most, only tangentially. Without a scientific theory to bolster their speculations, they guessed that the subjective element had to be granted far greater significance in any satisfactory theory of male nervous breakdown than the medical profession had thus far been able, or willing, to do. They sensed what E. M. Forster wryly suggested in *A Room With a View* (1908): "Life is easy to chronicle, but bewildering to practice, and we welcome 'nerves' or any other shibboleth that will cloak our personal desire."[80]

The personal devils that could drive a man into deepest depression made occasional appearances in the accounts written by some of the victims themselves. No Victorian portrayal of such numbing despair is more celebrated, more frequently cited, nor more problematic than J. S. Mill's description of his crisis in 1826, when, at twenty years of age, be began to realize that his father's utilitarian philosophy and Benthamite program of reform were not the all-sufficient system of thought that he had been raised to believe. When he wrote his autobiography decades later, he provided what appears to be a remarkably candid self-examination of his state of mind at the time. Whether the insights arrived with the wisdom of age or had occurred to the miserable young man himself, we cannot know. His surviving letters from the 1820s shed no light at all on the problem. At whatever stage in life he came to interpret his illness, however, it is clear that he utterly rejected comfortable medical platitudes.[81]

Although Mill did not place his interpretative emphasis on generational conflict, it was implicit throughout the analysis of his descent into depression and gradual recovery. He stressed how much the methods employed in his education contributed to his suffering, because he had been trained, virtually from infancy, to "the habitual exercise of the power of analysis." Under the tutelage of Bentham and his father, James Mill, his capacity to feel had atrophied. He could calculate what was conducive to the greatest good of the greatest number, but he could experience no pleasure in imagining its attainment. The ends for which the father strove "had ceased to charm" the son, and their downfall left nothing but a terrible void in Mill's life. Nor could he turn for advice to his father, as Mill normally would have done, for "he was not the physician who could heal" the young man's suffering. "I seemed to have nothing left to live for," he confessed; his well-disciplined analytic habits had become "a perpetual worm" undermining his capacity for passion, desire, and pleasure. It goes without saying that he brought to this denunciation of calculation and analysis the full breadth of his analytic powers. It was a prison from which he could never entirely break free. Nonetheless, as he recounted in his autobiography, he discovered that his feelings were not altogether dead when he burst into tears while reading Marmontel's *Mémoires*—the passage relating the father's death and the son's reaction to it. The brief incident relieved Mill enormously. "The oppression of the thought that all feeling was dead within me," he recalled, "was gone. I was no longer hopeless: I was not a stock or a stone." It was the beginning of his recovery. "I again enjoyed life," he exulted, "and though I had several relapses, some of which lasted many months, I never again was as miserable as I had been." In future, he did not slight "the cultivation of the feelings."[82]

Of the many difficulties that complicate our response to this compelling narrative, not the least is the fact that Mill did not suffer the kind of incapacitation that marks clinical depression. As his biographer Michael St. John Packe has rightly observed, it was not "a breakdown in any complete sense of the word: he went on with his normal work: none of his family or friends observed anything unusual about him: until he himself told of it, nobody knew there had been anything the matter with him." When, as an older man, he pondered his intellectual and emotional awakening in early adulthood, he cast the experience into a more coherent and intelligible pattern than it had doubtless assumed at the time. Whether consciously or not, he followed, in secular terms, the classic format of spiritual autobiography, centered around "a reassessment of the subject's education, a crisis, and a recovery or a discovery of a new self."[83] Unfortunately, the model did not quite fit and led Mill to considerable literary misrepresentations of his life after the crisis.

Although Mill referred to "several relapses," he devoted no further space in the autobiography to his depressive states and managed to convey the impression that the insights he gained into his inner self preserved him from ever suffering again as he had in the 1820s. His subsequent life was, however, far less emotionally tranquil than he suggested. The crisis had not really been surmounted at all; the tension between James Mill's utilitarian faith and his own mounting criticism of it, most of which he suppressed in public, had not dissipated. Ten years later, a second crisis occurred, which he did not discuss in his autobiography, although the symptoms were far graver than any in 1826. In 1836, his father was dying of tuberculosis, and Mill himself became so ill that his doctor sent him to Brighton. It was, Bain explained, not very informatively, "an obstinate derangement of the brain," which manifested itself, among other ways, as "involuntary nervous twitchings in the face." Shortly after James Mill's death in June, his son set off for the continent, needing "a complete change of scene," as he himself acknowledged. Yet even in Italy, the dreadful symptoms continued to plague him, with "disagreeable sensations" in the head, which he could not shake off. Bain's book makes it clear that, in addition to the tuberculosis which was eventually arrested after partially destroying a lung, J. S. Mill's mental health continued to worry his friends and family for years. He was so depressed in 1842–43 that "his doctors advised him to rest his brain"—advice that he ignored, believing that "work was the only thing to counteract melancholy." In 1848–49, his "prostration of the nervous system" prompted an acquaintance to suggest hydropathy, also without success.[84] Perhaps Mill chose to suppress the record of these later disorders because he believed that they were connected, not just with ambivalent emotions toward his father, but with the strains and frustrations of his deepening friendship with a married woman, Harriet Taylor, whom he met in the early 1830s but could not marry until twenty years later. What he offered in his autobiography, then, was not so much an attempt to dismantle conventional assumptions about shattered nerves as a poetically truthful account of a young man's coming of age. That was the period of his life on which he wanted to focus, the time when he began both to achieve some measure of economic independence and to discover himself as a person—albeit a troubled one—distinct from his father's ideas and aspirations.

A much briefer and, as far as one can tell, more straightforward analysis of his own depression came from Robert Lytton, son of the novelist Edward Bulwer-Lytton. Lytton, the son, shared Mill's views concerning the psychological nature of melancholy and the need for work to counteract it. His explanation of the depression he experienced in 1868 was remarkably similar to Mill's autobiographical account of his mental anguish in 1826. Like Mill, Lytton had ceased to believe in the hitherto guiding inspiration of his life. In Mill's case, it was the utilitarian blueprint for reforming society that no longer excited him; in Lytton's, it was faith in the power of his poetry. Although a diplomat by profession, eventually to serve as Viceroy of India from 1876 to 1880, Lytton fancied himself a poet by vocation and had, for some years, been publishing poems under the pseudonym of "Owen Meredith." At last, when he was in his late thirties, his father gave him permission to publish a volume of verse under his own name, and in 1868 *Chronicles and Characters* appeared. It attracted little attention, to Lytton's dismay. "In an evil hour," he wrote to the Comte de Gobineau,

I began to ask myself a host of foolish and fatal questions as to the nature of my own faculties, till the doubt of one thing became like despair of all. What had hitherto been the most cherished purpose of my whole life now appeared to me only as a phantom formed out of the refuse of undetected failures; and, in resolving to abandon for ever the pursuit of it, the motive power of labour left me. I lapsed into a lethargy of despondency, from which it became daily more and more difficult to extricate myself. . . . I had really lost heart in life altogether. I knew the only corrective to a state of mind so unwholesome lay in methodical and serious mental labour—labour in some new direction for the attainment of some new object. But, whilst I retained the wish, I had lost all energy for work of any kind. Daily I took up some new subject of study, and nightly I abandoned it, in sheer disgust at my own inability to be interested by it.

In a telling sentence that revealed how much his state of mind had made him feel impotent, he confessed: "Disbelieving in my power to reproduce, I had lost the desire to acquire."[85] There may have been some slight hyperbole in this cry of despair; Lytton was given both to self-pity and self-dramatization. His depression of 1868 was, nevertheless, a serious one, and it reflected something that doctors almost never discussed in their journals—the devastation that ensues when the goals shaping a person's life are destroyed.

The most daring, and conscious, attempt to break with social and medical conventions concerning male nervous prostration was the work of John Addington Symonds. His *Memoirs,* which he wrote in 1889, four years before his death from pneumonia and advanced tuberculosis, were both a sustained attack on the narrowness of the Victorian sexual code and an attempt to explain himself to himself. *Apologia Pro Vita Sua* would not have been an inappropriate title for a work that belongs among the pioneering studies of homosexuality. This eloquent effort to articulate a homosexual sense of identity was, needless to say, not intended for publication during the author's lifetime. Symonds bequeathed it, together with his diaries, to his literary executor, Horatio F. Brown, who made such good use of the material in his biography of Symonds, published in 1895, that Brown's book is little more than a compilation—with all of Symonds's self-revelatory passages suppressed. On Brown's death in 1926, the *Memoirs* were left in the keeping of the London Library, but the diaries had apparently been destroyed. Brown stipulated that the *Memoirs* should be placed under embargo for fifty years, and thus, although individual scholars were able to consult the document at the London Library, it was not available for publication until very recently.[86]

Symonds set out to explore the meaning of his own sexual nature at a time when homosexuality was becoming prominent both as a social scandal and as a medical controversy. It is obviously not true that sexual relations between men were only discovered in the late nineteenth century. Included within the category of sodomy, what we now call homosexual behavior had been a capital crime under statute law since 1533 and formally remained so until 1861. Until the 1830s, furthermore, the death penalty for sodomy was applied in England with a rigor no longer fashionable in other western societies.[87] That criminal classification, however, encompassed the other "unnatural offenses" of bestiality and anal copulation between a man and a woman. Although by the end of the eighteenth century the term *sodomy* was being used more and more narrowly to designate sexual intercourse between men, it was still not employed exclusively with that meaning in Victoria's reign. Indeed, there is some evidence that the label of *onanism* was invoked more often than sodomy to denote homosexual deviance. It is clear, at any rate, that the concept of a homosexual person, as distinct from a mere sex offender, was utterly absent from the late Georgian and early Victorian considerations of sodomy. This may help to explain social approval of deep emotional friendships—virtually indistinguishable from romantic love—between schoolboys and even between young men for the first three quarters of the nineteenth century. Such bonds, perceived in innocent and idealistic terms, betrayed no sinister features until the end of the period, because they were not believed to influence a boy's adult sexual identity. By the turn of the century, these highly sentimental attachments were no longer acceptable to late Victorian concepts of manliness, and the fact that they raised suspicions of homosexuality was not the least of the reasons why.[88]

During the last twenty-five years of the Queen's reign, a variety of converging developments molded British attitudes toward the homosexual as a man lacking normal instincts and as an object of public loathing. Headmasters and teachers were openly addressing the problem of immorality among schoolboys. The Criminal Law Amendment Act of 1885 declared any "act of gross indecency" between men a misdemeanor punishable by a maximum sentence of two years' imprisonment with hard labor, thereby not only extending the arm of the law to the sexual activities of consenting adults in private, but also specifically underscoring the criminality of homosexual practices among the other forms of sodomy. The Cleveland Street scandal of 1889–90 revealed that the patronage of a male brothel in London extended high up the ranks of society, and, as the coup de grâce, the trial of Oscar Wilde in 1895 resoundingly confirmed the public association of homosexuality with effeminacy and decadence. It was both an affront and a threat to English manliness.[89]

At the same time, a new international vocabulary of homosexuality was finding expression, steeped in implications of disease. This is not the place to discuss in any detail the variegated literature that explored the homosexual personality in the second half of the nineteenth century. Dominated by contributions from French and German authors, including Paul Moreau, Karl Ulrichs, J. L. Casper, and the extremely influential Richard von Krafft-Ebing, it debated the vexed question of innate or acquired pathology: was the sexual preference some men showed toward other men a congenital condition or the fruit of their own depravity? And if congenital, was it or was it not proof of a degenerate inheritance? The dominant opinion, not surprisingly, stressed that homosexual desire was abnormal and pathological, a form of sickness as well as a crime and a sin.[90] Initially, England did not contribute much to the European exploration of homosexuality in its medical and allegedly scientific aspects. Alexander Morison, it is true, had dealt with the practice, as he encountered it among asylum patients, under the heading of "monomania with unnatural propensity," but he established no British tradition of inquiry into the subject. Symonds's own pamphlets—*A Problem in Greek Ethics* and *A Problem in Modern Ethics*—were privately printed in 1883 and 1891, in tiny editions of ten and fifty, respectively.[91] In the early 1890s, however, Symonds began the collaboration with Havelock Ellis that led in 1897 to the publication of *Sexual Inversion*.

This volume, the first of Ellis's *Studies in the Psychology of Sex,* was the most significant early work on homosexuality to be written in English. It was the book that introduced British readers to the term *homosexuality,* a German-language invention dating from 1869, as well as to *inversion,* a frequently used synonym. Symonds, who died in 1893, is not widely associated with this pioneering work, partly because Ellis later minimized his partner's contribution, but also because Symonds's family, friends, and literary executor, after trying to buy up the whole first edition, sought to conceal evidence of his involvement in subsequent ones.[92] It is clear, nonetheless, that the same impulse to self-exploration that led Symonds to write his *Memoirs* inspired his work with Ellis. Both men wanted to establish, not the pathology of homosexuality, but its blamelessness. It was an innate condition, they believed, biologically imposed from conception, for which the individual was no more responsible than for his hair color. If it was abnormal, deviating from the standard pattern of heterosexual relations, it was not unnatural, and it represented proof neither of degeneration, nor of disease. It was simply the result of unknown hereditary influences affecting some people, but not others. Ironically, however, the joint work of Symonds and Ellis, who had studied medicine for eight years, helped significantly to establish homosexuality as a medical problem, the particular province of the psychopathologist.

The late Victorian uproar over inversion, in which schoolmasters, legislators, and doctors joined with much of the general public, drew substantial force from contemporary fear of male sexuality when deflected from safe and productive channels. The point hardly needs belaboring that the Symonds–Ellis view of homosexuality did not prevail and that British opinion continued to repudiate the invert as peculiarly unnatural, unmanly, and despicable. Like masturbation, inversion wasted a man's semen to no purpose except the satisfaction of animal lust, sapped his physical and moral strength alike, and advertised the overthrow of his will. It was antisocial for all these reasons, but, at a time when the family was being glorified ever more lyrically and unrealistically as the source of stability in a rapidly changing society, homosexuality posed a particular threat to the happiness and security of the home. As if that were not reason enough for alarm, middle-class arbiters of social morality condemned homosexuality on yet another count: it typically featured fraternization in sin between men of the upper and lower classes.[93] From whatever aspect the late Victorians and Edwardians regarded the practice, it appeared evil and menacing to a society that heard promoters of national efficiency and social purity crusaders preaching the inevitability of national decline, if vice and immorality were not driven from British shores.

Long-standing British hatred of sodomy, sharpened by the developing image of the modern morbid homosexual, formed the background against which Symonds wrote his *Memoirs* and interpreted his diverse nervous disorders. The overwhelming impression left by the document is that Symonds was made physically, and seriously, ill by the sustained attempt to suppress his homosexuality. Even the tubercular condition of his lungs, he believed, was aggravated by what he called "the forcible repression of my natural inclination for the male sex." That it was an innate bias of his nature, "constitutional" and "ineradicable," he was certain, and to deny it, to attempt to find peace in marriage, as he did, was only to magnify his sufferings. At

Oxford, he was sure that his "suppressed emotional life" had hindered him from greater academic and literary achievements. "It absorbed an enormous amount of time and engaged the larger part of my nervous energy," he insisted. Sexual frustration paved the way for the devastating breakdown that he experienced in 1863, not "overwork and religious perplexity," as his doctors—including his father—maintained. Indeed, like Mill and Lytton, Symonds directly confronted Victorian medical convictions by insisting that work was the only thing that preserved his sanity in the terrible months that ensued, when, with "aching eyes and dull pain-shotten brain," he turned to his writing, composed an essay on the Renaissance, which he dispatched to Oxford, and won the Chancellor's Prize. The success did not eliminate his pain; a year later, he wrote to a friend: "Every nerve seems as if it had been stripped of its integument & opened to the influences of the world." At least, however, he proved himself capable of resisting utter apathy. His will was not totally inoperative. Later in the 1860s, when his "nerves gave way" again, Symonds once more invoked "the goddess Drudgery," but found "particular source of misery" in the fact that, on this occasion, he was incapable of working. Like Benson during his worst depressions, Symonds was in a "state of entire negation," where even the satisfaction of accomplishing some slight labor was denied him. It was only after he had "yield[ed] to the attraction of the male" that he, at last, achieved real "self-mastery and self-control."[94] Victorian moral platitudes could not have been more completely overturned.

For all their frontal assault on Victorian sexual hypocrisy and restrictive views of manliness, however, Symonds's *Memoirs* reveal that he was unable to evade the powerful grip of conventional morality. He made every effort to do so, particularly after his father's death in 1871. Despite real bonds of attachment between the two men, Symonds knew that he had been a very keen disappointment to his father. Dr. Symonds represented to his son all that was honorable, upright, and wise in the culture of his class and era, but he also stood for the point of view that could only condemn, utterly and irrevocably, the sexual deviance that was threatening to ruin his son's life. Symonds frankly acknowledged that his father's death released in him literary energies and ambitions that could never have flourished under the doctor's "watchful supervision." It also freed him to participate in homosexual relations. By moving to Switzerland, as Symonds did in 1877 to stall advancing tuberculosis, he distanced himself even further from the mores that so disgusted him at home. Yet many of the attitudes toward health and disease that his father endorsed found an echo in Symonds's *Memoirs*. He shared, for example, his father's loathing of excess and wrote, in surprisingly dogmatic tones: "He who overworks any organ, whether brain, heart, lung, stomach or sexual apparatus, sins." Admittedly, this pronouncement was intended to echo the Hellenic ideal of humanity's balanced wholeness, but it was written with the pen of a Victorian moralist.[95]

In the final paragraph of his *Memoirs,* Symonds bore the fullest testimony to the unremitting authority which the Victorian moral canon never ceased to exercise over him. "Few situations in life are more painful than this," he wrote:

> that a man, gifted with strong intellectual capacity . . . should sit down soberly to contemplate his own besetting vice. In pleasant moments, when instinct prevails over reason, when the broadway of sensual indulgence invites his footing, the man

plucks primroses of frank untutored inclination. . . . But, when he comes to frigid reason's self again, when he tallies last night's deeds with today's knowledge of fact and moral ordinance, he awakes to the reality of a perpetual discord between spontaneous appetite and acquired respect for social law. By the light of his clear brain he condemns the natural action of his appetite; and what in moments of self-abandonment to impulse appeared a beauteous angel, stands revealed before him as a devil abhorred by the society he clings to. The agony of this struggle between self-yielding to desire and love, and self-scourging by a trained discipline of analytic reflection, breaks his nerve.[96]

No matter how congenital or how natural, homosexuality remained for Symonds his "besetting vice."

Symonds remained imprisoned, too, within the prevailing gender stereotypes of late Victorian culture. He vigorously repudiated the notion that any taint of effeminacy discredited his homosexual practices, and in the information he gave to Ellis concerning his own case history he stressed that point. As Ellis reported in *Sexual Inversion,* referring to Symonds only as Case XVIII, "he himself always plays the active masculine part," when engaging in sexual relations with other men. "He never yields himself to the other." To a man schooled in the classics, as Symonds was, this distinction assumed particular significance, for ancient Greek attitudes toward homosexuality had attached no shame to the practice if a man assumed the active role. (The other classical stipulations for untarnished masculinity in homosexual relations—that the partner be either a slave or an immature youth—were harder for Symonds to satisfy.) Ellis continued by observing that Case XVIII possessed "strong power of will and self-control," and that, in boyhood, he "was only non-masculine in his indifference to sport, was never feminine in dress or habit."[97] It was obviously important to Symonds to perceive himself as manly. No matter how much he detested narrow Victorian views of sexuality, he had been deeply indoctrinated by them.

We have become familiar in recent years with the idea that the lives of countless Victorian women were made unhappy by the restrictive models of femininity that society prescribed for them, but the pain inflicted by late nineteenth-century dictates on manliness has received little attention from today's scholars—no doubt because those prescriptions do not provoke the same degree of anger as Victorian pronouncements on womanhood arouse. Yet it is clear that British men in this period were no different from men at other times: they felt anxiety about their masculinity, as defined by their culture, and about society's expectations for them. Particularly in the final decades of Victoria's reign, as "The Woman Question" came to the fore, the emphatic definition of manliness in terms of physical and emotional toughness, predicated on iron nerves, created an ideal almost impossible to realize. Uneasiness on this score disguised itself in bold declarations, like the novelist Grant Allen's heavy-handed attempt in 1889 to explain why a woman was not the equal of a man, but it also emerged in much subtler ways. Mary Paley Marshall, a former lecturer on political economy at Newnham and wife of the economist Alfred Marshall, recollected, for example, that when her husband was diagnosed with kidney stone in 1879 and, forbidden exercise, found solace in knitting stockings, Andrew Clark stopped him, on the grounds that knitting "might cause some nerve trouble." It is hard to imagine Clark issuing such an injunction to female patients, and one suspects that he found the pursuit too feminine for the then principal of University College, Bristol.[98]

Benson specifically addressed the issue of gender stereotyping through the thoughts of the autobiographical "Hugh," in *Beside Still Waters*. Having described himself earlier in the volume as "rather on the feminine side" because "he valued delicate and sincere emotions . . . above practical activity and organisation," toward the end of the book he pondered the meaning of "effeminate" and "masculine" at great length. He fully realized that, with his belief "in books, in art, in music, as sources of tranquil enjoyment, instead of regarding them as slightly unwholesome and affected tastes," he was considered the "champion, not only of an unpopular cause, but of an essentially effeminate system." It distressed him to acknowledge that, by contemporary standards, "a man who lived in a cottage, occupied in quiet and intellectual pursuits, would be held to be a failure, even if he lived in innocent happiness to the age of eighty." It upset him deeply that the cultivation of art, once deemed perfectly compatible with manliness, and even heroism, had become "rather a dilettante business," which no self-respecting man would pursue, except as an amusing hobby.[99] He did not discuss the degree to which, by the early twentieth century, artistic or "aesthetic" men were suspected, not merely of effeminacy, but of homosexuality, nor the extent to which his own lifelong bachelorhood contributed to doubts about his manliness. Intensely close male friendships were certainly essential to Benson's emotional well-being, but we have no evidence to prove that they were sexual relationships. Whether frustrated sexual desires contributed to his breakdowns was not something he chose to confide to posterity.

Benson's spells of depression lifted for long periods of time, so that, while a fellow of Magdalene, Cambridge, after 1904, he was able effectively to play the busy man of affairs, "dashing off for a day of business in London," serving on educational committees, presiding over the Modern Languages Association, and much else.[100] Samuel Greg was not so fortunate. The son of one of the great early cotton manufacturers, Greg suffered a severe breakdown in 1847, after a strike at his Cheshire mill and the hard times that followed. By the end of the decade, his business was as bankrupt as his nerve force. Indeed, neither ever recovered, although he lived for nearly another thirty years. His was, apparently, a case of the total destruction wrought by the wreckage of a life's dream; he had nurtured many benevolent schemes for his workers, including a model village, that were based on the trust binding millhands to master—on an old-fashioned paternalism, in short, that was no longer in touch with reality by the mid-nineteenth century. The strike shattered that illusion, just as economic depression shattered his business. He suffered "a terrible attack of illness, affecting the spine and nervous system, . . . [and] felt that he had been struck down in mind, body, and estate, at one blow. The hopes and plans that had made his life worth living, seemed suddenly swept away into darkness." During the ensuing years, he and his wife lived in retirement. "Often he did not seem to have power or courage left to give the most ordinary directions about the garden or grounds." His friend Arthur Penrhyn Stanley, Dean of Westminster, recollected in the preface to a posthumously published collection of Greg's writings how the former mill owner once described to him "the exquisite pain that he experienced on hearing . . . some preacher enlarging on the details of the Passion. 'I could not bear it—it was too sad to hear of the infliction of those terrible sufferings on One so innocent, so tender, so good; I rushed out of the church.' '' Such conduct was scarcely manly, and it was precisely this element in his nature that served as the central explanation for his life's disappointments, according to the anonymous memoir that accompanied Greg's collection of prose and verse:

> There was much of the feminine element in his constitution. He rather lacked that
> harder, tougher fibre, both of mind and frame, which makes the battle of life so easy
> and so successful to many men. He had nothing *hard* about him, and was not made
> for conflict. . . . He was tender-hearted to an unusual degree—perhaps because he
> knew so well what suffering was. His compassion was most readily awakened,
> especially for children or young animals. A family of little motherless partridges, a
> brood of half-drowned ducks, a wounded hedgehog, &c., were, on different
> occasions nursed and cherished by him back to life and health.[101]

With his compassionate, nurturing, and motherly qualities, Greg would have been a much loved and admired Victorian woman, but as a man, who could not compete in the world, who had no tough, combative instincts, he was an utter failure, in the eyes of the memoirist writing in the late 1870s. We have no way of knowing how heavily a realization of his own inadequacy weighed on Greg, adding to the mental pain inflicted by the collapse of his philanthropic projects, but we may certainly suspect that the necessity to achieve, to outdistance rivals, to prove one's hardness, must have been burdensome indeed to men of Greg's and Benson's nature. To feel obliged to suppress and disdain their emotions, for fear of being thought effeminate, may well have contributed to the neurotic illness of those late Victorian and Edwardian men whose virtues failed to shine in the light of contemporary masculine stereotypes, and for whom nervous breakdown was the ultimate measure of how far they had fallen short. When medical wisdom urged them to summon the will to recover, the advice must have sounded like mockery to men who had been told that will was precisely what they lacked.

6

Neurotic Women

The burden of sexual stereotyping bore down even more heavily on Victorian women whose lives were plagued with nervous illness. With many of these women, it is difficult to speak of nervous breakdown as a specific event that interrupted the course of their normal daily activities. Their depression was more likely to be a chronic than an acute condition, similar to prolonged mood or anxiety disorders rather than a discrete, identifiable crisis. While we can usually recognize such crises in men who had work to perform and who were unable to fulfill their responsibilities for a given period of time, with affluent women whose lives were not defined by their occupation, the task of designating a particular phase of incapacitation is often impossible. They may have dragged themselves around for years, just managing to function as wife, mother, sister, or daughter, but always shrouded in hopelessness and emotional pain.

Much of the problem of definition arises from the fact that Victorian and Edwardian medical advisors typically subsumed their diagnoses of nervous maladies in female patients under the general category of "feminine disorders," related to menstruation, pregnancy, or lactation. This theoretical merger of the female nervous and reproductive systems was an integral part of the medical assumption that biology dominated women's lives, utterly beyond the regulatory power of the individual will. Unlike male nervous breakdown, the element of personal choice or responsibility was rarely granted much influence when doctors explained severe depression in women. Some medical writers found it simplest to deal with female nervous collapse under the great catch-all classification of hysteria, still the archetypal feminine functional nervous disorder in the nineteenth century. While the more grotesque physical symptoms of hysteria—the full-scale paroxysm, temporary convulsions, palsies, motor and sensory impairments, respiratory obstructions, and speech disorders— bore no resemblance to the manifestations of depression, the less dramatic ones certainly did. Hysterical women might abstain from food, suffer sudden fits of weeping, and experience chronic lassitude in a manner that was indistinguishable from profound melancholy. How a medical practitioner diagnosed the affliction was a purely individual decision on his part, but whether he labeled it hysteria, gynecological disturbance, or nervous exhaustion, he played an important contributory role in constructing the nineteenth century's model of womanhood, partly from new materials and partly from old ones merely refurbished in an up-to-date style.

At the heart of virtually all medical attitudes toward women's nerves, health, and character was the presumed weakness of the female will. It was implicit in the notion

181

of woman as a creature who reacted rather than initiated, and whose feelings dominated her intellect. It found expression, too, in numerous aspects of Victorian culture that were far removed from the realm of medical expertise—such as the Common Law principle, prevalent throughout most of the nineteenth century, "that married women were legally incapable of individual action."[1] The conclusions to be drawn about women's capacity for rational conduct were hardly complimentary to the female sex, but they were not the novel product of Victorian opinion. The alignment of woman with irrationality and emotion, in contrast to man's command of reason and logical analysis, goes back to Aristotelian theory, and assertions of female inferiority have circulated for at least as long a time. The Victorian era is noteworthy, not because many scientists and doctors joined enthusiastically in the denigration of female intelligence, for their professional ancestors had typically done the same, but because in the second half of the nineteenth century the apparently irrefutable authority of evolutionary biology gave credence to venerable suspicions concerning the imperfect development of the female brain.

At the very time when groups of middle-class women were organizing to claim the right to vote, to hold public office, to enjoy equal property rights with men, to gain access to economic independence through professional training and university education, and to stimulate a reevaluation of the laws governing marriage, evolutionary theory seemed to furnish undeniable reasons why the status quo should not be radically altered in response to these demands. The unfolding saga of evolutionary change, as applied to the human species, was summoned to prove the perfect appropriateness, not only of woman's subordination to man, but also of her consignment to domesticity. Coinciding chronologically, but clashing ideologically, evolutionary thought and feminism marshaled all the possible arguments in the controversy of nature versus nurture. For the advocates of women's rights, the apparent lack of intellectual achievement by women in the past and present was merely the product of social conditioning and adverse environmental influences. For their opponents, the mind of woman was the result of nature's inexorable laws, aided and abetted by the rigorous demands of humanity's social development. Throughout the second half of the nineteenth century, the argument extracted from evolutionary biology, ably seconded by social anthropology, made its strident voice overpower the soberer reasoning of the environmentalists.

The evolutionary explanation of woman's subservience to man was established by Darwin and Spencer themselves, the two giants of Victorian evolutionary thought. Their writings on sexual differentiation powerfully confirmed centuries of popular prejudice, imparting both a veneer of scientific expertise and a sharper focus to ideas that had been current in more inchoate form. It did not, of course, take Darwin's keen powers of observation to conclude that the natural female function was reproduction, not ratiocination: Victorians knew that motherhood was woman's "destined end on earth"[2] without any help from the theory of natural selection. Darwin's contribution, elaborated by Spencer, was to explain *why* women generally lacked the mental capacities of men, why they were incapable of abstract thought, sustained analytic reasoning, or even great creative works of the imagination. After the profound impact of *The Origin of Species* in 1859, Darwin's pronouncements in *The Descent of Man* twelve years later commanded reverent public attention, although his comments on the mental differences between men and women resembled more a parade of pre-judices than a scientific demonstration. They were, nonetheless, received as a re-sounding rebuttal of the environmentalist position forcefully argued by J. S. Mill in *The Subjection of Women* (1869).

Women were what they were, and men possessed their masculine traits, Darwin explained, because a complex interaction of natural and sexual selection had worked to that end. In the primitive struggle for existence, it was the man with mental perspicacity as well as physical powers of endurance who had triumphed over his rivals, attracted a desirable mate, and lived longer to produce more offspring. Since he defended his female, she did not need to develop similar qualities. As part of this process, Darwin believed that the inheritance of acquired traits was helping to distance male intelligence from female. In the late eighteenth and early nineteenth centuries, it was widely assumed among naturalists that physical and mental characteristics, acquired during life, could be passed on from parent to offspring as usage strengthened the importance of those traits in the relationship of the organism with its surrounding environment. Although now dubbed Lamarckian inheritance, after Jean-Baptiste Lamarck, the eminent French botanist and zoologist who en-dorsed the theory, it was, in fact, a relatively common feature of evolutionary thought at the end of the Enlightenment. Darwin accepted this hereditary mechanism and considered it compatible with his own hypothesis of natural selection, based on chance variations in the hereditary substance transmitted from one generation to the next. It seemed obvious that the more vigorously primitive man had to use his wits, the more he developed his brain, and his ever-expanding intellectual prowess descended to his sons after him. (Both Darwin and Spencer believed that traits acquired by men in adulthood were passed primarily to their sons, while those that mature women acquired were principally inherited by their daughters.) Over the millennia, an enormous intellectual gulf had developed between men and women that could never be bridged: although they no longer had to fight to win mates, modern men still had "a severe struggle in order to maintain themselves and their families" and thus would never cease improving mentally, even while modern women assiduously cultivated their own mental capacities. Those intellectual abilities that women possessed in excess of men, such as "powers of intuition, of rapid perception, and perhaps of imitation," only proved that woman was stalled at a less lofty stage of cerebral development than man, for those talents were found among the "lower races" of humanity and therefore indicated "a past and lower state of civilisation."[3]

As part of his lifelong effort to base the study of human society on the methods and laws of the natural sciences, Spencer embraced both natural selection and Lamarckian evolution in his illumination of female intellectual inferiority. There is a nice irony in the fact that the two men most responsible for the "scientific" confirmation of womanly weakness were themselves invalids for most of their adult lives, but their personal health problems in no way invalidated their status as Victorian sages. Already in the 1860s, Spencer had misapplied the first law of thermodynamics—the principle of the conservation of energy—in order to illustrate how the finite supply of energy available to any organism restricted the choices open to the female half of the human race. In the 1870s, he reformulated his argument in the context of Darwin's revelations about women. Spencer's *Study of Sociology* (1872—

73) blended energy and evolution to shed further light on the deficiencies of female development over the ages. Since woman's natural role was reproduction, a process requiring enormous resources of energy, she was incapable of pursuing any other activity that required equally heavy output. Science, after all, dictated that a given amount of energy could only be used in one form at a time: women had to choose between reproductive or intellectual achievements, for they could not enjoy both. The body had to conserve its energy for its principal tasks, Spencer reminded his readers. With women, both individually and generically speaking, reproductive responsibilities were paramount, and mental growth assumed a merely secondary significance; nature *intended* the female mind to cease developing at an earlier stage than the male, in order that a woman's reproductive organs might be fully and robustly developed.

Spencer recognized that social, as well as biological, forces had molded sexual differentiation. The need to placate wild and aggressive primitive man, he contended, had set in motion the evolution of specifically feminine traits through Lamarckian inheritance. From their mothers since the dawn of human history, women had acquired their intuitive insights, their keen discernment, their submissiveness, and also their powers of deception. In the first volume of his *Principles of Sociology* (1876), Spencer extended his argument to assert that the patriarchal, monogamous family was the natural social pattern of civilized humanity. Nature, in other words, favored the emergence of this pattern, for only when the man worked to support one wife and her children—and when the wife had no task but to raise their progeny—could healthy offspring be nurtured to maturity with maximum efficiency and greatest likelihood of success.[4]

Nothing less, therefore, than the inexorable processes of evolution had deprived woman of a strong, controlling will, as a formidable array of Victorian psychiatrists, physicians, physiologists, and social commentators concurred. Because the "general development" of the female gender as a whole had "been arrested by the special activity of her sexual system,"[5] woman had clearly missed out on the very final stages of cerebral evolution. She lacked the most intricately developed nervous structures, the so-called highest nervous centers that the will was thought to occupy, and which appeared only at the very pinnacle of the evolutionary scale. Victorian evolutionists assumed that ontogeny followed phylogeny: the maturation of every individual from embryo to adulthood (ontogeny) was supposed to duplicate, or recapitulate, the historical evolution of its species (phylogeny), and, more specifically, of its gender within the species. Each separate Victorian woman accordingly manifested the arrested mental development characteristic of woman's growth from primitive times. Among numerous nineteenth-century authorities in the fields of biological science, health, and education, this derogatory perspective on female intelligence became accepted as a "given" that required no further demonstration. In 1883, Crichton-Browne could simply assert, without substantiation, that "girls are in all countries more precocious than boys, but they stop at a lower point in mental evolution. . . ." In the same decade, the physiologist George John Romanes confidently maintained that the female mind could only with difficulty concentrate attention and pursue extensive specialized studies. It was, he explained, characterized by indecision, an unstable quality that betrayed "comparative weakness of will." The assumption that women's capacities were limited by the demands of reproductive physiology was so widely accepted by the end of the Victorian era that it even figured, as a throwaway line, in boys' literature. Woman, Kipling observed in *Stalky & Co.*, was "made for one end only by blind Nature, but man for several."[6]

For several decades beginning in the late 1860s, nothing was believed to underscore the biological basis of female mental inadequacy more resoundingly than craniology, "a collection of techniques for measuring all possible angles and dimensions of the skull."[7] Having already demonstrated the inferiority of the black to the white race, the findings of craniology were invoked to bear witness against women's brains. When the era of statistics was just dawning, with its naive, but settled, belief that numbers do not lie, craniological quantification appeared to offer pure facts, divorced from all passion and prejudice. The numbers derived from measuring skulls in the late nineteenth century all pointed to the smaller average size of the female skull compared with that of the male, a conclusion that was pregnant with meaning for anthropologists, alienists, and comparative psychologists on both sides of the Channel and the Atlantic. Their enthusiasm for taking cranial measurements was predicated on the phrenological assumption that the contours of the skull were an accurate indication of the size of the brain within. Equally central to their work was the equation of brain size with intelligence. It was only thanks to this facile and erroneous correlation that craniologists, after calculating the lesser bulk of the average female brain from cranial capacity, could proceed to announce that they had therefore certified the inferior mental prowess of the female sex. Over the decades, problems arising from faults in the craniologists' basic hypotheses forced them constantly to propose different ratios and angles of measurement, until, at length, it became apparent that intelligence could not be ascertained from a study of the skull at all. In England, Karl Pearson, professor of applied mathematics and mechanics at University College, London, played a large part in destroying the foundations of craniology early in the twentieth century. Using sophisticated statistical methods, he and his students dismissed once and for all the presumption of scientific accuracy behind its pronouncements.[8] By then, of course, a great deal of damage had been done.

While physical anthropologists had to extrapolate information about brains from the bones that once encased them, some psychiatrists had access to the organs of thought themselves. Performing autopsies on the inmates at Wakefield in the 1870s, Crichton-Browne, as we have seen, had the material on hand to reach sweeping conclusions about female intelligence. A comparison of his data with that of Robert Boyd from the Somerset County Asylum and John Thurnam from the Wiltshire County Asylum—both of whom weighed the brains of patients who died under their supervision—enabled Crichton-Browne to claim that the average female brain weighed significantly less than the average male specimen. Furthermore, he insisted that "the greater weight of the brain in man as compared with woman is not in relation merely to his greater bulk but is a fundamental sexual distinction." Without actually marshaling any evidence, but merely citing the opinions of Paul Broca, the famous Parisian surgeon, cerebral physiologist, and anthropologist, Crichton-Browne calmly insisted that woman's relatively small brain "is not to be accounted for by deficiency in stature or weight, but depends, as Broca has argued, as much on her intellectual as on her physical inferiority."[9]

Over the following years, Crichton-Browne found that woman's deficient intelligence could be demonstrated by numerous aspects of cerebral physiology. Sometimes he focused on the comparative paucity of convolutions in the frontal cerebral lobes of the female brain, on the shallowness of their gray matter, the restricted branching of their ganglion cells, or the poor quality of the blood flowing into them. It seems easy today to dismiss his calculation of corpuscles and convolutions as a blatant example of science, so-called, twisted out of shape for ignoble ends. In the late nineteenth century, however, the declarations of the Lord Chancellor's Visitor in Lunacy carried weight, particularly because they were joined by a chorus of other voices singing the same song. A consensus emerged that, on the average, the female brain weighed about five ounces less than the male. In those missing ounces lay all the mental vigor that women lacked, especially the power of rigorous self-control under the will's sovereign direction.[10]

The manipulation of measurements, whether cranial or cerebral, allowed scientists, medical doctors, and ethnologists to posit a fundamental similarity between women and children. Since cerebral evolution had come to an early stop for women, they preserved something distinctly childlike in their nature. In their uncurbed emotions, craving for sympathy, gifts of mimicry, and "deep sense of dependence," among other traits, "the feminine and the child-mind" were analogous, both revealing "peculiarities . . . such as belong to an inferior grade of mental evolution."[11] Whereas male children—white male children, that is—in due course grew progressively to a superior grade, female children never did. Evolutionary biology provided novel and effective means of justifying old prejudice, and medical practitioners were not reluctant to incorporate these arguments into their work. Science and medicine generally look for answers to questions that society raises, or to the needs articulated by the dominant segments of society. As it became more urgent to explain why women belonged in the home, in subordinate roles to their husbands, Victorian scientists and doctors came up with revised answers, producing the proof that bolstered "preconceived notions" about "the different moral, intellectual and physical worth" of men and women. The generalized image of womanhood thus depicted became a "fact 'in nature,' "[12] which medical men could cite when treating their female patients' nerves.

The confirmation of woman's inferior mental development by evolutionary biology in the second half of the nineteenth century thus powerfully buttressed the "separate spheres" ideology that emerged in the first half, and about which so much has been written in recent years. The evangelical celebration of woman's spiritual mission in the home itself had coincided with fundamental changes in patterns of labor that identified the workplace in industrial rather than domestic terms and consigned a significant number of middle-class women to lives of leisure, maintained in comfort by male relatives at the office and by servants in the home. Biological truths, in short, were made to conform to economic realities. When medical authorities affirmed that nature intended woman for domestic responsibilities devoted to bearing and raising children, however, they neglected the fact that these particular economic conditions defined the lives of only a limited segment of the female population. They were obviously irrelevant to working-class women, for whom labor, paid or unpaid, was the prime fact of life. They were likewise inapplicable to those aristocratic wives who were financially independent of their husbands, and whose menfolk, in any case, often enjoyed an equally leisured existence. Indeed, the unrestricted lives of many aristocratic women in the nineteenth century made a mockery of the feminine stereotypes paraded so relentlessly in medical texts.[13] Nonetheless only a few Victorian and Edwardian doctors recognized that diverse life experiences might render suspect their generalizations about women's health.

They certainly saw no reason to hedge with exceptions their pronouncements concerning the female nervous system, which derived its characteristic traits, they believed, both from the limitations of the woman's brain and from the excesses of her reproductive organs. It was a medical truism that female nerves were highly unstable. Not only was hysteria a common female neurosis, but women were believed to suffer from minor nervous disorders, such as headache or the fidgets, far more frequently than men. "Woman, as compared with man, is of the nervous temperament," Laycock commented in the 1860s. "Her nervous system is therefore more easily acted upon by all impressions, and more liable to all diseases of excitement." A contributor to Quain's *Dictionary of Medicine* made the same point in 1882. In defining the nervous temperament, he explained that "an organisation of this kind characterises children rather than adults, and, amongst the latter, females more than males."[14] The reason was not difficult to find: not only was there little will to control the activities of a woman's lower nervous centers, but the entire female nervous system was inextricably associated with the reproductive organs whose malfunctions gave rise to the vast majority of feminine maladies. Nerves, ovaries, and uterus bound women in a stranglehold of sickness, unlike anything that men experienced. While Victorian medical practitioners acknowledged the significance of the life cycle in the health or illness of their male patients, it never controlled their understanding of masculinity the way it overwhelmed their vision of femininity. For most doctors, the female reproductive functions, in their sequential phases, were the key to comprehending woman. They were, without doubt, the principal cause of her nervous ailments.

The medical juxtaposition of female nerves and reproductive organs in order to explain women's peculiar nervous excitability had a venerable history. Hysteria was, of course, traditionally associated with the uterus, and although the hypothesis of a wandering womb, which spread disorder throughout the female body, had lost all credibility by the late Georgian era, early nineteenth-century British medicine still credited the uterus with a formidable power to disrupt the workings of the nerves. Thomas Addison of Guy's Hospital, for example, published a volume in 1830 that explored the manifold deleterious effects of "uterine irritation," a particularly insidious female disorder that could exist "without either inflammation or organic lesion being *necessarily* present." What betrayed its existence to the discerning medical man was persistent menstrual irregularity accompanied by pain, as well as the nervous, melancholy disposition of its victims. A woman suffering from uterine irritation, he reported, tells her medical attendant that, without any assignable cause, she gradually declined in health and spirits; that she has lost her wonted alacrity, has become indolent, and is easily fatigued by comparatively slight exertion; that she is readily flurried; that her heart often beats, flutters, or palpitates; that the impressions made upon her mind are altogether disproportionate to the causes producing them; that she is very prone to weep, and occasionally experiences sudden and transitory feelings of alarm and dread, especially during the night, without being able satisfactorily to account for them; in short, that both body and mind are in a morbidly sensitive condition. . . .

Samuel Ashwell, obstetric physician at Guy's in the following decade, agreed that irritable uterus—or hysteralgia, as he dubbed it—could eventually confine a woman to her sofa, without producing the slightest change of organic structure.[15] In effect, medical practitioners in the first half of the nineteenth century were so certain of the connections binding a woman's nerves to her uterus that signs of severe anxiety attacks or depression were routinely ascribed to uterine disturbances, despite the frequent absence of corroborating evidence.

Not the uterus alone, but every aspect of the reproductive role significantly affected women's nerves, medical wisdom maintained. Like frogs "just before the period of copulation," mused the gynecologist E. J. Tilt in 1853, women "subjected to increased ovarian action" revealed nerves "endowed with a most remarkable degree of irritability."[16] Other doctors, omitting the frogs, offered the same observations over and over again, with regard to diverse phases of the female reproductive cycle. What was different in the final three decades of the nineteenth century was the monotony with which medical spokesmen commented on the feminine nervous and reproductive systems in the context of evolutionary choices involving limited supplies of nerve force. Having discovered that woman's nervous system was not as completely evolved as man's, owing to the needs of her reproductive organs, late Victorian and Edwardian medicine possessed an impressive theory to explain why nervous disorders so frequently accompanied the critical epochs in a woman's biological life. If men were prone to nervous collapse from time to time, in response to professional burdens and financial woes, women were liable to exhaust their nervous energy on the regular, periodic basis that nature decreed.

At puberty and menopause, during pregnancy, childbirth, and lactation, not to mention her monthly uterine upheavals, a woman was at great risk, for all these biological events demanded heavy payments of nerve force. Any additional exertion at these periods, so the medical theory argued, had to draw on other bodily reserves and could thus bankrupt her nervous resources altogether, consigning her to invalidism. "Periodicity," remarked the *London Journal of Medicine* in 1849, "is . . . more indelibly marked upon the female than upon the male constitution; and periodic tendencies are as distinctly seen in the diseases, as in the functions, of the female economy."[17] A flood of medical literature hammered home the point after mid-century. Countless books and articles urged women to take extreme precautions during their menstrual periods and warned them how easily they could drain their nervous energy during the active years of childbearing. It was no coincidence, from the medical point of view, that these were the years in which women were likeliest to fall prey to neurasthenia, or that women were most subject to serious bouts of depression at the very times when their reproductive system was most active. "At the period of puberty,'' Mercier wrote in 1892, and ''at the time of the other momentous changes, of pregnancy, childbirth, suckling, and the climacteric, all of which deplete the activities of the nervous system by making large draughts upon its energies, melancholia may appear.'' In grave cases, suicide might provide the tragic finale in this drama of exhaustion.[18] Melancholia, a comparatively mild form of mental alienation, came in many feminine varieties—melancholia of puberty, of pregnancy, and of lactation, for example, whose very names told the story of their origins. Even more alarming were the advanced forms of madness associated with childbirth, often gathered under the single name of puerperal insanity, or the climacteric insanity that awaited some women at the end of their childbearing years. Victorian medical men informed their female patients that even menstrual irregularities and uterine disease could end in lunacy.[19]

With hormones and the endocrine system a medical mystery until the start of the twentieth century, doctors in the nineteenth struggled as best they could to make sense out of the mood swings that they often witnessed in their female patients. Their theories were reasonable deductions from the existing state of medical knowledge about the nervous system. They also accorded so well with Victorian attitudes toward women that many Edwardian doctors were reluctant to abandon them, even when new information became available. Crichton-Browne may not yet have heard about hormones when he wrote in 1903 that Jane Welsh Carlyle was ''the very woman in whom the physician would expect a nervous breakdown at a critical epoch of life,''[20] but such attitudes took a long time to disappear in any case. It must have been terrifying for a young woman, embarking on adult life, to learn that the path ahead of her was fraught with menace. If she survived the physical ordeal of pregnancy and childbirth, she could go mad while nursing her baby; the strains of producing a family might relegate her permanently to the sickbed, or, at the end of it all, the cessation of her reproductive functions might prove as harmful as their fullest activity.

Much of the medical discussion that traced female nervous illness to the reproductive organs focused on menstruation in particular. While only some women experienced pregnancy, the vast majority experienced the monthly menstrual cycle, and this was unquestionably the dominant feature of female adulthood. As Tilt declared in 1851, the proper management of menstruation was *''the only sure foundation of the health of woman,''* both physical and mental.[21] The proper management, however, was no easy task, as Tilt and his gynecological colleagues conceded, underscoring how very readily menstrual trouble could occur to throw a woman's body and mind into complete disarray. Victorian texts on women's diseases offered such an alarming list of potential problems with the menses that they made it appear as if this manifestation of woman's God-given reproductive role was nothing short of a catastrophe for her. Yet nineteenth-century medical men knew almost nothing about the monthly female function that they deemed a kind of sickness. All sorts of hypotheses, some of them contradicting each other and some exploring analogies between human menorrhea and animal heat, were credited with explaining the relationship between ovulation, menstruation, and conception. The subject remained the focus of intense medical controversy until the 1930s, when the role of hormones in triggering the monthly cycle was finally well enough understood to provide the missing pieces of the puzzle. During the nineteenth century, medical advisors routinely told women that they were likeliest to conceive directly before and after their menstrual periods, the very times, in fact, of minimum fertility. Medical misunderstandings of this sort doubtless played a part in the production of large Victorian families, as many women believed that the middle of their menstrual cycles was safe for intercourse without conception.[22] It is no wonder that doctors and female patients alike associated nervous exhaustion with frequent pregnancies. After bearing six to eight children in a decade, as some women did, delicate health, low spirits, and frequent recourse to the invalid's couch hardly seems an inappropriate reaction.

Information of only dubious accuracy did not stop Victorian medical men from portraying menstruation as the chief reason for the physical fragility and nervous irritability that placed women at such a disadvantage in comparison to men. Under the best of circumstances, uterine activity subjected women to an exhausting drain of nerve force every month; under the worst, they might endure violent, ravaging gynecological disorders that amounted to serious illness. Menstruation was not a healthy release of plethoric body fluid, as it had sometimes been viewed in past centuries, but a condition that definitively marked women's morbidity. Maudsley's comments on this score, widely quoted ever since he published them in the *Fortnightly* in 1874, encapsulate the predominant medical point of view:

> If it were not that woman's organization and functions found their fitting home in a position different from, if not subordinate to, that of men, she would not so long have kept that position. . . . This is a matter of physiology, not a matter of sentiment; it is not a mere question of larger or smaller muscles, but of the energy and power of endurance of the nerve-force which drives the intellectual and muscular machinery; not a question of two bodies and minds that are in equal physical conditions, but of one body and mind capable of sustained and regular hard labour, and of another body and mind which for one quarter of each month during the best years of life is more or less sick and unfit for hard work.

Maudsley's statement was characteristically blunt and tactless, but the overall conclusion was one that the majority of his profession accepted uncritically. The voices of common sense that pointed to the nameless crowds of women who went through life without ever visiting a doctor or succumbing to nervous collapse could not compete against the heavy guns of evolutionary, neurological, and psychiatric theory combined. As Mary Wollstonecraft had observed eighty years before, "What a weak barrier is truth when it stands in the way of an hypothesis!"[23]

For female patients, the message was daunting. It proclaimed, not merely that menstrual difficulties could lead to nervous and mental disorders, but that menstruation itself was pathological. In fact, Victorian medicine insisted that *all* the biological phases of a woman's life resembled ill health. Pregnancy and childbirth, the very times when a woman was fulfilling her divinely ordained purpose, were equally suspect. Laycock was articulating a prevalent opinion when he described the adult female's "menstrual, gravid [pregnant], and parturient periods" as "closely allied to morbid states." Similarly, the physiological manifestations of menopause were frequently dubbed "the climacteric disease in women."[24] There can be no doubt that, generally speaking, the nineteenth-century medical profession considered women's bodies to be defective—suitable companions for their inadequate minds.

Just as the Victorians inherited venerable attitudes toward women's minds, so were they scarcely the first to stress the imperfections of the female body, to consider menstrual bleeding morbid, or to call pregnancy a disease. Such prejudices go back to ancient taboo. The impurity of a woman's body during menstruation, pregnancy, and childbirth was proclaimed both in the Old Testament and in the venerable "church-ing" ritual, still practiced in some twentieth-century parishes, which symbolically cleansed a new mother while welcoming her back into the religious community. The extraordinary aspect of the Victorian perspective on women's innate sickness was that it appeared alongside a sustained glorification of maternity, particularly after the mid-nineteenth century. When women were being told how much the future of the nation and the race depended on their fecundity, they were also hearing that the physical processes attendant on motherhood were somehow unnatural, abnormal, and diseased. Furthermore, in the century when physiologists confirmed that the nerves formed the organizing and directing system of the body, women learned that their nerves, far from being in control, were really at the mercy of their reproductive organs.

While this was the orthodox medical opinion, however, it was not the only one. A number of late Victorian doctors, some of them highly influential, dissented from the arguments that traced female neuroses to reproductive origins. In 1882, Playfair expressed regret that, in previous writings, he had linked uterine disease with nervous prostration and hysteria, for he had come to realize, he confessed, that there was no "necessary or constant connection" between disorders of the womb and neurotic illness. For his part, Dowse "utterly repudiate[d] the idea that the ovaries and the uterus are the main sources of every nervous state which a woman or girl gets into." Allbutt humorously raised the same objections when he berated gynecologists for their uterine obsessions. "*L'utérus c'est la femme* is a proverb which has received a new development in these days," he lamented; "for if by courtesy, rather than conviction, woman be granted the possession of a few subsidiary organs, these, at best, have no prerogative nor any order of their own." More seriously, he charged gynecologists with making women extremely "apprehensive and physically intro-spective," preoccupied with a part of their bodies that often had no effect whatsoever on the disorders for which they sought relief.[25] The paramount role of reproduction in determining the state of a woman's health, however, occupied too central a place in Victorian medical ideology for Allbutt, or anyone else, to dislodge it with a few wry comments.

It was not that his colleagues ignored other causes of nervous prostration affecting their female patients. Doctors knew that domestic life could produce severe anxieties and tensions, and that nursing a child, husband, or parent through prolonged illness, for example, could heavily tax a woman's nerve force. They acknowledged that romantic disappointments were potent sources of nervous illness in unmarried women and that, whatever her marital state, a woman's nervous power could often barely withstand the emotional trauma of bereavement. Nor did they minimize the impact of physical trauma, usually arising from accidents, on female nervous exhaustion, as on male. While crediting the harmfulness of all these situations, medical writers were nonetheless convinced that a woman was particularly liable to break down under their strains because the female constitution was perpetually weakened by uterine and ovarian activity.

It takes no special insight to realize that the loyalty of Victorian medical practitioners and evolutionary biologists to the concept of faulty and inferior womanhood,
dominated by reproductive functions, did not arise from careful examination of
statistically significant data. Whenever such evidence as was collected led to
contradictory conclusions, a little snipping and trimming allowed the learned tailors
to alter the public presentation of the information. Again and again, Victorian
medical texts about women betray, by their confused and convoluted arguments, their
authors' emotional investment in a set of misogynist attitudes incapable of actual
verification. During Victoria's reign, the internal inconsistencies in these writings
may have done nothing to undermine the prevalence of the opinions they promulgated, but they bear witness today to the ideological impetus that inspired them.

In the Victorian literature on women's mental limitations and nervous vulnerability, it is not unusual to find the author's own evidence running counter to the
general assumptions that frame his argument. On occasion, the medical writer seems
oblivious to this problem. James Gully, claiming that the "predisposition to neuropathy" was "attachable to the female rather than the male sex," offered sixteen cases of
nervous disability to support his contention: ten involved men and six women. Where
the author realized his difficulty, he went to considerable exertion, often tying himself
in intellectual knots, to explain it away. Crichton-Browne had to admit that his own
experience at Wakefield asylum indicated that diseases of the nervous system were
more fatal to men than to women, but he was able to account for the statistical
disadvantage in a way that reinforced male superiority. The larger size of the male
head, even at birth, he pointed out, entailed greater risk of damage to the brain during
delivery. Romanes encountered similar troubles in his disquisition on the mental
differences between men and women, published in the late 1880s. Reporting on the
results of his experiment in speed reading and memory retention with "well
educated" members of both sexes, Romanes confessed that women could not only
read more quickly, but "they were better able to remember what they had just read."
These results, however, did not challenge his basic belief that "the female mind
stands considerably below the male." "Rapidity of perception," he added, echoing
Darwin, "is no evidence of what may be termed the deeper qualities of mind—some
of my slowest readers being highly distinguished men." At the end of the century,
Dr. Harry Campbell, a London physician and pathologist who considered woman
"an undeveloped man," likewise belittled women's particular intellectual gifts when
he tried to "account for the fact that women acquit themselves as brilliantly as, or
more brilliantly than, men in examinations open to both sexes." He, too, stressed
female mental precocity, in unfavorable contrast to male mental substance.[26]

Beneath the surface foolishness, there was a fundamental confusion inherent in all
the Victorian literature that made the female nervous system a key feature in sexual
differentiation. As the evolutionary scenario of human development gained acceptance, complexity of structure became equated with advancement along the evolutionary scale. Particularly with regard to the nervous system, the most detailed
elaboration of the branching network of nerves was seen as marking the most highly
evolved creatures—and, therefore, those of greatest intelligence. Since woman's
nervous development, according to esteemed opinion, never attained the final stages
of cerebral growth, it should have followed that her nerves were less intricately

interconnected, her whole nervous system less refined and sensitive than that of man. Yet over and over again, scientists and doctors who subscribed to this evolutionary theory spoke of the delicacy and complexity of women's nerves. James Pollock, consulting physician to the Brompton Hospital for Consumption, was sure that "women are gifted with a more highly sensitive nervous system than men." Crichton-Browne compared schoolgirls' "sensitive and highly-strung nerve centres apt to be damaged by pressure" to those of boys "who are more obdurate and resistent." Romanes emphasized that "the whole organisation of woman is formed on a plan of greater delicacy, and her mental structure is correspondingly more refined: it is further removed from the struggling instincts of the lower animals, and thus more nearly approaches our conception of the spiritual." Clouston, too, was certain that woman's "nervous and mental organisation is more delicate and more complicated than that of a man."[27]

Examples of this mentality could be multiplied indefinitely, but the extent of medical befuddlement over the female nervous system should already be clear. To proclaim that woman's nervous and mental structures were more refined and complex than man's—further removed from animals lower down the evolutionary scale—was to make nonsense of the assertion that feminine cerebral evolution stopped at an incomplete stage and that female intelligence was, consequently, less acute than male. Victorian and Edwardian theorists of sexual differentiation never addressed this colossal contradiction in the component parts of their ideology. On the one hand, the eighteenth-century cult of sensibility, subjected to withering criticism by the mid-Victorian era where men were concerned, remained widely applicable to the middle- and upper-class woman who was depicted as delicate, decorative, and fundamentally idle, in deference to her husband's powers of financial support. The more fragile a woman seemed, the more manly appeared the husband, or father, who looked after her. As sensibility and excitability, both hallmarks of refinement, were clearly functions of the nerves, it was necessary to assign women a fully—even excessively—developed nervous system. On the other hand, a host of old cultural biases and current threats combined in the second half of the nineteenth century to dictate support for an evolutionary explanation of female mental inferiority, plausible only on the grounds of arrested nervous development. There was no way to reconcile these two lines of thought. The best that the medical profession could do was to reiterate that a woman's nervous instability was closely related to her reproductive system. In tracing female nervousness to the uterus or ovaries, doctors were diverting attention from the possibility, implicit in much of their writing, that a woman's brain might, in fact, be highly complex and fully evolved.

The jumbled strands of reasoning about woman's fragility, nervousness, and mental immaturity, all associated with the paramount significance of her reproductive responsibilities, came together with particular urgency to counter the feminist crusade for higher education in the second half of the nineteenth century. Much has recently been written about this aspect of Victorian misogyny, and women's attempts to enter the medical profession at this time are often cited as one reason for the virulence of some doctors' reaction to their efforts.[28] Few male medical practitioners, it is true, welcomed the intrusion of women in their midst, not only because "lady doctors'' threatened to lure away female patients, but because their presence was perceived to jeopardize the still precarious respectability of the medical profession. Obviously, however, the tenacity with which many late Victorian and Edwardian doctors opposed rigorous secondary and university education for women reflected anxieties that went far deeper than professional jealousy. Only a few women were seeking to become medical practitioners, but a far larger number were putting forward claims that challenged the ideology of separate spheres. Like other professionals in these decades, doctors sensed that they were being asked to rethink the basic pattern of bourgeois society in general, and sexual relations in particular. The only way to preserve that pattern, if not intact at least in some recognizable form, was to demonstrate its foundation in the biological essence of manhood and womanhood, and thus to underscore the absurdity of legislating changes in what nature had ordained. Unlike other alarmed and baffled Victorian men, doctors and scientists spoke on the issue of women's health and education with an authority that most of the general public assumed could not be questioned. Even the opinions of clergymen who marshaled scriptural dogma to uphold women's domestic role could not rival medical utterances in this respect.

Nineteenth- and early twentieth-century medical practitioners typically opposed the entry of women into the universities, and even into rigorously academic secondary schools, on the simple grounds that women faced crucial physiological choices, which were not at issue with men. If a woman strained her nervous resources on intellectual endeavors, for which she was not naturally well endowed, she risked seriously damaging—if not destroying—those reproductive capacities that nature meant her to exercise. Few doctors doubted that brain exhaustion frequently led to "an arrest of the ovarian and uterine functions,"[29] for, as we have seen, medical orthodoxy stipulated that the body could only accommodate excessive exertion of one organ by draining nerve force needed by others. Great intellectual effort, furthermore, channeled blood to the brain that should have carried nourishment to the ovaries and uterus. Thus at a time when a gradually increasing number of young women were choosing to extend their education well into the years of physical maturity, they directly confronted medical advice that warned them not to. From a doctor's perspective, the choice was very simple, as Clouston succinctly phrased it in 1882: "Why should we spoil a good mother by making an ordinary grammarian?"[30] It was particularly hard for feminists to dismiss these kinds of questions, which were frustratingly open-ended and impossible to disprove once and for all. A woman with a university education could enjoy blooming health and rosy children for years, and then develop a uterine tumor, or give birth to a defective baby, only to validate medical fears.

Victorian and Edwardian medical practitioners often appeared to favor advanced female education in general terms. They said they were delighted when women trained their minds to curb their emotions, and they assured their female audience that such self-discipline would lend stability to sensitive nerves. They applauded an education, such as Romanes envisioned, that would "tend the better to equip a wife as the helpmeet of her husband, and, by furthering a community of tastes, to weave another bond in the companionship of life." Higher education could be helpful, too, in preparing "a mother for the greatest of her duties—forming the tastes and guiding the minds of her children at a time of life when these are most pliable, and under circumstances of influence such as can never again be reproduced.'' Learning that tended in these directions was commendable in a woman and deserved to be encouraged. This conservative twist to feminist aspirations, similar to arguments already aired in the eighteenth century, could not, however, condone women who sought academic accomplishments for their own sake: such achievements were simply useless and damaging. Above all, the attempt to apply the principles of male education to women was utterly disastrous for creatures whose cerebral hemispheres were not as fully evolved as men's. Romanes may have described modern British womanhood as ''the sweetest efflorescence of evolution,'' but it was arrested evolution nonetheless, and could not compete with the male variety. For a woman to ignore nature in pursuit of unrealizable goals was to destroy her chances of succeeding where nature had designed her to excel and to destine herself for mediocrity, at best, in fields where women were never meant to wander. ''The essential difference between male and female cannot be obliterated at a stroke of the pen by any Senatus Academicus,'' Crichton-Browne averred in 1892. ''To essay such work is to fly in the face of evolution.''[31]

Medical literature abounded with tragic tales of intelligent young women rendered invalids (if not corpses) by their determination to obtain academic honors intended for men. Indeed Clouston and Crichton-Browne seemed engaged in a competition of their own to provide the most chilling examples of this object lesson in female perversity. One of Clouston's best specimens was a young woman who suffered torments from the most trivial thoughts and could not escape from a constant ''watching of herself,'' as she described an acute self-consciousness that left her no peace. She could endure hardly any physical exercise, and sustained reading or thinking caused mental confusion and pain at the crown of the head. Clouston immediately understood the symptoms. She ''had no surplus stock of nerve energy'' and ''had used up in school-work the energy that ought to have gone to build up her . . . body.'' She would have progressed to full-fledged nervous breakdown and total incapacitation had not Clouston quickly intervened, withdrawn her books and relegated her to life in the open air. He knew that she was recovering when she wrote to tell him that she had immersed herself in ''feminine pursuits,'' like painting, drawing, gardening, and poultry keeping. She was among the lucky ones, Clouston implied. Another young woman, twenty years old, after ''a school career of unexampled success,'' ended up insane at the Royal Edinburgh Asylum over which he presided.[32]

Crichton-Browne's hostility to women's departure from domesticity arose from his certainty that the home was the well-spring of all true happiness, the invaluable defense against individual and social breakdown alike. Only from domestic affections, he was sure, could true contentment and emotional stability arise. (In his opinion, even Cardinal Newman would have been happier had he been ''a family man.''[33]) In order to protect family life from all the dangers that he saw menacing its integrity in the modern world, Crichton-Browne produced endless variations on the theme that women's nerves were fitted for motherhood, not careers outside the home. Pride of place among his examples of blighted womanhood belonged to Ellen Watson, a brilliant young mathematician at University College, London, who died of consumption at twenty-four years of age. In 1885, three years after the German microbiologist Robert Koch had identified the tuberculosis bacillus, Crichton-Browne speculated at length about the ways in which nervous overstrain and studious habits in young women were particularly liable to result in consumption. Conceding the persuasiveness of the mounting evidence that tuberculosis was "directly due to a microbe or germ," he nonetheless insisted that the new etiology in no way excluded "the influence of states of the nervous system in conducing to [the] development" of the disease. It was not so impressive to argue that a microbe destroyed Ellen Watson, and Crichton-Browne preferred to contend that her "merciless intellectual discipline," her "incessant and strenuous exertions towards advancement," and "her speculative anxieties" could "account for the incursion and rapid progress of lung decay."[34]

The female, as distinct from the feminist, reaction to the elaborately articulated theory of woman's enslavement to her reproductive organs and incapacity for arduous intellectual work is difficult to ascertain, since ladies seldom wrote explicitly about such matters. The records kept by Victorian and Edwardian doctors leave the undeniable impression that countless women were bothered by disorders and discomforts accompanying menstruation, but whether the women themselves perceived their monthly periods as adequate reason to remain bound to hearth and home is another matter altogether, about which their medical advisors were silent. The slowly increasing numbers of women who attended university suggest that medical warnings were not taken seriously in certain middle-class families, but these were precisely the ones likeliest to harbor feminist sympathies, at least among daughters if not mothers. It would be comforting to think that even larger numbers of women paid little heed to medical misinformation—that the power of ideas unsupported by facts was, for once, negligible—but in the absence of specific information from their mothers, many young women probably did accept what their medical attendants told them about menstruation, until experience suggested otherwise.[35] Those attendants, by the end of the nineteenth century, might well have been female themselves, for the pioneering "lady doctors" ministered exclusively to women and children. One might anticipate that a woman who had successfully survived the ordeal of medical training could set the record straight about female ability to study and menstruate simultaneously.

Elizabeth Garrett Anderson, whose struggles to gain a medical degree launched the campaign to open the profession to women in the 1860s and 1870s, provided such a declaration in her eloquent reply to Maudsley's notorious article in the *Fortnightly*. In 1860, at the start of her efforts, she had written to her friend and fellow feminist Emily Davies, founder of Girton: "Every one seems to fear that my health and nerves will break down. Therefore I am determined by God's help to keep in good health if care can do it."[36] Fourteen years later, when she refuted Maudsley's position on female education, she knew that no physiological barriers needed to stop a woman from the professional training or higher education she sought. Systematically, sensibly, and for the most part dispassionately, she addressed the points in the antifeminist argument, proving them to be grounded not on a fair consideration of the evidence, but merely on masculine misconceptions. Women had reason to know otherwise. "When we are told," she wrote, "that in the labour of life women cannot disregard their special physiological functions without danger to health, it is difficult to understand what is meant, considering that in adult life healthy women do as a rule disregard them almost completely. It is, we are convinced, a great exaggeration to imply that women of average health are periodically incapacitated from serious work by the facts of their organization.'' Working women, she noted, were not exempted from their jobs, or given lighter loads, during those periods when Maudsley alleged them to be sick. In her own experience with female patients, she found that ''the break-down of nervous and physical health seems at any rate to be distinctly traceable to want of adequate mental interest and occupation in the years immediately succeeding school life. Thousands of young women, strong and blooming at eighteen, become gradually languid and feeble under the depressing influence of dulness. . . .'' In her conclusion, Anderson scornfully exposed the motives behind Maudsley's work:

> Dr. Maudsley appends to the physiological argument others which do not press for immediate attention. They are already familiar to all who are interested in noticing what can be said in support of the policy of restriction, whether as applied to negroes, agricultural labourers, or women. They remind us more of an Ashantee fight than of a philosophical essay; so abundant is the powder used in their discharge, and so miscellaneous and obsolete are the projectiles.[37]

Valuable data supported Anderson when she insisted that the personal experiences of educated women gave the lie to medical alarms. In the 1880s, two projects that collected specific information about the health of female college students should have silenced the canard that higher education interfered with reproduction. One, undertaken in the United States through the auspices of the Association of Collegiate Alumnae, inspired a similar survey in England, carried out under the direction of Eleanor Balfour Sidgwick, treasurer and future principal of Newnham. The Sidgwick study, published in 1890 as *Health Statistics of Women Students of Cambridge and Oxford and of their Sisters,* compared the physical condition of women who had attended university with that of the sister or female cousin, closest to them in age, who had not. Involving more than 1,000 students and relatives, it found nothing to support the contention that female university students experienced poorer health after their education than other women of the same age and economic background. In fact, the childbearing record of married, college-educated women compared favorably with that of their relatives. Although the data suggested that they bore fewer children, it also indicated that their offspring were healthier than those born to the control group, according to infant mortality rates. Statistics, however, simply could not unsettle fixed medical and scientific convictions, steeped in cultural biases and lavishly nourished by prejudice and fear. If Romanes could acknowledge that he had ''met with wonderfully few cases of serious breakdown'' among female students, while continuing to argue as though he had encountered many, evidence obviously counted for nothing in this debate.[38]

Anderson's views did not, by any means, command the support of all female doctors. So powerful were the myths that relegated women to the production and nurture of children that they even gained strong approval from women who were proof of their absurdity. Dr. Arabella Kenealy, for one, relied on all the old arguments about finite funds of energy and depletion of constitutional capital when she asserted in 1899 that "the whole question of evolution turns indeed on the function of child-bearing." To amplify this pedestrian observation, she added that nature had no interest in female mathematicians, nor in female athletes, for that matter. Mary Scharlieb, a prominent gynecologist around the turn of the century, likewise assured her readers that she would have "no difficulty in finding plenty of illustrations" among young women to prove "the evil influence of mental overwork on the whole organism."[39] The participation of women doctors in the late Victorian and Edwardian crusade to bolster the sagging ideology of separate spheres makes it impossible to dismiss female opponents of feminist goals as frightened creatures, subconsciously fleeing from freedom back into slavery—into the safe, known sanctuary of the home. The allegiance of female doctors to beliefs that they themselves knew to be invalid can, perhaps, best be explained by reference to their professional position. Working as medical practitioners in an environment saturated with antifeminist assumptions, they doubtless experienced considerable pressure to embrace their colleagues' point of view. They may have felt the need to conform as a matter of professional survival, or they may have succumbed to a kind of indoctrination that enabled them to bracket themselves as exceptional, while leaving unchallenged the denigration of the female sex in general. Even today, such a frame of mind is common enough among professionally accomplished women.[40]

Successful female writers likewise often betrayed the strength of cultural conditioning on those rare occasions when they discussed the biological circumstances that influenced their lives. Margaret Oliphant, to cite an extreme case, blamed herself, quite unjustifiably, for the deaths of two of her young children. She had been warned by Mary Howitt, another prolific female author, that babies could be born with defective hearts if their mothers performed "too much mental work" during pregnancy. Oliphant knew that it was foolish to believe such things; yet so strong was the contemporary prejudice against intellectual women when she wrote her autobiography, over several decades during the second half of the nineteenth century, that she imbibed some of its poison and burdened herself with guilt over her indefatigable literary endeavors, on which her family was financially dependent. It was another female novelist, journalist, and essayist, Eliza Lynn Linton, who wrote in 1886: "Strong emotions, strained nerves, excitement, anxiety, absorption, are all hurtful to the unborn child. They tend to bring on premature birth; and if not this, then they create sickly offspring, whom the mother cannot nourish when they are born. . . . The mental worries and the strain of attention inseparable from professional life, make the worst possible conditions for satisfactory child-bearing."[41] Whatever the psychological impetus behind the repudiation of feminist aspirations by women who themselves had broken free from the constraints of pure domesticity, the significant point is that female readers were hearing from many female writers the same message that male doctors conveyed to them—and some female doctors, too. There were even late Victorian women who, having earned a university degree, nonetheless publicly proclaimed their own mental inferiority to men.[42]

Men and women, feminists and antifeminists, could at least concur about one aspect of female education that bore directly on women's nerves. Virtually unanimous Victorian opinion called for girls and young women to enjoy more opportunities for physical exercise, preferably outdoors. Although most of the discussion focused on girls' secondary schools, the place of athletic activities and team sports at the women's colleges was, obviously, a related subject. Indeed, the women's colleges at Cambridge and Oxford led the way in organizing their students for competitive sports such as field hockey. Gymnastics, swimming, horseback riding, and vigorous walking were also popular. The move to engage women in physical exercise formed an integral part of the wide-ranging feminist campaign against female invalidism, but it also addressed the antifeminist goal of making young women physically fit for motherhood. It expressed, too, the slowly growing inclination to liberate women from long, heavy skirts and tightly laced corsets, which were no boon to female health. By the 1890s, grown women might be seen playing tennis or riding bicycles with a freedom their mothers could never have imagined. W. E. H. Lecky, the historian and essayist, was all in favor of these developments, as he wrote enthusiastically in 1896: "The beauty of perfect health and of high spirits has been steadily replacing, as the ideal type, the beauty of a sickly delicacy and of weak and tremulous nerves which in the eighteenth century was so much admired, or at least extolled."[43]

There was, admittedly, considerable disagreement over the extent to which female athleticism should be encouraged, and even at the end of the century one school of thought considered team sports too unfeminine for women. Prolonged and intense physical activity, this viewpoint maintained, could prove just as deleterious as excessive intellectual effort, for it was equally demanding of nerve force and equally dangerous to the reproductive organs as a result. Kenealy regarded "any extreme of muscle-power in a woman as in itself evidence of disease," for muscularity was not the "province" of women. By unduly developing her muscles, the modern woman was not only "squandering" the birthright of her unborn babies, but she coarsened herself in the process, destroying the basis for that "delicacy, tenderness, and virtue," which had so gloriously distinguished womanhood in the past. Clearly, when muscular athleticism had become a hallmark of masculinity, the idea of women competing for athletic laurels struck the advocates of strict sexual differentiation as inappropriate and socially undesirable.[44] No one, however, questioned the value of milder forms of exercise, like calisthenics, for women. By the end of the century, at least one of Mill's assertions in *The Subjection of Women* commanded general support. Examining "the greater nervous susceptibility of women," he had insisted in 1869:

> Much of all this is the mere overflow of nervous energy run to waste, and would cease when the energy was directed to a definite end. . . . Moreover, when people are brought up, like many women of the higher classes (though less so in our own country than in any other), a kind of hot-house plants, shielded from the wholesome vicissitudes of air and temperature, and untrained in any of the occupations and exercises which give stimulus and development to the circulatory and muscular system, while their nervous system, especially in its emotional department, is kept in unnaturally active play; it is no wonder if those of them who do not die of consumption, grow up with constitutions liable to derangement from slight causes, both internal and external, and without stamina to support any task, physical or mental, requiring continuity of effort.[45]

Medical men could have hardly objected to Mill's contention, for they had been foremost throughout the first half of the nineteenth century in lamenting the harmful system of education imposed on young women of the affluent classes. Repeatedly, they criticized the sedentary life at ladies' seminaries, with its overstimulation of the senses and emotions to the neglect of the intellect, its cultivation of fashionable refinement to the exclusion of healthful activity. It would be far better, the *Family Oracle of Health* argued in 1826, for young ladies to learn botany in a flower garden than card games in a drawing room, for then they might avoid "the sickly frame and miserable existence of a nervous patient." A few years later, Conolly sharply criticized a form of education that trained young women to nurture delicate sensibilities at the expense of brain and muscles alike: ". . . the improper expectations, the vain rivalries, the restless and frivolous pleasures of fashionable life, are but too well calculated to produce all varieties of nervous disorders in young persons whom an affected refinement has debarred from active and natural exercises, and whose minds have never been accustomed to the exercise of self-controul." Doctors complained that women brought up under such tutelage thought life consisted of attending balls and reading novels, while the overexcitement of the sensory organs, through music, perfume, and rich food, or the overstimulation of the emotions through sentimental literature, could indeed, as Tilt warned, "give an undue activity to the nervous system."[46]

The early Victorian medical profession, deploring hysteria and other nervous maladies in young women, recommended that they invigorate their minds through the cultivation of moral wisdom and their drooping bodies through moderate exercise. Medical practitioners well understood what Anderson stressed in 1874—that an empty mind becomes a potent source of illness through sheer tedium. As Marshall Hall once wrote to a female patient, with regard to managing her health: "I advise you to take up some systematic *mental* occupation during the rest of the day. Nothing is so injurious as unoccupied time. The mind then dwells on every ailment, the tongue becomes white, and the stomach deranged from mere emotion." Other medical advisors underscored the impact of boredom on the nerves, rather than the tongue or stomach, but the message was still the same: "Vacancy of mind and debility of body go hand in hand, and mutually increase each other."[47] In short, intellectual curiosity in women was no bad thing.

In the second half of the nineteenth century, doctors did not cease to regret the "dreary, aimless vacuity of mind that is hysteria's favourite soil,"[48] and feminists had no argument with them on that account. The difference between the medical and feminist perspectives was, nonetheless, fundamental. The first thought that educators could tinker with the curriculum at girls' schools without making any further changes in the lives of middle-class women. The second believed that to alter the assumptions behind female education meant, in effect, totally to reevaluate women's role in modern British society. In the face of such a challenge, the medical profession qualified its earlier counsel that women should exercise their minds. Just as doctors had previously stressed the dangers of mental underemployment and physical inertia, so now they marshaled evolutionary arguments to caution against intellectual overexertion and excessive physical strain. Caught in the midst of this modification of medical theory, middle-class women faced grim alternatives. They were told that they could become ill through idleness, but they faced equally certain punishment, in the form of nervous collapse, if they denied the natural differences between the sexes and attempted to compete with men. Breakdown from overwork was not a socially excusable failure in a woman, but loomed rather as a kind of retribution for ignoring both her reproductive duties and her responsibility to help, not rival, the men in her life. There was a very fine line between the acceptable and the unacceptable where women's intellectual endeavors were concerned, between "mental development," which could be beneficial, and "intellectual specialisation," which no woman could acquire without damaging her health.[49] It was women's misfortune that doctors not only claimed the exclusive right to draw that line, but, as circumstances altered, they drew it differently.

Implicit in the volumes of medical pronouncements concerning the female nervous system and reproductive cycle was profound medical confusion about women's sexuality. The subject occasioned tremendous uncertainty, bewilderment, and hostility among some medical men, sparking debate among all. It was a vast topic, which necessarily encompassed a smaller one—the extent to which female nervous disorders might be attributed, not simply to the dominance of a woman's sexual organs in her physiological constitution, but to sexual activity itself, whether insufficient, excessive, or unnatural. Among the general middle-class public, a similar ambivalence shrouded the question of female sexuality. While it was widely accepted that the male sexual drive was a potent force whose aggression had to be curbed by manly self-control, there was no such unanimity of opinion concerning female sexual feeling. The controversy, needless to say, was merely one aspect of the ongoing attempt to define woman's nature and, accordingly, her rightful place in society.

It is widely believed today that Victorian men (especially doctors and husbands) expected women to experience neither sexual desire nor pleasure, and that, owing in part to utter ignorance about their own bodies, women did, in fact, go through life in a state of sexual anesthesia. A few medical men doubtless promoted the image of the passionless British lady, whose deep maternal feelings enabled her to submit to marital relations that would otherwise have been highly distasteful to her. The principal proponent of this viewpoint was William Acton, the mid-Victorian surgeon without a medical degree who wrote on the subjects of prostitution, venereal disease, urology, and the reproductive organs of men and women. It was Acton who contributed the now much-quoted and reviled opinion: "I should say that the majority of women (happily for society) are not very much troubled with sexual feeling of any kind. What men are habitually, women are only exceptionally." He was, of course, referring to ladies of the leisured classes, for the sexual depravity—potential if not actual—of working-class women was rarely questioned by middle-class men.[50]

Acton was not, however, a highly regarded member of the Victorian medical profession, and although his vision of female frigidity confirms late twentieth-century assumptions about sexual repression 100 years ago, he did not speak for the majority of his colleagues.[51] Among the most vocal publicists for his point of view were, not medical men in good standing, but writers of advice for middle-class mothers and daughters. Women themselves in many cases, these authors implied that ignorance on all matters concerning human sexuality was an essential trait for young ladies of impeccable social respectability. The animalism inherent in, and even synonymous with, sexual desire should find no encouragement in the pure-minded female around whom the Victorian home revolved. A number of British feminists in the second half of the nineteenth century also warmly endorsed the theory that women did not experience sexual arousal. In their crusade against the male sexual predacity that victimized women and children, they sought to elevate the presumed model of female asexuality into an ideal for both men and women, in a utopian world devoid of sexual violence and domination.[52]

Victorian moralists of both sexes found comfort in the notion of women's sexual passivity because it seemed to guarantee female contentment with domesticity. Without urgent sexual desires, a woman was likely to accept the more placid emotional gratifications of family life, never experiencing the restlessness and dissatisfaction that sometimes drove a man to infidelity. The chaste wife-mother stood at the very center of middle-class social relations. Endow her with sexual needs, some alarmists believed, and the whole structure would collapse. It was, indeed, "happily for society," as Acton observed, that women lacked such passions. It was also a happy situation for husbands who did not want to worry about the paternity of their children and heirs. A woman's lack of sexual ardor helped her husband in other ways as well, for she did not tempt him to incontinence, but rather helped him to master his own debasing instincts—or so the theory went. For those who worried about nervous drain and the decline of masculine efficacy through abundant loss of semen, the sexually indifferent wife was the perfect mate.[53]

While such attitudes were implicit in much nineteenth-century literature on the home, on womanhood, and on marriage, they were by no means the dominant theme in *medical* texts about these subjects. The contrast between Georgian and Victorian views of female sexuality was less extreme than historians often suggest. If "there was no Georgian Dr. Acton," there was certainly a Georgian Pamela, the heroine of Richardson's novel (1740) and a paragon of female sexual anesthesia.[54] More significant than these isolated examples is the fact that a sizeable body of Victorian medical literature acknowledged the normality and acceptability of women's sexual desire, if satisfied within marriage, as freely as eighteenth-century medical opinion had done. Nor did all Victorian doctors agree that women should remain in utter ignorance of their bodily functions, particularly with regard to sexual relationships. Sir James Paget thought that sex education would help women, as well as men, to understand that sexual gratification contributed to good health, rather than otherwise.[55]

Recognition of female sexuality was reflected in all manner of Victorian medical writing, from the most elevated moral disquisition to the humblest piece of commercial puffery. Elizabeth Blackwell esteemed the strength of women's sexual desire as an essential element in married happiness and an "immense spiritual force of attraction." Clearly, a woman's ability to enjoy marital love also mattered to the doctors who, in the 1880s, opposed ovariotomies on the grounds that the operation might destroy the patient's sexual appetite. In keeping with his own unflattering view of human nature, Maudsley affirmed the presence of animal sexuality, albeit restrained, in women, while the purveyors of medical advice for a popular audience and the producers of cures for sexual disorders, like Dr. Solomon's "Cordial Balm of Gilead," had no doubts whatsoever that women possessed as ready a capacity to enjoy sexual relations as men.[56] It is highly inaccurate to maintain that medical tolerance of female sexuality in the first half of the nineteenth century, partly inspired by the commendation of married love within such influential dissenting sects as the Unitarians, Quakers, and Congregationalists, responded to feminist agitation in the second half with a punitive abrogation of feminine claims to sexual pleasure.[57] Throughout the century, many doctors accorded women, across the social spectrum, the right to sexual feelings and hoped that they would be sexually satisfied.

In the absence of extensive material explicitly confirming such a conclusion, historians today can only suppose that the numerous examples of successful, happy, mutually supportive and companionate marriages, which we find in Victorian diaries, letters, and memoirs, rested at least in part on sexual bonds that were gratifying to both partners. The fact that women were brought up never to mention the sexual side of marriage does not allow us to assume that they detested it. An exceptional case like Fanny Kingsley, who was totally unrepressed in her avowal of sexual yearnings, cannot provide the basis for sweeping generalizations, but the fact that Queen Victoria both purchased nude artwork for herself—paintings and drawings of naked men and women—and gave similar presents to Prince Albert suggests a lack of inhibitions about sexuality that we rarely ascribe to Victorian ladies.[58] Nor was the Queen representative of the sexual license that many aristocratic wives enjoyed, for she disapproved of the immorality and hedonism at the apex of society as heartily as did her middle-class subjects. While it is doubtless true that large numbers of Victorian women could not find happiness in sexual relations so long as the likelihood of pregnancy loomed as an ever-present threat in their lives, it is equally clear that they did not, therefore, peremptorily reject the idea of female sexual desire. The group of educated women who joined the Men and Women's Club, founded in 1885 by Karl Pearson to explore all aspects of gender relationships, believed that women would be freer to express their sexual feelings if there were no element of compulsion in marital intercourse, and if they did not have to bear the consequences of pregnancy as a frequent result. Pregnancy, they agreed, had done much to curb women's innate sexuality. Annie Besant, too, in the neo-Malthusian phase of her life before Theosophy claimed her, asserted that women experienced sexual passion, which it was both cruel and unhealthy to suppress—hence the need for contraception.[59] It seems fair to question, furthermore, how many Victorian husbands really wanted cold, impassive wives, and to speculate that, when medical men upheld the naturalness of female sexuality, they were providing precisely the information that many of their middle-class patrons wanted to hear.

The wide-ranging debate over female sexuality bore directly on the medical interpretation of women's nervous illnesses, because doctors typically expressed their belief that sexual relations within marriage were healthy for women by suggesting the damage wrought in their absence. Laycock's remark in 1840 concerning "females who . . . suffer from repressed feelings in civilized communities" betrayed an awareness of the toll taken on women's health by the suppression of natural sexual instincts. Medical writers conveyed this viewpoint repeatedly throughout the Victorian and Edwardian eras, particularly stressing that disappointed love and "the mortifications of celibacy," in Conolly's phrase, gave rise to hysterical symptoms. Much as they prided themselves on their up-to-date causative theories, doctors who traced hysteria to sexual frustration were, in fact, echoing the ancient notion of uterine depredations, according to which the manifestations of hysteria appeared when an empty, unsatisfied womb, deprived too long of sexual satisfaction, rampaged destructively throughout the body. Although nineteenth-century medical men officially rejected this venerable interpretation in favor of hysteria's nervous origins, they still frequently assigned a major role to the female reproductive organs or sexual feelings, because these could so violently agitate the nerves. Among the varied reasons doctors proposed for female hysteria, from menstrual irregularity through religious frenzy, many continued to find sexual abstinence the most plausible.[60]

Repression of sexual feeling could, of course, account for a range of female nervous disorders, in addition to hysteria. Although Clouston maintained that it was the emotional, not the sexual, side of marriage and maternity that spinsters missed, Schofield had no illusions on that score and, like numerous other medical men, insisted on the role of "enforced celibacy" in promoting the diverse nervous disorders of unmarried women. Lacking the opportunities to satisfy their sexual needs outside of marriage, respectable women suffered more from abstinence than men, Schofield felt sure. He blamed his professional colleagues for handling the subject with a certain lack of "refinement and sympathetic feeling," and he hinted that to emphasize this one particular cause of female nervous afflictions was a "coarse and unscientific view." Yet he, too, focused on this cause, identifying frustrated sexuality as a source of profound suffering in the lives of countless women.[61]

While willing enough to trace female nervous disorders to unrelieved chastity—a virtuous, if possibly unhealthy, condition—Victorian and Edwardian doctors were not eager to discuss sexual deviance as a potential cause of women's neurotic ill health. They were certainly not blind to the existence of female masturbation, and some credited it with the power to cause, not merely menstrual problems, but depression, hysteria, infertility, and ultimately insanity. The secret sin, in other words, was judged as dangerous to women as to men, but the female variety did not occupy anything like the space in medical texts that male indulgence in onanism claimed. As for female homosexuality, it figured even less noticeably in British medical literature before World War I. Although Havelock Ellis called attention to lesbianism in *Sexual Inversion*, a general sense that close female attachments were abnormal, and threatening to society, only began to emerge during the war years. Throughout the Edwardian era, female sexuality continued to be defined in terms of responsiveness to masculine overtures. So uncomfortable were Edwardian men with the notion of female sexual deviancy or aggressiveness that, under the Incest Act of 1908, only men could be prosecuted for sexual acts with close blood relatives, while women's role remained that of victim alone.[62]

Nineteenth-century doctors were as reluctant to believe that respectable women indulged in excessive sexual activities as they were anxious to ignore the possibility that ladies participated in deviant ones. While they warned that "excess in connubial intercourse"[63] could cause uterine irritation, nervous instability, and hysteria in an otherwise healthy married woman, they always assumed that her husband was to blame. Even those medical spokesmen who acknowledged women's ability to experience sexual desires never intended to condone immodest female conduct. Where sexual desire in a woman was too assertive to ignore, they could only assume that she was unhealthy and suffered from nymphomania, a term that came into use during the eighteenth century to designate an allegedly abnormal sexual appetite in women. This form of insanity might be attributed to undue excitation of the female reproductive organs—hence the proliferation of such diagnostic subspecies as uteromania and ovarian madness—but medical experts more frequently considered it a manifestation of moral insanity. To employ "indecent expressions" in place of female reticence, to betray "without reserve unbecoming feelings and trains of thought,"[64] and to appear preoccupied by carnal relations were all deemed so utterly unnatural in a woman of good breeding, raised to accept male sexual dominance, that they became comprehensible only in the light of lunacy, even if the offender appeared otherwise sane. The Victorian medical profession, and the British bourgeoisie in general, obviously preferred to think that aggressive female sexuality was alien to their own level of society. It might flourish among the lower ranks of the working class, indifferent to all notions of respectability and schooled in criminality; it might characterize women of different races and nationalities. It was not supposed to taint the flower of British womanhood.

The concept of female sexuality, needless to say, never managed to remain in the neat categories to which medical men tried to consign it in the nineteenth and early twentieth centuries. Not only did class prejudices constantly intrude on gender stereotypes, but the categorizers themselves were plagued by a host of quandaries that involved medical theory and masculine sentiment alike. In theoretical terms, the problem was simple and glaring. Sexual relations within marriage had to be good for women, since the main responsibility facing middle-class wives was to produce children and raise families. The future of the race, furthermore, required hefty numbers of strapping babies. At the same time, however, doctors were busy promulgating a vision of innate female weakness based on the dominance of women's reproductive organs over their nerves. Thus medical practitioners were simultaneously reassuring female patients that sexual relations with their husbands were healthy and gravely informing them of all the illnesses that followed pregnancy and childbirth. What is more, women were not supposed to be preoccupied with their sexual functions, yet medical advisors constantly reminded them that reproduction was the biological purpose of their lives. The pervasive ambivalence that doctors felt as men when they contemplated female sexuality led them, on the one hand, to spiritualize womanhood, elevating it far above the sensuality in which man was regrettably wont to wallow, and, on the other, to refer generically to all women as "the Sex." While respecting women as quasi-celestial beings, medical men also harbored the suspicion that these lovely creatures were actually closer to nature, and more in touch with natural desires, than were the civilized masculine members of the human race.[65] With these contrasting images and emotional inconsistencies to sort out, it is not surprising that some Victorian doctors chose to ignore the existence of female sexuality or to label it pathological. Others, never even recognizing the dilemma, simply continued to issue pronouncements that amounted to nothing more than medical muddle.

Conflicting attitudes toward women's innate sexual qualities were hardly restricted to the medical profession, but troubled Victorian men and women throughout the middle and upper classes. Nor did the ambivalence exclusively relate to the challenge of the "New Woman" in the second half of the nineteenth century, since it was implicit in writings on women throughout Victoria's reign. It went deeper than the age-old "wife and whore"[66] dichotomy, for even the Victorian vision of the good, pure woman was riddled with contradictions. Whether for a single decade or for the entire period, it is far harder to generalize about prevailing stereotypes of femininity than about models of masculinity. In medico-scientific texts, as in literature for the general public, the image of woman was shifting and fluid, one picture merging almost imperceptibly with its opposite. Those opposites invariably surfaced with any discussion of female nerves.

The stereotype of Victorian womanhood most familiar today is that of the extremely fragile creature, cursed by her biological nature with great liability to nervous illness. In Victorian fiction, "the cult of the invalid wife," daughter, or sister bears unambiguous testimony to the prevalence of this ideal among the reading public.[67] Such women were, of course, in no position to compete with men, on whom they relied utterly for protection and support, and whose power, in effect, defined their lives. Even before evolutionary science "proved" that the development of the female brain was incomplete and therefore childlike, a prevalent picture of sheltered, sickly femininity underscored the infantile quality of the adult woman, a portrayal that Wollstonecraft had rejected as early as 1792. Indeed, science was as much influenced by popular prejudices and literary stereotypes in this respect as novelists and poets were impressed by the findings of science. In *David Copperfield* (1849–50), Dickens produced two memorable child-women—Clara Copperfield, David's mother, and Dora Spenlow, his first wife. Dora's childishness became explicitly intertwined with invalidism after she suffered a miscarriage and gradually declined in health, until her death freed David to find a more mature spouse. (It was no coincidence that her illness was closely related to her reproductive role, for which the child-wife was obviously unfitted.) Poetry, too, perpetuated the view of under-developed femininity, although not always linked with ill health: for example, both Tennyson's *The Princess* (1847) and Coventry Patmore's now infamous *Angel in the House*, published in sections during the 1850s and early 1860s, glorified the child within the woman. Nor were such wives confined to the pages of literature. When Margaret Oliphant moved to Ealing in 1861, she was struck by the behavior of her neighbors, the Blacketts, an affluent family in the publishing business. "Mrs Blackett was about my age," she reported, then in her early thirties, "and a fine creature, very much more clever than her husband, though treated by him in any serious matter as if she had been a little girl. . . ." What surprised Oliphant most was that Mrs. Blackett in a sense connived at her own infantilism.[68] It is certainly true that, by the end of the nineteenth century, the partial success of women in challenging legal, political, and economic restrictions had modified this model of helplessness, but the general view of female passivity still found widespread endorsement. For many late Victorians and Edwardians, a woman who failed to evince the traits of submissiveness and dependence had doubtless been unsexed by too much education and had become a sort of freak.

Superimposed on the image of immature and debilitated women was the related, yet different, one of selfless wives, mothers, and daughters. Victorian women were told over and over again that they existed to serve others, that their goals were subsumed in those of their families. This characterization arose partly from the old belief that women were at the mercy of their feelings. As Forbes Winslow observed in 1840 "a woman's life is said to be but the history of her affections," and it was a Victorian commonplace, within and outside the medical profession, that women who lacked a satisfactory outlet for these emotions were not only incomplete, but likely to be ill. Crichton-Browne was very much part of that tradition when, commenting on George Eliot's recurring spells of severe depression, he suggested that "motherhood and the laughter of children of her own might have kept the demon at bay." Female altruism was further elucidated after mid-century by the realization that evolutionary processes had deprived woman of five crucial cerebral ounces. This critical shortcoming explained not only her childishness, but also her selflessness; lacking a well-developed will, she necessarily lacked a strong sense of her own self.[69]

What strikes us as so obvious today—that the attributes of the invalid and the child are particularly incompatible with the idea of selfless service to others—posed no problems for Victorian conceptions of womanhood. These were not, in any case, the product of reasoned analysis, as the hopeless confusion about woman's moral sense amply illustrates. From one perspective, she was deficient in moral character, possessing as much capacity for exercising moral choice as a child, or as her limited mental development permitted. (It goes without saying that the moral sense stood in Victorian estimation among the highest achievements of evolution.) From another perspective, however, woman was deemed capable of the greatest moral action, that of self-sacrifice for the good of others.[70] There is almost a "stream of consciousness" quality to nineteenth-century British writing on femininity, as if one idea about women simply engendered another, without concern for logical sequence or plausibility. The supposition that strength of affection and selflessness underlay the female nature became, in fact, the foundation of another model of womanhood diametrically contrasted to that of the passive, weak-willed, nervous, frail, and childish character paraded in countless diverse texts.

When middle-class Victorians thought about woman in the abstract, they may have chosen to emphasize her delicacy and dependence, but when they thought about her actually married and raising a family, they stressed very different qualities. Then she became nurse, nurturer and comforter, the embodiment of kindness, of tenderness, but also of moral rectitude. The evangelical vision of woman's sacred domestic work exerted a powerful influence on middle-class wives, who were inspired to try transforming the home into a haven of peace and spirituality in an increasingly turbulent and secular world. The ideal of domestic life that they embraced taught them not to relegate the upbringing of their children to servants; a mother was responsible for her child's early lessons, in religion and ethics, as in numbers and letters. Long before church, chapel, or school, she began the arduous work of transforming bawling infants into disciplined social creatures. She was also supposed to be an efficient manager, able to supervise the housekeeping, to handle the finances, and to keep the domestic ship of state sailing as smoothly as her husband captained his business affairs. Finally, or perhaps firstly, she was to be his companion and helpmate. These were all demanding tasks that required considerable capabilities, intelligence, and spirit. In Victorian writing about the home, the wife-mother, or sister-daughter on the verge of becoming a wife and mother, was not only the pillar of domestic life, but a fountain of strength as well, to mix architectural metaphors. She was the source of virtue in the family, teaching the meaning of goodness by her own example. Noble women of this genre grace the plots of countless Victorian novels, whether as the devoted sister Kate Nickleby in *Nicholas Nickleby,* the all-suffering daughter Agnes Wickfield in *David Copperfield,* the wise mother Mrs. Bretton in *Villette,* or numerous other examples. The Victorian glorification of the wife and mother, participating actively in all aspects of domestic life, was a social philosophy to which many women of the middle class, and of the upper-working class as well, could proudly subscribe, no matter how blatantly they failed to attain its standard of perfection. Its hold on nineteenth-century British culture goes far toward illuminating the virulence of much female opposition to feminism.[71]

Although the Victorians themselves were not apparently bothered by the fact that the vision of strong, capable womanhood effectively canceled out the notion of frail and nervous femininity, the historian in the late twentieth century who *is* disturbed by the egregious contradiction may find some comfort in the observation that the two conceptions were less diametrically opposed than they now seem. The strength of women, even when cast in its most positive light, was exerted to help others. It was a kind of fortitude at once supportive, obedient, and utterly self-denying. Although one image of womanhood implied inadequacy and the other competence, neither granted the Victorian woman independence. She existed primarily, if not solely, within the context of family relationships and could never achieve the autonomy that her husband enjoyed. Even at the end of the nineteenth century, when alternative female roles were beginning to gain acceptance for those unfortunate women consigned to spinsterhood, only the most advanced feminists questioned whether marriage and motherhood were still the finest destiny for a woman.

Yet another set of assumptions about womanhood rejected the premise that women were guileless, either as angelic invalids or domestic saints. Often existing alongside one of the more flattering portraits—or, indeed, lurking beneath it—was the manipulative female, who had to "resort to petty arts and petty ways" to secure her aims.[72] In particular she used her nerves in the daily negotiations of family life, to gain sympathy, attention, and a kind of power. Doctors encountered the type regularly in female invalids whose maladies appeared far less grave to medical wisdom than the patients themselves believed, or than they wanted their loved ones to believe. William Baly, a well-known London physician at mid-century, learned the lesson early, just after he had established himself in private practice in 1836. Writing to his mother about a mutual friend whom he had attended professionally, he explained that "her complaints are entirely nervous, but she has some unfortunate fancies with regard to them. *Do not* mention her illness as a serious one when you write." Crichton-Browne recalled that Sir James Simpson was known to prescribe a placebo for "nervous and fidgety" female patients, who benefited from the delusion that he had given them "a new and potent remedy" for their troubles.[73] It was not that doctors never encountered similar attitudes in male patients, but when they did, they considered the condition aberrant and, by the second half of Victoria's reign, unmanly. Where women were concerned, they tended to perceive it as all too characteristic of the female sex.

One suspects that literary sources encouraged medical men in this frame of mind, for the invocation of nervous debility to gain some personal advantage provided a recurrent motif in nineteenth-century fiction. With rare exceptions, such as Mr. Fairlie, the characterization applied to female figures who, if not actually deceitful, attempted to control those around them through the indirect means of sickness. Male authors were not alone in remarking on this tendency in women. Jane Austen mocked it, at the very start of the century, in *Pride and Prejudice* (1813). When Mrs. Bennett accused her husband: "You take delight in vexing me. You have no compassion on my poor nerves," his reply suggested how often she had tried that ploy before. "You mistake me, my dear," he reassured her. "I have a high respect for your nerves. They are my old friends. I have heard you mention them with consideration these twenty years at least." Dickens excelled at caricaturing professional nervous invalids, of whom Mrs. Wititterly in *Nicholas Nickleby* is the very epitome of the species. The least exertion or excitement exhausted her nervous resources and inevitably produced "a sinking, a depression, a lowness, a lassitude, a debility." The regular appearance of female nervous manipulators in Victorian novels suggests that readers recognized the type and associated women with the exploitation of ill health. Even Queen Victoria was not spared insinuations of flaunting her nerves when it suited her to evade royal responsibilities after Prince Albert's death.[74]

It was a short step from someone like Mrs. Wititterly, preying on Kate Nickleby, to a representation of womanhood that was even more sinister and menacing. Whether this final Victorian image of femininity was a projection of male fears or fantasies, it was the only one that explicitly acknowledged female sexuality. It was, in fact, predicated on the deadly power of woman's sexual appetite, for the angel in the house had not expelled an older vision of woman as lascivious temptress, the femme fatale who used alluring wiles to destroy, or unman, the opposite sex. Here was no spirituality, but only rampant sensuality; in place of morality, this siren, sorceress, witch, vampire, harpy, or other monster of choice was all immorality.[75] Woman's seeming innocence was merely a cover for seduction, part of her program to entrap man and reduce him to impotence. The vampire sucked his blood; the whore squandered his semen; the wife wasted his money. The images were interchangeable. Victorian iconography could, of course, go back to the classical world for vivid evocations of monstrous women, or to early Christian imagery for the juxtaposition of Magdalene and Madonna within a single conception of womanhood. No neat chronological progression traces the nineteenth-century interpretation of woman from the angelic to the diabolic; the picture of femininity painted by Victorian society always conjoined purity and depravity, sometimes featuring one in the foreground, sometimes the other. Nonetheless, the man-devouring symbolism became harsher and more overwrought at the end of the nineteenth and the start of the twentieth century, as it reflected both the fin de siècle cult of decadence and male recoil from the New Woman. Yet while paying a sort of tribute to woman's devastating power, even this Victorian stereotype of femininity denied her any autonomy. If she was a monster, she was monstrous in relation to men.

The predatory female menacing the pages of Rider Haggard's *She* (1887) or Bram Stoker's *The Lair of the White Worm* (1911) did not frequent medical texts on women's nerves, but the tension between the good and the bad woman, the helpless and the harmful, nonetheless informed medical attitudes toward female neuroses, both old and new, throughout the nineteenth century. With the ancient diagnosis of hysteria and the novel one of anorexia nervosa, doctors were particularly torn between two fundamentally contrasting points of view. On the one hand, the conviction that woman was defenseless in the face of her emotions explained female vulnerability to hysteria—an illness that defied reason—even if no scientific theory before mid-century actually elucidated how strong feelings could produce hysterical symptoms. That problem, however, vanished after evolutionary speculation proclaimed the insufficiencies of female cerebral development, for lack of a well-established will left women particularly prone to the onslaughts of hysteria. Without the dominant will to exercise supervisory and inhibitory duties, lower nervous centers in the female brain were free to function independently, creating the chaotic sensory and motor dysfunctions characteristic of hysteria. Thanks to weakness of will, Romanes commented in 1887, women's emotions tended "to break away, as it were, from the restraint of reason," and to find expression either "in the overmastering form of hysteria, or in the more ordinary form of comparative childishness. . . ." J. M. Clarke and Seymour Sharkey elucidated the situation in more dispassionate, but basically similar, terms. Clarke reminded his readers in 1894 that "six times as many women as men are affected with hysteria, and that the distinguishing features of the female mind as compared with the male consist of a weaker will, and greater predominance of the emotional over the purely intellectual faculties." The results, as far as Sharkey was concerned, were "two sets of phenomena" in the brain of the hysterical person: "one a too active and uncontrolled nerve discharge, the other paralysis of various kinds, sensory and motor."[76]

On the other hand, however, Victorian doctors always suspected that a different interpretation of hysteria was possible, one they hinted at more than announced. According to the alternative view, a hysterical woman evinced, not too little will, but far too much. By an act of will, she imposed fraudulent symptoms of disease on her body. "It is quite certain," Conolly observed in the 1830s, "that the unhappy temper and violent irritability of hysterical females . . . is in some instances sufficient to bring on, almost at the will of the patient, attacks which occasion much concern to their relatives or friends. . . ." For his part, D. H. Tuke believed that hysterical paralysis could result from exertion of the will's influence over the voluntary muscles, making them incapable of movement. A woman who manufactured hysteria in this fashion opposed her own will to that of her doctor, rejecting his sagacious counsel and refusing to recover. Not a few medical advisors conflated this behavior with sexual assertiveness and judged the patient all the more reprehensible as a result. Willful women, embodying the denial of womanhood, were objects of loathing, but also of fear, because they challenged medical authority. If, in the ensuing power struggle, the doctor could sometimes manage to use a soft touch, there were occasions, Albutt insisted, when the "steel glove" was requisite.[77]

For obvious reasons, medical practitioners were uncomfortable with this alternative theory of hysteria. They preferred to attribute hysterical seizures to some innate female defect than to acknowledge that women could be just as willful as men. To conceptualize hysteria in terms of women's weakness not only fitted a set of long-standing assumptions about female inferiority, but, after mid-century, invoked an impressive somatic explanation based on the structure of the female brain. By contrast, to present hysterical women as supremely willful had no theoretical justification at any time in the Victorian era. The dissenting medical interpretation may, nevertheless, have derived some of its tenacity from popular literature, where the willful woman, falling into hysterical fits whenever she failed to get her own way, was a stock comedy figure. Over the decades, in any case, there were instances when, all evidence militating against a diagnosis of inoperative will, doctors were obliged to denounce hysterical female patients as exemplars of selfish willfulness.

These diametrically opposed interpretations of hysteria underscore the dilemma in which Victorian and Edwardian women could be caught. Self-mastery, the hallmark of masculinity, was presumed foreign to the female sex. Women were affectionate and impulsive, without a strong will to curb their feelings. Therein lay the source of much charm, but also of much infirmity. Yet a woman who demonstrated fully developed powers of self-control risked being labeled "strong-minded," a pejorative adjective synonymous with "unfeminine." If she were guilty of self-assertion, particularly in conflict with masculine authority, she might find herself stigmatized as hysterical. Clearly, overt signs of an actively functioning will were no more admirable in a woman than all the indications of a feeble one.

The battle of wills implicit in much of the nineteenth-century medical literature on hysteria became more explicit when Silas Weir Mitchell's treatment, the rest cure, was applied. The American neurologist first outlined his therapeutic program for certain kinds of neurotic patients in 1873, and it rapidly became associated with the cure of highly nervous, undernourished women whose maladies had resisted all other means of treatment. Imported into Great Britain in the early 1880s through Playfair's enthusiastic and persistent promotion, it became for many medical practitioners the treatment of choice whenever the symptoms of severe neurosis were accompanied by emaciation and a refusal to eat. Since women have, it seems, always vastly outnumbered men in this form of self-punishment, the Weir Mitchell treatment has gained in medical history a virtually exclusive identification with female patients. It *was* applied to the treatment of men on rare occasions, but its principal efficacy was asserted to lie in the treatment of depressed or hysterical women who were starving themselves.

It was no accident that the development of the rest cure and the recognition of anorexia nervosa as a grave medical problem coincided chronologically. Within the British, American, and French medical communities, the nineteenth century witnessed a gradual realization that rejection of food by adolescent girls and young women was not necessarily a manifestation of religious exaltation, nor merely an attempt by deceitful females to gain attention and status by pretending to exist without food. By the 1870s, these earlier assumptions about self-starvation were yielding to a typically nineteenth-century effort to establish its diagnostic contours as a specific, and purely secular, form of sickness.[78] In England, William Gull, the leading figure in the exploration of anorexia nervosa, was a skillful diagnostician who fully appreciated the mind's contribution to somatic distress. In 1868, his first passing reference to a state of extreme emaciation in women clearly distinguished it from any morbid physiological condition of the intestines or lungs. Initially, he dubbed this disorder *hysteric apepsia,* but the implication that problems of digestion were involved made him shortly abandon *apepsia* for *anorexia,* a term already in medical usage to indicate "lack of appetite." By 1873, when he read a paper on the subject to the Clinical Society of London, he had tentatively adopted the name which designates the illness today. Although, when published, the paper was awkwardly entitled "Anorexia Nervosa (Apepsia Hysterica, Anorexia Hysterica)," his comments made it clear why he favored the first of these labels:

> The want of appetite is, I believe, due to a morbid mental state. I have not observed in these cases any gastric disorder to which the want of appetite could be referred. I believe, therefore, that its origin is central and not peripheral. That mental states may destroy appetite is notorious, and it will be admitted that young women at the ages named [16 to 23 years] are specially obnoxious to mental perversity. We might call the state hysterical without committing ourselves to the etymological value of the word, or maintaining that the subjects of it have the common symptoms of hysteria. I prefer, however, the more general term "nervosa," since the disease occurs in males as well as females, and is probably rather central than peripheral.[79]

Gull's reiterated distinction between "central" and "peripheral" was important, for he used it to underscore his conviction that anorexia nervosa was a form of mental illness, not a neurological disorder. Treatment, he believed, should be appropriate "for persons of unsound mind," but he did not intend the phrase to suggest that anorectic women were insane. In all the cases he described, the women could eventually be reasoned with and nursed back to "plump and rosy" health. When first examining a presumably anorectic patient, Gull determined, not only that organic disease was absent, but that the invalid should not, in fact, be sent to an asylum. Persistent refusal of food by a working-class woman might be grounds for committing her to the county institution, but for female members of the affluent classes other means of treatment were available. These ladies were, in Gull's opinion, not madwomen, but "wilful patients" definitely in need of medical treatment. He was sure that some deep distortion of the personality, or "perversions of the 'ego,'" lay at the base of their conduct.[80]

Despite Gull's high standing in the late Victorian medical profession, few British doctors shared his certainty that anorexia nervosa was a distinct disease, entirely separate from either hysteria or neurasthenia. By the end of the nineteenth century, a growing willingness to acknowledge the psychological element in all the functional nervous disorders meant that the classification of anorexia nervosa as a form of mental illness did not disqualify it to fit under the broad heading of hysteria. Indeed, many British doctors, not to mention the leading French writer on the subject, simply assumed that anorexia nervosa *was* a kind of hysterical disorder. Tuke's *Dictionary of Psychological Medicine,* for example, fused the terminology on at least two occasions.[81] The fact that anorexia nervosa and hysteria struck the same population— primarily young women from the beginning of puberty through early adulthood—lent credence to their close identification. So, too, did amenorrhea, or lack of menstruation, which was an almost invariable feature of anorexia, for menstrual disorders, as has been noted, were still widely associated with manifestations of hysteria. The prominence of depressive moods in anorectic patients supported the opinion of those who interpreted self-starvation as a symptom of neurasthenia. Playfair illustrated the connections among all three neurotic categories when he described a twenty-nine-year-old female patient, incapacitated since the age of twenty, as "wasted to a skeleton," suffering from "intense nervous depression" combined with "absolute anorexia," and altogether representing the "typical hysteric."[82]

In his paper to the Clinical Society, Gull merely sketched the lines along which treatment of anorexia ought to proceed, but the implications of his comments were clear. "The patients should be fed at regular intervals," he maintained, "and surrounded by persons who would have moral control over them; relations and friends being generally the worst attendants." For Gull, therapy centered on the struggle to dominate the "unsound mind" of the patient. If she were allowed to continue having her own way where denial of food was concerned, her morbidity would only increase until death intervened. Family and friends made terrible nurses because, loving and sympathizing with her, they could not be severe enough to challenge her. A medical attendant who understood what was at stake, however, would not hesitate to exert "moral control," forcing her to recover, until at last unsoundness of mind yielded to soundness, and she became an active partner in her own recovery. A man who, by all accounts, exerted a tremendous influence over his patients, Gull revealed in his suggestions for treatment the extent to which he perceived the anorectic woman's deplorable willfulness as deeply pathological. The only way that he could think to cure it was to make her submit to the doctor's even more powerful will.[83]

Weir Mitchell was designing his rest cure at the same time that Gull was exploring and defining anorexia nervosa in the context of burgeoning international medical interest in the problem. The principal elements of the cure—enforced rest and nearly constant feeding—were obviously designed to counter the physical fatigue, extreme debility, and severe malnutrition that were the most life-threatening aspects of anorexia. Gull, Playfair, and other doctors who treated the disorder observed in their patients a "peculiar restlessness, difficult to control,"[84] and Mitchell intended to break the pattern of exhaustion from hyperactivity, as we call it today, by confining the patient to bed for lengthy periods of six to eight weeks. For much of that time, absolute rest was prescribed. In extreme cases, the patient could not talk, read, write, or sew; she was not allowed to turn over in bed without assistance; attendants washed and fed her. Food, of course, was as important as rest, and milk served as the major ingredient in a readily digestible diet designed to add fat to the patient's frame as rapidly as possible. (One patient gained fifty-one pounds in four months of virtually around-the-clock feeding.) Mitchell did not shrink from the brutality of forcible feeding, through rectum or nose, when patients would not voluntarily take nourishment.[85]

The other elements of the rest cure were only slightly less central to Mitchell's strategy. He considered total isolation from the patient's family and friends to be essential, because, like Gull, he realized how much their doting care could hinder recovery. Often Mitchell would not allow the patient even to receive letters during the crucial first month of treatment. The ideal situation was to remove the patient to a rest home, under the strict care of a professional nurse trained to carry out the rest cure in every detail. Where that was impossible, the patient might be treated at home, but only if a nurse were installed to maintain a barrier between the sick woman and her environment, and to guarantee that Mitchell's rules were unswervingly observed. Massage and electrotherapy were included to make sure that the patient's muscles did not atrophy through disuse and to hasten the production of waste matter—thereby facilitating the patient's ability to absorb the vast amounts of food shoveled into her. Neither Mitchell nor his British supporters emphasized that the administration of galvanic or faradic currents was an occasional weapon in the fight to curb hysterical attacks or aggressive sexual conduct in women,[86] but the reputed success of electricity in those cases could have only recommended it to doctors who treated supposedly hysterical anorectics.

With varying degrees of efficacy, medical men had been using the separate aspects of the rest cure for some years, as Playfair observed in 1883, but it was Mitchell, the British doctor insisted, who deserved full credit for putting the parts together into a "regular, systematic, and thorough attack" on the problems of neurasthenia, hysteria, and anorexia combined. Donkin, Allbutt, and Gowers were only a few of Playfair's colleagues who joined him in recommending Mitchell's methods, and Dowse actually dedicated his *Lectures on Massage & Electricity* (1889) to "Dr. Weir Mitchell."[87] Nonetheless, the rest cure was never received as gospel in Great Britain, nor was there unanimity within the British medical community concerning its strengths and weaknesses. Modifications were demanded and made by many doctors who accepted the principles behind the therapy, but refused to apply them inflexibly. They did agree, however, that the Weir Mitchell treatment was useless, not only when somatic disease was involved, but also whenever mental illness progressed over the borderline into insanity itself.

Although Mitchell, unlike Gull, emphasized the physical aspects of anorexia, particularly the anemia of skeletal women and their urgent need for fat and blood, the will was never far from the heart of his theories either.[88] He commanded his patients to place unquestioning faith in his judgment, utterly surrendering themselves to his control until their cure was effected. His occasional employment of force-feeding starkly illustrates how convinced he was of the need to break the self-destroying will of the female anorectic. How better to do so than by forcing her to gain weight, thereby demonstrating that the doctor's power even encompassed the capacity to alter her body? Mitchell may well have been motivated by the best of medical intentions— to save lives—but his limited vision did not permit him to see beyond the immediate personal contest. His British admirers followed him in underscoring the doctor's obligation to establish complete "moral influence" over the patient and to place her "under thorough physical and moral training." While Charles Lasègue in France took some significant preliminary steps in analyzing the dynamics of family relations within the anorectic woman's domestic circle, medical interest in Britain focused predominantly, if not exclusively, on the struggle to make her gain weight.[89] If British doctors were aware that family tensions frequently pervaded the atmosphere in which anorexia flourished, they did not belabor the point. When they insisted on the patient's removal from home, they primarily sought to distance her from the permissiveness of family and friends, although they may have also wished to separate her from painful associations, as they did with many victims of shattered nerves. In any case, distrust of the female character always colored their attitude toward anorexia before World War I. What Victorian and Edwardian medical practitioners suspected all along about the feminine mind and body, including the capacity of the female will to challenge male authority out of sheer perversity, seemed definitively confirmed by the anorectic women they studied.

Weir Mitchell's rest cure and the fundamentally enthusiastic response to it, in the United States, Great Britain, and continental Europe, bear sad witness to the cross-purposes that, all too often, soured the relationship between nineteenth-century medical men and their female patients. Mitchell, Playfair, Dowse, and many other doctors who treated anorexia were certainly anxious to help desperately sick women, but their concept of help revolved around the restoration of invalids to domestic life, where they presumed that a woman's deepest contentment lay. Even Donkin, an "advanced thinker" among medical men thanks to his friendship with intellectuals and feminists, shared most of his profession's stereotypical assumptions about women's fundamental needs. If accounts in the medical press can be trusted, numerous women actually benefited from the rest cure and *were* restored to what their culture considered normal feminine roles, but independent-minded women who resented masculine domination were rarely among them, for obvious reasons. Indeed, Weir Mitchell is probably best known today because of the searing short story, "The Yellow Wallpaper," that one such patient, Charlotte Perkins Gilman, wrote in order to regain her mental balance after enduring the tortures of his treatment. Reducing a woman to the dependence of an infant, as befitted the Victorian identification of femininity and childishness, did nothing to help her become emotionally strong and self-reliant. Clearly that was never the goal of Weir Mitchell or his followers. They either thought of their patients as monstrous hysterics whose wills had to be crushed or as helpless neurasthenics who needed a doctor's invigorating will in order to recover. Whichever of these mutually inconsistent interpretations they espoused, proponents of the rest cure were certain that the impetus to restored health came from outside the female patient, from the commanding personality of the medical man. Medical women, Mitchell noted, could not effect such lasting cures.[90]

Apart from a handful of prominent women, like Gilman, Virginia Woolf, and Jane Addams, the pioneering American social worker, who recorded their highly critical views of the rest cure, most of those who suffered through its rigors never had a chance to make themselves heard in support or disapprobation of their treatment. We do not know what drove them to self-starvation in the first place. Whether, in individual cases, the patient was obsessed by the image of ethereal ladies with birdlike appetites so prominently advertised in Victorian culture, we cannot say. Nor can we tell how much the early stirrings of sexual desire may have driven frightened young women initially to repudiate the animal flesh they associated with carnality and then to deprive their bodies of nearly all nourishment. Psychiatrists today stress the anorectic person's desire to achieve total self-control and absolute autonomy, a goal that would have appealed poignantly to many Victorian and Edwardian women who so often heard and felt that it was beyond their grasp. In choosing to practice self-mastery through self-starvation, however, they only seemed to underscore, in the eyes of the medical profession, women's startling incapacity to act reasonably.

By the final quarter of the nineteenth century, the ambivalent messages concerning femininity that permeated British culture could painfully contribute to the emotional distress of young women suffering from serious depression, with or without anorexia. If they described their state of mind, the salient note in their writing was uncertainty about themselves, their goals in life, and the roles they were best suited to play. They wanted the sense of attachment to others, or the sense of being needed by others, which they had been told was one of woman's great rewards in life, but they longed for the freedom, the right to make significant choices, which feminism taught belonged equally to both sexes. The widening of women's sphere in the late Victorian decades did not necessarily make the tension between personal goals and public expectations any the easier to bear, for no conceivable form of employment could rival the status or, it was said, the emotional satisfaction that came with marriage and motherhood. As census figures revealed the inadequate numbers of potential husbands for all the adult women of the country, much public interest focused on the so-called surplus, superfluous, or redundant women of British society. The realization that many of these spinsters and widows were going to need to support themselves helped to fuel feminist demands for greater educational and professional opportunities. If a certain degree of sympathy came to be shown to members of the superfluous category, however, few late Victorian or Edwardian women voluntarily placed themselves in its midst.

Beatrice Webb pondered these issues at great length during the decade of the 1880s, while she was herself a single woman—Miss Potter—working to establish her credentials as a commentator on contemporary social and economic questions. Unlike many of those who addressed the female redundancy problem, she acknowledged that a lifelong sentence of celibacy figured prominently among a spinster's sources of anguish. As she wrote frankly in her diary: "I must check those feelings which are the expression of physical instinct craving for satisfaction; but God knows celibacy is as painful to a woman (even from the physical standpoint) as it is to a man. It could not be more painful than it is to a woman." To herself, she openly acknowledged her own sexuality, but she equated it with her "lower nature" and feared that to indulge it in matrimony would be the end of her professional aspirations.[91] Yet at the same time, as the friend and disciple of Herbert Spencer, she could not help but have serious doubts about a woman's capacity for substantial intellectual achievement.

Thus, while Beatrice Webb appeared in some respects as the archetypal New Woman of the late nineteenth century, smoking cigarettes, enjoying male companionship, and working as an equal with men in her social investigations, she was not, in fact, a feminist. There is no need to rehearse again her decision to endorse the "Appeal Against Female Suffrage," published by more than 100 women in the June 1889 issue of the *Nineteenth Century*. She later described her signature as "a false step" and publicly recanted. It remains true, nevertheless, that she shared many of the principal assumptions of the appeal, including the claim that "the emancipating process has now reached the limits fixed by the physical constitution of women, and by the fundamental difference which must always exist between their main occupations and those of men."[92] While she did not articulate her views quite so baldly, she suspected that women *were* intended for domesticity, and she persistently denigrated female intelligence. The inevitable corollary of belittling woman's mind was emphasizing her emotional character, and Webb had no doubts on that score either. "I cannot maintain my reason as the ruler of my nature," she lamented in 1881, "but am still constantly enslaved by instinct and impulse," a regret she expressed repeatedly throughout the decade.[93]

She was strongly attracted, furthermore, to the idea of women consecrating their lives to others. In 1874, at the age of sixteen, she had piously concluded "that the only real happiness is devoting oneself to making other people happy," and she never ceased to cherish the vision of woman as care-giver and comforter, surrounded by her loving family. As she grew older and feared that her own chances of ever enjoying "the holier happiness of a wife and mother" were vanishing, Webb became noticeably preoccupied with the maternal role. Images of pregnancy and mothering crept into her prose over and over again, as when she described herself, exhausted by several months of social research, as nonetheless contented with her life and "satisfied, like the child-bearing mother, to wait for returning strength." She conceded that the maternal "part of a woman's nature dies hard. It is many variations of one chord—*the supreme and instinctive longing to be a mother.*" Even her deepening fondness for Sidney Webb in the early 1890s was, she explained in her diary, partly "the growing tenderness of the mother," mingled—significantly enough—"with the dependence of the woman on the help of a strong lover.""[94] Well into the 1890s, after her marriage, she continued to find the image of the mother far more attractive than that of the professional brain worker.

An intensely introspective woman, Beatrice Webb recognized her own "duplex personality" and the unremitting struggle between her sensual and intellectual natures.[95] It was not just a contest between her desire for sexual fulfillment, which was unthinkable outside of marriage, and her longing for intellectual achievement, which she feared was unthinkable within marriage. The fight involved Webb's entire perception of a woman's relationship with her family. After her mother's death in 1882, Beatrice became hostess and housekeeper for her father, and, while she rejoiced in her new-found importance, she chafed at the time taken away from her own research on social questions. She believed that her scholarly efforts could serve a valuable public function, but she was honest enough to admit that they gave her profound personal satisfaction as well. She knew that work was as important to her as sleep, and, for all her idealization of wifehood and maternity, she could not bear to be relegated to the domestic sphere. Her own aspirations for freedom to think and work as her abilities allowed clashed with her deep sense of duty to serve her family. She had so thoroughly imbibed her culture's rigid stereotypes of masculine and feminine that she could only describe the purposeful, ambitious side of her nature as manly and the dreamy, emotionally dependent, affectionate side as womanly. Between the two, she assumed there inevitably existed an unbridgeable gulf, or an incurable wound within herself.

Throughout the 1880s, she suffered from periodic depression, sometimes of paralyzing intensity. During childhood and adolescence, her life had been marked by ill health and nervous debility, and the pattern followed her into adulthood, to be exacerbated by her own persistent questioning of motives and goals. The 1880s were, however, a particularly painful period in Beatrice Webb's life because they witnessed her passionate, unhappy love for Joseph Chamberlain, the prominent Liberal politician whom she met in 1883. She knew that they were temperamentally as unsuited to each other as two people could possibly be and that marriage to him would wreck all hopes of using her mind to good, independent purpose, but she could not stop thinking, daydreaming, and fantasizing about him for the rest of the decade. They saw and wrote to each other infrequently, but her vivid imagination provided all the material she needed to torment herself. Already in May 1884, she wrote: "Strength too fails me now. I look hopelessly through the books on my table and neither understand nor care to understand what I read. My imagination has fastened upon one form of feeling. . . . There is glitter all around me and darkness within, the darkness of blind desire yearning for the light of love. All sympathy is shut from me." During the following years, she often experienced the strange "feeling of life being *ended,*" try as she might to find relief in service to others. Hopelessness, pain, and exhaustion filled her diary with recurrent expressions of despair. She thought she had reached rock bottom in the winter of 1885–86, when she literally dreaded madness, but November 1888 held more punishment for her, when Chamberlain married Mary Endicott, the daughter of an American statesman. When Beatrice learned the news of the upcoming event, she remarked, in an apt metaphor for a chronic sufferer from neuralgia: "The blow has come. I thought the nerve was killed: it was only deadened. . . ." She intended to be strong and throw herself into her work, but instead she lived through "a week of utter nervous collapse." Four months later, she was still too depressed to concentrate on any research or writing: ". . . no work worth speaking of finished or even begun. These last months have been full of silent suffering. I have been unable to raise myself from a state of intellectual torpor, from a certain indecision and indifference."[96]

The only other event in these years that was able to distress her at all comparably involved the implication of inaccuracy or dishonesty in her work. In May 1888, she was summoned to give testimony to a Select Committee of the House of Lords that was investigating sweated labor. She had recently undertaken some inquiries of her own on that subject, trying to pass herself off as a seamstress and actually working briefly in a sweatshop to gain firsthand evidence. In giving her testimony, she misstated the number of days she had been employed, leaving the impression that she had worked longer than was, in fact, the case. Although the mistake was venial, occasioned by nervousness, her conscience tormented her when the exaggerated figure was widely reported. To rectify the situation, she erred in the other direction when correcting the proof of her testimony, prior to the publication of the committee's report, and "scrupulously reduced the number of weeks to less than the truth. This double sin of saying what was not true, and then altering it in what seemed a sly way," she recollected in *My Apprenticeship,* "caused me many sleepless nights." In fact, she endured a kind of ongoing panic attack, as though terrified of being exposed as a rank amateur whose social investigations could not be trusted. A few months later, she vividly described her state of mind at the time:

> . . . throughout a horrible pain was gnawing at my consciousness. I tossed about during the night, if I sank into a doze I woke up in a cold perspiration. All day I rushed from my own thoughts only to meet them at every corner. At last, . . . I had become a prey to mania. I lost all control and the laudanum bottle loomed large as the dominant figure. . . . In the end of course I bear the signs of extreme physical

strain written on my face, but no one could tell that the physical strain arose from mental misery.[97]

Beatrice Webb did not subscribe to any of the medical theories that attributed woman's nervous instability to her reproductive functions. She was convinced that mental misery always precipitated her attacks of nervous prostration, which she continued to suffer intermittently after her marriage in 1892. She was cursed, she felt, with an intense self-consciousness that would not leave her in peace and sometimes drove her nearly crazy. Her diary does, indeed, suggest a haunting preoccupation with the impression that she made on other people. She never ceased thinking about Chamberlain; a casual encounter with him could rekindle all the old despairing love and ensuing depression. Slightly deceptive dealings with her fellow members of the Royal Commission on the Poor Law in 1907, concerning her correspondence with medical officers of health, could agitate her and provoke what she called "a bad nervous breakdown." This, clearly, was not a severe crisis, for she was back at work in two weeks.[98] It was probably similar to the panic attack of 1888, prompted by fear of exposure and a guilty conscience. The narrative of her whole life reveals an almost constantly troubled woman, longing for religious certainty and a guiding creed, and disturbed by physical desires that she scorned but could not suppress. Around the turn of the century, she began persistently and dangerously to reduce the amount of food she ate, a habit that explains her frequent spells of exhaustion. It also suggests that her childless marriage to Sidney Webb did not provide a happy ending to her story, for all her loving tribute to him as "The Other One."[99] Their relationship proved to her that close intellectual companionship could coexist with matrimony, but it failed to address her deeper needs. Beneath her renowned arrogance lay perpetual doubt; she never ceased wondering whether she had made the right choices—whether she would not have been happier as "Woman" than as "Thinker."[100] Nothing in her personal experience or cultural milieu told her that she could successfully be both.

Late Victorian women with more pronounced feminist sympathies were not necessarily spared the pain of coming to terms with the meaning of womanhood. Olive Schreiner, Maria Sharpe, Eleanor Marx, and Amy Levy, all acquainted with each other and situated in or around London's radical intellectual circles, grappled in the 1880s with the same questions that troubled Beatrice Webb. For Olive Schreiner, the South African novelist who desperately wanted to see women break away from their subordination to men, the great obstacle was female sexuality. Women's need for sexual fulfillment, she believed, kept them enslaved. They could be free or they could be sexually satisfied, but, like Webb, she did not see how the two great desiderata could be combined. Far more than Webb, however, she stressed the limitations imposed on women by the prevailing stereotypes of femininity and was far less attracted to the idealized domestic role assigned to women. They needed complete independence, she insisted, to find their own selves. Yet she, too, yearned for the experience of motherhood and dwelt on the idea of a passionate sexual relationship with a strong, dominant man, even while she recoiled from its implications. In the 1890s, back in South Africa, she married Samuel Cron Cronwright, an ostrich farmer and politician, and they tried unsuccessfully to have a family. Never really at peace with herself or her society, her life was full of physical and emotional pain that helped to fuel the anger with which she drew connections between the dependent position of women and the oppression of blacks, courageously denouncing both.

In England, where her celebrated novel *The Story of an African Farm* was published in 1883 and where she lived for most of the decade before returning to South Africa, Schreiner tried to establish friendships with men on the basis of equality and the open exchange of views. She succeeded with Havelock Ellis, whom she met in 1884 and with whom she soon established terms of the closest, although platonic, intimacy. He recognized her "physically passionate temperament which craved an answering impulse," and "she swiftly realised that [he] was not fitted to play the part in such a relationship which her elementary primitive nature craved." That Havelock Ellis could label a woman with the capacity for strong sexual passion "elementary" and "primitive" says a great deal about the late Victorian and Edwardian sex reformers. Nonetheless Schreiner freely confided to him her most private fears and feelings, and he tried to help her through her frequent terrifying illnesses. Her attempts at frank friendship with another man, Karl Pearson, were not so happy. She joined his Men and Women's Club, where she dared to second Donkin's contention that suppression of sexual desire could harm a woman's health, and she had the misfortune to fall in love with Pearson.[101]

Bryan Donkin, her doctor and failed suitor, maintained that the total breakdown of Schreiner's health in December 1886, when he believed she had reached "a state of complete temporary madness," was due to the unbearable strain of repressing her feelings for the undemonstrative, domineering Pearson. She vigorously denied that causative theory, and although she offered no compelling alternative explanation, a recent biographer of Ellis has provided one in suggesting that Schreiner's sickness was bromidism. The condition, which arises from an accumulation in the body of potassium bromide, could well have grievously exacerbated her physical troubles. She had ingested large amounts of the drug for several years, apparently in the hopes that it would lessen her sexual desires.[102] The symptoms of bromidism include the kind of depression and mental disorientation that she described in her letters to Ellis from 1884 through 1886. "On Thursday night my head got so bad I thought it was going to burst," she told him in June 1884, explaining that she had mistaken Eleanor Marx for her own sister. (Donkin diagnosed "nervous prostration" at this point.) A few days later, her head was going "round and round," while in September, "sudden wild outbreaks of crying" added to her physical exhaustion. "I shall go mad," she wrote to Ellis that month. "I never felt like this before. It's so awful. Harry, what does make me feel like this? It's as much my mind as my body that is ill." In January 1885, she reminisced to her loyal friend: "I used to have that feeling of a power bearing me up, that would lead me. Now I have a kind of feeling that it has done; a blank wall now." Two weeks later, after reporting on her chest and legs, she burst out, "Oh, it isn't my chest, it isn't my legs, it's I myself, my life. Where shall I go, what shall I do?"[103] Month after month, the correspondence continued in this vein, with reports of utter despair illuminated by occasional glimmers of hope, with accounts of varying pains and weakness in chest, throat, legs, and head, until the situation attained the terrible finale of December 1886.

Heavy drugging doubtless bears a large responsibility for much, but not all, of

Schreiner's misery during her years in England from 1881 to 1887. In addition to bromide of potassium, she took numerous other forms of medication in reckless abundance, including quinine, morphia, chloral, and nux vomica, a drug related to strychnine.[104] She often prescribed medication for herself, without consulting a doctor, sometimes to ease the symptoms of asthma from which she suffered acutely. Her biographers make it clear, however, that Schreiner's emotional turmoil began long before she started taking bromide, or any other drug, on a regular basis. While still in South Africa, she had felt isolated and alienated, entertained thoughts of suicide, and experienced a numbing sense of failure. She had hoped that her life would change dramatically when she reached England in her mid-twenties; when it did not, she embarked on a program of self-starvation and medication that caused her severe physical harm. Whatever the reasons why someone initially becomes a victim of depression, the intensifying elements in Olive Schreiner's case were many and potent during the 1880s: promiscuous drugging, malnutrition, loneliness for much of the time, writer's block, and, finally, frustrated love. Behind all these immediate precipitants, her despair over the feminine condition and her inability to escape from the confines of the female body provided an ongoing source of torment.

Maria Sharpe, Schreiner's colleague in the Men and Women's Club, was also deeply disturbed by the nature of female sexuality and feared its fundamental incompatibility with women's intellectual ambitions. The club itself stirred some of those ambitions in her; in preparing papers for club discussions she had learned the pleasures of historical research. More important, as she wrote in some unpublished autobiographical notes about the club: "I had also to a certain extent exercised a control over my mind in doing them [the papers], which was reassuring to me. I felt that I could if I tried teach myself much." Gradually, she even gained the confidence to withstand Pearson's intellectual bullying. Initially Sharpe, who was in her early thirties, belonged in the feminist camp that celebrated women's sexual indifference— the social purity feminists who believed that female continence should serve as an inspiring example for the opposite sex. She bridled in December 1885 when a Dr. Louisa Atkins informed the club that "she had reluctantly come to the conclusion that much of the 'little health' of unmarried women came from their not being married." Sharpe "could not bear to consent to this."[105]

As the discussions unfolded in the club, and especially as Sharpe began to articulate her own thoughts about prostitution, a topic that the club kept gnawing on like the proverbial dog with a bone, she had to revise her assumptions. In May 1887, she still objected to the view that sexual desire was equally strong in women and men. "I said," she later recollected, "that the fact of prostitution, & the need men claimed to have of women, would appear to point to men's sexual desires being stronger, but that I did not then see clearly on the point." After reading intensively for her own paper on the subject, however, the issue presented itself in a strikingly different, if very confused, aspect.

> That study brought women before me in a new light, not as always the seduced but often the seducers; and also called up a picture before my mind of disorderly licentious women whom society had for its own safety to control and force into a degraded class. In the second half of my paper I made some remark on "the *greater strength* of women's sexual nature" as compared with man's. I am not sure if this is

the right way of putting it, but I do think that everything points to the fact that as the affections and especially the affections in marriage [are] the chief interest of woman's life it is in that sphere that she ought to have the greatest freedom of action, that freedom at least which goes along with deep sense of responsibility. The slave cannot be said to be a responsible person.[106]

Although she still subscribed to stereotypical thinking about women as creatures of affection rather than intellect, she was discovering that questions of personal freedom and responsibility were more complex than she had at first realized. Prior to joining the club, Sharpe "had always considered the best way to keep one's independence was to avoid the society of men and keep to one's own sex." Now she came to realize that such an attitude was merely evasion, not independence. If she was willing to condemn men for their shallow knowledge of women—"their general attitude either of adoration or contempt"—she knew that she must be willing to take a hand in educating them.[107] She educated herself in the process.

These years of questioning and of intellectual development for Sharpe were also years of recurring ill health. Throughout her notes covering the period 1885 through 1889, she referred to her physical and emotional condition in ominous terms. In the summer of 1885, she "was not very well and went to Switzerland," where she pondered the work that the club had undertaken. "I was particularly anxious to look at our subjects in their general setting. I felt the danger there must be to one's health, mental and physical, of treating them from a narrowly sexual one. I did not then know whether I should find myself strong enough mentally to carry the work on without its getting too much hold of my mind, but I meant to give myself a trial and watch myself closely." In moments of exhilaration, she felt "how healthful hard mental work was for both [her] body and mind," but such moments vanished rapidly. A careful reading of the debate over the Contagious Diseases Acts was "very depressing." She became increasingly certain that a knowledge of their past history could only arouse in women of the late nineteenth century

a consciousness of a side of their nature which they had long been taught to think of as non-existent or if existent to be condemned. To feel that strength of sexual passion might possibly go along with strengths of other kinds, that faithfulness in marriage or a close marriage tie had also come with greater subjection, and other thoughts, it seemed to me must necessarily work disturbingly on women who grasped them at all. I very seldom lose faith in my own sex, but I confess I shuddered sometimes then.

She also sometimes "sat down on the floor . . . and cried," when she contemplated the forces aligned against women who tried fully to express themselves as individuals. In the summer of 1888, she "was thoroughly tired in mind, besides being physically much below par," and well into the following autumn, she remained "in a very dejected state," "too stupid to feel or think at all."[108] This was also the time in her life when Sharpe was breaking away from the Unitarian faith in which she had been raised, and the severance of old ties that had contributed so much to her moral development augmented her emotional exhaustion.

By December 1888, her mind was at last "beginning to move without pain after a long period of depression," and she could rouse herself to respond to Pearson's contemptuous reference to "the apathy of middle-class women." Indeed, the drama that lies underneath Sharpe's autobiographical notes is her unfolding relationship with this overbearing but stimulating man, who goaded her into action and infuriated her. She, who "had never in [her] life attempted to write anything," found that she had things to say that were worth hearing. She even published a paper on Ibsen's male and female characters in the *Westminster Review,* in June 1889. Always, however, one senses in her autobiographical notes that it was "Mr. Pearson" to whom she was responding. She was both attracted to him and terrified by the idea of surrendering her newly discovered selfhood to him. If she had come to accept the idea that heterosexual passion was natural to women, as many late Victorian feminists were willing to acknowledge, she nonetheless shared Schreiner's conviction that it vitiated women's capacity for genuine independence from men. Specifically where Pearson was concerned, she recognized that their relationship, if continued, would move beyond the purely intellectual exchange of ideas. When he proposed to her in 1889, she accepted him, but then suffered the nervous breakdown she had just held at bay the year before. They were married in 1890, but marriage was no more a resolution of Maria Sharpe's troubles than it was of Webb's or Schreiner's. Unlike the other two women, Sharpe had children, but in embracing the role of wife and mother, she lost the sense of her own voice and ceased to write for publication.[109] What she had learned about femininity upset and alarmed her. It seems to have driven her to accept the traditional womanly roles that she had been so vigorously questioning.

For Eleanor Marx and Amy Levy, the resolution was even more tragic. Marx's long-sustained refusal to eat, extreme physical exhaustion, and profound emotional distress in the fall and winter of 1881–82 may have partly reflected sexual frustration, as Karl Marx, her father, insinuated, but her own explanation suggested a less specific cause of tension in her life. In January 1882, she explored her anguished state of mind in a long letter to her sister Jenny from the Isle of Wight, where she was supposed to be caring for her invalid father:

> What neither Papa nor the doctors nor anyone will understand is that it is chiefly *mental worry* that affects me. Papa talks about my having "rest" and "getting strong" before I try anything and won't see that "rest" is the last thing I need—and that I should be more likely to "get strong" if I have some definite plan and work than to go on waiting and waiting. If I really were needed just now to nurse Papa—as for instance when he was so ill—I should not feel this—but he does not really want me now, and it drives me half mad to sit here when perhaps my *last* chance of doing something is going. . . .
>
> . . . (For a long time I tried various drugs—this quite *entre nous,* and am loth to try them again—it is not much better, after all than dram-drinking, and is almost if not quite as injurious.) *Since I have been here I have not slept six hours.* You may imagine—even without counting other things—that this is killing—and I really do fear a complete breakdown—which for Papa's sake I would do anything to avoid. What I most dread is the consulting of doctors. They cannot and will not see that mental worry is as much an illness as any physical ailment could be.[110]

Like Beatrice Webb at this time and J. A. Symonds twenty years before, Eleanor Marx was convinced that some definite, regular work was essential for her sanity. Desperate for purposeful activity, she was fundamentally protesting against the thankless role of unmarried daughter left at home to care for elderly parents. She had just watched her mother die of cancer, and now she envisioned years of emptiness as her father's health steadily declined. Deeply as she loved him, she was in her late twenties and resented the sense of time slipping ever more rapidly away from her. In her agitation, doctors' sermons on bodily needs, like rest and food, struck her as ludicrously irrelevant. There was, furthermore, an emotional crisis centered around the figure of Hippolyte Lissagaray, a veteran of the Paris Commune, seventeen years older than Eleanor, to whom she had become engaged in 1872. Her parents had disapproved strongly, not because of his politics, needless to say, or even because of her extreme youth, but because of his none too sterling personal reputation. By 1882, the engagement had dragged on for a decade, and the situation had become a source of torment to her. She wanted to be released from her commitment, but felt remorse for wasting ten years of Lissagaray's life. At last she made the break, but the decision to do so added much to her emotional troubles at this time.[111]

Longing for independence and, at this point in her life, the chance to pursue a theatrical career, Marx scornfully rejected the notion that she was too debilitated for either. Yet starving herself, she firmly buttressed male opinion of her physical and mental fragility. Her ultimate expression of independence from late Victorian bourgeois society—the establishment of a common-law marriage—had equally ironic, and far more devastating, implications for her. The partner she chose in 1884, after Karl Marx's death, was the socialist Edward Aveling, a man whose personal amorality and contempt for women, she later learned, were limitless. In the end, the humiliation of her emotional dependence on so repulsive a human being contributed to the frame of mind that drove Eleanor Marx to commit suicide in 1898, at the age of forty-three years.

Although Amy Levy's life was much less amply recorded than Eleanor Marx's, it is clear that she shared the same concerns about freedom, selfhood, and womanhood. Alone among the group of women portrayed here, Levy received a university education, at Newnham. At twenty years of age, she published a volume of verse entitled *Xantippe and Other Poems* (1881), in which Socrates' wife finally had the chance to say her piece, and a few other collections of poetry followed in subsequent years. Her greatest success, however, was her novel *Reuben Sachs* (1888), which offered a probing look at the values of London's wealthy Anglo-Jewish community. Strongly affected by the book, Eleanor Marx translated it into German. Perhaps she was drawn, not merely by an interest in her own Jewish origins, but by the character of Judith Quixano, a poor relation of the Sachs family, who was deeply in love with Reuben. Although her love was reciprocated, she realized that Reuben would never propose marriage, for she lacked money and position in society, and he harbored political ambitions. Reluctantly, she agreed to marry another man, although it nearly broke her heart. Yet, Levy wrote, "she was so strong, so cruelly vital that it never for an instant occurred to her that she might pine and fade under her misery." The men in the novel are nervous and delicate, but Judith is unbreakable. Sadly, Levy, who apparently suffered from severe depression, was not. In the summer of 1889, Schreiner, a close friend, tried to cheer her up by suggesting she read "Have Faith," in Edward Carpenter's *Towards Democracy*. Levy thanked her, but found the author's philosophy of human freedom no help in her despair. "I am too much shut in with the personal," she explained, in what could have served as a late Victorian gloss on the dangers of introspection. Shortly thereafter, Levy committed suicide, for reasons that have not become part of the historical record.[112]

The encounters with depression that scarred, or terminated, the lives of these women seem to demand due acknowledgment that an entire cultural milieu can potently contribute to nervous breakdown. The problem was not just that the boredom and emptiness of many women's lives, spent without intellectual stimulation or meaningful work, could end in melancholy, apathy, and physical malaise, as many commentators, both male and female, pointed out before World War I. It was that attempts to rectify the situation often involved struggles against social expectations, cultural stereotypes, and family practices, which left the fighter physically exhausted and mentally depressed, thereby earning her the diagnosis of nervous collapse. A case like Anna Lloyd's further illuminates this sad scenario. Lloyd, a member of the first tiny class of students at Girton (still located at Hitchin) in 1869, was already in her early thirties when the chance for higher education presented itself as the "raison d'être" that her life had lacked. Her family, however, was shocked by her dereliction of duty to married sisters, bachelor brothers, nephews, and nieces. The pressure on her to abandon her studies was intense, and at length she yielded to the argument that she was wallowing in "self-indulgence and self-satisfaction," while ignoring "the plain duties that lay before her." College life had been the perfect solution for a lonely single woman without the financial resources to keep a home of her own, after her parents' death had left the family house in the hands of a married brother. It is hardly surprising that, during her last term at Hitchin, and after leaving, she experienced "deep depression and discouragement." Numerous similar stories tell of women's personal hopes at odds with family plans, although many have a happier denouement. These accounts support the speculation, popular among feminist scholars today, that much of the vague, recurrent ill health, borne by some Victorian women who challenged the ideology of separate spheres, "was symptomatic of unresolved conflicts."[113]

As much as we can know about the psychological springs of illness long after the fact, this seems a judicious, if uninformative, conclusion. The hypothesis that profound uncertainty over goals and responsibilities can make someone sick does not, however, necessarily imply any motive on the part of the sufferer. If we can surmise that nervous disorders, ranging from headaches through complete breakdown, were the outward manifestation of an inward turmoil, we cannot assume that the women who fell ill had any particular intention in doing so. Yet thanks to Freud, if not to Dickens, the idea of exploiting illness—consciously or subconsciously—for personal advantage is a familiar one today, and a long list of potential reasons could be cited for the infliction of sickness on oneself: to gain attention or time, to avoid unpleasant decisions or painful situations, to exercise a certain kind of control, to express resentment against people or circumstances. For men and women alike, the elusive and protean qualities of nervous maladies make them particularly useful in this regard. Charles Darwin, Florence Nightingale, Elizabeth Barrett Browning, and Harriet Martineau are only a few of the Victorians, eminent and otherwise, about whom some such explanations for chronic invalidism have been offered over the decades.[114] In recent years, the paramount psychological theory with regard to nineteenth-century women has fastened on the concept of rebellion. The contention is now almost unquestioned among feminist scholars that middle-class Victorian women subconsciously turned to illness to vent their rage against limited, unsatisfying lives, devoid of personal significance and imposed on them by the tyranny of a male-dominated society. Through sickness, the argument claims, their rebellion allowed them to escape from endless service to others by forcing others to serve them, while society could not condemn a form of insubordination that confirmed standard expectations of female weakness. It was the refusal of these women "to adjust to the 'inevitable' conditions of their lives" and their "rebellion against their sex roles" that "led to an unprecedented wave of nervous disorders" in the second half of the nineteenth century.[115] The emotional satisfaction that this claim affords late twentieth-century feminists should not obscure the fact that real historical problems mar its explanatory value.

In the first place, it is not at all clear that an "unprecedented wave of nervous disorders" did, in fact, wash over the British Isles in the latter half of Victoria's reign. In the seventeenth century, after all, Sydenham had declared hysteria to be the commonest disease in England after fevers of various sorts. Scarcely any woman, except those who led "a hard and hardy life," could hope to escape hysterical complaints, he asserted.[116] Even if Sydenham reached his conclusion by conflating symptoms of what Victorian doctors considered other nervous and mental disorders (including melancholy) with those of hysteria, it remains clear that nervous illness was common in his day, and prevalent among women. Medical men in the late nineteenth and early twentieth centuries certainly expressed alarm over what they perceived as a mounting tide of neurotic afflictions, but lacking statistical records of such ailments outside the asylum, historians have even less evidence about this question than about the possible increase in the incidence of insanity. The Victorian medical profession had numerous reasons for concentrating attention on ambiguous nervous disorders. Every year, physiological research was revealing the role of the nervous system in an extraordinary array of pathological conditions. Medical eagerness to pin down and classify diseases, furthermore, led to the multiplication of diagnostic labels, of which neurasthenia is only the most familiar. These trends alone could create the impression of vastly augmented numbers of neurotic women merely because doctors showed more interest in cases formerly considered unworthy of note.

The rebellion hypothesis is misleading, too, in its implication of broad applicability to all middle-class Victorian women who suffered from serious nervous complaints. Whatever validity it may have for undetermined individual cases, it cannot serve as an overarching theory to elucidate female nervous collapse among the British bourgeoisie in the nineteenth century. Its most serious failure, as with general psychological explanations of male depression, is to neglect the consideration of possible organic disease, an oversight that medical men themselves tried not to commit. Donkin, for one, recognized anemia, mercury poisoning, enteric fever, pneumonia, malaria, syphilis, brain tumor, and uterine cancer among the potential somatic precipitants of hysterical symptoms, and all medical writers on the subject of nervous disorders urged their colleagues first to ascertain what, if any, physiological disturbances could be identified before proceeding with treatment. Medical examinations in the Victorian era, however, were more decorous than instructive—as late as the 1890s, the reputable obstetrician who delivered Jeannette Marshall Seaton's baby physically examined the prospective mother only when she went into labor. Under the circumstances, it is safe to assign at least some of the cases of alleged female neurosis to prolapsed uterus, fibroids, hemorrhoids, or other tangible ailments that went undetected. When the prolific journalist Harriet Martineau became confined to a sofa from 1840 to 1844, it was not to protest against the role of spinster daughter and sister, but because she was painfully incapacitated by uterine displacement and a tumor.[117] If Victorian and Edwardian doctors knew that depression could follow in the wake of influenza, mononucleosis, which can also occasion symptoms of depression, was a mystery to them. Similarly, many glandular disorders and vitamin deficiencies produce a depressive effect, which could well have been attributed to shattered nerves in the nineteenth century. None of this is to imply that physiological and psychological causes cannot coexist where depression is concerned, but only to insist that their interaction must be taken into account.

It is important to remember, too, how much female depression in the nineteenth century was a physiological response to pregnancy and childbirth. Victorian medical men, as was noted, fully appreciated the connection between low spirits and the reproductive cycle, even acknowledging what is today called *postpartum psychosis* under the name of *puerperal insanity*. Her doctors were probably not surprised, therefore, by the appalling blackness of mood that descended on Catherine Symonds, John Addington's wife, during and after each of her four pregnancies.[118] The chronic invalidism, as distinct from temporary depression, of some married women may well have reflected the physical exhaustion that came from too many pregnancies in too few years. No doubt purely psychological causes *were* also at work when depression accompanied pregnancy and parturition. Ignorance about the whole process must certainly have increased its terrors for some women, while fear of death in childbirth loomed as a very real threat to all. Where marriages were unhappy, as in Catherine Symonds's case, the discomforts of pregnancy could easily have seemed a punitive burden to bear for an unloving or emotionally distant husband. Before the widespread use of birth control by middle-class couples, the time often came, even in happy marriages, when wives cultivated nameless maladies in the hopes of avoiding marital demands and further pregnancies. What needs emphasizing is simply that any interpretation of Victorian depression associated with childbearing that looks only at women's fears and resentments, neglecting the physiological factor of hormone levels, skews the argument too sharply on behalf of ideological purposes. The role of the cultural environment in stimulating postpartum depression is, in any case, very unclear. Recent research had found as high a rate of postpartum depression in rural Africa as in western industrialized countries.[119]

Even in those cases where psychological causes seem to make the best sense of a Victorian woman's nervous breakdown, the rebellion hypothesis is not particularly serviceable. In fact, the severe depression suffered by some nineteenth-century married women, quite apart from childbearing, could reasonably be interpreted in a diametrically opposed way—not as a rebellion against the institution of Victorian marriage in general, but as an expression of crushing disappointment that one particular marriage had failed to live up to expectations. Sarah Austin, for example, wife of the self-pitying depressive John Austin, was a devoted spouse who used her considerable literary gifts to supplement the family income up to her husband's death in 1859. Within a few years of her marriage in 1819, she was already wondering whether John's chronic melancholy reflected indifference to her. They had one child, a daughter born in 1821, but one can readily surmise that their relationship was neither sexually close nor emotionally fulfilling for Sarah. In the early 1830s, while she was translating Prince Hermann Pückler-Muskau's *Tour in England, Ireland, and France in the Years 1828 and 1829* from German into English, she allowed herself an extended epistolary romance with the prince, expressing feelings that would have ruined her had he ever been enough of a cad to publish his correspondence. She knew that the literary exchange of passion was a fantasy that could not be realized, but her willingness to indulge in such indiscretion was a measure of her misery in those years. When her translation was completed and their correspondence drew to a close in 1835, Sarah Austin was in the process of packing up her home in London and moving to Hastings, as a preliminary to relocating the household in continental exile, since they could no longer afford the expense of living in England. The combination of circumstances brought her as close to complete breakdown as she ever came. She could not control her weeping and wrote to a friend that she felt quite ready to die.[120] When Jane Welsh Carlyle endured a long period of agony with "diseased nerves" during the mid-1850s, her grievance was not with the married state, but with what she interpreted as her husband's egregious neglect. These were the years when Thomas Carlyle spent much of his leisure time in the company of the cultured and gracious Lady Harriet Ashburton, to Jane's deep distress. That her marriage itself was not at the root of her depression seems clear: her despondency lifted within weeks of Lady Ashburton's death in 1857.[121]

Still other likely causes of depression for Victorian and Edwardian women have even less relevance to the notion of feminine rebellion against cultural constraints. Loneliness and isolation could be cruelly effective precipitants, as Charlotte Brontë learned at Haworth, and psychiatric studies repeatedly confirm today. Death in the family—the loss of husband, children, siblings, or parents—could drive a woman to the verge of nervous collapse and sometimes across. Whatever other terrible agents were also at work, Virginia Woolf's earliest breakdowns, in 1895 and 1904, followed the deaths of her mother and father respectively. Lant Carpenter's daughter Mary lost all interest in life for a full two years following her father's mysterious death at sea in 1840. For married women, however, it was the loss of a child or spouse that proved particularly devastating, since their emotional lives were so entirely bound up with the care of both. Rachel Grant-Smith, in her disorientation and despair following her husband's death, offers an eloquent picture of a woman who lost, not just her emotional center, but all sense of connectedness as a result. Concerns about economic security and social status in the absence of the breadwinner often added a cruel element of anxiety to the sense of abandonment that widows experienced. The loss of long-cherished religious beliefs could also exert a nerve-shattering influence. It contributed to Maria Sharpe's distressed state of mind in 1888, and to Annie Besant's in 1871. In Besant's case, a mounting crisis of faith was intensified by brutal marital discord with her clergyman husband, but religious anguish was undoubtedly prominent among the elements that contributed to her breakdown. She had begun to question God's goodness, an axiom by which she had hitherto guided her life, and the strain of her thoughts finally became intolerable. Unable to turn to a loving God or a loving husband, Besant "lay for weeks helpless and prostrate, in raging and unceasing head-pain, unable to bear the light, . . . indifferent to everything."[122]

The varieties of emotional crises that may trigger profound depression are not, in many instances, specific to one gender or the other. Victorian men suffered from loneliness and grief; they struggled with religious doubt; they even coped with intense self-consciousness, a form of torture that most people associate with a feminine desire to please the eye of the beholder. The contexts in which men and women wrestled with their demons certainly varied, but the underlying problems frequently did not. An unrelenting emphasis on the gendered nature of experience is not always a help in solving historical puzzles. It does not tell us, for example, why one Victorian woman, driven by ambition to succeed beyond the feminine sphere but sincerely attracted to the ideal womanly type, could successfully negotiate her way among these tensions, as did Anne Jemima Clough, the first principal of Newnham, while another facing the same dilemma, like Beatrice Webb, became enmeshed in nervous illness. Perhaps only a geneticist can answer the question, but a historian surely will not unearth any clues by glossing over the extreme diversity that characterized the lives of Victorian middle-class women. As much variety, in short, distinguished the causes of depression among women as among men in nineteenth-century Britain. Both sexes were deeply affected by social tensions and cultural prescriptions, but these reacted with widely varying individual circumstances and personalities to make each case unique. Just as we should reject any blanket explanation for all male examples of shattered nerves, we should judge equally insufficient the oversimplified generalizations applied to women. On close scrutiny, historical arguments that rely on something as vague as the cultural or social milieu for explanatory purposes invalidate themselves by their indiscriminate ability to account for everything. Like theories that depend on subconscious processes at work in the past, such arguments offer no real answers to historical problems, for they can neither be disproved nor corroborated.

What is particularly unfortunate about the rebellion interpretation is that, ironically, it appears to confirm the Victorian medical equation of femininity and sickness. To argue that large numbers of intelligent, sensitive women had to embrace neurotic illness in order to protest against an unsatisfactory social environment suggests that they could not achieve a sense of self-worth in healthier ways, and that retreat into invalidism was the prevailing method by which nineteenth-century women dealt with their frustrations. It implies, furthermore, that women manipulated sickness, even if unknowingly, quite as much as many doctors and novelists suspected. It fails to acknowledge and celebrate the countless thousands of women, in all ranks of society, who soldiered on in the face of discouragement and found meaningful work to fill their days. Most distorting of all, it leaves the impression that Victorian and Edwardian women who were contented with their lives were either dupes or dullards. In fact, as far as we can tell, the experience of matrimony and maternity *did* satisfy innumerable wives and mothers in the nineteenth century, not because they lacked the wits to realize their subordination, but because they invested their domestic roles with a sense of dignity and personal significance that may be hard for the late twentieth-century consciousness to recapture. If Englishwomen's private diaries from this period, as from earlier ones, on the whole reflect highly positive attitudes toward marriage and motherhood, it is unfair to dismiss that frame of mind as the product of "masculinist cultures" using maternal indoctrination of daughters to "promulgate their doctrines."[123] Nor should we forget that a woman's domestic sphere included, not just her own household, but the community of which it was a part, and that Victorian women were encouraged to take an active and variegated interest in the affairs of that world. Even within their undoubtedly patriarchal culture, women were able to express their personalities and create outlets for their talents that reveal ingenuity and resilience, with seriousness of purpose and humor combined. Far from the passive (or passive–aggressive) victims that the rebellion theory depicts, many Victorian women found they could, to a significant degree, shape their own lives.[124] Whether their options would satisfy us today is not the issue.

In the midst of these Victorian women—some strong, some weak, some challenged by adversity, some devastated by it—the medical profession occupies a highly ambiguous position. We hear a great deal about the misogyny of the scientific and medical communities today, and abundant evidence reveals how vigorously that outlook flourished in the nineteenth and early twentieth centuries. The physiological theories on which medical attitudes toward women were predicated could not have been more disparaging, although it is worth remembering that the theoretical coup de grâce was delivered by Darwin and Spencer, not by medical men. The assumption that women suffered from constitutional nervous instability and that their reproductive functions trapped them in an endless round of sickness could only have encouraged doctors to promote female invalidism, no matter what they said to the contrary. It was financially advantageous to stress female nervous liability, in any case, for neurotic women were "a class of invalids who really do a great deal to support the doctors," as Dowse wryly observed, and Playfair told of one such female who saw no less than twenty-five medical practitioners before consulting him. Yet profits from such patients did not necessarily endear them to doctors. Playfair's fundamental dislike of women who became chronic nervous sufferers was palpable when he remarked to his colleagues: "Nothing could possibly be more hopeless than the experience of all of us of these wretched instances of broken and shattered lives, these bed-ridden, helpless creatures, who became a burden not only to themselves but to all around them, making happy homes miserable, and exhausting at once the patience, and the resources of those who are responsible for their care."[125]

That many Victorian feminists feared and hated the medical profession's intrusive power over women's bodies is more than understandable, in light of the battle over the Contagious Diseases Acts—which authorized the forcible examination of prostitutes for venereal disease while leaving their patrons untouched—and of the subsequent part taken by prison doctors in the forcible feeding of hunger-striking suffragettes. Force seemed the characteristic feature of the relationship between male doctors and female victims. The use of such grossly abusive surgery as ovariotomy, hysterectomy, and clitoridectomy to curb masturbation, hysteria, and sexual assertiveness in women, although never widespread or professionally condoned in England, would scarcely have allayed women's anxieties about medical procedures. Nor would other highly unpleasant means of treating the uterine and genital disorders believed to stimulate nervous complaints: leeches applied to the pudenda, cupping from the loins, or scarification of the vagina, in the first half of the nineteenth century;

vaginal electrodes in the second.[126] It would seem easy to conclude from this list of atrocities that some doctors were determined to control and punish female sexuality, except for the fact that they devised similarly ugly and humiliating means of dealing with male masturbators.

Before evidence from the past is used too enthusiastically in today's sport of doctor-bashing, however, the position of Victorian women and doctors needs to be examined more closely. At least when middle-class ladies were involved, female patients were not always powerless in relation to their medical attendant. Playfair's model neurotic, after all, had dismissed twenty-five of his professional rivals before turning to him, and other doctors regularly complained that female nervous patients were notoriously fickle. When family members joined forces with doctors, needless to say, the patient's control over the situation could be very much reduced, but the fact remains that women, as individuals, were not necessarily at the mercy of their medical men. When cooperating as a group, they could be formidable, as the medical profession found when it confronted organized and articulate women enraged over the Contagious Diseases Acts. The doctors ultimately lost that contest.

"Contest" is perhaps an unfortunate word here. Considerable diversity of opinion existed among Victorian medical practitioners on the subject of womanhood, and many would have been deeply distressed to perceive themselves locked in conflict with female patients. The family doctor was typically a friend, whom mothers and daughters trusted just as much as fathers and sons. Occasionally, he was the one who comfortingly explained menstruation to a terrified adolescent girl, when her mother was too embarrassed to help.[127] Nor was the doctor's assistance necessarily offered in a paternalistic and condescending manner. Dr. Lauriston Winterbotham of Cheltenham not only took the time to discuss anatomy and physiology with Annie Besant in 1871, when he was trying to help her recover her peace of mind, but eight years later he risked his professional reputation by testifying on her behalf in court, when she was battling her estranged husband for custody of their daughter. Even busy London psychiatric consultants could be supportive and reassuring to distraught women. When Rachel Grant-Smith sought out Dr. (later Sir) James Goodhart, an authority on neuroses, in his Portland Place office, he did not lecture her on female nervous instability. He explained instead that the shock of her husband's sudden death had dealt her a severe blow from which she would need months to recover, but that nothing was wrong with her that could not be explained by the tragedy, or that should cause her any anxiety. It seems from her somewhat confused account that Goodhart was the hero of her tale, while the villains, who incarcerated her in a lunatic asylum for twelve years, were her own sister and brother. No less eminent a doctor than Allbutt insisted in 1895 that women were immeasurably improved in recent years, thanks to the "freedom to live their own lives, and the enfranchisement of their faculties in a liberal education, which, physically put, means the development of their brains and nerves."[128] This was no formulaic approbation of gentle exercise and light learning for women, but a sincere expression of support for women's efforts to extend their horizons and exert control over their own futures. At every level of the medical profession, misogyny in theory was thus frequently, and substantially, modified in practice. Perhaps nothing so strikingly challenges our assumptions about male medical antipathy to women as the fact that the Medico-

Psychological Association voted to admit female psychiatrists—admittedly very few in number—to membership at the comparatively early date of 1893.[129]

Yet it is true that ideology blinkered the vision of even the best intentioned Victorian and Edwardian medical men where issues of gender were concerned. Their treatment of male nervous patients was molded by assumptions equally as rigid and repressive as those that shaped their response to female neurotics; they could be as high-handed with the former as the latter, as unwilling to listen carefully to the patient's own story and as eager to impose their own interpretative framework upon it. By the same token, they could expend as much genuine concern, individual attention, and therapeutic effort on women as on men. If the influence of the medical profession ultimately proved more harmful to Victorian women than to men, the reason may have partly arisen from sheer ignorance about the female reproductive cycle, which limited, if not eliminated, any real medical help to women concerning an aspect of physiology central to their health. Another part of the reason, however, surely lies in the double-edged sword that physiological theory handed to medical men when they confronted female illness.

The explanations that Victorian science and medicine constructed around female nervous disorders too closely resembled the "heads I win, tails you lose" game to have assisted women in deep distress of mind. On the one hand, doctors could explain all manner of physical and mental debility by the reproductive burdens that women bore. On the other, when they encountered unmarried or childless women suffering from neurotic illness, medical men could ascribe their condition to the thwarting of biological destiny. As Clouston observed about the female nervous patient in general: "If such a woman marries, she runs innumerable risks in pregnancy, childbirth, and lactation, and she is likely to have weakly children; if she remains single, she has nearly as many hazards in unused functions, hysteria, unsatisfied cravings, objectless emotion, and want of natural interests in life."[130] Furthermore, despite public attention to the problem of surplus women, medical wisdom throughout the late Victorian and Edwardian decades continued to categorize the single woman as an aberration and never seriously addressed her needs. It did spinsters little good to learn that marriage and maternity would cure their nervous ailments, just as it hardly helped wives to learn that the physiology of motherhood could throw their nerves into utter disarray. However much medical practitioners were constrained by professional insecurity from challenging the so-called truths by which Victorian society sought to govern human relationships; however much doctors themselves were subject to the dictates of cultural prejudices, the fact remains that medicine conveyed a particularly intimidating message to nineteenth-century women. Whichever way they turned, they heard that femininity was a deeply flawed condition.

7

Nervous Children

When Victorian and Edwardian doctors worried about the nervous instability of British women, they were often thinking about the children that neurotic females might produce. It was a medical platitude in the nineteenth and early twentieth centuries that nervous mothers bore nervous children. Although few medical men expected to find the symptoms of full-blown nervous prostration in the young, they all agreed that the observant practitioner could note, even in little children, the telltale traces of nervousness that foreshadowed future disaster. They hoped that, by calling attention to the early warning signals, they could help parents and teachers create a childhood environment conducive to healthy, stable adulthood. Leonard Guthrie was convinced that the "cerebral and gastric neurasthenia" that "trammelled" the talent and "embittered" the careers of Charles Dickens, Thomas Carlyle, George Eliot, and many others, could be traced "to want of sympathetic and judicious treatment in their youth."[1] He and his colleagues wanted to make sure, not only for the future intellectual luminaries of the country, but for the unexceptional men and women, too, that their lives would not be similarly blighted.

Although medical practitioners in the nineteenth century followed their Georgian predecessors in viewing childhood as a period of life utterly distinct from adulthood, with its own unique health problems, their frame of mind about youthful patients was not unlike the point of view they applied to fully grown neurotics. As with adult patients, doctors wielded the language of neurology and psychiatry to justify their intervention as moral managers of childhood. In doing so, furthermore, they accepted the underlying assumptions that guided their pronouncements as unquestioningly as they embraced those that informed their visions of adulthood. They rarely, if ever, stopped to examine the role of environmental agents in accentuating the differences between boys and girls, because they viewed those differences as innate—an integral part of the very order of nature. Equally, they revealed the same willingness to generalize about childhood as about manliness or femininity, without conceding that class distinctions rendered the very concept ambiguous. As many historians have pointed out, children of the affluent classes were receiving education, and financial support, for years after poor children of the same age had been hard at work, helping to feed their families. If, by the eve of World War I, fourteen years old was the age by which most children left school and the law ceased to regard them as juveniles, the medical profession never dated adulthood from such an early point.[2] The passage between childhood and maturity, in fact, remained shrouded in mystery, even for self-proclaimed authorities on childhood illness.

Most British medical men in the nineteenth century rejected the Lockean notion of the infant mind as a tabula rasa and accepted the existence of inherent mental differences that distinguished one child from another. Nonetheless they keenly believed that the primary adult task with *all* children was a moral one—to form character by training infant minds in self-discipline. After mid-century, this older approach to childhood behavior, heavily tinged with evangelical fears of covert sinfulness and exhortations to systematic self-scrutiny, joined forces with a new emphasis on the scientific study of childhood. This was the period when child psychology first emerged as a speciality, among philosophers and medical doctors alike. In 1895, James Sully, for example, followed his sweeping survey of the *Human Mind* with a specific scrutiny of the child's mental landscape, attempting to incorporate anthropological insights into his discussion of such standard psychological subjects as the origins of language and of morality.[3] These were the years, too, when the idea of mental testing took root, and experts in Europe and the United States began to consider that the workings of a child's mind could be encapsulated in a series of numbers.

The growth of child psychology was only one aspect of the gradual development of pediatrics as a reputable branch of medicine during the nineteenth century. As throughout western Europe and North America, the organic diseases of childhood became the subject of specialized medical attention in Great Britain; the first modern British hospital devoted solely to sick children, as distinct from eighteenth-century foundling hospitals, opened in Great Ormond Street, London, in 1852, soon to be followed by others, in the provinces as in the metropolis. With young people, aged fourteen years and under, never amounting to less than 30 percent of the entire population of England and Wales between 1801 and 1901, there was a desperate need for such institutions.[4] Even so, infant mortality rates remained appallingly high until the early twentieth century. The dreaded infant and childhood killers, including diarrhea, measles, scarlet fever, diphtheria, and whooping cough, proved terrible threats down to the end of Victoria's reign, and not only in working-class slums.[5] All aspects of children's health became the subject of increasing medical knowledge and expanding public interest. It was to encompass both that Clement Dukes, physician to the Rugby School and Hospital, expanded his volume on *Health at School* from a mere 324 pages in the 1887 edition to 606 in 1905.

With life-threatening infectious diseases still on hand to challenge medical skill, one cannot help wondering why so much attention was paid to childhood nervousness, a disorder of scarcely comparable gravity. It is clear that Victorian and Edwardian doctors did regard the signs of a nervous diathesis in children as extremely serious, largely because they believed it foreshadowed adult incapacitation unless timely preventive measures were taken. While modern studies may "have found that there is little association between neurotic traits in childhood and the development of neurosis in later life," alienists and neurologists before World War I were unanimous in their conviction that the opposite was true.[6] They acted on that conviction, waging vigorous war against any threat to the childish nervous system, wherever it might lurk. Even before Victoria came to the throne, alarms were being sounded against such practices as destroying children's nerves with doses of calomel, or applying leeches to the temples of drowsy, heavy-headed children, in the mistaken belief that they suffered from brain congestion, rather than "deficiency of nervous energy."[7]

The point of departure for all medical discussion of children's nerves in the Victorian and Edwardian periods was precisely the ease with which they could be drained of force. Like the adult female nervous system, youthful nerves were considered highly sensitive to impressions. Their ready excitability was supposedly apparent from birth, in the convulsive movements to which infants were prone. Children were "constitutionally and instinctively nervous," as Sully pointed out,[8] while the unremitting strain of sheer physical growth imposed further demands on their nervous resources. On all accounts, it was essential for adults to guard them from fatigue and reckless expenditure of nervous energy. The circumstances were, of course, particularly hazardous when a child evinced the signs of an inherited nervous temperament, but medical men were adamant in warning parents that no child could be judged immune from the incursions of nervous illness.

When doctors anxiously scanned young patients for what they called the "prodromata," or premonitory signs, of nervous disorders, they particularly focused on a cluster of symptoms: insomnia, nightmares, somnambulism, headaches, stammering, and daydreaming, or "dreamy mental states." "Night terrors" became so common a feature of medical commentaries on childhood nervousness that Tuke included an entry on this affliction in his *Dictionary of Psychological Medicine,* where it was described in some detail. "An hour or two after onset of sleep," the dictionary reported, in terms that betrayed the social class for which it was written, "the child affected suddenly screams out and wakes in a great fright, not at first recognising its surroundings or nurse. The child often has difficulty in getting to sleep again, the fright passing off gradually. As a rule there is no recurrence the same night, but there usually is on succeeding nights." Late in life, Symonds still recollected with startling vividness the recurring night terrors he experienced as a little boy. Particularly awful was the dream that a corpse underneath his bed had risen up to throw a sheet over him, or that a single finger "disconnected from any hand, crept slowly into the room and moved about through the air, crooking its joints and beckoning." When he was slightly older, he began sleepwalking, in order to escape the corpse that he dreamt lay in bed beside him. At puberty, the development of a stammer, which temporarily left him tongue-tied, provided further irrefutable evidence, according to medical opinion, that his nerves were in considerable disarray. In fact, since Cheyne's day, if not earlier, medical wisdom had categorized stuttering or stammering as a manifestation of "weak nerves" and "a great degree of sensibility." Victorian medicine likewise interpreted headaches as signs of a "mobile or irritable condition of the nervous system" that promised no end of trouble for the suffering child.[9]

Of all the nervous symptoms that young Symonds displayed, those that most alarmed the medical profession were the trancelike states into which he passed. Commencing some time before his eleventh birthday, and continuing with less and less frequency until he was twenty-eight years old, they obliterated all sense of "space, time, sensation and the multitudinous factors of experience which seemed to qualify what we are pleased to call ourself." While he was under the spell of this condition, he had no will of his own and no sensory contact with his surroundings. It was only when he regained "the power of touch" that he knew ordinary consciousness was returning. Victorian psychiatrists concurred that these were grave pathological conditions. If a child were allowed to continue in the practice of dreaming while awake, Maudsley warned, a habit could be established that would "in all likelihood ultimately issue in the degeneration of some form of insanity." The hallucinations experienced in this mental state, he announced, were frequently the result of some "morbid deposit" in the brain. Delivering an address to the West London Medico-Chirurgical Society in 1895, Crichton-Browne explained that dreamy mental states, such as Symonds experienced, consisted in "a feeling of being somewhere else—in double consciousness—in a loss of personal identity—in supernatural joyousness or profound despair—in losing touch of the world—in a deprivation of corporeal substance." The morbidity of that condition, he insisted, could "scarcely be questioned." Its affinity with the onset of an epileptic seizure, or at least of migraine, underscored its diseased nature. Crichton-Browne agreed with Maudsley that it could prefigure insanity, and it was, in any case, an "aberration of mind" signifying "a want of equilibrium in the nerve-centre." Symonds's adult life was strangely unfulfilled, Crichton-Browne explained, "because his highest nerve-centres were in some degree enfeebled or damaged by these dreamy mental states which afflicted him so grievously." The alienist concluded by urging parents to be unceasingly alert to signs of similar states in their children, for Crichton-Browne felt confident that, if detected at an early stage, they could still be remedied by rest and a nourishing diet.[10]

Although Maudsley and Crichton-Browne were referring to an unusual mental condition, quite distinct from the reveries in which most children customarily indulge, Victorian medical men suspected that any sort of daydreaming was unhealthy and should be systematically routed out of children. It was too close to morbid introspection to be condoned and encouraged in a child that confusion between reality and illusion that a was sure sign of mental illness. The advice that P. C. Smith, a Durham physician, gave in 1903, with regard to neurasthenic children, was standard medical counsel by the late nineteenth century: "Reading should be carefully supervised and limited, and all dawdling and day-dreaming rigorously repressed." Even Allbutt, generally a medical moderate, shared his colleagues' extreme viewpoint on this issue, emphasizing that "children must not think or dream, they must be made to do things with their hands." Medical attitudes colored the way many adult nervous sufferers looked back on their own childhood. Beatrice Webb was sure that her old habit of "building castles in the air" and creating fantasies in which she shone as the faultless heroine had been a severe obstacle to the development of her character. Sully, by contrast, was all the less prepared for his nervous breakdown in young adulthood because he was "a good healthy specimen" as a boy, "being unencumbered by any tendencies towards moping or dreamy abstraction."[11]

While most medical admonitions against childish castle-building and the more pronounced, trancelike states stressed the potential dangers for adult mental health, Crichton-Browne maintained that the boy or girl who indulged in prolonged, intense reveries might consequently experience mental depression and feelings of lethargy even as a child. From his earliest psychiatric work, he concerned himself with

childhood depression, insisting that even young infants could evince signs o
condition close to melancholia. "The buoyancy and gladness of childhood n
place to despondency and despair," he lamented, "and faith and confiden
superseded by doubt and misery." Some of his fellow alienists found the ide
genuine melancholia, as a mild form of insanity, difficult to accept in prepubertal
children, except under very rare circumstances, but others, including Maudsley, were
certain that the "insanities of early life" could encompass melancholia. Suffering
from "a constitutional defect of nervous element," melancholic children failed to
thrive, Maudsley observed; they cried all the time and would not be calmed. Whether
Victorian and Edwardian doctors found evidence of major depression, which
psychiatrists now believe can afflict children before puberty, or simply assumed that
their young patients were suffering from intensified versions of the anxieties and fears
common to childhood, they nonetheless concurred that feelings of hopelessness in
children were unnatural, an unmistakable index of serious trouble. "There are certain
mental symptoms," Clouston explained, "which, in a child, are undoubted danger-
signals. If a child ever shows depression or mental pain, then there is certainly
something wrong. . . ."[12]

Surprisingly, there was substantially less concern over childish manifestations of
hysteria. Sydenham had pointed to hysterical disturbances in children, and many
Victorian doctors did the same, in young boys and girls alike. Medical writers had no
trouble finding reasons to explain why this particular neurosis should disturb a
youthful clientele. Primarily, they relied on the belief that children, like adult
women, lacked an adequately developed will; the higher centers of their immature
brains could not completely control the lower ones, while the unstable nature of
childish nerves, with their tendency to spontaneous discharges, further promoted the
unpredictable symptoms of hysteria. Additionally, as Conolly pointed out in 1833,
"the proneness to imitation which is observable in all persons in early life" helped to
spread hysterical symptoms among children. Conolly was not accusing them of
conscious mimicry, but merely observing how stammering, nervous twitches, and
even more convulsive motions could become infectious among an impressionable
audience. Down to World War I, medical practitioners realized that "neuromimesis"
was common between the ages, roughly, of seven and twelve years, and they did not
alarm themselves unduly over it.[13]

One of the most ambitious attempts to collect precise data concerning the physical
manifestations of nervous instability in children was undertaken in the late 1880s and
1890s by Francis Warner, a doctor who wrote widely on childhood nervous
development and who viewed physiological "nerve-signs" as serious matters, not to
be lightly dismissed under the guise of "neuromimesis." In collaboration with a joint
committee of the British Medical Association and the Charity Organization Society,
Warner claimed by 1897 to have examined the physical and mental condition of
100,000 children attending elementary schools in and around London, according to
"the principles used in biological study and natural history." Despite pretensions to
scientific objectivity, however, his project reveals how relentlessly and confidently
medical men could impose their own definitions of health or morbidity. Warner's
methods were simple. Having decided, largely on the basis of previous research into
motor development, what constituted proof of abnormality in children of school age,

he entered a classroom on the lookout for any incriminating evidence. As the children stood in front of him, he particularly scrutinized "movements, action, balance, gestures, or other motor acts" that yielded information about the general cerebral condition of the child under review. Warner believed that these indexes fairly reflected the "modes of mental action" occurring within each youthful brain. "A boy whose eyes are wandering everywhere, with the head moving and the fingers twitching," he reported, "is asked to say what he knows about King Charles I, and replies that he had his head cut off at the battle of Waterloo. Such mental confusion often accompanies excessive nervous movements. . . ." Every child who presented suspicious "nerve-signs" was examined separately, with particular regard to facial expressions and body posture.[14]

In an educational system not known for its tolerance of slow learners and which still permitted corporal punishment as a regular tool of classroom discipline, Warner's survey served a useful purpose. He added his voice to the medical chorus that stressed the importance of recognizing incipient nervous disorders at an early stage, when treatment could produce happy results, and he urged that special educational provisions be afforded, not just for the blind and dumb, but also for children who were "feeble in make and constitution" and needed extra help. It was important for teachers to be made fully aware that numbers of their pupils struggled with defects that kept them from attaining the standard levels prescribed for their age group. Whether the problems stemmed from poor eyesight or hearing, from malnutrition, or from slight mental retardation, the people who directed the education of these children needed to hear that they merited additional attention, not punishment for dullness.

Warner's procedure, however, was so insidious as to undermine the potential benefits of his undertaking. Setting before his mind's eye the "normal or healthy type of development," he could at once spot "any point in form or action that is below the normal." The children filing past him were entirely at the mercy of his idiosyncratic ideal of physiological perfection. After her individual examination, one twelve-year-old girl was described as having a well-proportioned face, with entirely "normal" features. She was said to be "quick at lessons; recites well. Talkative in school, playful and often laughing. Is fond of the society of other children like herself." She sounded a happy, well-adjusted child in all respects. True, she was rather thin for her height, but nothing else could have provoked Warner's judgment that she was "likely to become an hysterical girl after leaving school at fourteen years," except the array of nerve-signs that he attributed to her. Her left shoulder was lower than her right; her eyes wandered (although they could "fix on an object if she is told to"); her head drooped slightly; her fingers twitched, and so on. There was no doubt in Warner's mind that this girl deviated egregiously from the normal type and required "careful training in physical exercises" to save her from serious nervous illness. From among all the schoolchildren he inspected, he designated 20 percent "subnormal in some point."[15] He no more questioned the validity of his diagnostic criteria than specialists today ponder the utility of the various "learning disabled" labels they stick on children so readily. In Warner's case, one suspects that his time would have been better spent in securing three square meals a day for most of the boys and girls he categorized with such assurance.

Whenever the Victorian and Edwardian medical profession considered the health of schoolchildren, they invariably worried about the effects of academic cramming, or intellectual force-feeding, on young nervous systems. Early Victorian delight in childish sagacity, which, again under evangelical influence, had set little boys to memorize Milton or study sermons while still in the nursery,[16] enjoyed no medical approbation in the second half of the nineteenth century. The similarities between mental precocity and genius were too striking to ignore; since psychiatrists generally judged the latter to be abnormal and pathological, they devoutly deprecated premature intellectual development in a child, whose physical growth ought to have primary claim to nervous energy. Crichton-Browne was in the vanguard of medical efforts to call public attention to the dangers of early mental maturity, stating his views at nineteen years of age, as we have seen, and prophesying that mentally precocious children "almost invariably die young." More than forty years later, he was still harping on the same point, when he cited the unhappy Jane Carlyle, plagued with functional nervous disorders, as an object lesson to prove the long-term dangers that result from provoking a child's brain "to put forth precociously its budding powers." It was obvious to mid- and late-Victorian doctors that to encourage gifted children in such a manner was virtually to consign them to future invalidism, if not a premature grave. Fothergill, too, assured his readers that precocious children rarely survived into adulthood, "being carried off by brain disease or some form of tubercle; in other cases by acute disease. The over-stimulated nervous system possesses little resistive power, and exhaustion setting in early in the disease is quickly fatal. They have used their nerve force too freely, instead of storing it up, and when the hour of trial comes that force is spent which would have enabled them to weather the storm."[17] The grim choice for the precocious child lay between early death or blasted talents, as medical men never tired of telling parents and teachers, with particular insistence after mid-century.

While bright children who showed early promise might be pushed to excel even in the nursery, doctors feared that academic pressure at school fell indiscriminately on slow and gifted students alike, at both state and private institutions. Believing that the unflagging effort required by the modern struggle for success compelled children to contend for scholastic honors virtually from the start of their education, the medical profession revealed predictably ambivalent attitudes toward the competitive examinations that began opening civil service careers to talent rather than patronage in the second half of the nineteenth century. Boon though these were to their own middle class, doctors saw in competitive exams an agent of that rampant individualism that drove men to overwork and menaced the well-being of society. They argued, moreover, that the exams posed a very direct threat to schoolboy nerves, for anxious parents and teachers tended to assume that an adult competitor could perform successfully only after thorough preparation during his youth. If a man expected to excel by his wits, the process of sharpening them could never begin too early. Hence the heavy demands placed on young children, which doctors deplored, but were often powerless to stop. As Frederick MacCabe observed with regret in 1875: "The claims of education are gradually and steadily infringing upon the years that formerly were devoted to exercise and school-boy's play. The shadow of future competitive examinations, which at first curtailed the sunshine enjoyed by lads in the higher forms of our public schools, next shortened the playtime in elementary schools, and now fairly darkens the threshold of the nursery." Of all the threats to the nation's collective mental health and nervous stability, "the illimitable folly of examining boards," in D. H. Tuke's phrase, was not the least.[18]

Medical writers were certainly not alone in lambasting the practice of academic cramming. A strong tradition of Victorian criticism could boast Dickens and Matthew Arnold among its most eloquent spokesmen. As Guthrie recalled in the Edwardian decade, when he made his own attack on "mental and educational overstrain in childhood," "no one was more strenuous than Charles Dickens in denouncing the principle of 'Gradgrinding'"–a reference to the famous schoolroom lecture on "Facts" at the start of *Hard Times* (1854). Dickens loathed the dryness of Gradgrind's approach to education, with its resolute repudiation of imagination, humor, and fancy, but he did not perceive it as placing excessive strain on the childish mind. It was in an earlier work, *Dombey and Son* (1846–48), that he exposed the dangers of forced learning, as in this description of Dr. Blimber's academy:

> Whenever a young gentleman was taken in hand by Doctor Blimber, he might consider himself sure of a pretty tight squeeze. . . .
>
> In fact, Doctor Blimber's establishment was a great hot-house, in which there was a forcing apparatus incessantly at work. All the boys blew before their time. Mental green-peas were produced at Christmas, and intellectual asparagus all the year round. . . .
>
> This was all very pleasant and ingenious, but the system of forcing was attended with its usual disadvantages. There was not the right taste about the premature productions, and they didn't keep well. Moreover, one young gentleman, with a swollen nose and an excessively large head . . . suddenly left off blowing one day, and remained in the establishment a mere stalk. And people did say that the Doctor had rather overdone it with young Toots, and that when he began to have whiskers he left off having brains.[19]

The father who could subject a six-year-old son to this regimen, in paternal zeal to have the boy "get on" rapidly, was even more the object of Dickens's wrath than the fatuous pedagogue. Matthew Arnold's anger was largely vented against a more impersonal force, the burgeoning educational bureaucracy of the British government, which adopted the system of "payment by results" in the early 1860s as a means of financing primary education. According to this method of subsidy, the parliamentary grant for each elementary school seeking support was calculated from the number of its students who passed a series of yearly examinations in reading, writing, and arithmetic. Teachers in the state elementary schools were consequently obliged to spend most of their time drilling pupils for the annual ordeal that determined every school's livelihood. Arnold's sustained protests against "payment by results" provided a bitter refrain throughout his reports as a school inspector charged with administering the exams.

Where a child was particularly delicate, like the young H. T. Buckle, family doctors especially emphasized the dangers of mental overstimulation, but they felt equally sure that healthy children could likewise suffer permanent debility from too much brainwork during the years of maximum physical development. When bones, flesh, and muscle needed vast amounts of nerve force simply to increase in size and strength, it was foolhardy to make them compete with the child's mental apparatus for that precious resource. The medical argument changed very little from the 1830s to the Edwardian era: childhood was a time for growing, not premature sagacity. Even during the decades up to mid-century, when evangelical attitudes were most influential and children were expected to mirror adults in serious intellectual pursuits, some doctors bemoaned any sustained pressure on young minds. James Johnson, warning that "a precocious development of the intellectual faculties" generally led to "an early failure of mental powers," claimed in 1831 that the modern system of education erred in forcing youth to learn too much too fast. In the following decade, J. T. Conquest, who specialized in the diseases of women and children, pinpointed "the unnatural urging forward of feeble youth" as "the bane" of his age, particularly among the urban middle classes. To overexercise the mind by setting it to achieve results beyond its grasp, he explained, was to punish the body and establish the foundation, "if not for dropsy of the brain, for that long and affecting train of nervous complaints which so frequently embitter the existence of those whose mental energies and acquisitions are the greatest."[20]

After mid-century, the message only gained in urgency, as the improvements in female education and the introduction of civil service examinations intensified medical fears for the nervous stability of girls and boys alike. Virtually every medical practitioner who treated children made a literary parade of cases like Thomas Savill's Agnes, aged eleven, and William, aged fourteen. The girl suffered from "attacks of crying and depression, two or three times a day, . . . and she often sat brooding for hours together, saying she thought everybody was 'against her.'" Broken sleep and bad dreams augmented her misery, and for a while her family feared insanity. Savill found that she needed eye-glasses, but most of all she needed to break the habits that had caused her symptoms to appear in the first place, namely "a too close application to study." William "complained of having been getting gradually more and more 'nervous' . . . and gradually losing his memory." Headaches plagued him, together with disturbed sleep, night terrors, "attacks of giddiness and faintness on returning from school." Having been a delicate child, often kept home from his lessons, he was academically backward, and "to regain the lost ground he had recently been working extremely hard. . . ." The result, of course, was illness, which began to improve when the doctor regulated his hours of schoolwork and supervised his diet. By the early twentieth century, authorities like Guthrie were insisting that "no school lesson should last for more than forty-five minutes."[21]

The leading figure in the late Victorian medical campaign against overpressure in schools was Crichton-Browne. He was a lifelong critic of payment by results and never forgave Robert Lowe (later first Viscount Sherbrooke), the Whig politician who, as vice-president of the Committee of Council on Education, was responsible for introducing the system. At ninety years of age, Crichton-Browne could not resist inserting into a volume of reminiscences "a teacher's epitaph on the Right Hon. Robert Lowe":

> Here lie the bones of Robert Lowe;
> Where he's gone to I don't know;
> If to the realms of peace and love,
> Farewell to happiness above;
> If haply to some lower level,
> I can't congratulate the devil.[22]

The crusade against academic force-feeding was for Crichton-Browne an integral part of his sustained attempt to make parents, teachers, and fellow doctors fully cognizant of the early warning signs of mental strain and nervous illness in childhood. Although he had earlier expressed concern over the dangers to children from physical overwork in factories and mills, by the early 1880s his interest had centered on the dire consequences that he was convinced must ensue from excessive mental labor by immature brains. In that decade, he played the central part in what one historian has called "the great 'over-pressure' row,"[23] which for a few years concentrated significant public attention on the physical and mental health of schoolchildren.

The issue came to a head at that time largely because the Education Act of 1880 imposed compulsory education on all English children to the age of ten, with the expectation that most boys and girls would stay in school for a few years thereafter as well, unless exempted by their local education authority. New regulations for determining primary school grants, issued a few years later, raised further queries about reasonable academic expectations for children. Gladstone's government found itself attacked both by right-wing Tories, who questioned the appropriateness of state interference in the field of education, and by the National Union of Elementary School Teachers, who wanted state aid without the existing system of subsidies.[24] The Education Department's every move became a matter of public scrutiny. In July 1883, Baron Stanley of Alderley rose in the House of Lords to ask the Lord President of the Council, the cabinet minister responsible for education, to reconsider compulsory homework for students in state elementary schools. The request was merely the opening end of the proverbial wedge, for Lord Stanley proceeded to air his concerns about increasing brain disease and other fatal results of academic overwork, in the context of compulsory education and "the increased severity of the Revised Code" for grant payments. He strengthened his case, significantly enough, by citing the opinions of two leading psychiatrists—Daniel Hack Tuke and Crichton-Browne. The earl of Shaftesbury, an octogenarian by this time and the veteran of numerous philanthropic campaigns, supported his colleague, insisting that "many people had begun to see that the forcing system in schools, and the burning competition for place and position among teachers, were producing much mental injury." Still another peer, Lord Norton, similarly denounced the Revised Code in the belief that it compelled teachers to overwork their pupils. In reply, Lord Carlingford, Lord President of the Council, articulated the Education Department's position throughout the controversy. He regretted the "gross exaggeration" that had been allowed to permeate all consideration of overwork in elementary schools. He conceded that "there were here and there cases of such a thing as overwork on the part of children, and more so on the part of ardent pupil teachers, who were anxious to distinguish themselves," but he was confident that, "upon the whole, there was very little ground for the wide and highly-coloured statements that had appeared in some of the newspapers.'' The code, he pointed out, set forth a modest requirement of twenty-five hours spent on school instruction per week, ''and any instruction to the children beyond those hours was entirely the doing of the local managers, and not under the authority of the Code.'' Nor did the Education Department ''lay down any compulsory rule with regard to home lessons.''[25]

With criticism coming from local school managers, doctors, teachers, and opponents of state intervention, the government was clearly on the defensive. Early in 1884, in an attempt to deflect hostility, A. J. Mundella, the vice-president of the Committee of Council on Education, asked Crichton-Browne to investigate the situation in several London schools. In some respects, Crichton-Browne was an excellent choice for the inquiry. His position as Lord Chancellor's Visitor in Lunacy gave him unquestioned authority as a public spokesman, and his earlier expressions of alarm about educational overpressure denied critics of government policies the chance to accuse Mundella of planning a whitewash. Yet if Mundella had wanted someone to report that overpressure in schools was a figment of the collective public imagination, he had selected the wrong man, for Crichton-Browne was sincerely convinced that state primary schools grievously overworked their students. As he had told members of the British Medical Association in 1880:

> Of the many conditions tending to the increase of mental disease I would specially direct your attention to education. . . . Injudicious haste or ill-considered zeal may work serious mischief among fragile or badly nourished children, by inducing exhaustion of the brain. It is a curious fact that, since the recent spread of education, the increase of deaths from hydrocephalous [*sic*] has not been among infants, but among children over five years of age.[26]

The lengthy essay that Crichton-Browne published in 1883, on ''Education and the Nervous System,'' had explored in great detail what he perceived to be the real risk inherent in pushing young students too far. He was sure that intense mental exertion caused insomnia, thereby depriving boys and girls of the sleep necessary for their physical development. Although preparing lessons at night was the most damaging work in this respect, any ''peculiarly painful and prostrating'' effort could have tragic effects, including death from inflammation of the brain. Such terrible consequences were likeliest, Crichton-Browne claimed, ''under a system of 'cram' or spurt teaching, with a view to a specific examination, or of learning by rote and by rule, without any real understanding of what is being learnt.''[27] With these convictions, he was not likely to exonerate London's state-aided elementary schools from the charge of child abuse through overwork.

Crichton-Browne's report to the Education Department, based on visits to fourteen state schools, was so critical that Mundella was reluctant to have it printed among the year's Parliamentary Papers. It was published only thanks to pressure from the opposition in the House of Commons.[28] Many of the points in the report merely elaborated what Crichton-Browne had already asserted in his essay of 1883. Very early in the document, for example, he aimed his criticism against the examination system enforced in the schools, a system that obliged the teacher to incite ''examination fever,'' with all its ''unpleasant *sequelae*,'' in the classroom. ''Examinations,'' he mourned, "instead of being tests of school work, have become to a great extent its one aim and guiding principle, and whatever educational fruits they may have yielded, they are producing, I am confident, a rich crop of nervousness." Even Crichton-Browne had to admit, however, that this crop did not flourish among the majority of pupils. He acknowledged that 20 to 30 percent of the students whom he saw were "bright, clever children, who can easily accomplish all the work required of them by the Code each year in seven or eight months." Another 40 to 60 percent, he conceded, showed "average intelligence" and were able to complete the necessary work by steady application through the allotted twelve months. It was the remaining percent that aroused his anger and anxiety—the "backward children" who could not work through the year's academic program in the given time and who, accordingly, had to be "hard pressed, in order to get as many as possible of them to make a passable appearance." These were the ones who faced permanent damage to their health so that "the great modern giant Examination [might] have a huge meal." Eating was obviously on Crichton-Browne's mind when he wrote the report, for he eloquently deplored the effort to force-feed knowledge into children who came to school with empty stomachs.[29]

As in 1883, Crichton-Browne maintained in his report that all manner of nervous and mental ailments followed in the wake of academic overpressure. Madness, hydrocephalus, tubercular meningitis, inflammation of the brain, habitual headache, insomnia, somnambulism, St. Vitus's dance or chorea—all could be laid at the door of excessive school work. In the report's concluding pages, the Lord Chancellor's Visitor urged that schools be allowed to make liberal use of a generally ignored provision in the code, which sanctioned "the withholding from examination of scholars on account of 'delicate health or prolonged illness; obvious dulness or defective intellect.'" This clause, if implemented by teachers rather than school inspectors, he argued, would spare the "backward children upon whom over-pressure operates most injuriously." He called, too, for the doctor to play as important a role as the school inspector, making periodic visits to check the sanitary conditions under which the pupils labored and to interfere on behalf of the children against overzealous instructors. He wanted each school to keep a logbook, recording at monthly intervals the "height, weight, head, and chest girth" of every child, in order to enable inspectors to apply different standards where the student population was obviously less robust than at schools in more prosperous neighborhoods. This was the great age of anthropometrical measurement, and Crichton-Browne was certain of its value to both medicine and education. Finally, he recommended that teachers be taught physiology; once they comprehended the laws of health, he believed they would themselves take the lead in abolishing overpressure in their schools.[30]

The Education Department not only disputed Crichton-Browne's findings; alleging that he had reached his conclusions even before the start of his inquiries, it entirely repudiated the report.[31] The author stuck to those conclusions, however, and tried to drum up support for them in influential places. In September 1884, he wrote to Herbert Spencer, whose opposition to premature forcing of the brain made him a likely ally, asking the philosopher to read the report and, if possible, "to say a few words, which might be quoted, condemnatory of 'over-pressure.'" In the same month, he corresponded with Dr. Norman Kerr, a physician well-known for his work as a temperance reformer, thanking him for a letter to the *Times* that endorsed the report's concerns. With characteristic self-aggrandizement, Crichton-Browne added: "As you will understand it has required some courage on the part of a servant of the government as I am to speak out boldly as I have done."[32]

Unfortunately, his courage outstripped his supporting data. It was easy for J. G. Fitch, chief inspector of schools, to demolish the report simply by demonstrating how slight was the evidence for Crichton-Browne's sweeping claims. "There is in Dr. Browne's paper much strong assertion," Fitch commented drily after taking it apart point by point, "but there is not a line which seems to me to deserve the name of 'proof,' either that the amount of intellectual effort required of children under existing regulations is excessive, or that youthful sickness, weakness, or any other evil is directly traceable to school-work." The report was, in fact, filled with dubious inferences from insufficient information, not unlike Crichton-Browne's conclusions about female brains. After visiting five Scottish primary schools, "all situated in a purely agricultural district of Dumfriesshire," for example, he drew broad comparisons between English and Scottish elementary education, concluding that the latter was healthier than the former. Repeatedly, he attributed to unreasonable academic burdens symptoms of fatigue and strain that were far more likely to result from the living conditions imposed on the majority of students in London's state primary schools. He knew that many young pupils held jobs before and after school to supplement family income by a few pence. He was aware that a number did not have proper beds to sleep in, proper meals, and proper clothes to keep them warm. He probably realized that sharing a room with several siblings, and perhaps parents as well, did not provide a quiet haven of repose at night. Yet he persisted in particularly blaming schoolwork, and—above all—home lessons in the evening, for the broken sleep that thousands of working-class children endured every night.[33] Much of "the over-work panic," as one teacher called it, might have abated sooner had the public carefully scrutinized the kinds of arguments being served up in the guise of scientific investigations. As it was, *overpressure* passed into the national vocabulary and by the Edwardian decade had become one of several "quasi-medical explanations" popularly invoked to account for suicidal behavior, among young people as among adults.[34]

At an official level, however, the furor died down within a year or two after Crichton-Browne's report. With the Conservatives back in power, a Royal Commission on elementary education was appointed in 1885, in a move to pacify public opinion about the overpressure controversy. Crichton-Browne was neither appointed as a commissioner nor called as a witness.[35] Presumably his views were too well known and too antagonistic for the commissioners to need or desire further familiarity with them. The snub hardly silenced the Lord Chancellor's Visitor. That same year he returned to the attack, in his lengthy introduction to the English translation of a Danish study on overpressure in high schools. Here he described an even heavier burden of stress on middle-class youth than he had found among London's working-class children, and he bluntly condemned "the vanity and cupidity of parents," British and Danish alike, for subjecting their offspring to the "relentless grasp" of crammers who squeezed them "into the approved form for satisfying the requirements of certain examiners." In 1892, he worked the same theme, with exclusive application to girls' education, in an address to the Medical Society of London. As late as 1920, in the first Maudsley Lecture to the Medico-Psychological Association, he insisted, yet again, that the British educational system had "been responsible for some disastrous consequences where it has over-strained immature, feeble and undernourished brains."[36] The tenacity with which Crichton-Browne clung to this argument, despite its application, at most, to a small percentage of British school-children, makes sense today only in the context of the mounting panic over racial degeneration and national decline that dominated public health concerns in the late Victorian years. For a social conservative like Crichton-Browne, it was far simpler to seek comparatively minor educational changes in response to these alarms than even to consider the fundamental economic and environmental alterations that London's working-class children really required. It was also easier to blame parents and teachers than to admit that the medical profession had badly failed to meet the children's needs.

Whatever their views on academic overpressure, Victorian and Edwardian medical practitioners concurred that fresh air and physical exercise were its antidotes. Medical theory considered these even more essential for children than for nervous adults, because outdoor sports not only provided a necessary change from school work, but also gave the body's nerve centers the activity necessary for vigorous health and growth. Throughout the nineteenth and early twentieth centuries, there was total unanimity among doctors on this point, whether they advocated organized games, calisthenics, "Swedish drill," or just romping. Generally speaking, they saw the same advantages in outdoor exercise for girls before puberty as for boys, for schoolchildren as for youthful mill hands. Fothergill, for example, insisted that prolonged physical labor in a factory was as deleterious to children's health as extended mental concentration "in an ill-ventilated school." Exercise, he explained, was essential to both sets of victims: "The action of the muscles leads to their growth directly, and the bones, ligaments, and nerves, grow *pari passu.*" (He could not resist adding, however, that many working-class children had to toil only because of the "thriftless habits and gross improvidence" of their parents.)[37]

For middle-class boys and girls whose parents were not thriftless and who had the time to play under the open sky, doctors prescribed large doses of this medicine whenever nervousness threatened. Medical consultants told Leslie Stephen, when he was a thin, delicate boy, that he "must do little work with his brain, but must ride and row and live in the open air, or, when that was impossible, have recourse to the gymnasium or the 'chest expander.'" The Potter family doctor regularly ordered fresh air and exercise for young Beatrice when she was suffering from one or another of her "indefinable" nervous maladies and told her to stay out of the domestic schoolroom. Evidently Ruskin attributed some of his adult misery to "the way he was brought up—not like other boys, no out-door games, etc." For pale, sickly, nervous children in Victorian and Edwardian fiction, cavorting out of doors likewise often proved more beneficial than any conceivable pharmaceutical concoction. In *Tom Brown's Schooldays,* frail George Arthur, who "seems all over nerves" on his first appearance, is spared the evil effects of "too much reading" thanks to his friendship with "strapping boys," who teach him to collect birds' eggs, to run through the fields, to swim, and, above all, to play cricket.[38] Both the hysterical Colin Craven and his thin, sallow cousin, Mary Lennox, in Frances Hodgson Burnett's pre-war classic, *The Secret Garden* (1911), gain health and happiness from facing the Yorkshire winds and, quite literally, cultivating their garden. While the story is primarily a text on overcoming selfishness, both children learn to think of others—to move outside of themselves—only as they become enchanted with the outside world. In most factual and fictional cases, open air medicine worked its magic only *after* the child's health became cause for concern. How much better, doctors contended, to forestall neurotic illness altogether, by making sure that school holidays were spent ''in bodily exercise as much as possible in the open air in the country,'' as Johnson recommended, or by guaranteeing that ''an interval of ten minutes to be spent in fresh air and exercise, not drill, should always elapse between each lesson'' at school, as Guthrie insisted more than seventy years later.[39]

Medical paeans to outdoor exercise did not, however, amount to a medical endorsement of rampant athleticism. Just as doctors who treated adult nervous patients stressed the importance of maintaining mental and physical development in a state of equilibrium, so a balanced regimen for children was similarly the goal of most family doctors and nerve specialists, with neither brain nor body cultivated at the other's expense. It was only when the two increased their strength together, in moderation, that a medical advisor could feel confident of his young patient's future nervous stability. Robert Farquharson, the medical officer at Rugby and formerly assistant surgeon to the Coldstream Guards, saw at first hand where the veneration of athletic skill might lead and in 1870 published in the *Lancet* a temperate warning against the growing emphasis on outdoor sports at the public schools. He worried that too much pressure on boys to participate in these activities would tax their physical powers, detract from their mental abilities, and in the end cause ''serious cerebral mischief.'' ''It may thus happen,'' he surmised, ''that a weakly lad, who is studious, and anxious about his work, feels that playing takes too much out of him; he finds his working power fail, perhaps he does not get enough sleep, and in the end he breaks down.''[40] Many Victorian educators voiced the same concerns.

Whether overpressure came in the form of parental demands for academic success, peer group emphasis on athletic skill, or a harassed teacher's anxiety over examination results, today's historians are hard pressed to learn how Victorian children themselves responded. Virtually everything we know about prepubertal childhood in the nineteenth century comes through the filter of adult recollections and judgments. By the time a boy or girl could articulate feelings about his or her own health and could record reactions to the treatment received from parents, teachers, and doctors, childhood was usually over, and the writer had reached adolescence, if not young adulthood. Memoirs of childhood, written long after the fact, abound, but the survival of actual childhood writings—letters to family members or early attempts at keeping a diary—is rare. Even where an unusually complete collection of family papers exists, such as that of the Bensons in the Bodleian Library, obstacles bar us from clearly hearing the children's voices. Although the documents in the Bodleian include letters written by Martin White Benson, the archbishop's eldest son, from the age of seven, the record of his life is cast almost entirely in Edward White Benson's terms.[41] Our views of this precocious and fluent boy, born in 1860, whose life became an object lesson in the risks of mental forcing, are formed more by his father's high hopes for him than by his own perceptions.

A devoted and loving father, E. W. Benson was, nonetheless, a difficult parent, as Martin's brother Arthur recollected in his many explicitly and covertly auto-biographical works. "Hugh's" father in *Beside Still Waters* had a taste "for the improving in literature" and was always urging the boy to read "the little dry books, uncouthly and elaborately phrased, that had pleased himself in his own early days."[42] Like many Victorians, the elder Benson hated to see children waste time, and, as both a clergyman and headmaster (at Wellington College during Martin's childhood) he had particularly definite ideas about teaching and learning. Any flights of fancy or lapses from earnest endeavor were not to be tolerated. He wanted his own children to be exemplary, both in moral rectitude and in academic distinction. The future archbishop had been deeply molded by the ideals of "godliness and good learning" that dominated Anglican education in his youth, and he expected his eldest son to embody that tradition in turn. Before he was two years old, Martin could point out Jesus in a Raphael painting; at the age of five, he was helping his mother define words, clearly and concisely, for his younger siblings. Remembered by his brothers as "a boy of extraordinary brilliance," possessing "the most singular gifts of thought and expression," he obviously showed exceptional promise.[43] After Martin's death at the age of seventeen, his father, then serving as bishop of Truro, wrote about him as if he had been faultless. In fact, however, E. W. Benson had had cause to criticize his son's academic performance at the age of ten and, over the years, had warned him repeatedly about inattention and daydreaming. "Your fault intellectually," he told Martin when the boy was almost fourteen, "is to be rather *dreamy,* and let the grass grow while you are turning round. It is a weakness which you should try to cure."[44]

Apart from this drift toward dreaminess and a stammer from which he always suffered, Martin evinced no worrisome "nerve-signs" and was perfectly healthy by any standards. His letters to his parents reveal an affectionate and happy boy. He matured intellectually as richly as his father could have wished, winning the top scholarship at Winchester, where he became a student in 1874, and developing his mind in breadth and depth through his studies there. Edward Benson never ceased to keep a vigilant eye on his son, but he had good reason to be pleased and very proud. Then in February 1878, Martin died of meningitis, or "brain fever." To the stunned and shattered bishop of Truro, the death seemed a terrible retribution for all the aspirations and ambitions that he had focused on Martin. After 1878, no longer feeling sure of God's purpose, he reacted vigorously against the kind of academic pressure he had lovingly, but relentlessly, pushed on his eldest son. In keeping with the widespread Victorian assumption that excessive mental strain could provoke a high fever in the brain, the whole Benson family became convinced that the precocious nurturing of Martin's intellectual gifts had played a major role in his untimely death. The bishop drastically altered his child-rearing tactics, sparing his younger children the paternal demands and criticism that Martin had borne so cheerfully. A. C. Benson clearly had his older brother in mind when he wrote in 1911 that Ruskin's "mental activity was perilously stimulated" in youth, suggesting that "perhaps the irritability of brain which worked havoc in [Ruskin's] later life was partly caused by his prodigious precocity."[45] Martin Benson's own writings reveal that his brain did *not* suffer from persistent overstimulation at too early an age, but that he was an extremely intelligent product of a thoughtful, serious family who derived tremendous pleasure from learning. The guilt that burdened Edward Benson for the remainder of his life after Martin's death can have done little to ease the moods of crushing despair to which he had always been prone. The medical profession was surely justified in seeking to protect the young from unreasonable academic expectations and unremitting pressures, but in labeling dangerous any mark of unusual intellectual distinction in children, doctors must have caused parents much needless suffering when tragedy struck.

Martin Benson's death occurred when he was, of course, closer to adulthood than childhood, in that indeterminate phase of growth which the late Victorians began to call adolescence. If the concept of childhood as a period of life separate from adulthood was secure by the nineteenth century, despite uncertainty over its terminal point, the concept of adolescence was only starting to assume coherence at the close of Victoria's reign. By then, it had become obvious to all who dealt with young people that children did not suddenly become emotionally mature when their bodies became physically adult and, furthermore, that sexual development did not, in fact, necessarily mark the end of bodily growth. It is certainly true that this realization effected no change in the experience of most British boys and girls; for the vast majority of them, leaving school between the ages of ten and fourteen years signaled their immersion in the adult world of long working hours. Yet adolescence was not a phase of life reserved solely for the affluent, whose daughters found shelter under the family roof until marriage and whose sons enjoyed the same security until the achievement of financial independence. As early as 1833, the Factory Act of that year distinguished workers aged thirteen to eighteen from full-fledged adults, and also, of course, from the younger children whose hours of labor were considerably more restricted. From the middle of the century, furthermore, social reformers were troubled by the distinctive culture of working-class adolescents and tried, through a variety of youth programs, church clubs, and sporting events, to channel it into socially useful directions.[46]

Although the Victorians seldom used the word *adolescent,* preferring the terms *young person* or *youth,* the idea nonetheless gained ground in the second half of the nineteenth century that a span of years, suspended between childhood and adulthood, presented physical and mental problems common to neither. No one was too precise about the chronological limits of this period. The common assumption was that it began at puberty, although Clouston, for one, chose to disagree. In an article contributed to the *Edinburgh Medical Journal* in 1880, he proposed regarding adolescence as a distinct stage, commencing at eighteen and extending until twenty-five years. "I should restrict puberty," he explained, "to the initial development of the function of reproduction," while adolescence, he believed, lasted until "the full perfection of the reproductive energy," when both the male and female bodies had attained their entirely adult appearance. Clouston acknowledged, however, that his system of dating was not likely "to change the accepted meaning of the present nomenclature," and most of his contemporaries would have designated as adolescents all boys and girls old enough to leave school, even if they did not have to.[47] The ending of adolescence was even more difficult to determine than the start, for there was no specific age by which medical men could say that all young people had attained complete physical and emotional maturity. Class considerations, as always, played a much more decisive role in hastening adulthood than most doctors wanted to admit. Legal definitions, furthermore, continued to pay little attention to medical views right down to World War I.[48]

If medical practitioners in Great Britain, continental Europe, and the United States remained divided over the actual timing of adolescence, they agreed on its distinctiveness within the life cycle. At the very start of the nineteenth century, Pierre-Jean-Georges Cabanis, the celebrated French physician and materialist philosopher, had specified certain mental traits as characteristic of the age of awakening sexuality, particularly a dominant imagination and a tendency to profound reverie. For the rest of the century, and into the twentieth, alienists and other medical men continued to stress the mental oddities and dangers that accompanied the development of the reproductive function in boys and girls. They emphasized that the years during and just after puberty were formative ones, when young people were in a highly volatile condition, extremely open to new experiences and reacting to them without emotional restraint. Subject to rapid mood changes, boys and girls at this stage of life were also visited by periods of utter lethargy, indecision, and listlessness. It was, in short, an age of antitheses and contradictions, as the American psychologist G. Stanley Hall noted in his pioneering two-volume work *Adolescence; its Psychology and its Relations to Physiology, Anthropology, Sociology, Sex, Crime, Religion and Education*. Published in 1904, *Adolescence* represented the culmination of more than twenty years of inquiry and speculation on Hall's part. By synthesizing the earlier, inchoate ideas about adolescence into a consistent and plausible theory, Hall gave the concept of adolescence, and the word itself, an official place in the international vocabulary of psychology. He contended that, above all else, adolescence was a time of "storm and stress," a period of turbulence and upheaval during which the individual personality redefined itself anew.[49] Although critics of a later period have faulted him for not recognizing the ways in which maturing youth normally adapts to new emotions and experiences so as to avoid damaging the self, and, most of all, for failing to realize how much his notion of adolescence was molded by specific cultural conditions, Hall's interpretation of adolescence has nonetheless proved extraordinarily tenacious and influential. It still deeply colors our approach to adolescence today.

The idea of adolescence articulated in the late Victorian and Edwardian eras was, indeed, the product of economic, social, and medical developments in the Western world during the preceding 150 years or so, which were confined neither to one nation nor, as we have seen, to one social stratum. With the concept finding fertile soil in countries as different from each other as republican America and imperial Germany, broad historical trends were clearly at work—including the shift from a predominantly rural to a mainly urban population, with greater concentrations of young people in close proximity, and the growth of professions that required extended periods of secondary and even tertiary education. Rising social expectations that delayed marriage among both the middle and the respectable working classes, until the groom could support his bride in their own home, intensified the problem families faced in trying to encompass a sexually mature but economically dependent member. The concept of adolescence both helped to make sense out of the fact that these young people were often centers of unrest within the family and served to justify parental authority when it denied them the full autonomy of adulthood. What is particularly striking about the medical depiction of adolescence by the eve of World War I is the willingness with which doctors embraced Hall's stress on inner turmoil as its preeminent feature. Yet it is hardly surprising that they should have found this vision of adolescence compelling: it mirrored, on the psychological level, what they had been saying for years about the massive physical disturbances that accompanied the transition from childhood to maturity.

In their extensive literature on the bodily changes that occurred during adolescence, British doctors in the late nineteenth and early twentieth centuries always paid especially close attention to the hazards threatening the nervous system. Girls were not alone in undergoing "large re-arrangements in the distribution of nerve energy" at puberty, they observed; similar readjustments agitated boys' bodies as well.[50] Much as medical practitioners sought to foster among younger children habits that promoted future nervous stability, they were chiefly concerned about adolescents, and, according to their theories, with good reason. "The problem of the whole future life as regards health is often settled in adolescence," Schofield explained in 1908:

> All hereditary pathological nervous tendencies seem to come out in adolescence. At this time, therefore, the child should be closely watched for any well-known ancestral idiosyncrasies; and everything should be done to combat any suspected or manifest nervous instability or weakness. Special note should be taken of the powers of the inhibitory centres, and these should be strongly fostered, developed, and exercised at this period. Self-restraint and self-control are not only valuable moral qualities, but invaluable prophylactics against nervous troubles.

Speaking specifically of the adolescent woman, Crichton-Browne commented, with his usual hyperbole, that puberty was the "great epoch" when, thanks to "momentous changes . . . taking place in her body and mind . . . a wave of irritability sweeps through her nervous system."[51]

With the attainment of sexual maturity straining the entire "nervous economy," it is no wonder that Victorian and Edwardian alienists associated several functional nervous disorders particularly with adolescence. Of these afflictions, the gravest by far was a form of insanity linked exclusively with puberty. "Mania of pubescence" figured in David Skae's system of classifying mental illnesses in the early 1860s. It was, he believed, "apparently dependent upon the changes affecting the circulation and nervous system" that characterized puberty. When Clouston wrote about "the insanity of puberty," or "the insanity of adolescence," as he also called it, he underscored the significant role played by heredity in its incidence, although he conceded that "some irregularity in the coming on of the reproductive or menstrual function" could serve as its precipitant. Despite his reference to menstruation, Clouston had no doubt that the "years of gradual coming to maturity are full of danger to the mental health of both sexes," and insanity, he was convinced, could strike equally in the male or female direction. "The mental symptoms," he pointed out consist most frequently of a kind of incoherent delirium rather than any fixed delusional state. In boys the beginning of an attack is frequently ushered in by a disturbance in the emotional condition, dislikes to parents or brothers or sisters expressed in a violent, open way; there is irrational dislike to and avoidance of the opposite sex. The manner of a grown-up man is assumed, and an offensive "forwardness" of air and demeanour. This soon passes into maniacal delirium, which, however, is not apt to last long. It alternates with periods of sanity, and even with stages of depression.[52]

To anyone reading this description in the 1990s, the immediate assumption is that the mid- and late Victorians simply used the label *adolescent insanity* to stigmatize unruly and defiant teenage behavior, just as they sometimes wielded the diagnosis of *moral insanity* to express disapproval of conduct that they judged aberrant. A British psychiatrist, Edward Hare, has recently suggested, however, that around the beginning of the nineteenth century some as yet unexplained biological change produced a form of mental illness that was substantially different from the previously existing types. The name eventually given to this malady in the twentieth century, Hare contends, was schizophrenia, but the earlier, nineteenth-century designation, *dementia praecox,* better reveals one of its most significant features—the fact that it typically appears in young adults between the ages of fifteen and twenty-five years.[53] While psychiatrists today no longer perceive the symptoms of schizophrenia as a form of premature dementia, they still emphasize its onset during the years of early adulthood and are probing its potential relationship to changes in cerebral physiology that occur during adolescence. It is probably impossible to counter or confirm definitively the hypothesis of schizophrenia's nineteenth-century novelty, but it suggests that the medical attention paid to "adolescent insanity" by the 1850s might not merely have been an expression of the psychiatric urge to police society.

Although recognizing adolescence as the first phase of life seriously threatened by the possibility of insanity, alienists found milder forms of neurotic illness to be much more common in the years during and just after puberty. They observed that hysteria, migraine, chorea, and epilepsy arose at this period, particularly among young women, while mental depression belonged prominently among the adolescent afflictions of both sexes, as Clouston thoroughly described it in his Edwardian text, *Hygiene of Mind:*

> It may consist simply of low spirits at times, especially in the mornings, and pessimistic views of life, which are quite unnatural for that period of life. Often the subjects of this depression are troubled with headaches and have neuralgic tendencies. The sleep is often neither so long nor so sound as it should be. The mental depression of which I am speaking is really more or less marked mental pain. . . . It is apt to be periodic in its occurrence. . . . Study or work of any kind cannot be properly engaged in while the depression lasts. Work is no longer a pleasure, as it should be. The social instincts are diminished. Friends are not so welcome. Games are not gone at with zest. The eye, the countenance, and the walking often show a lack of nerve and muscular energy.[54]

It goes without saying that, while late Victorian and Edwardian psychiatrists focused on the emotional symptoms of adolescent dislocations, they continued to attribute even the most disturbing of them to a physical cause, namely the underlying somatic condition of exhaustion arising from the rapid development of the reproductive organs and the consequent depletion of nerve force. Alienists were willing to acknowledge that other causes, such as poor nutrition or intellectual overstrain, could promote neurasthenia among adolescents, but their fundamental explanation always remained fixed on the maturing reproductive function in young men and women.

The centrality of that process as the key to understanding adolescence led medical practitioners to invest very different meaning in female and male development during puberty. Adolescence became for them the point at which boys and girls could no longer be treated as more or less undifferentiated children, but needed to be molded according to the cultural prescriptions for their respective genders. It was not, of course, the case that Victorian children entirely avoided the burdens of sexual stereotyping before puberty struck. If seven-year-old-boys at mid-century could be described as "bold, combative, muscularly active," while girls of the same age were portrayed as "retiring, timid, yielding,"[55] a distinctive sexual identity was clearly being imposed on them early in life. The fact remains, nonetheless, that both mothers and doctors enforced those identities far less rigidly when children had not yet reached puberty. "Before that time," Clouston pointed out in 1880, "there has been a general psychical likeness between individuals of the same and of opposite sexes," but all that changed at puberty, when "psychical energy" in man began to develop "far more in the direction of energizing and cognition, in the woman in the direction of emotion and the protective instincts." To explain the appearance of hysteria in young male children, Donkin made a similar point a few years later, contending that "the sexual distribution" of the disorder was "much less unequal in the earlier years" than after puberty, when hysteria became primarily, although not exclusively, a female affliction. As far as liability to neurotic illness was concerned, the approach or arrival of puberty marked the great separation between the sexes. While the male body at puberty began gradually gaining the physical vigor of its adult maturity, fragility and nervous instability emerged as the salient traits of the adolescent girl.[56] It came as no surprise to Victorian or Edwardian doctors that some female adolescents, like Elizabeth Barrett Browning, fell into patterns of invalidism that set the course of their lives, or that others first evinced at puberty those psychic powers of mediumship which, according to most medical authorities, betokened abnormalities of the nervous system.

Although a time of stress and risks for boys and girls alike, medical opinion argued that puberty posed particular problems for the latter, owing to the comparative intensity of the process in women. Mary Scharlieb succinctly pointed out the differences between male and female maturation when she observed: "Between the ages of 12 and 15 the girl undergoes a more or less rapid evolution from the common to the feminine type, while the boy remains more or less a child up to the age of 15, and even then alters both more slowly and less completely, gradually assuming the characteristics of manhood."[57] Male doctors, however, did not need a female colleague to belabor the point; they had been saying as much themselves for years. They always considered puberty more overwhelming for girls than for boys, not only for the reasons Scharlieb gave, but owing to their conviction that the reproductive organs occupied a far more dominant position in female than in male physiology. From the medical point of view, adolescent girls were, above everything else, potential mothers. By comparison, future fatherhood was not the paramount theme when medical texts discussed adolescent boys.

With menstruation commanding medical attention as the single most common source of female health troubles, it hardly needs observing that doctors viewed menarche as the most important event in an adolescent girl's life. Gynecologists and alienists joined forces to insist that the proper establishment of menstruation was utterly essential to the future well-being of the adult woman. In the 1850s, E. J. Tilt wrote with genuine dismay about the traumatic ignorance in which girls were allowed to commence puberty. A quarter of his patients, he found, were totally unprepared for their first menstrual period, and a number were understandably terrified, believing themselves to be wounded. Their shock contributed to menstrual irregularities and general health problems, including "excessive nervous susceptibility." With so much hanging in the balance, it behooved medical advisors and, more importantly, mothers to guarantee that the critical phase of female puberty passed serenely, with as little stress as possible on the developing woman. Emotional and physical strain were to be avoided at all costs, even to the point of barring the adolescent girl from piano playing and novel reading, should these prove too stimulating during her monthly periods.[58] Such admonitions merely foreshadowed the advice that doctors gave to adult women concerning the need to rest during menstruation, but medical practitioners pressed their case with particular urgency for the adolescent girl. In some medical texts, they actually seem to assert that girls should avoid excitement throughout the entire stage of puberty, not merely during their "monthlies." These beliefs explain, of course, Victorian medical hostility to the intellectually challenging secondary schools for girls that emerged after mid-century. A number of influential alienists and other doctors simply assumed that competition, whether in the form of academic examinations or team sports, was extremely perilous for adolescent women whose bodies could withstand virtually no agitation.[59]

An unsuccessful passage through puberty betrayed itself in manifold ways. In addition to menstrual irregularities, hysterical or neurasthenic symptoms were other obvious signs that a young woman had failed to sail safely through the dangerous channels of adolescence. Playfair reported such a case—a neurasthenic seventeen-year-old girl who "broke down from overwork at school" and suffered from "arrested menstruation," not to mention "excessive emaciation, cold and livid extremities, progressively increasing muscular debility, and inability to take any active part in the work of life." A variety of related behavioral patterns, including fasting, religious ecstasy, and "the simulation of disease," in Crichton-Browne's acerbic phrase, particularly revealed severe disturbances in the female adolescent nervous centers. Although highly emotional religious conversions were not unknown among adolescent boys, especially in Nonconformist working-class communities, medical men never included intense religiosity among the characteristic abnormalities of male puberty. In fact, they did not delineate a profile of deviancy for adolescent boys anything like their detailed and complex picture of aberrant female adolescence.[60]

Sham illnesses, excessive religious devotions, and morally reprehensible behavior recur repeatedly as very odd partners in medical descriptions of adolescent girls during the late Victorian and Edwardian years. Playfair, always ready with a case in point, described "a clever girl of highly developed nervous organisation" who, at fourteen years of age, while straining her mind over schoolwork, "had suddenly broken down, got complete hysterical hemiplegia, and for four years had never been out of bed or moved either of her lower limbs." A "loud barking cough," equally incurable, and anorexia complicated the situation. Playfair, who was consulted when the girl was seventeen, immediately applied the methods of the Weir Mitchell rest cure, separating her from her family and keeping her under his own strict supervision. The cough vanished two days later, the paralysis shortly thereafter. By the end of a month, she was able to walk a short distance to visit her parents. Playfair was not interested in probing the reasons why her body imitated the symptoms of severe disease for four years, nor why the illness suddenly vanished after the patient was removed from her home; his point was merely to demonstrate the efficacy of the rest cure. He labeled her disorder "aggravated hysteria," not adolescent insanity, but the distinction was usually a matter of the attending doctor's personal choice. With one of Clouston's youthful patients, "the physiological crisis of commencing menstruation," exacerbated by "study and the unnatural life at a boarding-school," manifested itself in perfervid religious observances. The depressed fifteen-year-old girl became obsessive in her spiritual devotions—"kneeling, uttering over and over again rhythmical expressions of prayer, swaying her body backwards and forwards, and wringing her hands at intervals." As was his fashion, Clouston "sent her at once to the country, to ride, walk, live in the open air, to take aloes, iron, and quinine, to read little, not to go to church for a short time. . . ." (He had to be careful here for, convinced though he was that her intense religiosity was unhealthy, he did not want to appear hostile to religion.) Eventually, "after a tour in Switzerland she returned fat, cheerful, and vigorous," quite cured of her "undue religious emotionalism." Another female adolescent of his acquaintance distinguished herself by "disobedience, lying, perversity of every kind and outrageous unconventionality of dress and conduct."[61]

"Adolescent girls," Mary Scharlieb remarked a few years before World War I, "are as anxious to have the control of their own individuality as was Phaeton to drive the chariot of the Sun, and, as a rule, they are likely to be as successful as he was!"[62] By the Edwardian decade, medical opinion had come to view the subject of Scharlieb's comments as not merely troubled, but fundamentally willful, seeking to impose their poor judgment about matters of health, diet, rest, work, recreation, and friendship, over that of their more experienced elders. It is not surprising, since hysteria was so closely associated with female adolescence, that the "contest of wills" interpretation of that neurosis heavily colored medical attitudes toward the age of puberty in young women. Ironically, adolescent boys—in whom the supervisory will was supposedly assuming its dominant role in preparation for adult responsibilities—were not subjected to this generalized explanation of their conduct. Most Victorian and Edwardian girls certainly had more occasion to experience and resent restraints on their "own individuality" during adolescence than did their brothers, who were likelier to escape from parental control, at least temporarily, while at school or at work. Adolescent boys of the middle classes, however, hardly enjoyed much freedom under the watchful eyes of schoolmasters or employers, and their challenges to these authority figures could not have been rare events. The absence of a pronounced theory concerning boyish willfulness at puberty makes medical suspicions about headstrong adolescent girls all the more revealing.

One of the best documented cases of female adolescent breakdown, that of Rose La Touche in October 1863, tragically featured the tensions between parental domination, emotional dependence, and a young woman's efforts to express her own personality, unfolding within a highly unusual context. At fifteen years of age, Rose was the frequent correspondent and confidante of John Ruskin, a famous man nearly three times as old. By the autumn of 1863, she must have realized that his attraction to her held more than an interest in teaching her art, the reason for their first meeting in 1858, when she was ten. He was, in fact, falling obsessively in love with her, and she was not emotionally prepared to deal with his devotion, despite a genuine fondness for him. Although high-spirited, she evinced the signs of a neurotic temperament, experiencing painful headaches and, from the autumn of 1861, strange spells when she briefly lost consciousness. She was, furthermore, intensely religious, sometimes spending hours in prayer and suffering agonies of perplexity when she heard the truth of the Gospels being questioned. That Ruskin was, by this stage in his life, one of the questioners tormented her. There were also mounting conflicts with her parents, as when, in the spring of 1862, they offered Ruskin a cottage on their Irish estate for part of the summer and then abruptly withdrew the invitation, for reasons that are not clear. Perhaps his religious views alarmed them; more likely, the nature of his feelings for Rose caused their anxiety, particularly since Maria La Touche, herself a few years younger than Ruskin, was apparently more than a little in love with him. In any case, Ruskin blamed Rose for not launching a greater campaign to keep the cottage for him, and the unfortunate girl found herself at the center of a quarrel between him and her parents that raged for much of that summer. In the autumn of the following year, Rose's religion provoked a severe crisis with her mother. On her father's urging, Rose decided that the time had come to take her First Communion. John La Touche, who had recently departed from the Anglican faith of his family to become a Baptist, saw no need for his daughter to undergo Confirmation before Communion. Maria La Touche, still firm in her Anglican beliefs, disagreed and, when Rose did not accede to maternal wishes, refused to accompany her daughter to First Communion on 11 October 1863. The following day, Rose suffered a severe breakdown.[63]

"I suppose," Rose La Touche later wrote in the autobiography she undertook in 1867, around the time of her nineteenth birthday,

> all the trouble of body, soul, and spirit had been too much for me, for on Monday morning I had a terrible headache and before evening was very ill. It was a strange illness . . . I know I suffered terribly. (I was in bed about four weeks.) *Everything* hurt me. People coming in and talking however kindly, used to give me tortures of pain—I seemed to *think through my head,* and every thought hurt me. I was only comfortable when I was not thinking . . . Light hurt me. Food hurt me (not my head). Sometimes I was hungry but had such terrible pain after eating. . . . I can only say again—I seemed to hurt myself. I got very weak and thin and the Doctors were frightened.

Like Eleanor Marx nearly twenty years later, Rose wondered at her doctors' resolute concentration on physical symptoms. "They seemed to think so much more about my body than about my head," she recalled. Throughout her month of agony, she constantly felt that her medical attendants did not understand what she needed in order to recover, nor would they listen to her. "They said I could not know, and went on their own way. This made me very unhappy and worse. . . ." Eventually her doctors did concede that some of Rose's "ideas were sensible," especially with regard to the food she ordered for herself.[64]

While the medical attendants justifiably concentrated their attention on her weakened and exhausted body, Rose's family and friends interpreted the illness as a kind of hysterical condition, brought on by extreme mental agitation. "It is one of her mysterious brain-attacks," Maria La Touche wrote to a friend a few days after her daughter's collapse, neglecting to mention her own role in the drama. "I am afraid she has *thought* herself into this illness, & I attribute it partly to the strong wish & excitement which resulted in her being admitted to her first Communion last Sunday. . . . Her brain is so terribly sensitive that all impressions give pain."[65] When Rose was sufficiently recovered to carry on a conversation, Maria persuaded her that religious perplexity, of her own childish creation, was at the root of her troubles. "She showed me," Rose subsequently recounted in her autobiography, "how wrong I had been, how He would so much rather I had been happy and not tired myself and made myself unChildlike for His sake. And I saw it all, and everything looked different. . . . I had tired myself out when He had not meant me to, and after all now I had only to learn His lesson and rest." Thus Maria La Touche left Rose with the firm conviction that her suffering was entirely her own fault. "I always thought *I* had done wrong," Rose confessed, "and got utterly confused in what was Right and Wrong, and what I knew I ought to do, and what I ought to do because they told me." Ruskin, too, was sure that Rose had made herself gravely ill by baffling "her poor little head" over great theological issues, which no woman was competent to unravel.[66]

One of the most fascinating aspects of Rose's breakdown in 1863 was the psychic power she seemed to possess during the most painful phase of her illness. "Being with her was like a Revelation to me," Maria La Touche wrote in mid-November to her correspondent of the previous month. "There was a sort of clairvoyance, both of spiritual & earthly things, which was startling. For the first fortnight of her illness she was able to tell beforehand every little thing that would befall her thro' the day. . . . The doctors were perfectly amazed & actually yielded against their judgment, in allowing her to follow this 'guidance' which never once erred. I do believe it— whatever it was—spared her much suffering, & saved her much 'treatment.' . . ." Subsequently Rose appeared to have lost all recollection of the last eleven years of her life, and, as if under deep hypnosis, could only converse about the people and things she had known at the age of four.[67] Ruskin may have had her in mind when he began investigating spiritualist seances the following year and concluded, at least initially, that the evidence of so-called spirit power was more pathological than prophetic. "In all the manifestations of this new power I have great sense of a wrongness and falseness somewhere," he wrote in August 1866. "It seems, in the *best* people, to mean some slight degree of nervous disease. . . ."[68]

Rose's nervous disease gradually improved, and over the next few years she had medical carte blanche to indulge her love of the outdoors. She reveled in the freedom to be a tomboy, enjoying the open air under doctor's orders. "The Wild Rose is very well but wilder than ever," her mother reported in September 1865. "I sometimes wonder if she will ever be a civilised being. . . . All day long she is in & out, let the weather be what it may, & not one single thing that girls do, does she do—except a *little* music when she pleases."[69]

The development of the saga over the next decade distressingly resembles a tug of war between Ruskin and Rose's parents for possession of her. Early in 1866, he asked her to marry him. She had just turned eighteen and requested a three-year delay in order to make up her mind. Throughout that entire period, she was barred from seeing him and, for much of it, from writing to him. To what extent parental pressure molded her decision to refuse him is impossible to say; it is entirely likely that a young woman in her early twenties had no strong inclination to marry a fifty-year-old suitor, particularly one whose previous marriage had ended so publicly. The whole question of Ruskin's impotence, which her parents made sure to bring to Rose's attention, doubtless raised the issue of sexual relations in a highly unpleasant way, guaranteed to increase her anxieties and suffering. John and Maria La Touche were probably right in thinking that Ruskin could not make their daughter happy, but they never granted her the independence to reach her own decision. In the peculiar circumstances of her story, it seems sadly appropriate that, when she died in May 1875, she was of unsound mind and had been placed under medical restraint in Dublin.[70] No matter how securely Ruskin's parents had woven their nets of suffocating love around him as a child and adolescent, he was able, as an adult, to slip away for a while, even if depression accompanied him wherever he went. The entrapment from which Rose never found the means to escape was physical as well as emotional. It held her in the "liminal" status of adolescence, even when she was fully adult.[71]

It was entirely characteristic of Victorian attitudes toward adolescence that the principal event in the unfolding relationship between Rose La Touche and Ruskin— her sexual development from girlhood to womanhood—remained largely unmentioned in all the masses of letters that passed among the numerous participants in the disaster. Genteel reticence about such matters was not the only reason for this omission. Even medical texts on adolescence, while fully discussing the growth of reproductive organs at puberty, did not linger long on the concomitant emergence of sexual desires and capacities. Medical practitioners were willing enough to deplore excessive religious emotionalism in adolescent girls and to denounce its morbidity, but they never more than hinted at its function as a substitute for frustrated sexual feelings. Yet it is clear that doctors well understood how much the first appearance of sexual passions contributed to the stress and tensions of adolescence. Indeed, their very concept of adolescence as a dangerous and disturbing time for both sexes derived much of its force from this realization. When they played down the strength of sexual needs before adulthood, they were pursuing a deliberate policy based, they claimed, on their insight into the immature nervous system.

All Victorian and Edwardian medical opinion agreed that the later a young person acknowledged his or her own sexuality the better. Premature experience of sexual feelings not only depleted large quantities of the nerve force required for physical and mental growth, but threw the individual's entire nervous system into disarray, jeopardizing future sexual development in the process. "It is very fairly inferred," the *Journal of Psychological Medicine* asserted in 1851, in an article dealing primarily with women,

> that a too early development of the sexual functions leads to disease—especially of the nervous system—or, if not to any well-defined form of affection, at least to that state of the nervous system termed "nervousness," the "hysterical temperament," "great sensitiveness," &c., and the leading characteristic of which is an exalted susceptibility of all impressions, . . . and a refinement of the feelings and intellect, such, that the individual is hardly equal to the ordinary wear and tear of life.

More than half a century later, Clouston was equally emphatic with regard to boys. "Proofs abound," he claimed, "as to it being a physiological law that neither reproduction nor sexual function should be exercised till full bodily development is completed. Neither desire nor a certain capacity is the test of fitness here but the organic completeness of the whole organism. Developmental nutrition should have ended before reproductive output begins." Decade after decade, medical wisdom informed parents and teachers that children's health and well-being depended on the gradual accumulation of experiences that kept pace with, but never outstripped, the sequential growth of their physical and mental strengths.[72]

If the educated public recoiled from the idea of *adolescent* sexuality, Victorian and Edwardian consternation over signs of sexual awareness before puberty was all the more intense. The middle and upper classes of society obviously preferred to believe in childhood innocence, but their optimism contended throughout the period with a more venerable belief in the inherent depravity of children, which the disciplinary agents of society had to restrain. The roseate views of childhood promulgated by Rousseau, Wordsworth, and Blake, among others, in the late eighteenth and early nineteenth centuries never vanquished the bleak image of sinful youth; toward the end of Victoria's reign, the writings of the Italian criminologist Cesare Lombroso—with their emphasis on the delinquent within every child—only reinforced that grim vision.[73] To the Victorians, nothing seemed more sinful in children than knowledge of the body's sexual functions.

Amid the conflicting interpretations of childhood that Victorians harbored, psychiatric opinion by the final third of the nineteenth century came down squarely on the side of corruption over purity, and alienists acknowledged, with considerable distaste, that even young children experienced sexual feelings. "Whoever observes sincerely what a child's actual mind is," remarked the childless Maudsley, "without being biased by preconceived notions of its primal purity, innocence and natural inclination to good, must see and own that its proclivities are not to good but to evil, and that the impulses which move it are the selfish impulses of passion. Give an infant in arms power in its limbs equal to its passions, and it would be more dangerous than any wild beast." Savage denounced "precocity of the animal passions" as nothing less than an indication of moral insanity, sometimes revealing itself before the age of five. In 1886, the French psychiatrist Charles Féré, reacting more calmly than his British colleagues, merely identified the "premature development of the sexual instinct" as a sign that the child in question was "predisposed to nervous disorders.''[74] Whatever the medical tone of voice, the presumed connection between childhood sexuality and nervous or mental derangement was clear.

The threat of sexuality in immature boys and girls was not, therefore, limited to the adolescent years, and much of the Victorian discussion of children's "animal passions" did not specify the precise age of the youthful offender. A sizeable segment of the British public found it an all too fascinating subject, as the abundant market in child pornography, sometimes thinly disguised as art, fully attests. Child prostitution flourished in a society that allowed the age of consent to remain at twelve years until 1871, and even then only raised it to thirteen, where it stayed until the Criminal Law Amendment Act of 1885 brought it up to sixteen. Incest likewise lurked in the Victorian consciousness, as ongoing witness to the child's potential and disruptive sexuality. Alarmed members of the middle classes chose to assume that incest only occurred in overcrowded working-class homes, where drunkenness and immorality set the tone for children as well as adults, and throughout Victoria's reign committees of inquiry carefully avoided examining the abuse in any detail. Whether between adults and children or between siblings, incest was anathema, a subject closed to discussion, for it represented a highly damaging case of dry rot in the family, the critical center of Victorian society. It too vividly illustrated how treacherously thin was the barrier of progress that modern western civilization had erected against the forces of inherent human bestiality.[75] Wherever it occurred—in homes, in schools, or in brothels—adult exploitation of children's sexual appeal was a shocking and sinister reality that very few Victorians, including medical practitioners, were prepared to confront. By couching their pronouncements in terms, not of children's sexual growth, but of their nervous development, doctors managed to blunt the impact of an extremely disturbing issue.

For all their denunciations of sexual activity in children before puberty, however, the medical profession understandably concentrated more of its attention on the question of adolescent sexual experimentation. Among middle-class children, this generally occurred at boarding schools and took the form of onanism, mutual masturbation, or homosexual practices. The "discovery" of homosexuality coincided chronologically with the emerging concept of adolescence: together they lent considerable urgency to the already profound medical anxiety over masturbatory habits among British men and boys. In the final quarter of the nineteenth century, doctors, clergymen, and educators joined forces to wage a vehement crusade against "immorality" and "vice," specifically perceived as unnatural sexual activities, at boys' boarding schools.[76]

Although they privately acknowledged widespread homosexuality in the schools, their emphasis in condemning schoolboy vice remained, throughout the Edwardian decade, the secret sin of masturbation. It was the form of premature sexual experience which doctors assumed to be most common among boys of the middle and upper classes, and which they exerted the most effort to suppress. Medical advice to parents and teachers abounded with hints concerning the ways to detect when a boy was practicing this solitary indulgence. Indeed, any sign of nervousness could be interpreted in a revealing light: pallor, clammy hands, acne, involuntary twitches, daydreaming, inability to look one in the eye or answer questions directly—all testified to the destructive impact of onanism on youth.[77] If masturbation could damage the health of adult men by draining their nervous energy, its effects on immature boys had to be utterly devastating, for the extreme nervous excitement promoted by sexual arousal, not to mention the exhaustion that followed loss of seminal fluid, caused far greater harm when physical and mental growth were still incomplete. Nor did masturbatory lunacy await adulthood to strike; onanism was a recognized agent in the onset of adolescent insanity, as Clouston, among many others, observed. Adults went to awful lengths to impress boys with this horrible lesson and resorted to all manner of threats to coerce them into purity. Perhaps the cruelest was the one devised by Coventry Patmore in 1861, when his first wife was dying of consumption and he wrote to his son at school: "Remember that you are not likely to have your poor Mama long so you should make the best of the time you have left to please her. . . . Although your learning well is very important, there are other things much more important . . . to be *pure* (you know what I mean). If you are not pure . . . you will not see your dear Mama any more when she is once gone." Schoolgirls, it would seem, were not subjected to the same kind of intense psychological warfare where masturbation was concerned, although they were certainly warned of its dread impact. By the eve of the war, lesbian relationships at boarding school were just beginning to attract some slight comment in medical texts, as yet another aberrration likely to occur at puberty. Adolescence was "the time beyond all others in life," Scharlieb warned, "when girls are apt to form overwhelming and most unhealthy attachments to each other, or to women of maturer years. Not unfrequently these absorbing friendships are carried beyond the bounds of sanity, and form one of the most serious difficulties to guardians and dangers to the young people."[78]

Guardians, parents, teachers, doctors, clergymen, and anyone else in a position of authority over adolescent boys and girls obviously brandished the allegedly dire consequences of early sexual activity as a weapon in the struggle to control youthful conduct at this perilous stage of life. Not only did they hope to nip nascent sexuality in the bud, they aimed to inculcate—particularly in boys—those habits of rigorous self-discipline that were essential for health and success in adulthood. Although we may find their methods appalling, they felt fully justified in marshaling the strongest arguments available, including the threat of eternal damnation, the fear of madness, and a boy's love for his dying mother. Since they believed that sexual experience before adulthood could destroy a boy's prospects, they had to take what measures they could to forestall its occurrence. While some medical men in the late nineteenth century were willing to minimize the evil effects of adult masturbation, they joined ranks to affirm its grave threat to children. Even radical critics of the medical profession who advocated unorthodox approaches to healing, like the spiritualist James Burns, condemned masturbation as a vice that could permanently injure young people.[79] The fact that no foundation of proof supported this rare unanimity of opinion did not undermine it at all. By blaming sinful habits for a range of childhood disorders, particularly those believed to involve the nerves, medical practitioners could simultaneously attempt to guide the young toward moral rectitude, try to curb adolescent misbehavior, and conceal from parents how much they did not know about childhood illness.

Medical and moral reasoning thus combined to create the frame of mind among adults that strongly favored prolonging sexual immaturity and ignorance. The counsel that Tilt issued in 1851—"to keep a girl in the nursery as long as possible"— echoed down the rest of the century, assuming ever greater authority as the dangers of adolescence impressed themselves more forcibly on the medical mind. Similar precepts, needless to say, were applied to boys; to read the literature about adolescent sporting heroes, cast in the late Victorian mold of athletic manliness, one could only assume that youths on the verge of leaving school were as asexual as their little brothers just commencing formal education. Indeed, the cult of eternal boyhood, which critics of the English public schools have accused these institutions of perpetuating among their alumni, threatened to extend that asexuality well into adulthood. Between Peter Pan who refused to grow up and Kipling's Stalky who, as a soldier in India, played the same tricks on Afghan tribesmen that had outfoxed obnoxious schoolmasters and overbearing prefects, Edwardian boys were given some strikingly immature role models.[80] Down to the outbreak of the war, suppression and denial remained the paramount ways in which most middle-class adults approached the subject of adolescent sexuality. When they talked to young people about "social hygiene," their aim was to highlight the dangers of immoral indulgence until the time when sexual activity could be channeled into the morally sanctioned, socially productive direction of marriage and children.

When Victorian and Edwardian doctors claimed that their attempt to restrain youthful sexuality was designed to spare boys and girls the miseries of severe nervous disability later in life, they were not prevaricating. During the course of the nineteenth century, they had become convinced that childhood health problems, particularly of the nervous variety associated with early sexual experimentation, reverberated resoundingly throughout adulthood. Yet other causes were also at work, which stemmed from deep-seated fears about the well-being, not of individuals, but of society at large, if children and adolescents were free to express their sexual feelings. Medical authorities were certain that, should boys and girls indulge in any sexual activity before maturity, they would irreparably destroy their chances of producing healthy offspring. Anxiety about the future of the nation was thus inevitably and inextricably entangled with concerns about the moral and physical health of children.[81] The uproar over national decline and racial deterioration, on the one hand, and humanitarian programs to improve the lives of British infants and children, on the other, provided two sets of motives for social reform that were by no means mutually exclusive. While official attempts on behalf of children in the late nineteenth and early twentieth centuries focused on national vitality in the years to come, they did not overlook puny, undernourished bodies whose claims on the national conscience at present could no longer be ignored.

Much was accomplished for children in these decades, by public and private agencies alike. From 1870, when the Elementary Education Act was passed, until 1914, Parliament enacted some sixty laws relating to children, with the greatest concentration of legislation emerging after 1900.[82] Acts were passed to extend education to children with physical and mental impairments, to provide free or low-cost meals to needy schoolchildren, to furnish medical examinations at state elementary schools, to enable more children to attend secondary school, to shield children from physical abuse, and to protect them at the workplace. The Children's Act of 1908 was a wide-ranging statute that consolidated the advances made thus far and covered a number of issues pertinent to the welfare of the young, including the treatment of juvenile offenders under the age of sixteen. Local government not only followed where Parliament led, but also took its own initiative, providing milk dispensaries, for example, and building municipal playgrounds. Voluntary organizations devoted their energies to all manner of crusades for children. The National Society for the Prevention of Cruelty to Children was launched in the 1880s. The Society for the Study of the Mental and Physical Conditions of Children boasted 100 members by the spring of 1904, including George Savage and Francis Warner among its vice-presidents.[83] The Infants' Health Society, the National League for Health, Maternity and Child Welfare, and the Women's League of Service for Motherhood, among other groups, joined with the older Ladies' Sanitary Association, dating from the late 1850s, to teach the principles of diet, cleanliness, and infant care to the poor. The Local Government Board sponsored conferences on infant mortality, while private groups organized trips to the country for slum children, and, in general, large numbers of middle-class "experts" became engrossed in the problem of how to teach hygienic child-rearing practices to working-class mothers. The "mothercraft" movement was well under way.[84]

Crichton-Browne's role in the child welfare campaign suggests how complicated the historian's job of attributing motives can become. His identification with the crusade against academic overpressure and, indeed, his interest since university days in the mental and nervous disorders of childhood made him an obvious participant in the growing public effort to assist children. At the 1902 International Congress for the Welfare and Protection of Children, he served as president of the Medical Section; he involved himself in the work of the Child Study Society, established in the Edwardian decade for the purpose of engaging parents, doctors, and teachers in the study of childhood developmental psychology, of a non-Freudian sort; he denounced the quality of milk available to children in London. There is no question but that he wanted childhood to be a happy, relatively carefree time, and he championed the rights of children to develop without needless tensions, just as he supported the rights of the elderly to have a rich and fulfilling old age.[85] At a time when the emotional life of children was at last gaining appreciation as a significant element in their general health, and when children were being recognized as "sentient beings" who could be permanently hurt, in mind and body, by brutal discipline and thoughtless cruelty,[86] Crichton-Browne was in the vanguard of polemicists on their behalf. As early as 1859, he severely criticized parents or nursery maids "who compel timid, nervous children to sleep alone in the dark, and who amuse them by narrating horrific tales." Although many of his professional colleagues, convinced that warm baths aroused sexual impulses in children, accordingly advocated the cold variety, Crichton-Browne recommended a warm bath just before bedtime, as particularly likely "to allay the nervous irritability which prevents sleep in children." When a child feigned or exaggerated illness, he did not heap verbal abuse on the malingerer and prophesy a bleak future for the moral reprobate, but assumed that the child was, in fact, not quite healthy. He loved to see children playing freely at their games, indulging in spontaneous, unregulated activity, for he firmly believed that "mere frolic is more conducive to bodily and mental well-being than formal gymnastics." He thought schooling should be a pleasant experience for children, with teachers endeavoring "to educate with as little pain as possible, to lead on gently and gradually, step by step, ever enlisting interest, and sparing violent efforts and harassing application." When Guthrie urged in 1907 that the doctor's responsibility to youthful patients included the recognition of "emotional sufferings," he was contributing to a school of pediatric thought that Crichton-Browne had helped to formulate.[87]

At the same time, Crichton-Browne was deeply preoccupied with questions of national fitness, both moral and physical, in the years before World War I. One cannot separate his zeal to abolish overwork in the schools and his plea for childhood happiness from his idealization of family life, the home, and motherhood; these, in turn, were inseparably associated with his efforts to combat the deterioration that he perceived threatening the British race on all sides. He showed real sympathy toward neurotic children partly because he dreaded to see the emergence of neurasthenic adults. It was entirely consistent with the dual nature of his involvement in the child welfare movement that his presidential address to the Medical Section of the International Congress in 1902 was entitled *Physical Efficiency in Children*.[88]

8

Nervous Degeneration

During the Edwardian decade, the ambiguous phrase "national efficiency" expressed diverse, but profound, concerns about British ability to compete in the modern world. Around the slogan of national efficiency gathered proponents of child welfare, housing reform, state support of motherhood, imperial expansion, and military preparedness alike. Strange alliances proliferated. Fabian socialists, or at least the majority of them, were as keen advocates of national efficiency, and as concerned about racial deterioration, as a Tory champion like Lord Roberts, the hero of the Boer War, who led the National Service League in the years preceding World War I. Feminists crusading for social purity—another slogan of equivocal import—voiced as much alarm over rampant immorality and vice as did their arch-opponents who sought to confine women to the home, in the interests of healthy babies. Implicit in this hodgepodge of anxieties were the conflicting claims of heredity and environment that challenged medical certainty about childhood nervous development throughout the nineteenth century. Since doctors were never sure how much of a child's nervous stability or instability was decided in the womb and how much depended on life's experiences, they hesitated between acknowledging the deterministic dictates of heredity and devoting redoubled efforts to environmental reform in a sustained effort to improve national efficiency. Although the spread of insanity, criminality, syphilis, alcoholism, and other dreaded scourges appeared to loom as particular social threats in the late nineteenth and early twentieth centuries, nervous weakness was not any the less deplorable by comparison. In 1905, when the *Strand Magazine* asked "Has the public schoolboy deteriorated?",[1] the idea of nervous degeneration was inseparable from the more overt discussion of moral degradation and physical debility. For a country beleaguered by worldwide competitors, hardy nerves were more than ever necessary to sustain the British people in their struggle to maintain international hegemony. If deterioration of the nervous system became part of the national inheritance, the future looked nothing short of hopeless.

So many Edwardians, embracing such strikingly different ideologies, participated in the campaign for national efficiency that the concept sometimes appears to dissolve into nothing more than a vague malaise about the future. The meaning of the catch phrase clearly varied with its audience. For the radical right, it contained a heavy dose of xenophobia. For army recruiters, it implied physical fitness that could be measured, weighed, and translated into national military clout. For the Webbs and their Fabian colleagues, it signified the abolition of poverty through the exertions of efficient administrators employed by an actively interventionist central government.

Crichton-Browne, who accompanied Lord Roberts to Downing Street in February 1914 to urge the imposition of compulsory military training on every eligible British man, understood national efficiency as the product of coordinated efforts on simultaneous fronts. For him the expression encompassed the cultivation of moral fiber and physical toughness, together with a concerted assault on "hooliganism, syndicalism, and other social aberrations." Lord Roberts's goal of national military service was as essential to Crichton-Browne's vision of an efficiently functioning, socially stable nation as were motherhood, carefree children, happy families, and religious serenity. In the clamor for national efficiency, conditions of body were inseparably intertwined with states of mind.[2] Over and over again, all manner of alarmists asked whether the British people had, not merely the stamina, but the will to triumph over their rivals. Never had the connotations of power, force, and energy associated with the nerves assumed greater significance in the public consciousness.

The very existence of commercial and military rivals, after decades of nearly unchallenged global leadership, goes far to explain the emergence of something close to a panic mentality in Great Britain by the close of Victoria's reign. The aggressive new style of scrambling for colonies, the challenge that Germany posed to British naval supremacy, and the threat, raised by both the United States and Germany, to British markets around the world created substantial uneasiness about the nation's future role in the international arena. The Boer War did nothing to allay those anxieties, and agitation over the alleged physical deterioration of the British people reached new extremes when high-ranking military officers in 1902 and 1903 claimed that as many as three-fifths of the men who either tried to enlist or actually enlisted in the army were unfit for service.[3] These assertions and the furor they aroused helped to place the mothercraft and child welfare movements at the forefront of public concerns, for it seemed ever more obvious that the rearing of a robust race was, in the long run, the paramount national priority.

At the same time, the size and social composition of the future British race was in itself the object of no slight alarm among members of the middle and upper classes, including academics and intellectuals, clergymen, politicians, social reformers, and medical practitioners. By the start of the twentieth century, the national birthrate had dropped steeply—from a peak of 36.3 births per 1,000 of the population in 1876 to 28.5 in 1901—and the implications of the decline frightened all those preoccupied with the country's potential military vigor, not to mention its capacity for imperial expansion, against the far greater population resources of Germany. To make matters worse, studies revealed that the birthrate was not slowing down uniformly across the social spectrum: the decline was considerably more marked at the higher levels of society than at the lower. Even when the greater incidence of infant mortality in the slums was taken into consideration, it nonetheless remained ominously probable, according to Edwardian prophecies, that the most impoverished and unhealthy social strata would, in the near future, beget a predominant proportion of the British population. Since these were obviously the segments of society that suffered from the greatest degree of physical debility and deformity, the other end of the social scale issued a discouraging prognosis for the British nation. The prospect of "race suicide," as it was called, did not stop affluent and educated couples from choosing to limit the size of their own families, but they nonetheless vociferously bemoaned the fecundity of the poor. As Grant Allen had already complained in 1889, "If the best and most intelligent classes abstain, the worst and lowest will surely make up the leeway for them." In the judgment of countless Edwardians, the worst and lowest included rapidly growing numbers of Eastern European Jews, whose influx into England after 1899 prompted the passage of the Aliens Act in 1905, to bar foreign undesirables from entering the country. The imposition of these immigration controls further reflected the exaggerated national anxiety over racial decline.[4]

The value judgments that permeated the late Victorian and Edwardian debate over physical deterioration reveal nothing but confusion where the concept of race was concerned. Whether it was a matter of ethnic identity, religious affiliation, national citizenship, linguistic determinants, or cranial measurements was never resolved in these decades, and many writers on the subject of race seemed unaware of the need even to grapple with such issues. At different times, and in different hands, the "race" whose purity was threatened by inferior outsiders was the Caucasian, the Anglo-Saxon, the British, the Protestant, or simply the prosperous and refined segments of society.[5] The anxiety and hatred that created the bugbear of "racial decline" focused on no single target, but created an enormous conceptual muddle in which all prejudices could flourish.

In the final quarter of the nineteenth century and the first decade of the twentieth, numerous crusades pursued such elusive goals as social purity, national morality, and mental hygiene. The indefinable nature of their objectives allowed the largely middle-class campaigners to turn their reformist zeal in all directions, channeling it now to suppress public school vice, now to sequester the feeble-minded, now to criticize overcrowding in the homes of the poor, and now to deplore the rising suicide rates that seemed to reveal the spread of degenerative tendencies among the population.[6] The difficulty they experienced in distinguishing between physical and moral causes seriously complicated their search for solutions to the supposed crisis of racial decline. Although there was no unanimous medical opinion on the question of national deterioration, British doctors were in the thick of all the controversies pertaining to physical or mental fitness. Some sought to assuage public worries, and others—like Crichton-Browne and Schofield, who was "an active member of two Purity Societies"—helped to intensify them. In either case, medical men grandiloquently presented themselves as "the guardians of the physical and mental qualities of the race."[7] In the confrontation between an optimistic emphasis on environmental reforms and an essentially pessimistic preoccupation with patterns of heredity, doctors who stressed defective inheritance believed that the key to the problem lay with the nerves. Indeed, most late Victorian and Edwardian psychiatrists envisioned national efficiency in terms of a nervous system able to withstand the pressures of modern life and to resist those retrograde forces that appeared to threaten their country, their race, and their class.

With all the emphasis on imperialism, military threats, commercial competition, and the falling birthrate, social commentators before World War I neglected to realize that the debate over the physical and moral deterioration of the British people had been brewing for decades. Long before late Victorian international rivalries provoked a pervasive sense of public insecurity, doctors had been tracing the links between nervous maladies and declining racial standards. In 1807, against the background of the Napoleonic Wars, Thomas Trotter had already commented:

> We meet with numbers of persons in the world, who, though obstinate in refusing advice for their own health, are nevertheless very ready to comply with every precept that may correct the hereditary predisposition to disease in their offspring. Much of my animadversions on these disorders, is with a view to the *prevention;* and if parents and guardians will only interest themselves in the business, my trouble cannot be in vain. It is indeed a task, in the present stage of society, that well deserves the attention of every friend of his fellow-creatures, and his country. Great Britain has outstripped rival states in her commercial greatness: let us therefore endeavour to preserve that ascendancy, which is so essential to our welfare in the convulsed condition of Europe, by the only means that can do it effectually. That is, by recurring to simplicity of living and manners, so as to check the increasing prevalence of nervous disorders; which, if not restrained soon, must inevitably sap our physical strength of constitution; make us an easy conquest to our invaders; and ultimately convert us into a nation of slaves and ideots [*sic*].[8]

Nor was a "convulsed condition" of European affairs necessary to prompt medical conjectures of this sort. In his early denunciation of academic overpressure on schoolboys, James Johnson advised that "tremendous competition and exertion of the intellect, at a period of life when Nature points to and demands exuberance of corporeal exercise, must have a deleterious influence on mind and body—and this injury, though acquired at first by external circumstances, will, in time, be propagated from parent to progeny hereditarily." A few years later, Edwin Lee observed that those groups in society, like the Quakers, "who adopt from childhood temperate and regular habits—whose education does not lead to the development of undue susceptibility of the nervous system, and whose passions are consequently more under control—are comparatively little liable to some diseases, which are of daily occurrence among other classes of the community, and as a necessary consequence are much longer lived, and produce healthier offspring."[9]

The anxious suspicion that hereditary processes were working against future generations buttressed cautious medical criticism of industrialization and urbanization in the early years of Victoria's reign. It was in 1843, not 1903, that Daniel Noble described factory labor as tending, "under present circumstances, to deteriorate the race." In language that would be used again sixty years later, he cited evidence to demonstrate that it was becoming more difficult to obtain army recruits "of the proper strength and stature" from big cities. So heavy was the toll that urban life took on its working-class male population, "so great and permanent [was] the deterioration" in their physical condition, that of 613 men from the Birmingham region who had recently sought to enlist, only 238 could be accepted for military service. When Noble advocated housing reform in urban slums, he defended his point of view simply and directly: "In this way, might the health and the strength of the productive classes to a considerable extent be maintained, and the race invigorated."[10]

Whether emphasizing academic overpressure on middle-class boys or the malign impact of urban life on working-class youths, medical concern for racial decline in the first half of the nineteenth century confronted the question of heredity. Long before Germany posed any challenge whatsoever to Great Britain or the British birthrate showed any indication of slowing down, medical men were grappling with the implications of the hereditary transmission of racially undesirable qualities. As with their theory of an inherited nervous temperament, early Victorian doctors had only the vaguest notions of how heredity might actually work to ''deteriorate the race.'' In this period of general optimism about sanitary reforms, many agreed with Noble that the unhealthy environmental influences threatening to wreak hereditary havoc could be countered effectively, and thus they saw no need to predict unalterable racial decline. Whatever their long-term forecast for the health of the British population, however, the great majority—in all branches of medical practice—subscribed to Lamarckian views of heredity; they were convinced that characteristics acquired by parents during the course of life figured among the inherited traits of the next generation, and of successive ones thereafter. Lamarckism was, in fact, essential to the fully developed theory of racial degeneration that came to flourish after mid-century.

A critically important aspect of Lamarck's work in the early years of the century, which subsequently played a central role in the articulation of degeneration theory, was his emphasis on the simplicity or complexity of the nervous system as the crucial feature defining an organism's place within the animal kingdom. The questions of morphological change over time and the structural differences separating one species from another that preoccupied the biological sciences in their infancy helped to focus attention on the nerves; it was precisely the accumulation of knowledge about the nervous system that helped revivify and transform the ancient concept of a great chain of being. Irrefutable scientific evidence at last appeared to demonstrate with precision the different gradations of animal life and to provide indisputable reasons why some species ranked high on the scale and others low. Everything hinged on nervous development: the more intricate the network of nerves an organism possessed, the more functions it was capable of fulfilling, and the higher it stood on the ladder of creation. The exercise of reason under the coordinating control of the will, for which the most complicated nervous system was necessary, represented the highest stage of all animal development.[11] With such commanding neurological proof, humanity's place at the head of the natural order became a matter of pure physiology, utterly removed from philosophical speculation or theological dogma. As Lionel John Beale, who later became a medical officer of health, explained at mid-century:

> There is . . . reason to think that different parts of the brain perform different functions; as animals ascend in the scale of instinct and intelligence, new parts are added to its structure, these additions being probably the instruments of the new functions and faculties. In man, the chief additions are—a great increase of size in the anterior and upper parts of the brain, and the presence of deeper and larger convolutions all over its surface; may we not, therefore, infer, that these are the parts of the brain which give to man those superior qualities of mind in which he surpasses all other animals.

On another occasion, Beale succinctly asserted that ''the position of an animal in the scale of being, is directly dependant on the degree of development of its nervous system.''[12]

If humanity's leadership over all of nature rested on the capacity to reason, loss of reason could only mean the absence of some essential quality of being human.

Ironically during the very decades when alienists were embracing the doctrine of moral management and attempting an appeal to the reasonable human inside the lunatic, psychiatrists were hearing from physiologists and early neurologists that madness did, indeed, represent a less than human condition, not too far removed from bestiality. At the start of the nineteenth century, Charles Bell argued in his *Essays on the Anatomy of Expression in Painting* (1806) that the physiognomy of the insane revealed the raw animality of the person who had lost his or her mind. Similar notions were expressed by many other students of the brain and nerves in the years when evolutionary thought was in the air, but had not yet been formulated into a coherent scheme of natural change. Clearly, the ideas that prompted Darwin to write to Crichton-Browne in 1869 had long been circulating[13] and in ways that had more immediate relevance for physiologists than the outdated theological vision of all human history as a saga of degeneration from Adam and Eve.

The terrible possibility of backsliding down the scale of animal life formed a dominant theme in the extraordinarily influential work of Bénédict-Augustin Morel. The chief medical officer at a lunatic asylum near Rouen, Morel published his *Traité des dégénérescences physiques, intellectuelles, et morales de l'espèce humaine* in 1857, and his *Traité des maladies mentales* in 1860, inspired by the apparent evidence for sharply rising numbers of French lunatics, unfit military recruits, and people suffering from neurotic complaints—all of which suggest that these precipitants of panic were not confined to the British Isles. Although French literature in this vein proliferated after the disastrous events of 1870–71, with the humiliation of defeat by Prussia and the mayhem of the Paris Commune, French medical consideration of potential racial decline, like its British counterpart, preceded by some years these obvious stimuli to national self-examination. Morel's *Treatises* were heavily speculative, but their emphasis on morbid deviation, or regression, from originally healthy stock reverberated throughout western Europe. With Morel, fears that had for years found unsystematic expression in medical literature began to coalesce into a coherent theory of degeneration.

Although Morel cited numerous external agents at work to produce pathological regression—such as poor nutrition, an unhealthy environment, and poisonous or addictive substances—it was his insistence on the exacerbating impact of the hereditary transmission of acquired defects that most impressed his contemporaries. The sins of the father, he claimed, were not only visited on the son, grandson, and great-grandson; they were magnified as they passed down through the family. The damage wrought to the nervous system of an alcoholic or opium smoker, for example, became progressively more destructive in each generation thereafter, until idiocy supervened and extinction of the line at length halted the devastation. Here was Lamarckism with a vengeance, although Morel kept it surprisingly compatible with the Biblical account of man's fall, for he believed that Adam was the ideal type from which humanity had morbidly deviated and that original sin itself made mankind vulnerable to the degenerating effect of adverse causes. If other alienists embraced Morel's degenerationist beliefs without their religious foundations, subsequent decades saw complete agreement among international psychiatrists that heredity was, as Morel had insisted, the linchpin of the degenerative process. The hereditarian emphasis of Morel's work received support in 1859, when his countryman, Jacques-

Joseph Moreau de Tours, published *La Psychologie morbide dans ses rapports avec la philosophie de l'histoire,* a volume that stressed the central role of inheritance in perpetuating pathological and regressive conditions of the nervous system.[14]

British psychiatrists responded promptly and enthusiastically to the ideas on degeneration emanating from France. The *Journal of Psychological Medicine* devoted a long review article to Morel's first *Treatise* as soon as it appeared, quoting from the work at length and judging it "able and philosophical." Morel's opinions were cited with respect, as when, for example, the alienist W. H. O. Sankey reported the Frenchman's view that insanity was "one form of degeneration 'transmissible and transmitted.'"[15] Even before he went to Paris in the early 1860s, Crichton-Browne had begun to ponder the likelihood of racial deterioration, drawing on degeneration theory to underscore his alarm. In his first contribution to the *Journal of Mental Science,* after noting that "the spermatozoid and the ovum convey to the progeny, in a manner as yet eluding all research, the physical and psychical qualities, not merely of the parents, but of the parents' parents for generations back," he made it clear that "acquired tendencies and liabilities to particular forms of disease" figured among the inherited characteristics. Of these, lesions and functional derangements of the nervous system especially concerned the future alienist. Already at this early stage of his career, Crichton-Browne subscribed wholeheartedly to the degenerationist belief that the vices of parents somehow worked their way into the germ cells to become a tragic hereditary bequest to descendants. In his next published article, he combined the moral strand in degenerationist thought with the environmental criticism expressed in earlier British warnings of future racial decline. Like Noble and many others, Crichton-Browne associated life in the crowded urban slums with the rearing of an enfeebled population, marred from birth. "Improper marriages, excessive exertion of body, impure air, badly ventilated houses; adulterated, scanty, and innutritious food; sedentary habits, unhealthy occupations, intemperance, and immorality," he enumerated in a somewhat ill-assorted list of causative agents, "are all busy in deteriorating our race and in rendering individuals more liable to psychical disorders." After his stay in Paris during 1862–63, when the ideas of Morel and Moreau were widely discussed in French medical circles, Crichton-Browne's conviction that hereditary degeneracy held an important clue to the modern study of the nervous system was irrevocably confirmed. At the start of his psychiatric career in the late 1850s and early 1860s, Maudsley, too, pondered the implications of Morel's hypotheses and began to think about insanity in terms of hereditary degeneration—a tendency only strengthened later, in his increasingly pessimistic work.[16]

Morbid conditions of the nervous system dominated British medical writings on degeneration in the latter half of the nineteenth century. In these decades, when evolutionary models of natural change informed all aspects of the physical and social sciences, British neurologists and psychiatrists were ready to furnish a scenario of pathological heredity passed from one generation to the next and predicated on the cumulative deterioration of the brain and nerves. Every field of inquiry that influenced late Victorian understanding of the nervous system, including the zealous measurement of skulls, was shaped in an evolutionary mold: the efforts of anthropologists, comparative physiologists, and animal psychologists, both to distinguish humanity from other animals and to separate civilized from primitive man, were part of an enormous nineteenth-century endeavor to trace the course of mental evolution and to discover, in the process, the true nature of mankind. When Victorian psychiatrists highlighted the role of degeneration in nervous and mental illness, they were staking their claim to a specific part in that enterprise.

It was the notion of change over time, intrinsic to the very concept of evolution, that marked the critical difference between the older hereditarian theories of nervous temperament and the idea of nervous degeneration that emerged in the third quarter of the nineteenth century. An inherited nervous diathesis did not worsen from one generation to the next; nervousness remained nervousness and did not automatically assume a graver pathological form in offspring. A nervous temperament was merely one trait among many passed from parent to child, and, while it often merited medical attention, it carried no shameful connotations for the recipient to bear. With the exercise of good judgment, furthermore, the legatee could lead a rewarding life, experiencing only minor inconveniences from his or her inheritance. Nervous degeneration was something altogether more frightening and more disgraceful. Once set in motion, virtually everyone assumed that it was an irreversible process, dragging entire families into an inexorable downward spiral of declining physical and mental powers. From the 1860s, the two forms of nervous heredity coexisted somewhat confusingly in medical literature.

The powerful hold that the theory of nervous degeneration managed to gain over the imagination of many late Victorian psychiatrists primarily rested on their conviction that civilized humanity was the product of nervous development. Keen intelligence, esthetic sensibilities, and moral sentiments all attested to the vast distance that separated the human nervous system from that of mankind's closest neighbors on the animal scale. Yet the very source of superiority also emerged as the cause of great weakness, for the most highly developed nervous system, with the greatest ramification of nerves and the most elaborate connections among all parts, was certainly the most liable to malfunction. The susceptibility to nervous afflictions and mental illness, which the medical profession considered characteristic of modern civilized populations, was the result of their much acclaimed neurological advancement. What was perhaps even more alarming to consider was the situation that, in societies developed far beyond the conditions of raw nature, the struggle for survival could not be relied on to check the tendency toward nervous maladies; people with faulty nervous organizations could reach the age of maturity and bestow their defects on the next generation. The message that late Victorian neurologists and psychiatrists publicized at large was not so much that the fittest survive, but that the evolutionary process was, in some critical respects, rendering modern man less fit. Here lay further reason for that fundamental ambivalence about modernity that permeated Victorian and Edwardian medical literature.

An involved and rarely articulated series of assumptions connected the medical conviction that modern nerves were especially fragile with the conclusion that degeneration—that is, reversion to a more primitive, less evolved type—was a possible consequence. The first step in the thought process involved an analogy between the human nervous system and extremely complex machinery. The analogy was an obvious one that occurred to victims of depression, or their families, as readily as to medical men and played on ideas of breakdown, organic or mechanical, for its particular effect. "As the rude implements of primitive life are to the marvellous machines of our present civilisation," Crichton-Browne wrote in 1871, "so is the brain of the savage to that of the civilised man; in both are there an infinitely higher intricacy, and combination, and refinement, and in both is there a greater liability to damage and derangement." More than twenty years later, G. F. Blandford, a prominent psychiatric consultant in London during the final third of the nineteenth century, made the identical point. In his presidential address to the Psychology Section of the British Medical Association in 1894, he explained that "by a well-known law of evolution the brain of civilised man increases in complexity," which meant that it could be "more and more easily put out of order as any very complex piece of machinery."[17] No great effort was needed to merge this assumption with the already well-established belief that disruption of nervous function could become a hereditary condition and, from there, to maintain that hereditary nervous dysfunction could signal degeneration. Convinced that the nerves held the key to all states of mind and body, late Victorian alienists understood advanced human thought and civilized human behavior to result from the close cooperation of all the manifold parts of the brain and nervous system. The breakdown of any piece of the gigantic structure meant a reduction in the individual's capacity to act as a civilized member of the human race. That person initially became a little less civilized—in the matter of exerting self-control, for example. If the process continued, however, his or her descendants would end by being considerably less human, for their nerves would have to work in the simpler ways characteristic of animals on lower rungs of nature's ladder.

These were the metaphorical and speculative foundations on which a prominent school of late Victorian and Edwardian medical thought constructed arguments that portrayed nervous exhaustion as a potential indication of "impending degeneracy."[18] The identification of a highly evolved brain with a nervous system prone to disease and the association of both with the ultimate threat of racial degeneration were widely accepted among nerve specialists, alienists, and neurologists, with only a few dissenting voices to point out the fallacies that supported the whole scheme. Clouston, who doubted "if any child is born in a civilised country without some inherited brain and mental weaknesses of some sort or in some degree," set his profession of medicine the special task of protecting the British "population . . . against . . . our becoming a nervous race. We want to have body as well as mind," he declared; "otherwise we think that degeneration of the race is inevitable."[19] The concept of neurasthenia gained rapid acceptance in the United States and Europe to a significant extent because it emerged at a time when much anxious public attention was already turned to the terrifying eventuality of race suicide by means of nervous degeneration. Doctors who used the new label of neurasthenia perceived the disorder as evidence of something dangerously wrong with the patient's nervous system, a condition that might be transmitted to offspring in the form of innate nervous debility and to later generations as still more disturbing neurological or mental states. "Let me tell you," Dowse thundered in 1889, "that neurasthenia, as I know it, is inseparably chained to, and indissolubly connected with, every retrograde, deteriorating, and degenerating process which alters the normal constitution of all animate matter. . . ."[20] In a century and a half, Cheyne's views on susceptibility to nervous disorders had been entirely up-ended. No longer an essentially admirable quality marking a superior sort of person, the late Victorians and Edwardians feared that such delicacy might be nothing less than an agent of racial degeneration and national decline.

Hughlings Jackson's theory of nervous dissolution, worked out during the 1870s and 1880s, bore further witness to the impact of evolutionary thought on late Victorian neurology and appeared to invest degeneration theory with impeccable scientific credentials, although that was not Jackson's particular intention. With greater precision than had distinguished earlier notions of cerebral growth and alteration over time, Jackson hypothesized that a three-tiered hierarchy of lower, middle, and higher levels had developed sequentially within the central nervous system during the course of animal history. The integration of each new higher level with already existing nerve centers created the capacity for more advanced coordination of impulse, thought, and action, so that the most complex activities of the human brain were made possible by the most recently evolved centers. What was important for degeneration theory in Jackson's argument was his contention that the highest, and most lately developed, functions of the nervous system were precisely those that first succumbed to decay in the presence of disease. Since the diversified activities of the nervous system were, in effect, a team effort, the faulty operations of the highest, coordinating centers in the cerebral cortex—or the suspension of their activities altogether—meant the eventual disintegration of the entire network. Jackson felt sure that this sequence of events explained widely disparate symptoms of neurological disorder, which, he believed, were attributable to the action of lower nervous centers functioning without restraint from above. Although psychiatrists and nerve specialists had long assumed that a breakdown of the will's supervisory role could account for many such symptoms, Jackson's theory of a developmental nervous hierarchy seemed to move the discussion beyond metaphysical guesswork, offering an elucidation of nervous dysfunction in apparently concrete physiological terms that neatly meshed with evolutionary concepts. As he made explicit in 1882, in a speech to the Pathology Section of the British Medical Association, he regarded nervous diseases "as examples of Dissolution—using this term as the opposite of Evolution."[21] While Jackson himself did not apply his theory to the burning question of racial degeneration, it clearly suggested a likely mechanism by which the process of slipping down the evolutionary chain might be initiated.

The rapid integration of Jackson's neurological hypothesis into degeneration theory arose in no small part from his adaptation of earlier approaches to the study of the mind. Although Jackson was not interested in the old faculty psychology that carved up the mind's functions into rather arbitrary mental powers, his grades of nervous development, from lowest to highest, transferred to an evolutionary context the hierarchy once beloved of faculty psychologists, who assigned ethical value to mental operations and, of course, placed the moral faculty in the topmost position. Before Jackson, Spencer had traced the evolution of mind in a way that allowed his disciples to equate the most recent development in time with superior worth, and he had inaugurated the use of the term *dissolution* to signify that mental illness and criminal behavior both represented regression to a more primitive state than was normal in civilized human society. James Sully was not alone in recognizing that some of Jackson's "most important ideas on the course of decay in the brain-organs showed him to have been a diligent student of Herbert Spencer's writings.''[22] The common debt to Spencer may explain the striking similarities between the work of Jackson and of Théodule Ribot, French synthesizer of philosophy, psychology, and neurophysiology, and a leading degeneration theorist in the late nineteenth and early twentieth centuries. Ribot's *Maladies de la volonté* (1883) drew heavily on Spencerian dissolution, but by the time he contributed an article on ''Disorders of Will'' to Tuke's *Dictionary of Psychological Medicine* in 1892, he sounded like a perfect Jacksonian. ''The will,'' he asserted,

> is therefore not an imperative entity, reigning in a world of its own, and distinguishing itself by its own actions, but it is the last expression of an hierarchical co-ordination of tendencies, and as every movement or group of movements is represented in the nervous centres, it is clear that with the paralysis of each single group, one element of co-ordination disappears. Dissolution of the will is absence of co-ordination, which terminates in an independent, irregular and anarchical action.[23]

Many British psychiatrists and neurologists echoed Jacksonian theory when they wrote about nervous degeneration after the early 1880s, for levels of nervous integration and disintegration proved a profoundly influential idea that seemed to account for physiological breakdown and psychological disarray at one and the same time. Maudsley found that the notion helped him to understand the innate criminal personality; Savage summarized and relied on ''the scheme of Hughlings Jackson'' for part of his etiological explanation of neurasthenia in 1894, while he insisted on another occasion that, among mankind's ''mental possessions,'' ''the last and highest acquisitions are those which are lost most readily''; in his presidential address to the Neurological Society in 1904, Seymour Sharkey retraced the argument that the most recently evolved portions of the human nervous system showed the least ''power of resisting causes which derange function.'' Much like the ''last in, first out'' dismissal policies of some employers today, the assumption that the most lately developed, and therefore most distinctively human, elements of the nervous system were ''the first to be lost'' became a virtually unquestioned ''fact'' of British psychiatry by the Edwardian decade.[24]

The diverse implications of the word *degeneration* inevitably obfuscated everything it touched. Like depression, irritability, sensitivity, and other attributes of the nerves, degeneration possessed a physical denotation and a moral connotation, which late Victorians and Edwardians found nearly impossible to keep distinct. When physiologists and medical practitioners spoke of nervous degeneration, they generally meant to discuss a somatic defect—in particular, a reduced complexity of the nervous system due to some pathological condition, such as inflammation, that affected the highest nerve centers in the brain. Hughlings Jackson, for one, intended no moral judgments when he supposed that various neurological disorders were the result of nervous degeneration. Nor did George Rennie, an Australian physician, when he explained that a ''degenerative process'' could be recognized by ''macroscopic or microscopic methods.'' Nor did Sharkey when he suggested that ''a real degeneration of nerve-cells has occurred in neurasthenia.''[25] Such straightforward neurological applications of the word are, however, misleading, for degeneration was, and remains, a concept saturated with moral implications. Like Morel, who claimed to employ the term solely with regard to morbid physical processes but included original sin among them, British psychiatrists before World War I could never leave the moral aspect of nervous illness alone for very long. They suspected that in the majority of instances what made a reasonably healthy person the parent of a degenerating line was conscious indulgence in vice or excess, and, with such cases, degeneration clearly implied disintegration of character as well as nerve tissue.

That degeneration also figured as the cultural phenomenon of decadence by the 1890s only added to the confusion of concepts. If the manifestations of decadence in British literature and painting were, on the whole, more restrained than the continental varieties, they nonetheless sufficed to outrage and frighten segments of the British public, who interpreted the amorality of a few artists and writers as proof of an entire culture in extremis. Public media events like the trial of Oscar Wilde spread the impression that spiritual decay threatened the British nation as profoundly as physical decline. While the second law of thermodynamics taught the harsh lesson of a slowly dying universe, British prophets of doom charged that some of their compatriots were unduly hastening the process at home. Men in a position to know better seldom scrutinized the flawed logic that allowed the conflation of literature and painting with pathology. The warning issued by Dr. Alfred Mumford, a thoughtful participant in the Edwardian controversy over racial deterioration, that "the making of analogies is a very uncertain and even dangerous pursuit" went unheeded by those who chose to believe that entire civilizations, like unfortunate individuals, could degenerate, or fall backwards in a regressive pattern of reverse evolution. Mumford was unusual, too, in the care with which he tried to give specific meanings to the words *deterioration, degeneration,* and *decadence.*[26]

For most of his contemporaries, within the medical profession or outside it, these were words for all seasons, indiscriminately useful for manifold purposes—whether to dismiss works of art, denounce individuals, deplore the decline of families, or mourn the downfall of vast, amorphous populations. The articulation of degeneration theory in the second half of the nineteenth century may have begun as a medical and scientific endeavor, but it rapidly outdistanced its creators. Indeed, as one of its most perceptive interpreters has argued, "the debate over deterioration always had much more to do with contemporary middle- and upper-class anxieties about economic, social, political, and cultural change than it did with quantifiable reality."[27] It certainly makes impossible any facile assertions about the Victorian response to evolutionary biology: naive optimism and glib confidence in ongoing human advancement hardly went unchallenged. Carlyle's query to Darwin, whether "there was a possibility of men turning into apes again," expressed with characteristic hyperbole a worry about future human progress that countless numbers of his compatriots shared.[28]

It was the widespread assumption of a neat parallel between the biological life of a human being and the development of a civilization that allowed social critics to pass back and forth at will between the faults of an individual and the fate of society, spreading the impact of degeneration theory far beyond the consulting rooms of psychiatrists and neurologists. That the presumed parallel rested on a profound theoretical misconception and the careless use of language never weakened its hold on late Victorian and Edwardian social, biological, and racist thought. Throughout the nineteenth century, while the primary scientific meaning of *evolution* was coming to signify the gradual emergence of new species from earlier forms over long periods of time, the word continued to harbor an older meaning that pertained to the growth of an individual organism from embryo to full adulthood. When Victorian medical men discoursed on evolutionary development, they often allowed these two definitions to mingle in ways that were not conducive to clarity. Francis Warner's reference to schoolchildren who "remained unevolved to the average type," for example, left it unresolved whether he was suggesting that they were merely immature for their age or hinting that they were not quite worthy representatives of the human race.[29]

The overlapping definitions of evolution lent plausibility to the law of recapitulation, to whose erroneous principle that ontogeny follows phylogeny the great majority of biological and social scientists pledged allegiance in the late Victorian and Edwardian periods, conjuring up for themselves the image of each human embryo *in utero* passing through piscine, reptilian, and lower mammalian forms before assuming the appearance of a human baby.[30] Although the Jacksonian concept of developmental levels within the nervous system did not mesh precisely with any particular stages of the recapitulation process, both theories clearly supported the hierarchical patterns of thought that cast all aspects of human society in an evolutionary drama featuring the constant struggle between progress and dissolution—between moving forward to higher, better forms and falling backwards to lower, worse manifestations.

Degeneration, allegedly spreading outward from the individual bearer of disordered nerves, placed the family in the very front ranks of its victims. At the same time that advocates of national efficiency were hailing the family as the guardian of social stability and the incubator of national virtue, many of them were also recognizing it as a potential powder keg of self-destructing forces. P. C. Smith, a physician from Tunbridge Wells, tersely explained the situation in 1906:

> The unit of degeneracy is the family. A degenerate family is one in which there is imperfect heredity, showing itself by a loss that tends to be progressive of racial characteristics, anatomical, physiological, and psychical. The losses in the anatomical sphere are manifested as malformations, usually of a minor order, affecting mostly the head, face, and hands. Of the physiological defects, the commonest are disorders of metabolism and vaso-motor instability; the most important is diminution of sexual or generative power, which leads to the extinction of the family. The psychical abnormalities are impulsiveness, irritability, instability, suggestibility, and a tendency to obsessions, tics, and phobias.

The idea of hereditary taint, pervading European psychiatry by the end of Victoria's reign, not only extended from parents to children, but also reached out to menace cousins, nieces, and nephews who might share in the pathological inheritance from common stock. For many a doctor in this period, particularly for alienists and neurologists, the family was demarcated not so much by shared values and memories as by the morbid traits circulating among its members.[31]

With its relentless insistence that the family was an institution at risk, degeneration theory lent moral urgency to the antifeminist campaign of the late nineteenth and early twentieth centuries. How much the degeneration scare was manipulated by opponents of higher education and professional careers for women is impossible to assess. Undoubtedly the threat of a deteriorating population proved immensely useful in bestowing a scientific-sounding rationale on deeply cherished and beleaguered prejudices, providing powerful ammunition to all those who denied that women could function successfully as breeders if their energies were wasted outside the home. Women's responsibility to "produce stalwart forceful sons and daughters"[32] became nothing less than a matter of national security, the best and most effective means to forestall the degenerative tendencies at work among the British population. Women could not, accordingly, think only of their own aspirations in chasing after dreams of academic glory, "for it would be an ill thing," Maudsley warned, "if it should so happen, that we got the advantages of a quantity of female intellectual work at the price of a puny, enfeebled, and sickly race." It was sheer selfishness for women to "shut their eyes to the good of society" in pursuit of unnatural achievements, admonished Eliza Lynn Linton. After all, she insisted, "a girl is something more than an individual; she is the potential mother of a race; and the last is greater and more important than the first." "We must do what we can in this life, not always what we would," she concluded didactically, "and the general interests of society are to be considered before those of a special section, by whose advancement will come about the corresponding degeneracy of the majority." Clouston, predictably prolific in his pronouncements on this topic, outdid himself in 1880, when he considered what might happen "if the education of civilized young women should become what some educationalists would wish to make it." In that dreadful eventuality, "for the continuance of the race there would be needed an incursion into lands where educational theories were unknown, and where another rape of the Sabines was possible."[33]

Assertions along these lines, if couched somewhat less aggressively, could be multiplied a hundred times over, and still the late Victorian and Edwardian literature linking race degeneration and higher education for women would not be exhausted. Male and female writers, with or without medical degrees, contributed to the argument, sustained over three or four decades, that feminist aspirations jeopardized the very survival of the British race. The emphasis in Germany before World War I on women's domestic and maternal roles only intensified the perception among conservative circles in England that any feminist tampering with those roles amounted to little less than treason. Some headmistresses at advanced secondary schools for girls in the Edwardian decade even found it advisable to encourage training in housewifery, which their pioneering predecessors would have scorned, in order to declare their sympathy with the effort to preserve family life, promote motherhood, and protect the vigor of the British race. With the vocabulary of racial degeneration at their disposal, the proponents of separate spheres for men and women could fight old battles with renewed force.[34]

The message that women had to subordinate personal goals to national needs occupied a central place in the writings of the Edwardian eugenists, an assortment of middle-class men and women who exploited the language of racial deterioration without subscribing to all the basic tenets of degeneration theory. For the most part, they rejected the Lamarckian view of inheritance intrinsic to that theory and insisted that hereditary processes worked with innate, not acquired, characteristics. The goals and program of the British eugenics movement place it largely outside the scope of this study, since the nerves did not figure in the forefront of its agenda. Nonetheless, its members' obsessive concern with the differential fertility of the affluent and the poor, as well as their confusion of poverty with biological degeneracy, gave them much in common with other social pessimists whose ideas derived from Morel rather than Galton. Although Galton had coined the word *eugenics* in 1883 and had been thinking about the subject since the 1860s, a national organization to further the so-called science of race improvement was not launched in Great Britain until 1907, four years before his death. The Eugenics Society, known as the Eugenics Education Society until 1926, always remained a small organization of less than 2,000 members, which never even captured a substantial body of enthusiasts from among the educated, professional middle classes. What support it did marshal, however, came from precisely that portion of the population. University lecturers, scientists, medical practitioners, lawyers, clergymen, and headmasters gave the society a voice far more authoritative than its numbers alone would have warranted.[35] Together they accumulated all manner of anthropometric and demographic data to justify their social prejudices.

Doctors occupied a highly problematic position within the Eugenics Education Society. Although they were numerically strong, amounting to one fourth of the society's officers and council members before World War I, they represented only a small proportion of the entire medical profession, for good reason.[36] A significant strain in eugenic thought roundly criticized doctors for extending the lives of men and women who could contribute nothing but weak-bodied and feeble-minded offspring to the future British population. Eugenists regretted, furthermore, that medical intervention enabled so many of these undersized children to survive in the adverse conditions of industrial urban life, to propagate mental deficiency, alcoholism, venereal disease, and criminality in their turn. Considering heredity, not environment, the decisive agent in an individual's moral and physical development, eugenists viewed urban slums more with an eye to halting the inhabitants' fertility than to fixing up the neighborhood. Such views aroused plenty of medical enmity, particularly among medical officers of health and doctors active in social reform campaigns, who were committed to the belief that ameliorating the conditions of life and labor could materially improve the race. Concern about national efficiency, which many of these doctors shared, by no means necessarily indicated sympathy with eugenic proposals; the environmental roots of sickness had long been acknowledged in Victorian medicine, and rectifying those sources of debility and disease appeared to a significant body of medical opinion a far more promising road to national efficiency than attempting to manipulate heredity. Even when public health officials recognized the possibility of racial deterioration, as they often did, they generally refused to concede that only selective breeding could arrest its advance. Most fundamentally of all, eugenic ideas challenged the responsibility of medical practitioners to use their healing skills wherever and whenever necessary.

Yet a comparatively small group of doctors saw no incompatibility between the eugenic program and their own professional conscience. It is not surprising that "specialists in pathological conditions and diseases thought to be hereditary in their transmission" numbered significantly among them,[37] for these physicians could endorse the eugenic assertion that the only way to halt the spread of such afflictions was to stop their victims from reproducing. Similarly, doctors active in the social purity campaign could find attractive the eugenic denunciation of indiscriminate breeding. Mary Scharlieb, author of *Womanhood and Race Regeneration* (1912), was one such purist who considered the Eugenics Education Society an appropriate forum for the articulation of her opinions. In the first volume of its journal, *The Eugenics Review,* she expressed her fervent desire "to place the well-being of the English race on a really satisfactory and stable foundation," conveying at the same time her conviction that the results of modern education for girls were not heading in that direction.[38]

Whether or not they officially joined the Eugenics Education Society, British psychiatrists who were particularly concerned about the hereditary nature of nervous and mental diseases tended to find many of its views congenial. Decades before the society even existed, Maudsley called attention to the dangers of allowing women, released from lunatic asylums, to bear children.[39] Clouston wanted "the breeding of a good race" to "become an operative political motive" and suggested that Parliament might make a start by modifying the local tax structure so as to encourage residence in the country, "especially outlying districts." These areas, he observed in 1906, were "the real breeding-places of the stable-minded, non-nervous element of our population." Crichton-Browne joined the Eugenics Education Society at its establishment and served as a vice-president for several years after 1910.[40] It was hardly coincidental that these alienists, all deeply worried about the implications of the Woman Question for nervous stability and national well-being, looked with favor both on the positive eugenic program to encourage the fertility of racially desirable stocks and on the negative one to discourage reproduction among those segments of society judged unfavorable to racial progress.

Crichton-Browne's involvement with the Eugenics Education Society not only illustrates the problems encountered by a Lamarckian in such company, but also suggests the variety of social viewpoints that managed to fit under the label *eugenist.* The eugenics movement certainly represented a natural outlet for his profound anxieties over the socially unbalanced state of the British birthrate—anxieties that also found expression in his membership, from 1913 to 1916, on the National Birth-Rate Commission, an unofficial body established by one of the leading Edwardian moral vigilance societies, the National Council of Public Morals. The fundamentally conservative outlook common to the vast majority of British eugenists when they pondered social change or political reform, furthermore, must have made their society a reassuring place for Crichton-Browne as he became increasingly disturbed by the spread of radicalism in various guises.[41] There is no doubt, too, that he liked the aura of scientific precision that surrounded eugenic studies and wanted psychiatry to be associated with them as closely as possible. Already in March 1905, he had written in response to a letter from Galton: "I do not know where you can get trustworthy data such as you desire relating to insanity in families, but if you would show the way the Medico-Psychological Association would, I am sure, take the matter in hand, issue circulars to all the asylums in the kingdom and procure very valuable and trustworthy information, for asylum medical officers now-a-days are thoroughly imbued with the scientific spirit and pursue scientific methods." Above all, he embraced the orthodox eugenic position that mankind could not indefinitely continue tampering with natural selection, preserving the unfit at the expense of the fit. By the end of his life, he was even ready to endorse "measures that are distasteful," should these prove the only way that society could protect itself from inundation by morons, imbeciles, and idiots.[42] It hardly needs to be said that he favored the eugenic selection of marriage partners and believed that a family history of nervous complaints—migraine, hysteria, and neurasthenia, as well as more serious neurological disorders like epilepsy—had to be weighed as carefully as insanity, alcoholism, or syphilis in the planning of eugenic partnerships. For Crichton-Browne, "eugenism" was nothing less than "the acme of evolution."[43]

Crichton-Browne's opinions were not, however, in all respects typical of the mainstream of British eugenic thought. At times, he almost regretted whatever influence it had on those educated members of the middle class whose fertility he was eager to promote. "May not eugenic prudence be carried too far?", he questioned Galton in the same letter of March 1905. "A man came to me the other day in a great state of trepidation," the psychiatrist continued, "fearful to carry out his engagement to marry a lady because he had discovered that an aunt of hers had died of diabetes— an aunt of his having died of the same disease. At that rate we should very soon have no marriages at all." His conviction that eugenics followed the trail blazed by phrenology must have offended a good many fellow eugenists, who would have seen no similarity between their own supposedly rigorous accumulation of statistics and phrenologists' outdated speculations about the mixing of temperaments and mental faculties. His most profound disagreement with the predominant strain in late Victorian and Edwardian eugenics arose from his loyalty to Lamarckian principles, for he sincerely believed that changes in the physical conditions and moral outlook of individual men and women could effect alterations in their hereditary transmission to offspring. When, as president of the Sanitary Inspectors Association early in the twentieth century, he eloquently denounced the inequity of housing facilities in Great Britain, with a few men enjoying "half-a-dozen houses of palatial size" while "half-a-dozen pinched families huddled into one mean hovel reeking with filthy effluvium," he sounded remarkably like the Lloyd George whose social policies would shortly become repugnant to the majority of Edwardian eugenists. Even if his anger over slum dwellings was largely inspired by a desire to foster happy domesticity among the working classes, which was an impossible endeavor without decent housing, he nonetheless joined ranks with environmentalists on issues that most eugenists considered a foolish waste of time and money.[44]

While the degeneration hypothesis generally complemented rather than informed eugenic pronouncements, it played a far more central role in the articulation of late Victorian and Edwardian racism. Indeed, it served as the "dark side" of evolutionary theory in providing a basis for that ranking of races implicit in almost all ethnological studies during these decades. A widespread fascination with the origins and distinctive traits of different races thrived in an atmosphere of imperial expansion, when international competition was couched in social Darwinian terms and colonial conquests were celebrated as the triumph of civilization over barbarism. Since western culture, with the science and technology that enabled it to dominate primitive peoples, was equated with advanced evolutionary development of the nervous system, a whole series of adjectives clustered together as diametrical opposites. "White" stared at "black" from polar ends of the racial scale, "sophisticated" at "natural," "intelligent" at "instinctual." "Moral" paired off with "brutal," "adult" with "infantile," "complex" with "simple," "higher" with "lower," and, above all, "superior" with "inferior." In between the extremes of black and white, races other than the Caucasian and the Negro corresponded with their appropriate adjectives. Thus Victorian ethnologists constructed their array of racial "types."[45]

While these stereotypical patterns of racist thought had taken shape long before the full articulation of degeneration theory, the idea of nervous degeneration contributed a special note of menace to them. It meant that deterioration, or incomplete development, of nervous tissue could reduce a civilized Caucasian to the status of a despised savage. If ontogeny recapitulated phylogeny in the forward evolution of the human species, then each white-skinned person not only underwent embryonic transformations, but during childhood progressed through the mental and moral conditions of primitive peoples. When Sully watched "the unfolding of the infant consciousness in [his] own children," he was especially keen to trace "an affinity between the ideas and impulses of the child and those of backward races." In "working out the analogies," he "found it necessary to look more closely into ethnological records of the mental peculiarities of savage peoples, and also to seek information from anthropologists."[46] There was nothing wrong with Sully's children; they were perfectly normal white babies in the early stages of their mental growth, and thus the implications of the common assumptions on which he acted were all the more noteworthy. Within every single member of the higher races skulked the features of the lower ones, ready to be exposed whenever nervous degeneration fueled the processes of regressive evolution, stripping away the attributes of civilization with the destruction of nerve cells. Inability to display the mental traits of fully developed humanity might relegate the incompetent or deranged Caucasian to the level of Negro, aborigine, or some other inferior race.

That "mental defects" were, in fact, "defects of evolution" was Laycock's contention as early as 1863. Writing in the *Journal of Mental Science* that year, he explained that "congenital defect and degeneration imply a standard of perfection as to both evolution of function of brain and of form of body, or, at least, of the head and face. . . . This kind of standard of comparison is based on the attributes of a complete adult of a given race; with us it is the European. . . ." "Inasmuch as the European passes during uterine and infantile life," he continued, "through stages of form which are the adult characteristics of other races, as the Mongolian and African, the defect in development may be manifested more or less in adolescence or adult life by Mongolian or African characteristics of mind, brain, and countenance." Just as the non-white races had stopped evolving at different stages of arrested development, so mental defectives and nervous degenerates represented, on the individual level, parallel examples of incomplete evolution. In the same decade, Dr. John Langdon Haydon Down, medical superintendent of the Earlswood Asylum for Idiots in Surrey, considered it thoroughly appropriate to draw comparisons between his patients and African, American Indian, and Oriental peoples. The particular syndrome associated with his name was, of course, long known as Mongolism. It would have stunned nineteenth-century ethnologists to learn that Down's Syndrome was caused by something extra in the victim's constitution—an additional chromosome, as twentieth-century research has discovered. The Victorians assumed, in orthodox racist manner, that the problem was one of pure deficiency.[47]

Against a conceptual framework constructed by the new science of neurology, the principle of recapitulation fused effortlessly with the notions of arrested development and atavistic throwback to flavor the unsavory blend of distorted science and blatant bias that composed Victorian racist thought. The network of associated ideas had richly varied uses, from justifying imperial annexations, to elucidating tribal customs, and explaining a wide range of aberrant behavior, including the "primitive" sexuality of prostitutes.[48] "Primitive," of course, was one of the most loaded words in the Victorian vocabulary, imposed on dark-skinned races, criminal offenders, and the undeserving poor alike. Nowhere was the confusion of individual and racial development, characteristic of degeneration theory, more noticeable than in this sweeping application of a highly pejorative label. Respectable women were not even safe from its malign reach, for they, too, with their incomplete cerebral equipment, were less than fully evolved human beings. Although gentlemanly theorists did not belabor the resemblance between fair-skinned ladies and black savages, or specifically compare their intelligence, the similarities between them were evident in the literature on mental evolution. Both were cast in the role of irrational, childish creatures, incapable of functioning as fully mature human beings who practiced self-mastery under the will's supervision. Just as Crichton-Browne charted women's inferiority in terms of brain weight, shallowness of gray matter, and comparative smoothness of cerebral convolutions, so he underscored the gulf separating white Europeans from Africans, Asiatics, American Indians, and Australian aborigines. Brain weight, cranial capacity, and the folds and fissures of the cerebral hemispheres, he insisted in a variety of formal and informal texts, all told decisively against the latter peoples. The evidence on which he based his findings was no more impressive in the case of the "lesser" races than in the indictment against women, but misogyny and racism powerfully helped to buttress each other in a cultural context all too supportive of both.

There is no doubt that degeneration theory positioned its adherents in the very midst of late Victorian and Edwardian social controversies. Yet it is also clear that the initial enthusiastic response to the theory from members of the British medical profession, particularly alienists, in the 1850s and 1860s was scarcely influenced by the crises of confidence that disturbed their countrymen at the end of the century. Psychiatric acceptance of degeneration theory first emerged in the period of mid-Victorian prosperity, between the unrest of the 1840s and the Great Depression of the 1870s, 1880s, and early 1890s. Economic, imperial, and demographic trends at the end of Victoria's reign certainly increased the credibility of the theory; the opportunity to hobnob with generals and other pessimistic celebrities may have augmented its appeal after the turn of the century; but these reasons only bolstered already existing support for the theory. They cannot alone make sense of the resolve with which a vocal segment of the psychiatric profession for several decades emphasized the threat of accelerating physical and moral deterioration on a national scale.

That resolve is all the more puzzling when one considers how insubstantial a foundation upheld the British degeneration scare. Dispassionate observers pointed out that, without earlier anthropometric studies for purposes of comparison, the crop of statistics produced in the 1880s and 1890s was meaningless and would remain so until identical measurements were taken, on the same demographic groups, some decades in the future. As for the supposedly decreasing bulk and height of military recruits, voices of calm reason argued that enlistment in the army varied with conditions of the labor market and that, over the years, military records did not deal with a homogeneous sample of the population. The declining mortality rate among the population of London as a whole and the extended life expectancy of all males in recent decades were, furthermore, reasons for exultation.[49] The statistical evidence for a declining birthrate, and for a different rate of decline at opposite ends of the social spectrum, was admittedly incontestable, but only class prejudice and deeply ingrained fears enabled prophets from the affluent ranks consequently to determine that, in a couple of generations or so, the typical British man and woman would be a feeble-minded, sunken-chested midget.

There were late Victorian and Edwardian psychiatrists, it is true, who refused to be stampeded by panic into the degenerationist camp, until they had more compelling data to defend that position. George Edward Shuttleworth, for example, formerly the medical superintendent of an asylum in Lancaster and the author of a highly regarded study on *Mentally-Deficient Children* (1895), told the Society for the Study of the Mental and Physical Conditions of Children in 1904 that he "disavowed the pessimistic views held by some as to the extensive prevalence of degeneracy in the nation." Reviewing "the alleged evidence of physical deterioration," he insisted that "even if it were proved it would apply only to the lowest stratum of the community," and he remained confident that a determined assault on environmental problems could significantly combat the "physical deformity" of the urban laborer.[50] Savage's equivocal stance in his Lumleian Lectures to the Royal College of Physicians in 1907 was particularly revealing. On the one hand, he was convinced both that the numbers of the insane in Great Britain had steadily grown during the nineteenth century and that the increase was definitely related to "the progress of civilisation." On the other, he cautiously eschewed the grimmest conclusions. "I do not myself think that this estimation necessarily implies the hopeless degeneration of the race," he ventured, "nor do I think that it furnishes an authentic basis for dread as to the future of the minds and bodies of our successors. With the multiplication of rules and regulations it becomes more and more difficult to fall into all varying social requirements, and my own particular experience indicates that many cases [of insanity] are attributable rather to social misfits than to material brain disease."[51] By this remarkably frank acknowledgment of society's ability to produce deviants through its changing definitions of acceptable conduct, Savage implied that mental illness resulted more from a failure of adaptation to an altered environment than from morbid physiological processes.

Despite hesitation on the part of individual alienists, however, no group within the medical profession so thoroughly incorporated degeneration theory into their work as the psychiatrists. Since the theory was predicated on Lamarckian concepts of evolution, it allowed them to acknowledge environmental forces that molded the acquired traits passed along to future generations. Like Crichton-Browne in the Eugenics Society, they could genuinely support all attempts to create an environment less favorable to the initiation of irreversible degeneration. But the fatal power of heredity, once set in motion, eclipsed the influence of environment in degeneration theory, and most British psychiatrists in the decades before World War I paid far more attention to biological inheritance than to sanitary reforms. The problems confronting them, they managed to imply, were far vaster in scope than a polluted water supply, open sewers, or poorly ventilated homes. The Royal College of Surgeons in 1903 may have issued a report that minimized the threat of hereditary nervous degeneration and emphasized the goals to be won through hygienic improvements;[52] the Medico-Psychological Association would not have published such arguments, for degeneration theory, in all its ramifications, had proven its worth to British psychiatry well before the start of the twentieth century.

It was no coincidence that Victorian alienists embraced Morelian views of degeneration in the late 1850s and 1860s, at the very time when therapeutic pessimism was beginning to sour the outlook of asylum superintendents and medical officers. The failure of moral management to effect curative miracles among the insane, together with continuing frustration in the search for cerebral lesions proportionate to the mental disorder of lunacy, created increasingly awkward obstacles for psychiatrists eager to demonstrate the importance of their medical specialty. The hypothesis of a morbid hereditary process, worsening with each generation, possessed unique value for them in this embarrassing situation, as they quickly realized. In its lengthy article on Morel's ideas, published in early response to his degeneration treatise, the *Journal of Psychological Medicine* quoted the following significant passage from the volume:

> In proportion as I advanced in the career which I had adopted as a speciality, I was not long in perceiving that the curability of mental affections became a problem more and more difficult of solution. The strange complications supervening upon very simple cases of delirium, . . . the *almost constant want of relation between the gravity of the symptoms and the anatomical lesions,* and the ever-increasing proportion of incurable cases—all these became to me facts too often repeated not to have their reason in the intimate nature of the evil to be combated. . . . Never since the origin of medical institutions had such strenuous efforts been made for the interests of the insane. How was it, then, that, in reference to cures, these efforts were so disappointing? . . . I only saw one mode of accounting for the fact, which was, to consider, in the generality of cases, mental alienation as the final result of a series of moral, physical, and intellectual causes, which, by determining in man successive transformations, connect him with the morbid varieties of the race, which we have called degenerations.

As the anonymous British author of the article immediately explained by way of commentary, "in cases representing so deplorable an ancestry as this, medicine will do little in altering the condition of the individual, which may be considered virtually unmodifiable."[53] Degeneration theory, in effect, absolved alienists from criticism for their failure to cure insanity and, indeed, all the other severe disorders of the nervous system that were now depicted as the product of a pathological inheritance far more potent, and more relentless, than a mere nervous temperament. No matter how devastating the imminent onslaught of degeneration might prove among the British people, Victorian psychiatrists welcomed a theory that held out the promise of rescue from impending professional disgrace.

The likelihood of such humiliation intensified during the second half of the nineteenth century and the first decade of the twentieth, as the isolation of pathogenic microbes improved the chances of eventual triumph in the fight against infectious diseases. With few exceptions, such as tracing general paralysis of the insane to the syphilis spirochete, psychiatry reaped no benefit from these advances and risked looking all the more backward by comparison with other branches of modern medicine. Degeneration theory, however, made it obvious—or so alienists hoped—that the problems of mental and nervous illness were substantially different from those of infectious diseases and would not be readily subdued by the same kinds of medical intervention. What psychiatrists could do, and here their indispensability became patent, was to inform the public about the degenerative process, calling particular attention to the way in which the terrible downward plunge commenced within a family. "There remains a noble part to play in the enunciation of principles which, when carried out, will tend to the removal of those causes to which so many of these evils are attributable," the *Journal of Psychological Medicine* had informed its readers in 1857. Down to World War I, British psychiatrists continued to echo the claim that their particular mission was "to point out the source of these evils, and the mode in which they first act upon individuals, and, through them, upon society at large."[54]

Although degeneration theory helped alienists out of a professional impasse, its overt influence on psychiatric thought appeared entirely negative. For all their assumption of "a noble part" in the campaign to halt the inroads of nervous degeneration, a note of barely concealed defeatism nonetheless became more and more audible in the writings of British psychiatrists during the final quarter of the nineteenth century. It was evident in the therapeutic nihilism that many embraced. Without meaningful alternatives, they continued to rely on the same range of treatments for nervous and mental illness that they had employed before, but with increasing conviction that all methods were futile in cases where, they assumed, degeneration of nervous tissue had already commenced. Who knows how much this pessimism limited their ability to help the insane? It may even have curtailed their efficacy with only mildly neurotic patients.[55] Defeatism was implicit, too, in the late Victorian and Edwardian category of degenerative "stigmata," those physical traits that identified the individual man, woman, or child whose nervous system had begun to regress in evolutionary terms. The characteristics in question were many and varied: narrow jaws, flattening at the back of the head, malformation of the ears, pupils of unequal size, irregular teeth, enlarged tonsils, hernias, stunted growth, paroxysmal coughing in infants, defective metabolism, rapid pulse, and much else.[56] Unlike Warner's nerve-signs among schoolchildren, many of which were considered remediable through increased physical exercise and decreased academic pressure, the stigmata of nervous degeneration never disappeared. They were permanent marks designating incurable defects.

Yet, even in their message of despair, the concept of nervous degeneration and the telltale stigmata assisted alienists by shifting the focus of psychiatric inquiry from specific lesions of the brain, which were proving elusive, to a far more generalized notion of nervous malfunction and disintegration. In fact, the whole idea of a lesion, as the manifestation of morbidity, underwent significant redefinition in light of degeneration theory. From the late 1850s, when psychiatrists spoke of a hereditary lesion, they typically meant, not a pathological alteration of particular tissue, but ''a diffuse condition'' of the nerves, which no one could expect to pinpoint at an autopsy.[57] In any case, autopsies were unnecessary where the stigmata of degeneration were involved, for these highly visible signs proclaimed the fact that psychiatrists dealt with real somatic disease. Nor did the utility of degeneration theory end there for psychiatry; in describing the simultaneous dissolution of nervous complexity and mental ability, the theory seemed to contribute compelling new insights into the ancient enigma surrounding the relationship between body and mind.

The very term *stigmata,* furthermore, encouraged alienists in that tendency to moralize which the ambiguous concept of degeneration invited. Of the word's several meanings, the pathological one, which signified the identifying characteristics of a disease, had far less currency than the connotation of a stain on one's good name. Psychiatrists may also have been drawn to the religious resonance of stigmata, so appropriate to their moral-pastoral role,[58] but nothing remotely Christ-like or saintly clung to the miserable people who bore the stigmata of nervous degeneration. As embodiments of evolutionary atavism, these creatures represented deviation from normalcy, health, and progress, and they could not be regarded with sympathy. Indeed, their moral failings assumed the proportions of degenerative stigmata just as readily as their misshapen ears or jagged teeth. Thus, while confirming that psychiatrists performed the work of physiologists, degeneration theory bolstered their moral authority at the same time.

It is distressingly obvious from the extensive literature on the subject in the late nineteenth century that degeneracy, like the earlier concept of moral insanity, was in the eye of the beholder. Depending on the writer's purpose, any physical deformity or ugliness, any mental or nervous disorder, any deviant, antisocial, or simply eccentric behavior, even any serious illness, such as tuberculosis, that confounded the medical arts might be labeled a stigma of degeneration. Since degeneration theory catered to class hostility as effortlessly as it propped up racist views, it was often invoked for no apparent reason other than pandering to middle- and upper-class anxiety about the lowest echelons of the working class. Alienists were certainly not the only members of the bourgeoisie who used the theory in blatantly discriminatory ways when they denounced that destitute segment of British society for harboring the greatest concentration of hereditary degenerates among its vagrants, paupers, mental defectives, drunkards, and criminals. In the overwrought imagination of countless men and women, unsettled by socialist agitation, rising crime rates, and chronic unemployment during the long years of depression, reproductive fecundity invested the most impoverished and desperate ''residuum'' of the population with a destructive potency utterly lacking in reality. It is hardly surprising, under these circumstances, to find significant British contributions to the idea of an inherited ''criminal personality,'' which Lombroso called to international attention at the end of the century. Galton had even worked on its composite photographic portrait in the late 1870s.[59] Although few British psychiatrists imitated Lombroso in measuring ''the bodies of criminals for signs of apish morphology,"[60] they fully accepted the assumptions on which he proceeded.

While they portrayed the "dangerous classes" at the bottom of society as the prime location of degeneracy in the country, British alienists admitted that it flourished at other levels, too. Indeed, their self-appointed responsibility to prevent the spread of nervous degeneration among families as yet unscathed required vigilance in all ranks. The sins of excess that frequently initiated the process lurked in the homes of the affluent as of the humble, and it gave psychiatrists considerable moral ascendancy over their private patients to remind them of that fact. The potential precipitants of nervous degeneration closely paralleled the ones held responsible for inducing a nervous temperament, where that was acquired rather than inherited: certain organic diseases, overwork, alcoholism, morphinism, and unnatural sexual behavior were the chief among them. While no blame fell on an individual who succumbed to the first of these causes, all the others unleashed varying degrees of censure on the perpetrator, regardless of social position. Yet psychiatric evaluations were always nicely attuned to the class of the sinner. Alcoholism, for example, looked much more degenerate when combined with indigence than with wealth. Where sexual deviance was concerned, psychiatrists emphasized the degenerative impact of incest among the working classes, while they bemoaned the similar effects of masturbation at a higher social level. Overwork appears in late Victorian psychiatric texts as the only exclusively middle-class vice, but it likewise merited moral condemnation when signifying the selfish motives of aggressive individualism. Maudsley was particularly vehement in lambasting the "single minded pursuit of riches as a cause of moral and mental degeneracy."[61]

According to degeneration theory, moral deficiency and nervous disintegration advanced together through the combined force of individual choice and inexorable heredity. Except for the innocent victim of disease, environmental poison, or an accident that destroyed nerve tissue, the person who initiated degeneration within a family did so by choosing unhealthy and immoral habits that damaged the nerves. The acquired trait of damaged nerves was then passed on to offspring, for whom incomplete nervous development became an inherited characteristic. Since the moral sense represented one of the final stages of human evolution, it soon vanished as deterioration of the brain and nervous system proceeded apace. What started as conscious immorality in a grandparent or great-grandparent thus became inherent amorality three or four generations later. The moral judgments implicit in this story were by no means unconnected with biological reality, particularly when they dwelt on the dire hereditary implications of alcoholism, drug addiction, incest, and sexual promiscuity that could end in syphilitic degeneration. Still speculating about the actual means of hereditary transmission, however, late Victorian and Edwardian alienists were not so much aiming to reveal a physiological pattern as to tell a moral tale.

The moral power of degeneration theory was, fundamentally, the principal source of its appeal to alienists, and it was a power that rested as much on optimism as on defeatism. Paradoxically, the Lamarckian beliefs embedded in the theory enabled alienists to embrace both attitudes, evincing hope even while expressing discouragement. The very incurability of nervous degeneration, once begun, threw psychiatrists back on preventive tactics, which were founded on the belief that people could be persuaded to follow expert advice. To alter habits and lifestyles, even without administering a single pill, was perceived as a significant medical accomplishment, for it not only ameliorated the health of the individual, but, thanks to the inheritance of acquired traits, could in time work extensive improvements among the population at large. Although medicine had nothing to offer the men, women, and children already in the grip of familial degeneration, it had plenty to say that was hopeful and forward-looking to everybody else. That message was predicated, not so much on the possible benefits of environmental reforms, as on the vast potential of individual moral reform. Unlikely as it may seem, a progressive outlook occupied the very center of degeneration theory: if people could set the downward process in motion, they could equally choose not to. In the eternal contest between good and evil, the decision was, as ever, a personal one. Exhortations to spurn vice in all its guises could just possibly enlist the individual man or woman in the crusade for moral hygiene and the effort to halt racial decline before it spread throughout the population.

Everything depended on the inheritance of acquired traits. Not only was that evolutionary mechanism responsible for the devastations of nervous degeneration, but it supported the psychiatric hopes that individual effort could effect positive change in the opposite direction, spreading increased vigor from parents to children in ever expanding circles. Lamarckian theory maintained that those members of a species who adapted best to their environment were likeliest to survive and to produce numerous offspring, who, in turn, possessed the newly altered characteristics so well fitted to their habitat. In the human species, such adaptation required conscious effort—the exercise of volition and intelligent choice. The ability to accommodate personal initiative, purposeful action, and, above all, the power of the will goes far to explain the enduring popularity of Lamarckian thought in Victorian science, medicine, and philosophy. Its emphasis on the degree to which a person's own decisions profoundly affected both private and public health helped to guarantee it an especially warm reception among psychiatrists. The Lamarckian strain in degeneration theory made that body of ideas particularly palatable to alienists who were wary of determinism in biological thought and eager to maintain the efficacy of self-help.

The Lamarckian and determinist aspects of degeneration theory were perfectly compatible so long as precious little was actually known about genetics. Until the 1880s, biologists generally assumed that anything affecting a person's body and mind became stamped, by means that eluded scientific investigation, on the individual's germ, or reproductive, cells, which were not perceived to be qualitatively different from the general body, or somatic, cells. The theory of pangenesis, which Darwin proposed in his *Variation of Animals and Plants under Domestication* (1868), fully reflected this point of view and was based entirely on Lamarckian assumptions. According to Darwin's hypothesis, every component part of the body "throws off gemmules [infinitesimally small material particles], each of which can reproduce itself, and a combination of these gemmules forms a sexual element.''[62] Thus Galton explained a theory that stimulated him to typically inventive and fertile speculations of his own, and ultimately to the repudiation of pangenesis. The notion that all body cells contribute representative particles to the content of the germ cells could be traced back to ancient Greece, but Darwin's advocacy of pangenesis gave his version of the venerable concept a certain brief notoriety. The idea that the blood stream collects these contributions as it circulates through the body and deposits the accumulated material in the sexual cells had the virtue of apparent simplicity and could, at least, be readily imagined. It also seemed to explain how somatic changes that occurred during a person's life could be transmitted through gemmules to the sexual cells and become characteristics inherited by the next generation. In maintaining that an individual's germ material underwent constant modification during the course of a lifetime, however, pangenesis raised more questions than it answered. Darwin himself dubbed it his "well-abused hypothesis," but the very fact that he proposed it is telling. The man whose theory of evolution by natural selection is widely understood to have stressed accidental variation and random change, which made individual effort irrelevant, actually incorporated into his work evolutionary models capable of encompassing the inheritance of acquired traits.[63] Down to the end of the century, natural selection and the inheritance of acquired characteristics coexisted as plausible alternative explanations of evolutionary change, both attracting staunch adherents and acerbic critics. The point to stress is that Lamarckism was never eclipsed by Darwinism during the Victorian era because there was no tidy distinction between the two.

During the 1880s, the work of the German biologist August Weismann took the first substantial step in discrediting the plausibility of Lamarckian evolution. Weismann's view of heredity acknowledged no evidence for the constant interjection of somatic material into the germ cells. He argued instead for a germ plasm that was unalterable; changes in the body, whether arising from injury, illness, or purposeful adaptation, did not work their way into an individual's reproductive matter, which was formed early in the fetal stage of life from parental germ plasm and remained utterly distinct from all somatic cells thereafter. The germ plasm, according to Weismann, formed a virtually closed system, into which external influences could not penetrate, and such a system possessed no means for transmitting acquired characteristics to the next generation. Environmental adaptation that helped an organism was not inheritable; neither were harmful responses to environmental change. Weismann contended that germ plasm always arose from that of the preceding generation; it was never formed *de novo* by new combinations of altered particles from the body cells. In 1900, the rediscovery of Gregor Mendel's experiments with plant hybridization, published in the 1860s but ignored, made biologists aware of persistent patterns of inheritance according to discrete "elements," or genes as we now call them. Like Weismann's germ plasm, these elements, located in the male and female reproductive cells, were impenetrable to external, fortuitous forces, at least of the sort that Edwardian science could command. With the long overdue recognition of Mendel's investigations, biologists at last had a clue to the way heredity worked, and that was clearly not the way Lamarck had supposed.[64]

The Lamarckian interpretation of evolution did not, however, immediately fall into disrepute. No single explanation of heredity swept scientific opinion before World War I, and as the new ideas gradually gained disciples, the old ones continued to find loyal defenders. In the heated debate over the workings of heredity, which engaged British scientists, social theorists, philanthropists, doctors, and intellectuals of all variety through the Edwardian decade, Lamarck's views held their own against

Weismann's and Mendel's, as well as those contributed by Galton and other eugenists, particularly Karl Pearson.[65] In fact, the Lamarckian perspective was not definitively discredited until the 1940s. While some Edwardian eugenists, vitalized by the infusion of Mendelism, contended that the evidence indubitably pointed to the need for selective breeding now that the negligible impact of environmental reforms on race improvement had been demonstrated, other spokesmen still found reason to appeal to the moral sense of their compatriots by insisting that individual effort continued to matter. Psychiatrists, particularly those old enough to have been exposed to the gospel of moral management early in their careers, generally preferred the latter point of view.

In jettisoning Lamarckian assumptions, the new accounts of hereditary transmission undermined the notion of personal responsibility fostered by the belief that acquired traits could prove a boon or curse to one's offspring. Neither Weismann's germ plasm nor Mendel's elements were susceptible to moral exhortation, and therefore Crichton-Browne, for one, rejected them. Like his great reluctance to accept the microbic origin of tuberculosis, he was loath to endorse a genetic theory without moral value. Although he was only in his forties when Weismann's ideas began to circulate in Great Britain, he refused to reconsider his position and remained true to Lamarckian beliefs for the remainder of his life. He never ceased warning that the damage unhealthy habits could work on the nervous system was, in fact, passed on to progeny. "Notwithstanding all Weismann's arguments," he declaimed in 1892, "I would say, 'Woe betide the generation that springs from mothers amongst whom gross nervous degenerations abound!'" In 1905, he told the Sanitary Inspectors Association that the modern urban population of Great Britain "under the stress of competition undergoes mental modifications, which (*Pace Weismann*) it passes on to its successors." As an elderly man, he was excited by Pavlov's experiments, which proved to his satisfaction, not only that "new neural connections" could be irrevocably established by acquired habits, but, further, that these new connections could "be so deeply impressed on the organism as to become hereditary." Despite the fact that Pavlov's work illuminated the neural reflex function, without bearing on questions of purpose and choice, Crichton-Browne cast its meaning in a different light. For him, the experiments confirmed the hope that "the precept and example by which we modify the behaviour of our children may beneficially influence their descendants," although he was candid enough to add that "evil tendencies may equally run on."[66]

For all the pessimism that shrouded late Victorian and Edwardian psychiatry, alienists raised in the nineteenth century wanted to continue believing in the possibility of progress. They wanted the comfort of thinking that, when they taught by "precept and example," they were causing meaningful changes in their patients' lives, and in the lives of their patients' descendants. A faith in mankind's malleability—for the good, one trusted—was a precious bequest from the Enlightenment to the Victorian era, expressed in Lamarckian evolutionary thought, as in countless other ways. Degeneration theory did not, in fact, make a mockery of this optimism, although it certainly seemed to deny, and even ridicule, the fondest beliefs of the early Victorian asylum reformers. Thanks to its Lamarckian foundation, degeneration theory, too, rested on the ultimate bedrock of individual moral endeavor. The struggle against animal instincts and base habits, which every member of the human race inevitably possessed, could end in victory, and the Victorians were sure that the successful outcome of each individual fight furthered the advance of society as a whole. Curiously enough, degeneration theory prolonged the life of the mid-Victorian certainty that private exertions were the key to public progress.

CONCLUSION

The Psychiatric Dilemma

In 1840, a friend of John and Sarah Austin could no longer conceal his frustration over the jurist's chronic incapacitation and wrote tartly: "I think Mr. Austin is the *Opprobrium Medicorum*. Nothing and Nobody seem to do him any good." In 1920, in the first Maudsley Lecture to the Medico-Psychological Association, Crichton-Browne recalled Maudsley's "moment of bitterness," when he "imagined a physician who had spent his life in ministering to the mind diseased looking back sadly on his track, recognising the fact that one-half of the diseased beings he had treated had never got well, and questioning whether he had done real service to his kind in restoring the other half to reproductive work." Crichton-Browne felt sure that this was not Maudsley's final frame of mind about the psychiatric endeavor and that he subsequently regained "hope in the future of psychological medicine";[1] yet toward the end of his own life, Crichton-Browne himself expressed a mordantly pessimistic attitude toward the work he had pursued for more than six decades. In *The Doctor's Second Thoughts* (1931), he abandoned all professional reserve and issued a scathing indictment against chronic nervous patients, whom he dubbed "the half-mads." These were the people, he insisted, who caused the most misery in the world. The "out-and-out lunatic" can be restrained, he pointed out, but the "half-mad is practically unrestrained and free to go abroad broadcasting trouble and perplexity." Echoing Weir Mitchell's portrayal of hysterical women as "the pests of many households, who constitute the despair of physicians," Crichton-Browne extended the denunciation to *all* nerve patients:

> There is, I believe, scarcely a family in these days that does not include some psychopathic or neuropathic member, not certifiable, passing muster as a self-regulating human being, often as one who is injured and misunderstood, but who is more or less or from time to time abnormal, difficult, irritable, depressed, suspicious, capricious, eccentric, impulsive, unreasonable, cranky, deluded, and subject to all kinds of imaginary maladies and nervous agitations, thus diffusing discomfort and perturbation all around.

There was little that doctors could do to help, he conceded. Change of environment, of climate, and of companionship, bed rest, bromides, electricity, and sunshine were alike useless, although the nursing home offered "welcome relief" to the patient's family for a while. "It must be a long wait," Crichton-Browne concluded, "but Eugenism must do something toward the elimination of these half-mads."[2] Over

293

nearly a century, psychiatry had apparently made very little progress in treating people like John Austin.

Crichton-Browne's admission of defeat was clearly much more than a reflection of the general postwar anxiety that afflicted British literary culture in the 1920s and 1930s, often finding expression in images of impotence.[3] It revealed the crisis of confidence that disabled British psychiatry, from the collapse of professional optimism in the third quarter of the nineteenth century through the horrific challenges of World War I. Although individual doctors might wax enthusiastic about particular treatments for a time, the psychiatric profession as a whole remained unable to resolve the fundamental uncertainty that had hindered its efforts throughout the Victorian era. Alienists were no closer to deciding whether they treated physiological or psychological disorders than they had been in the 1830s; in fact, they were less so, for the assurance of yet undiscovered somatic causes behind neurotic illness, which lightened the psychiatric task in the early nineteenth century, raised far fewer hopes by the start of the twentieth. Freud's solution of the problem in favor of psychological factors was vehemently rejected by most of the British psychiatrists who had been practicing medicine since the 1860s or 1870s, but they also sensed that allegiance to somaticism was leading psychiatry nowhere more novel than talk of depleted nerve force or more promising than the negativity of degeneration theory. While military victory over Germany in 1918 may have put an end to the most ominous predictions of British racial deterioration, it did little to give the psychiatric endeavor the unequivocal sense of direction that it so noticeably lacked.

Late Victorian alienists did not need the *Times* to remind them in 1889 that their understanding of insanity had scarcely advanced during the preceding century, and they keenly felt how little interest the rest of the medical profession showed toward psychiatry. Three years later, a contributor to the *Dictionary of Psychological Medicine* commented on "the want of knowledge of mental science among physicians"—a situation that arose largely because most medical practitioners still considered mental science a contradiction in terms. Playfair, an authority on female nervous disorders although not an alienist himself, used another article in the dictionary to remark on the glaring inadequacy of medical information concerning "the course and symptoms of the functional neuroses." "We are satisfied," he asserted, "that there is no department of medicine so little understood, and so much requiring study."[4]

The same observations echoed down the first decade of the twentieth century. "Mental therapeutics [was] still the Cinderella of medical sciences," in Schofield's apt phrase, with nervous invalids "the pariahs and outcasts amongst patients and doctors." In his Harveian Oration to the Royal College of Physicians in 1909, Savage offered to explain the widespread medical disdain for psychiatry:

> The general feeling, certainly among the seniors of our profession, is that experimental psychology is hardly likely to reward those who are devoting their lives to it, and I have heard some good and thoughtful physicians express regret that men of promise were, as they thought, wasting their energies on what will be of little service either to psychology or to medicine. They look upon the two as incompatible, and consider that physics and the imponderable are not to be brought together.

From such a perspective, medical psychology was an utterly futile enterprise, yet Savage nonetheless insisted, albeit forlornly, that "we have no right to stop investigation because we cannot see any immediate prospect of material result, or because we cannot see the lines on which advance is to be made." Sir Arthur Hurst, an eminent physician between the wars, remembered from his student days at Guy's Hospital in the opening years of the Edwardian era that, "if no evidence of organic disease was discovered, it was assumed that the symptoms were 'functional' or 'nervous' in origin. The case was then regarded as of no further interest, and the possible cause of the illness and its treatment were not discussed." It was only while he worked in Paris, during 1907–08, that Hurst "learnt what a fascinating study the investigation and treatment of the neuroses presented."[5]

Even after the war, British medical circles continued to harbor deep pockets of prejudice against psychiatry. In 1920, C. Hubert Bond, a former lecturer in psychiatry at the Middlesex Hospital, deplored both the inadequate facilities currently available for the mentally ill and "the insufficiency of attention paid at medical schools to this important branch of medical science with its consequent ill-effects both to patients and to the medical profession. . . ." Crichton-Browne echoed Bond's sentiments that same year in his Maudsley Lecture. It was unfortunate, he told his fellow psychiatrists, that "the nature of the medium in which we work and the legal restrictions under which that work is carried on have in the past kept us to some extent aloof from the main body of our profession." As a result, he feared, "gross misconceptions of our status and performances are prevalent in some quarters," and hostile critics were able to spread the picture of backward, negligent, and ill-informed British alienists plodding through their asylum chores in stark contrast to the up-to-date, research-oriented psychiatrists of France, Germany, Switzerland, and the United States.[6]

Although they repeatedly asserted their aim to steer psychiatry into the mainstream of modern medicine, however, late Victorian and Edwardian alienists frequently underscored, both explicitly and implicitly, their distance from the rest of the medical profession. It was not just that their willingness to impose degeneration theory on mental and nervous disorders in these years tended to cut them adrift from all medical disciplines preoccupied with the germ theory of disease. The problem went deeper than that, as Crichton-Browne acknowledged in 1880, when he observed that the "scheme of mind" to which he and his fellow psychiatrists clung was an artificial construct, which failed to "harmonise with any scheme of brain" accepted by neurologists, anatomists, or pathologists. About the same time, Charles Mercier emphasized the "fathomless abyss" separating "the facts of consciousness" from the workings of the nervous system. While endorsing the theory of psychophysical parallelism and considering that some alteration in the nervous system inevitably accompanied mental change, he was unable to conceive how either could cause the other. "Why the two occur together, or what the link is which connects them, we do not know, and most authorities believe that we never shall and never can know."[7] With statements like these to challenge the standard psychiatric assertion that medical psychology was a branch of physiology, it is no wonder that "neuropsychiatry never really flourished in Britain."[8]

While somaticism remained the ideology that officially inspired British psychiatric thought down to World War I, it was honored more as a matter of routine than
conviction. Its practical utility had long been in doubt, not only where insanity was
concerned, but where lesser forms of neurotic illness flourished as well. Exhaustion
of nerve force as an explanation for nervous breakdown left too much unanswered to
remain satisfactory forever. It could not account for someone like Faraday, whose
muscles often showed no signs of prostration even while his mind was shut down to
all but the most mundane tasks. It shed no light on those victims of nervous collapse
who never regained strength of purpose, despite generous opportunities to replenish
nervous energy. Nor did anyone ever elucidate how the will commanded nerve force
to execute its orders. Difficulties like these suggested that incapacitating depression
had less to do with the body's nervous resources than with a troubled mind. By the
close of Victoria's reign many alienists were, in fact, relying more and more on
psychological terminology to make sense of the neuroses, even though they also
continued to parade old images and metaphors in their writings. Furthermore, as the
medical application of psychology, psychiatry in Great Britain was hardly encouraged by its parent discipline to undertake laboratory research into the physical
workings of the brain. Ontological questions and ethical concerns retained a prominent place in British psychological texts throughout the Edwardian decade and
contributed to a prejudice against physiological inquiries centered in laboratories,
such as invigorated German psychology and psychiatry during the final quarter of the
nineteenth century. British academic institutions showed no interest in psychology
laboratories until the late 1890s, when both Cambridge and University College,
London, established theirs; the facility at Cambridge was inadequate, however, until
the eve of the war, and Oxford did not choose to set up any sort of psychology
laboratory until 1936.[9]

Institutional obstacles merely underscored the deeper philosophical differences
that, around the turn of the century, were starting to distance British neurology and
psychiatry from each other. Not only did existing evidence fail to provide support for
a purely physiological explanation of mental illness and neurotic distress, but
alienists were more uncomfortably conscious of the fundamental challenge that such
an explanation posed to any psychiatric model of mental health constructed around
the supremacy of the will. Few late Victorian and Edwardian psychiatrists would
have taken issue with David Drummond, the Newcastle physician who made
neurasthenia his speciality, when he wrote in 1906: "What we want to secure is a
central will, reassured, instructed, strengthened, and set free from worrying trammels
to play its proper part as director-general of the personality."[10] Without the concept
of will, as we have seen, there was no focus to the therapeutic process in psychiatric
treatment, no means of appealing to the patient's own desire to recover, no target at
which to aim the artillery of moral suasion. To embrace an etiology of the neuroses
that dealt solely with brain tissue or nerve currents minimized the significance of a
separate force for orderly, stable, and rational conduct—the very thing that psychiatrists were supposed to be fostering in their patients.

Belief in the efficacy of the will was as important to those who suffered nervous
collapse as to their doctors, for it gave patients the sense that some initiative to recover
remained under their control, that they were not the utterly helpless victims of blind

physiological forces, or of deterministic "antecedent circumstances," as Mill wrote in his *Autobiography*. While gradually recovering from his first prolonged experience of depression in the 1820s, Mill discovered "that what is really inspiriting and ennobling in the doctrine of freewill, is the conviction that we have real power over the formation of our own character; that our will, by influencing some of our circumstances, can modify our future habits or capabilities of willing."[11] If patients accepted a measure of responsibility for having shattered their own nerves by violating nature's laws of health, they also wanted to know that they might play a major part in restoring themselves to vigor. The possibility was important in a culture committed to the idea of punishment for making the wrong choices and reward for the right ones.

Drummond's definition of neurasthenia as "a disorder or disease of the mind"[12] proclaimed his psychological interpretation of the malady; indeed, medical men who emphasized the will could not help but deviate from a strictly somatic approach to the neuroses. The will might be located in the highest nervous center of the brain, and it might be unable to function if the center deteriorated, but it was not identical with the neurons that composed that structure. It was the metaphysical core at the center of psychiatric thought, and so long as British alienists adhered to theories of mental health and illness that revolved around the presence or absence of will, they were fundamentally committed to the idea of mind as distinct from brain, even though they recognized that the workings of the former required the material foundation of the latter. Alone among medical practitioners, alienists were professionally obliged to grapple with the mind, the most elusive of all subjects. Doctors in other branches of medicine could fix their attention on somatic disorders without thereby passing any judgment on human nature, but an alienist who ignored the patient's will in prescribing therapy was, in effect, doubting the human capacity to exercise responsibility, to exert self-control, and, by implication, to make moral choices. Despite all their formal disavowal of philosophical speculations, psychiatrists' profound involvement with ethical and even religious questions most starkly underlined the contrast between their work and the rest of modern medicine at the end of the Edwardian era.

In no field of medicine was it necessary by then to make a public show of religion in order to have loyal patients. The inroads of agnosticism had demonstrated that people of principle could remain in doubt about theological matters without threatening social stability or public morality. The growing acknowledgment that professions of faith were not essential to the conscientious performance of occupational duties certainly represented a striking departure from early and mid-Victorian attitudes. For all that, however, doctors confronted with the manifold forms of mental illness remained deeply influenced by the Christian doctrines on which they had been raised. Even those who abandoned conventional religious practices fully understood that questions about the will's existence could not be separated from the issue of independent mind and, ultimately, immortal soul. The psychiatric interpretation of nervous breakdown reflected that comprehension; morally neutral somatic explanations in terms of depleted nerve force or the commencement of tissue degeneration in the nervous system never obscured the psychological aspects of the story that encompassed the will.

During the final quarter of the nineteenth century and the first decade of the twentieth, as the bodily basis of nervous breakdown appeared an ever less fruitful subject of investigation, British psychiatrists and nerve specialists paid increased attention to the value of psychotherapeutics in neurasthenic cases. The most common form of psychotherapy, as was noted, featured the doctor's own strong personality attempting to revive the patient's desire for health. Yet alienists generally deployed this strategy in conjunction with various forms of physical treatment, for they were never willing in these years to embrace purely psychological theories of nervous collapse. Any explanation of depressive states that failed to take somatic conditions into account was as unsatisfactory to the psychiatric viewpoint as was the strictly material interpretation, and alienists continued their old policy of trying to treat debilitated bodies together with disturbed minds. Their conduct was not inspired merely by the need to advertise their status as medical practitioners, in contrast to psychologists, metaphysicians, or other laymen who might claim expertise in handling the immaterial side of the problem; it was prompted, too, by their reaction to the principal forms of pure psychotherapy available in these years—hypnosis and psychoanalysis.

British medical attitudes toward hypnotism went through two distinct phases, in neither of which it ever enjoyed widespread esteem among psychiatrists as a therapeutic tool. During the first stage from the 1830s through the 1850s, when it was called animal magnetism or mesmerism, it was linked with the grandiose notions of the Viennese doctor Franz Anton Mesmer, who claimed to have command over the curative powers of a universal, invisible, imponderable magnetic fluid. Animal magnetism was only one of numerous pseudosciences that merged with occultism in the late eighteenth century, but in Mesmer it boasted a particularly creative publicist. His theory maintained that a force analogous to the effect produced by magnets coursed throughout the human body, causing illness when unequally distributed or blocked from flowing freely; the mesmerist's task was then to restore the superfine fluid to its proper state by touching the sick person with his hand, by rubbing the afflicted portions of the patient's body, or by simply making passes in the air above them. Despite the striking results Mesmer achieved at his fashionable Parisian clinic during the last years of the Ancien Régime, a French royal commission in 1784 denounced his pretensions and found no evidence whatsoever for the existence of his magnetic fluid. True, the commissioners attributed many of Mesmer's more spectacular cures to the patient's expectant imagination, but the psychological implications of animal magnetism aroused no medical interest at the time, and orthodox medical opinion generally dismissed the work of animal magnetists as mere charlatanry. The results of the official French inquiry appeared to place the subject beyond the scope of legitimate scientific investigation.[13]

Medical men in Great Britain were, for the most part, slow to take heed of these continental developments, and when they did, it was primarily to dismiss the untenable concept of an imponderable magnetic fluid. "Concerning animal magnetism," John Conolly scoffed in 1833, "we shall only express our hearty disbelief of most of the circumstances related by its supporters, and our conviction that the rest admit of explanation without having recourse to the principle the magnetisers so anxiously desire to establish."[14] In the late 1830s, some eminent doctors, like

Herbert Mayo, did express interest in mesmeric phenomena, and John Elliotson, a highly successful physician, actually gave up his post as professor of the practice of medicine at University College, London, in order to pursue unrestricted inquiries into the workings of animal magnetism. The disapproval expressed by his former colleagues at University College Hospital, however, was far more typical of British medical response to mesmerism than Elliotson's boundless enthusiasm. When James Braid, a Scottish surgeon practicing in Manchester, tried to present a paper on the subject to the annual meeting of the British Medical Association in 1842, he was refused permission.[15]

Braid was nonetheless responsible for substantial changes in British medical attitudes toward mesmerism, as the occasional subsequent use of the label *Braidism* in place of *hypnotism* reveals.[16] Whereas Elliotson, to his own professional detriment, continued to uphold the existence of an invisible magnetic fluid, Braid sought other ways to interpret the processes that cast the mesmerized subject into a profound somnambulistic trance. At first, in the early 1840s, he suggested a strictly physiological explanation that involved the mesmerized person's circulatory, respiratory, muscular, and nervous systems, all deranged by the rigid stare and fixity of attention needed to bring on the trance. In order to distinguish this form of induced sleep from the fluidist theories of animal magnetism, which he dismissed, Braid called his version "neurohypnotism," from the Greek word for "sleep," *hypnos*. The neologism was later shortened to its current form. As his investigations continued, however, Braid's emphasis shifted from the physiological to the psychological. By the early 1850s, he was sure that the hypnotic trance resulted from a mental state of such intense concentration that all external distractions were excluded. He became convinced that the hypnotized person was an active partner in the production of the hypnotic state and that no one could be hypnotized against his or her will. The introduction of will into the discussion profoundly influenced the future of hypnotism as a tool of psychotherapy in Great Britain.[17]

At mid-century, Braid's work ignited few sparks of curiosity among his compatriots in the medical profession. His reinterpretation of hypnotism seemed to provide no compelling reason for doctors to devote time to a subject that, without demonstrable material foundations, lacked scientific credibility. Furthermore, doctors who *had* experimented with mesmerism pronounced it at best "an uncertain and somewhat dangerous agent."[18] The fact that it was eagerly embraced by unorthodox medical practitioners, like James Gully, and flourished among a range of alternative medical therapies, on which orthodox medicine severely frowned, scarcely improved its reputation. During the 1860s and 1870s, British medical men accordingly wrote very little about the therapeutic possibilities of hypnotism. Hack Tuke tried to keep the topic alive in the Medico-Psychological Association, but his lack of success may be gauged by the evident frustration with which he insisted, as late as 1883, that research into hypnotism *did* fall within the association's jurisdiction and *was* appropriate for consideration at the association's meetings.[19] Despite his efforts, the interesting studies of hypnotism were proceeding elsewhere, in Germany, Holland, Switzerland, Italy, the United States, and, especially, France. There, from the late 1870s, Charcot's use of hypnosis in treating hysterical and epileptic patients at the Salpêtrière brought it within the charmed circle of academically respectable subjects, while the development of a rival approach to hypnotism, centered around the work of

Ambroise Liébeault and Hippolyte Bernheim at Nancy, suggested the wealth of psychological questions that could be explored by means of hypnosis.[20]

Renewed interest in hypnotism at length manifested itself across the Channel in the 1880s. This second phase of British medical attention to the effects of hypnosis received much stimulus from the inquiries undertaken by members of the newly founded Society for Psychical Research, including Dr. John Milne Bramwell and Dr. Charles Lloyd Tuckey. Tuckey traveled to Nancy in 1888, to observe Liébeault in his dispensary, and was painfully struck by the difference between his own country's ignorance of the benefits available from hypnotic therapy and its widespread use on the continent. During the next decade the situation improved enough for Bramwell to acknowledge, early in the twentieth century, that his medical colleagues at home treated hypnotism fairly, even generously. *Psychotherapeutics* had, in fact, become widely accepted as a synonym for treatment by hypnotic suggestion.[21] Nonetheless, only a few alienists worked to incorporate hypnotism into their standard therapeutic armory, for the medical prejudice against it was still too firmly entrenched to allow most psychiatrists to greet "hypnosis redivivus," as Tuke called it, with anything but suspicion.

Much of the lingering bias against hypnotism arose from the company it had once kept, for psychiatrists eager to validate their own professional respectability could not readily forget its disreputable past. What was worse, a taint of quackery and occult nonsense still clung to hypnotism in the present, and men with medical degrees were quick to denounce the untrained healers of both sexes who claimed to achieve medical cures through the hypnotic arts alone. When nervous patients, despairing of traditional therapies, resorted "to mesmerists and unqualified practitioners," as Dowse complained in 1880, they did not endear hypnosis to psychiatrists protective of their own good names.[22] "Unqualified" usually meant "unscrupulous" in Victorian medical parlance, and the opportunities for unprincipled behavior were legion among popular mesmerists, or so psychiatrists declared; but they also voiced fears that bona fide medical men could abuse the power that hypnotism gave them over their patients. This particular anxiety, needless to say, focused on defenseless women, who might, while under hypnosis, be subjected to sexual advances of which they were subsequently unaware. Alternatively, since the feminine nature was considered highly suggestible, the hypnotized female patient might reveal secrets that jeopardized her doctor's ability to sustain the role of confidant and counselor. French doctors, it is true, articulated these concerns far more vociferously than their British counterparts: the tradition of public mesmeric performances was less well established and less widely disseminated in Great Britain than in France, where the conflict of amateur versus professional, centering around mesmerism, assumed epic proportions in the late nineteenth century. In England, where medical interest in hypnotism remained limited, professional possessiveness was similarly muted. British psychiatrists perceived little need to fight for control of something they did not value, and their rhetoric stayed comparatively cool. Nevertheless, uncertainty about the conduct of wives and daughters under hypnosis, and the possibility of misconduct on the hypnotist's part, counted heavily against that form of psychotherapy in the eyes of British medical men.[23]

Even more damaging in the opinion of British psychiatrists, however, was the close affiliation of the hypnotic trance with a whole cluster of pathological conditions. Foremost among them was hysteria, for Charcot's amply publicized work underscored the similarities between hysterical and hypnotic states. Indeed virtually all the manifold features of hysteria could be imitated in the hypnotic trance and were amenable to treatment by hypnotic suggestion. The suspicion that hypnosis was more an illness than a cure had actually been mounting for several decades before receiving apparent confirmation in Charcot's investigations. Between the 1850s and 1880s, what little discussion of mesmerism or hypnotism appeared in British medical literature was largely directed to its morbid implications, as, for example, in the writings of Maudsley and of William B. Carpenter, a distinguished physiologist with medical training.[24] According to this school of thought, any entranced condition was a pathological abnormality.

In the three decades before World War I, British psychiatrists generally concurred that suggestibility to hypnotism was in itself an indication of nervous instability, if not outright disease. The great majority of late Victorian and Edwardian pronouncements on the subject adopted the Salpêtrière position that hypnosis was a form of neurotic disorder, which could only be induced in people who harbored hysterical tendencies. By contrast, Liébeault, Bernheim, and their followers at Nancy worked on the assumption that hypnosis was not a pathological, but a normal, state; they believed that, although induced artificially, it was analogous to sleep in important respects, with possible therapeutic benefits for a wide array of sufferers. According to the Nancians, a patient did not have to be hysterical or neurotic, but only somewhat impressionable, to be hypnotized. This moderate approach, however, seemed far less plausible to leading British alienists than Charcot's point of view. "Notwithstanding the recent teaching of the school of Nancy that all human beings are potentially hypnotisable," Donkin remarked in 1892, "it is certain from general experience that human beings are hypnotisable in direct proportion to their nervous instability."[25]

From the British psychiatric perspective, what was especially worrisome about hypnotism as a means of psychotherapy was its impact on the patient's own will. Even Hack Tuke, who in his *Illustrations of the Influence of the Mind upon the Body* (1872) had urged his fellow alienists to harness the curative role of the imagination through the methods of Braidism, subsequently had to admit that the will was entirely "abrogated" in the hypnotic trance. Merely "reflex cerebral action" remained, as Laycock and Carpenter had already contended, to reveal some trace of intelligence in the hypnotized subject, but Tuke conceded that "the highest cerebral functions" were in a state of "suspension or negation." On another occasion, using the term *ego* as synonymous with the will, he described "the essential and striking characteristic of hypnotism" in terms that would have sent a chill along any Victorian psychiatrist's spine: "It is as if all that directing, controlling, originating, and regulating power, which we attribute to the *ego* were annihilated." In its place, the hypnotized person was plunged into a state of "mental slavery to the expressed or implied will of the operator."[26] For that very reason, Maudsley argued, any medical practitioner who repeatedly hypnotized a nervous patient was guilty of serious professional irresponsibility. "It is not a mere harmless amusement for one who is susceptible to the hypnotic trance to suffer himself to be frequently practised upon," he cautioned, "for there is danger of his mind being weakened temporarily or permanently. Indeed were his will strong and well-fashioned the operation could not succeed, for its success is a surrender of the subject's will to the will of the operator. . . ." Perceiving in hypnosis the ultimate loss of self-control, most alienists, neurologists, and nerve specialists judged the risks inherent in such a surrender too great to condone. The neurologist William Thorburn expressed a common attitude among all these doctors when he explained in 1913 that he had stopped hypnotizing patients long ago because, despite some temporarily promising results, "the effect of designed and elaborate hypnotization was to intensify the mental deterioration and increase the general nervous condition."[27]

If hypnotism only exacerbated the very deficiency of will that alienists aimed to correct in their neurotic patients; if a person's nervous instability and vulnerability to suggestion, which increased the likelihood of successful hypnosis, were themselves powerful reasons *not* to employ that form of treatment,[28] then, from the viewpoint of British psychiatry, hypnotism as psychotherapy had nothing to recommend it. The psychiatric response to hypnosis at the end of the nineteenth century in fact makes it clear that professional snobbery, self-interest, and social prejudice were not the only motives molding the medical rejection of mesmerism in earlier years. What emerges from the late Victorian and Edwardian psychiatric literature is a genuine fear that hypnotism, under whatever name, would prove exceedingly harmful to the very people who were likeliest to be exposed to it. Little effort was accordingly made to work out the precise limits of its therapeutic efficacy or to study systematically the methods of its employment that furnished the best results.[29]

This is not to deny that British medical practitioners who treated neurotic disorders occasionally made unsystematic use of hypnotism on an experimental basis. With illnesses that taxed their ingenuity to the utmost, doctors were sometimes driven to try any kind of therapy that might produce even temporary improvement in the patient's condition or, better yet, turn the course of illness around, but, not surprisingly, there was no unanimous opinion concerning the results of such experiments. From the Salpêtrière came the message that hypnosis could be effective in treating hysterical cases, but Charcot himself cautioned, in the *Dictionary of Psychological Medicine,* that hypnotism actually figured among the innumerable "occasional causes" of hysteria and asserted that the "inconsiderate use or abuse of hypnotism" on hysterics had "been followed by very serious complications." Allbutt considered hypnosis useful in dealing with hysteria, as did Savage, particularly with cases involving "hysterical spasms and palsies," but Schofield warned that hypnotism often aggravated the hysterical condition. British medical attitudes were equally mixed concerning the application of hypnotic therapy to other neurotic maladies. With regard to neurasthenia, for example, Allbutt dismissed hypnosis altogether, while Savage reported on several cases that responded well to hypnotic treatment, with significant improvement in the lassitude, indecision, sense of weakness, and severe depression characteristic of the ailment.[30]

Out of desperation, some medical practitioners seized on the slight evidence in favor of hypnotic therapy and applied the treatment to particularly intractable cases of shattered nerves. Benson had suffered in the grips of his tormenting depression for one year—had tried nursing-home care, travel, veronal, and ocean climate to no avail—when, in October 1908, Ross Todd sent him to a specialist in hypnotic therapy, one Dr. Oulterson Wood. Benson was not impressed when Dr. Wood pompously informed him that "mental depression . . . involves a considerable degree of discomfort," for the patient knew that all too well already. Wood did not himself hypnotize Benson, but sent him to another specialist, with whom Benson had five sessions. These primarily consisted of stroking his midriff and forehead with a comforting hypnotic hand, an effort that the patient likened to quenching "a conflagration with a drop or two of scent." Yet the following year, in September 1909, when Benson began experiencing a strong desire to be well and tossed away his medicines, it was to hypnotism that he turned, again on Todd's suggestion. This time he went to Dr. Bramwell, and also to a Dr. Wright (the tenth medical man whom Benson had consulted during his two years of illness). Both men, radiating confidence, dismissed his fears of incipient insanity, and, after a few sessions, he had to admit that "the gloom [was] a little lightening." It embarrassed him to think that the "absurd treatment" actually improved his condition, and it is, of course, possible that his bout of depression had run its natural course by the autumn of 1909. At least, however, hypnosis offered itself as an alternative to drugs of doubtful efficacy and potential danger; in the hands of skilled practitioners, it had done Benson no harm. He could not be sure that it had not helped.[31]

The controversy surrounding hypnotic suggestion as a method of treating neurotic illness was inextricably intertwined with the reevaluation of the neuroses that late Victorian and Edwardian psychiatry gingerly undertook. The growing belief that, whenever hypnotism proved beneficial, the nervous disorder under treatment was psychological in origin mirrored rising doubts about the neuroses' somatic foundations. There were, admittedly, some attempts to provide a physiological theory for the workings of hypnosis. Carpenter speculated that the trance state arose from reduced circulation of blood in the brain, while Tuke wondered whether some kind of cerebral blockage was involved, with the overstimulation of a sensory nerve possibly inhibiting the action of the highest nerve centers in the cortical substance of the brain.[32] These suggestions, however, could not obviate the paramount importance of the will, or its absence, in permitting the hypnotist to exert absolute control over the hypnotized subject. Whatever happened to the highest nerve centers under hypnosis, the events were significant because they affected the subject's will. No matter what somatic channels were employed, hypnotism apparently succeeded when it matched a dominant will against an enfeebled one.

It was precisely the power of hypnotism to alter the mind that frightened many British alienists, for the process threatened to destroy the safe buffer zone between the perishable body and the incorruptible mind that the theory of psychophysical parallelism had conveniently constructed. Even if they recognized the limitations of the old theory and conceded, like Mercier, that it could serve no heuristic function for psychiatry, the idea that, through hypnosis, they could tamper so directly and substantially with the immaterial essence of the human personality troubled them. Disillusioned though they were by the failure of somatic hypotheses to elucidate the ailments they examined, Edwardian psychiatrists were not prepared to accept the psychological solutions that hypnotism proposed.

With these attitudes, British psychiatry at the end of the nineteenth century and the start of the twentieth was not likely to prove receptive to the theories of another Viennese doctor, Sigmund Freud. Although psychoanalysis was a form of psychotherapy free of discreditable connections with quackery, the majority of British alienists in these years repudiated it even more emphatically than they dismissed hypnotism. Freud himself, as is well known, trained as a neurologist and began his study of the neuroses with the almost universal medical assumption that they derived from physiological conditions, in which heredity played a central part. By the early 1890s, however, his thoughts were straying from their neural grooves into the uncharted terrain of the unconscious mind, and his first use of the term *psychoanalysis* in 1896 signaled his departure from the orthodox approach to neurotic illness.[33] Thereafter no one played a more significant part than Freud in transferring the neuroses from a putative physiological to a supposed psychological basis.

Many of Freud's early ideas were stimulated and clarified by the use of hypnotic suggestion with hysterical patients, whose cases were presented to the psychiatric world in his pioneering collaborative effort with Dr. Josef Breuer, *Studies on Hysteria* (1895). An early statement of their joint endeavor appeared as a "Preliminary Communication" in 1893,[34] and the enterprise soon became known in England. Although first publicized in the *Proceedings of the Society for Psychical Research,* it almost immediately attracted some attention in more professionally established journals as well. In reviewing the current literature on hysteria and neurasthenia for *Brain* in 1894, J. M. Clarke mentioned the Breuer–Freud work with hysterics and singled out for comment its use of hypnosis to ascertain "the causes and the phenomena immediately preceding the onset of the hysterical symptoms."[35] Hypnosis, however, retained no permanent place in Freudian practice; before the end of the 1890s, Freud had abandoned it in favor of nothing more remarkable than allowing his patients to talk. His rejection of hypnotism and adoption of the "talking cure" or *catharsis,* first utilized by Breuer in the 1880s, did not increase British esteem for Freud's ideas. His articulation of an unequivocally psychological approach to psychiatric questions in *The Interpretation of Dreams* (1900) and *Three Essays on the Theory of Sexuality* (1905) only persuaded the most vocal of British alienists that he was a menace to his profession.

Psychoanalysis did, nonetheless, attract a small core of devoted medical advocates in Edwardian Britain. Ernest Jones, born in 1879, became the best known of them in international Freudian circles. Although he was in Canada from 1908 to 1913, serving as director of the University of Toronto Psychiatric Clinic during the years that confirmed his commitment to psychoanalysis, he returned to London before the war to join forces with the handful of doctors who had discovered Freudian ideas in his absence. Chief among these was David Eder, Jones's partner in launching the London Psycho-Analytical Society in 1913, initially with seven other members. Eder had become impressed with Freudian theory partly because his work with children at a school clinic in the slums made him receptive to Freud's writings on childhood sexuality. By 1912, he had set up the first psychoanalytic practice in Great Britain, while the year before he had led the way in exposing the British Medical Association to psychoanalysis. The reception of his paper on the subject would have been devastating to a less fervent enthusiast: when Eder finished talking, his entire audience expressed its outrage by trooping out of the room.[36] It was exceedingly difficult for the generation of British alienists born between 1835 and 1855, and trained before 1880, to accept Freud's revision of the old psychiatric orthodoxies, no matter how inadequate these were to explain the workings of the mind. Younger medical psychologists, less constrained by the values of their mid-Victorian predecessors, were freer to try Freudian psychoanalytic methods in an effort to liberate themselves from the frustrations and negations of contemporary psychiatry.

In the midst of the contradictory, confused, and often apparently haphazard theorizing about mind and body that had embroiled psychiatrists for decades, Freud's Edwardian disciples found in his work clarity and consistency. To their way of thinking, his interpretation of the neuroses broke through the vacillations and evasions of their professional colleagues with one bold thrust of his overarching explanatory theory, which asserted a sexual etiology at the core of all neurotic disorders. Although he divided the neuroses into two groups—the actual neuroses and the more numerous psychoneuroses, with different sexual problems at their origins—Freud was far less concerned to categorize illnesses than to explore what have subsequently been called psychodynamic processes, like repression, conflict, defense, and transformation. In the actual neuroses, among which he included neurasthenia, "the pathogenic agents are operative at the actual time when the symptoms are being manifested, . . . while in the psychoneuroses they always precede them in time—commonly by many years; the ultimate causes of the former lie in adult life, of the latter in childhood." As an actual neurosis, Freud argued, neurasthenia arose concurrently with unhealthy sexual practices, which caused the physical exhaustion and weakness that he considered neurasthenia's outstanding features. Because masturbation was typically accompanied by an "intense moral conflict," as draining in its way as the excessive loss of sperm was alleged to be, it ranked in Freudian theory as the cause *par excellence* of neurasthenia.[37] As a psychoneurosis, by contrast, hysteria had its roots in the patient's past; according to Freud, it was the manifestation of a person's unconscious efforts to deal with the devastating effects of traumas experienced in childhood, which had adversely influenced the patient's developing sexuality. Throughout his career, the psychoneuroses engaged Freud's interest far more fixedly than the actual neuroses, but in his hands both were molded to illustrate the central tenet of his sweeping psychological hypothesis: the fundamental force of sexual energy, or libido, to which civilization could not allow free rein, had to be repressed and redirected to other ends, but if the unconscious conflicts fostered by this process from infancy did not achieve a satisfactory psychic resolution, neurotic illness inevitably resulted.

Here was a single plausible explanation of hysteria, such as nineteenth-century medicine had always lacked. It emphatically dismissed the suspicion that hysterical patients were simply feigning illness, and it readily accommodated male hysteria as well as female. Indeed, it managed to include hysteria, and all neurotic disorders, among the possible varieties of human behavior in such a way as to minimize their morbidity. To a certain extent, Freud removed the neuroses from the category of pathology, although he did not thereby incorporate them into any definition of normalcy. As Jones commented in 1913:

It is highly important to realize that, strictly speaking, neuroses are not diseases in the medical sense at all, but only in the social sense. In the former sense a disease is the product of the interaction between a given individual and an injurious, non-human environment, whether the latter be a physical trauma or an invasion of microörganisms. On the other hand, a social disease is the product of the interaction between a given individual and a certain human environment. Put a little figuratively, it may be said that neuroses are the result of a conflict between the individual and society, whereas other diseases are the result of a conflict between the individual and nature. This fundamental distinction is often not grasped by members of the medical profession, who commonly regard all disease from the one standpoint, and the failure to grasp it is an important reason why the pathology of the neuroses has in the past been investigated with such signal lack of success.[38]

The leading Edwardian spokesmen for British psychiatry did not accept Freud's resolution of the long-standing medical puzzle created by the neuroses. They did not relish the dismissal of their life work as a "signal" failure, nor were they responsive to a causative theory that appeared to implicate society together with the individual violator of society's moral laws. What did not fuel their rejection of psychoanalysis, however, was sheer Victorian prudery. They were not recoiling in horror from the critical place of human sexuality in Freudian theory, for British alienists, nerve-doctors, consulting physicians, and general practitioners were no strangers to the force of sexuality in human relations. Even Freud's explicit focus on infantile sexuality, distasteful though it might be to British medical men and women, struck them as nothing new. They had heard as much from Maudsley, Savage, and others, native and foreign. The difference was, of course, that British medicine regarded sexual precocity in a pathological light, as proof of moral insanity, degeneracy, or at the very least a nervous diathesis, while Freudians accepted infantile and childhood sexuality as a normal aspect of human development, albeit one that merited careful attention. Furthermore, since British psychiatrists and nerve specialists had always included sexual excess among the possible causes of nervous collapse, Freud's selection of masturbation as the chief instigator of neurasthenia appeared to confirm much of their own outlook, but here, too, the similarities were merely superficial. What caused the physical exhaustion and extreme mental fatigue of neurasthenia, according to psychoanalytic theory, was not merely the excessive loss of semen attendant on prolonged sexual arousal, but the insupportable tension between the masturbator's desire for sexual gratification and civilization's voice of moral censure. Psychoanalysis cast the perpetrator in the role of victim as much as sinner, an ambiguity that Victorian psychiatrists could not accept, especially since Freud identified middle-class society as the locus of repression. The sexual aspect of neurotic illness was, nevertheless, a familiar enough concept in British psychiatry to mean that Freud's variation on that theme need not have provoked the hostility that greeted psychoanalysis in Great Britain before the war.[39]

If numerous British, as well as continental, psychiatrists in these years regarded psychoanalytic literature as little better than pornography, their attitude arose, not because Freud paid close attention to sexuality in examining the neuroses, but because he concentrated on nothing else. Whereas most alienists weighed a variety of interacting causes behind hysteria, neurasthenia, phobias, obsessions, and other neurotic afflictions, Freud seemed interested in one alone. His theory proclaimed that the force of the sexual drive and its repression were the primary reasons for the neuroticism of the times. To make matters worse, his work struck critics as little more than an unremitting spotlight on the most perverted forms of human sexuality. Worst of all, Freud not only blamed middle-class moral values for imposing the sexual self-restraint that promoted neurotic illness, but he also depicted the family, that most cherished of middle-class institutions, as a proverbial viper's nest. The sexual desires and tensions that Freud relentlessly probed all seethed within the family: sons hated fathers as they lusted for their mothers; daughters directed their sexual energy toward their fathers, creating fantasy sexual attachments that engendered countless cases of hysteria. Incest, real or far more often imagined, seemed to dominate familial relations, as depicted by Freud. No form of sexuality repelled the Viennese doctor, nor fell outside the scope of his tolerant explanations. Just at the time when the psychiatric profession was recognizing the existence of homosexuality and interpreting it as a particularly insidious threat to domestic and social order, Freud used his *Three Essays on the Theory of Sexuality* to elucidate how a child's sexual development could follow a path different from that leading to adult heterosexual preferences. He regarded homosexuality as a neurosis—not the innate condition that Symonds proclaimed it, but far from the crime that English law labeled it. He did not even consider homosexuality a vice. While it remained an arrested stage of development to his way of thinking, he could accept it as one among many possible ways in which human beings dealt with the imperious power of the libido. At the height of the moral and social hygiene crusade in Great Britain, such notions were utterly unthinkable.[40]

To men who had become medical psychologists in the third quarter of the nineteenth century, psychoanalysis seemed to violate the alienist's most fundamental responsibility: to help patients master their problems and to provide the moral guidance needed to steer each patient's wavering will back to fixity of purpose. Freudian psychotherapy, by contrast, evidently encouraged men and women to wallow in the very miseries that obsessed them. It either dredged up recollections that were better left buried or allowed the doctor's potent suggestions to create alleged memories that tormented patients more cruelly than their own thoughts ever did. In the years preceding the war, Allbutt expressed these attitudes most thoughtfully and Mercier most persistently.

Allbutt understood how much he instinctively shrank from the psychoanalytic approach to neurotic illness, for everything in his medical training told against it. "To me," the former commissioner in lunacy confessed in 1910,

> possibly from personal prejudice, the recent introspective and confessional methods are odious; if so, this prejudice may disqualify me from equitable judgment, as it certainly repels me from exact perusal, of certain modern books. . . . We are hearing enough and to spare of suggestion—but what about the doctor's suggestions to his marionettes, these morbid women and effeminate men, enticed to heat up sophisticated autobiographies, egotisms, and fictions? . . . For these secret introspective dramas, inflamed by reminiscent curiosity, are more than half facti-

tious. . . . If the human heart is deceitful above all things, if before the Father of Spirits we all dissemble, what conceits will not these disconsolates, craving even for scientific sympathy, imagine before the self-ordained confessor of the flesh? Is this by precept and example to develop self-command, to regenerate the faded self-respect?

To emphasize "the sexual passion beyond, and even to the neglect of other emotions," Allbutt contended, was a false and dangerous method; it entirely ignored the paramount fact that "in the calling of medicine especially, moral values have always held their pre-eminence." "If then," he continued, "medical influences are to be kept sweet and wholesome, we must consider the wiles of the human heart, conscious and half-conscious, with a decent reserve and in general terms, and in general terms brace the patient to rise superior to them; but this is not to be done by dabbling in them. The sickly person who analyses his sentiments for exhibition to his doctor begins inevitably to pose." Although he used the pronoun "his," Allbutt nonetheless believed that "these medical penitents are mostly women," all the likelier, by virtue of their sex, to suffer from "the very loss of self-control which we seek to repair." The only psychotherapy that Allbutt could justify to himself was what he called "'moral education' or re-education."[41] Mercier's attacks, by contrast, contained no shred of self-analysis. They were more in the nature of sledge-hammer blows against the pornography and immorality that he saw infecting the psychotherapeutic literature from the continent.[42]

Crichton-Browne withheld most of his comments about psychoanalysis until he had retired from professional life, after the Great War had made Freudian methods and principles reasonably familiar to the medical profession and the general public alike. In the 1920s, he was surprisingly moderate in tone, saying that the value of psychoanalysis was a "moot" point about which it was better to maintain "a prudent reserve." Unlike his colleague, Sir Robert Armstrong-Jones, the recently retired medical superintendent of Claybury Asylum, who in 1920 pronounced "'Freud-ism . . . dead in England today,'" Crichton-Browne was slow to articulate an overtly hostile point of view.[43] He hesitated largely because he feared that all forms of psychotherapy might suffer from the sweeping condemnation of Freud's work. In recent years, he believed, neurological investigations into the physiology of the brain had eclipsed "the mental symptoms of cerebral disorder," which had consequently received less close study than they merited. He insisted that there was "room for psycho-analysis of the right sort, involving no hazardous probings or questionable suggestions." He was sure that "the personal influence of the physician" mattered to a psychiatric patient and that "psychological means" could, in some instances, effect the cure that eluded "physiological methods."[44] For fear of throwing out the baby with the bath water, he refrained from roundly abusing Freudian psychoanalysis, at least for a time.

In the final decade of his life, however, as Freud's methods infiltrated more deeply into private psychiatric practice, Crichton-Browne's opinions grew more unequivocally adverse. He became certain that "unburdening the mind of traumatic memories" often led the patient to feel a "wounding sense of shame for having divulged . . . conduct or inclinations of a discreditable kind." Echoing the assertions that Allbutt had made twenty years before, Crichton-Browne cautioned that "the morbid mind under psycho-analysis sometimes comes to revel in its own wrongdoing, and invents transgressions that were never committed." Psycho-analysis, in brief, achieved the exact opposite of psychotherapy's proper goal—"to withdraw the patient's mind from the contemplation of an objectionable and painful past . . . and to occupy it with prospective duties and wholesome pursuits, and sure and certain hopes." With less restraint, he subsequently dismissed "the Freudians, with their dirty and dominating Œdipus complex" and protested that "passages in Freud's writing" were "capable of creating profound nausea."[45] He intensely disliked Freud's interpretation of dreams, calling on "decent people" to reject the claim that elements of sexuality are "seldom lacking in dreams." "Astonished and disgusted by all this jargon and quest of the unclean," Crichton-Browne was convinced that "any right-minded father who found out that his daughter had been subjected for an hour to dream interpretation of this kind" would subject the analyst to a well-placed kick. From time to time, a psychiatrist inevitably had to hear "painful confessions and elicit unsavoury truths," but that did not oblige him to "go boring in search of veins of pruriency or suggest it in every simple case." If any psychoanalyst tried to claim that the Socratic instruction to "Know thyself" was "a sort of forerunner of Freud," Crichton-Browne was ready to retort that the Austrian doctor's theories represented a "perversion of the dictum of Socrates, whom Freud resembles as much as a toadstool does a British oak."[46] Freudian psychotherapy was, in the end, utterly repugnant to the ninety-year-old veteran psychiatrist because it sent an intrusive searchlight into the most private recesses of human nature, from which Crichton-Browne had always preferred to avert his gaze, and because it mocked his celebration of domestic affections as the source of lasting health.

The small circle of Freud's admirers before 1914 expanded during the war as cathartic methods of treating shell-shocked soldiers proved valuable. Yet the employment of psychoanalytic techniques by some members of the Royal Army Medical Corps always proceeded in the face of entrenched psychiatric opposition and probably achieved some measure of success only because the military doctors who used Freudian insights to treat distraught servicemen largely ignored the sexual foundations of the therapeutic program. There was no need to probe a soldier's infancy for early sexual trauma in order to understand why the experience of the Western front had almost literally shattered his nerves. The conflict between overpowering fear and the demands of duty seemed to offer adequate enough explanation. Freud's work was, in fact, eviscerated for its first significant application in Great Britain and, no doubt, that operation helped make it more palatable to a suspicious public, ready to reject "Teutonic science" out of hand.[47] The reception of Freudian psychiatry among British medical psychologists born in the 1860s and 1870s—such as William H. R. Rivers, Hugh Crichton-Miller, Robert Henry Cole, William H. B. Stoddart, and Charles S. Myers—lies beyond the scope of this book, since it mainly reflected wartime experiences. Clearly, however, these men were willing to read in the lessons of the war the message that psychological forces alone could cause the breakdown of body as well as mind.

Although they had suspected as much for years, senior alienists and nerve specialists before the war not only rejected the bald assertion of a strictly psychological interpretation of neurotic collapse, but particularly disliked the Freudian elucidation of it. The priority granted to unconscious drives and repressions toppled all the props that had supported Victorian psychiatry and painted a shockingly hideous picture of human nature in the bargain. Although initially influenced by the prevalent late Victorian emphasis on hereditary taint, Freud's maturing ideas soon dispensed with the role of inheritance as a factor in neurotic illness.[48] They thereby eliminated the foundation for degeneration theory, which rendered psychiatry so many convenient services, and threatened to make irrelevant the evolutionary context that confirmed the alienists' pose as biological scientists. Indeed, Freud rendered irrelevant for psychiatry nerve force itself, which, despite its explanatory inadequacies where nervous breakdown was concerned, connected Edwardian psychiatrists with the inquiries of physiologists and neurologists. In dismissing an entire tradition of neuropsychiatric explanation, Freud threatened to expose precisely how much psychiatry was drifting away from somatic medicine. To alarmed alienists of Crichton-Browne's generation, it seemed that Freud's theories might undermine the very legitimacy of their own work, especially since the slight evidential basis for Freud's vast generalizations hardly upheld their contention that the methods of psychiatry were rigorously scientific. In the early 1890s, when Pierre Janet, the eminent French psychiatrist and former student of Charcot, examined the cases of 120 hysterical patients, he found four in which sexual desires played a significant causative role. British alienists could accept that kind of statistical evidence, which did not make the figures bear greater importance that they could justifiably carry. Freud based his epochal conclusions on a handful of cases, which offered grounds for speculation, according to his critics, but no reasons for certainty. It is understandable why Donkin, born in 1845, declared after the war that the "Unconscious Mind" featured in psychoanalysis was merely an assumption, part of an unscientific methodology that gave psychotherapy a bad name.[49]

The men who constituted a psychiatric "establishment" of sorts in the late nineteenth and early twentieth centuries may have been right to repudiate psychoanalysis, which has proven to be more theoretically provocative than therapeutically reliable. Its expense and the length of time necessary to complete treatment limit its usefulness for mental health specialists. Whether or not the response was valid, however, it underscored the reluctance of leading British psychiatrists in these years to confront psychological pain directly. They preferred to address its physical symptoms and treated the possible mental causes of depressive illness primarily by trying to rally the patient's will. From their perspective, to acknowledge that destructive and irrational urges were perfectly normal aspects of human nature seemed tantamount to sanctioning social chaos. World War I, in revealing the primacy of violence and brutality in human affairs, increased the readiness of younger British psychiatrists to accept some, or all, of Freud's theories, but their professional predecessors could not follow suit. It is ironic that the perception of their moral responsibilities, which were themselves purely psychological constructs, blocked these older men from sympathetically evaluating both of the exclusively psychological therapies—the hypnotic and the Freudian—that emerged in the late Victorian and Edwardian periods.

The irony is particularly striking in the case of psychoanalysis, for Freud offered British psychiatrists a potential solution to the problem they faced in identifying their own domain of medical practice, extending beyond the asylum but safe from the competition of neurologists and nerve-doctors. Freud's neuroses were not "nerve problems" at all, but riddles of a disordered mind that only specially trained psychiatrists could fathom. Having applied modified psychoanalytic techniques to shell-shocked soldiers during the war, C. S. Myers, an experimental psychologist with medical training, pronounced the emergence of a new species of doctor. The so-called functional nervous disorders, he explained in 1918, to an audience at the Royal Institution, are

> essentially of mental origin and demand treatment, not by those who have merely specialised in the effects of specific injuries of the brain, cord or nerves and in movement and sensation; . . . nor by asylum doctors whose life is largely spent among cases of advanced and more or less hopeless insanity. A new class of medical men, educated in the psychological theories and practice which I have described, is being trained. One centre of instruction has already sprung into existence during the war and others must be instituted.

Myers argued that "the treatment of cases of nervous breakdown," which concerned neither neurologists nor asylum officers, had to become the province of "specially trained physicians, in specially allocated hospitals." Three years later, T. S. Eliot, on the brink of nervous breakdown, could find no such consultants or facilities in England. Seeking "a specialist in psychological troubles," as he wrote to Julian Huxley in October 1921, he encountered only specialists "in nerves or insanity" and had to travel to Lausanne to find the kind of doctor he desired.[50] Nerves, he realized, were the least of his problems, nor was there anything seriously wrong with his mind; he was severely depressed and exhausted, with his emotions in disarray, and British medicine, he felt, was ill-equipped to relieve his specific condition.

For any alienist who wanted to become "a specialist in psychological troubles," psychoanalysis opened a door between neurology and asylum psychiatry. With its own vocabulary methodology, and rationale, it not only offered disciples an arcane branch of medicine, accessible only to the initiated, but also convinced them that they alone could heal the deep wounds of those whose psychological distress did not cross the boundary into madness. The great majority of British alienists before the war, however, were unwilling, and indeed unable, to perceive psychoanalysis in this advantageous light. Not only did it contest their notion of scientific credibility and medical legitimacy, but, like hypnotism, it invested its practitioners with a power over patients that Edwardian psychiatrists generally viewed with alarm. Never worrying that their own dominating personalities might create emotional dependence in the men and women who sought their help, they were quick to find such dangers in the psychotherapies they deplored. While confident that they always acted in the best interests of their patients, promoting autonomy and self-discipline as a matter of course, they contended that Freudian psychoanalysis degraded its patients just as thoroughly as hypnotism enslaved its victims.

In their frustrating attempts to create a psychiatry that both did justice to the psychological aspects of mental illness and commanded the respect of physical scientists, British alienists in the twenty-five years or so preceding the war registered the changes in terminology and classification that signified the efforts of their

European colleagues to distinguish more precisely between mental illness and neurological disability. Long before Freud expressed his dissatisfaction with the undifferentiated classification of the neuroses, other continental doctors had toyed with various terms and labels to underscore their growing realization that, despite frequent assertions to the contrary, a somatic etiology could not always explain mental afflictions. Hence the gradual acceptance in British psychiatric parlance of the word *psychosis,* which originated in Vienna in the 1840s, but only began to appear regularly in English during the 1870s and 1880s. Although there was considerable diversity in its usage, by the turn of the century it was generally employed to designate severe mental derangements affecting the powers of thought and reason. Since late Victorian psychiatrists no longer always found it plausible to ascribe an organic foundation to these disorders (or at least had given up hopes of finding one) they stressed instead their characteristic psychological aspect. Psychotic illness was, accordingly, separated from the class of functional nervous disorders, such as neurasthenia, for which some sort of physiological account was still offered in the pre-war years. The psychoses were recognized as far more severe and intractable than the neuroses. As Tuke lamented in 1881, "It must be frankly granted that Psychological Medicine can boast, as yet, of no specifics, nor is it likely, perhaps, that such a boast will ever be made. It may be difficult to suppress the hope, but we cannot entertain the expectation, that some future Sydenham will discover an anti-psychosis which will as safely and speedily cut short an attack of mania or melancholia as bark an attack of ague."[51]

In the early twentieth century, the stumbling block for those who worked to restructure psychiatry's scheme of classification was not so much mania, or other unmistakable signs of madness, as the less dramatic afflictions still labeled neurotic. Particularly with hysteria and neurasthenia, the pretense that they stemmed primarily from disturbances or deficiencies of the nervous system was wearing thin, but how to categorize them remained baffling to medical ingenuity. In both, the psychological manifestations were of obvious significance, yet they were not of psychotic proportions. The variations among the many cases of hysteria and neurasthenia further complicated the classifier's task, for some featured physical symptoms more prominently than mental ones, while in others the emotions alone appeared deranged. Freud's answer to this difficulty was severely to limit the characteristics of what he considered *real* neurasthenia—the actual neurosis—and to move all the other so-called neurasthenic manifestations, together with hysteria, into the more inclusive category of the psychoneuroses.

Pierre Janet handled the problem differently, by creating the disease category of *psychasthenia* to designate those neuroses in which the patient's perception of reality became impaired and the mind fell prey to obsessions, phobias, anxiety, and agitation. Although rooted in a physiological state of cerebral weakness, the symptoms of psychasthenia, according to Janet, were psychological, unlike the physical lethargy and exhaustion associated with neurasthenia. Janet, however, abandoned the whole concept of neurasthenia; because it corresponded to no specific somatic condition that he could identify, he considered it useless. His diagnostic system for the neuroses included only psychasthenia and hysteria, the former affecting the conscious mind, the latter working through the unconscious. He did not appear to realize that the same criticism he aimed against neurasthenia could be leveled against psychasthenia, which encompassed every bit as much diversity in its features as Beard's diagnostic invention managed to include. Psychasthenia nonetheless enjoyed a brief international vogue.[52]

In Great Britain, a few psychiatrists and nerve specialists adopted psychasthenia alongside, and not instead of, neurasthenia. W. H. B. Stoddart, for example, devoted a chapter to each in his textbook on *Mind and its Disorders* (1908). A few years later, Stoddart became a full-fledged Freudian, but in 1908 his vocabulary was closer to Janet's. In psychasthenia, he explained, "the mental state is such that some particular instinct is so uncontrollable and predominates to such a degree that it becomes a real annoyance to the person possessing it." While psychasthenia featured "irrepressible thoughts, fears and impulses," neurasthenia was marked chiefly "by an increased susceptibility to fatigue on slight exertion, mental or physical."[53] Schofield saw a real need for some such diagnostic classification as psychasthenia precisely in order to distinguish between the two main types of nervous collapse. "It is surely inadvisable," he reasoned just before the war,

> to place under the same category cases of ordinary nervous breakdown where the principal manifestations are emaciation, muscular debility, and incapacity for physical exertion with those other cases of asthenia of a cerebral type in which there may be no emaciation or muscular debility, but in which the manifestations consist almost entirely in diminished functional activity of the higher psychic centres, and [are] characterized by deficient will power and self-control, defective judgement, and a general incapacity for mental work.

It was a tidy division, but few cases fit neatly into one category or the other, and the new classification was never generally adopted in Great Britain. It encountered the opposition of influential medical men, like Clouston and Allbutt, as Schofield ruefully admitted, and remained more an indication of what was wrong with psychiatric categories in the early twentieth century than a way of fixing them.[54] The concept of neurasthenia, as an all-inclusive net designed to catch a rich assortment of physical and mental symptoms short of actual insanity, was simply disintegrating at the seams.

British alienists in the Edwardian decade demonstrated that they read German psychiatric literature as well as French. In particular, the efforts of Emil Kraepelin to refine the concepts of a manic-depressive psychosis and of dementia praecox worked their way into British discussions of the ongoing attempt to separate psychological afflictions from those of presumably nervous origin. Mercier remarked waspishly in 1914 on the "fashionable titles of dementia praecox and manic-depressive insanity that have of late become so popular," but Clouston, a few years earlier, had provided a more analytical commentary on Kraepelin's work. He praised the German psychiatrist for elucidating "the essential relationship between the conditions of morbid depression and elevation," but nonetheless insisted:

> It is in their practical treatment and management that their real mental distinctiveness and the importance of distinguishing the two states come in. The precautions against accident require to be different in each. The management of the one commonly differs from that of the other. The moral and mental treatment of each also differs.

> The medical treatment is mostly different too. Even if Kraepelin's scientific
> conception is a true one, they require to be differently regarded by the physician who
> has charge of them.[55]

Clouston, in short, valued a pragmatic approach to the needs of different patients over
a scientifically convincing argument for the union of mania and melancholia into a
single psychosis.

One senses that the collective heart of British psychiatry in the years just before
the war was not really committed to the international enterprise of reclassifying the
neuroses. British alienists did not contribute significantly to it, and there are more
than a few hints that they found it fundamentally irrelevant to their task of curing
unhappy men and women. In fact, much of the British literature on nervous and
mental ailments from this period largely ignores continental refinements and complications. Certainly for the general practitioner, the precise distinctions between
neurasthenia and psychasthenia, or among neuroses, psychoneuroses, and psychoses, were too subtle to be helpful in the daily round of medical care, but even
psychiatric specialists, as Clouston illustrated, tended to regard the continental
disputes over diagnostic terminology with a detachment bordering on indifference. If
they were superficially responsive to French and German ideas drifting across the
Channel from the 1880s through the early 1900s, they were also stubbornly resistant.

The effort by prominent Edwardian alienists to avoid making a deliberate choice
between somatic or psychological interpretations of nervous breakdown was doubtless sensible, given the state of their medical knowledge, but it helped to prolong the
professional identity crisis that had curtailed the growth of British psychiatry
throughout the nineteenth century. Nearly eighty more years of research into the
functions of the brain and the workings of the mind have not altered the situation as
much as one would like to think. Terminology has changed, it is true; people no
longer have nervous breakdowns, a label considered meaningless now that nerve
force has gone the way of animal spirits. Unfortunate men and women suffer instead
from varying degrees of depression, a category of illness that surely begs as many
questions as nervous exhaustion. The effort neatly to sever neuroses from psychoses
has collapsed, but new diagnostic distinctions, as confusing, ambiguous and unreliable as the Victorian and Edwardian ones, have multiplied. Psychiatrists today debate
the differences between adjustment disorders, anxiety disorders, and mood disorders,
as if some curative power resided in these elaborate taxonomies themselves. They
probe the contours of the chronic fatigue syndrome and create seemingly infinite
varieties of schizotypal, schizoaffective, and schizophreniform afflictions, not to
mention the frequently invoked "borderline personality disorder." No readier
solutions to the anguish of depression arise today than they did a century ago; no
omniscient guide through the mysterious realm where mind and body interact has yet
emerged.

The psychiatric profession continues to debate the respective merits of somatic
and psychological therapy, while still looking in vain for definitive solutions to the
puzzle of depression's etiology. Although late twentieth-century medicine is much
enlightened about the chemical bases of the disorder, which were unknown at the turn
of the last century, psychiatrists are by no means willing to dispense with psychologi-

cal modes of treatment, for antidepressants alone do not cure most cases of depression. The emotional and social triggers of this complex illness also receive their due recognition among the numerous agents that psychiatrists evaluate, and therapy, as in the nineteenth century, is designed to incorporate both physical intervention and psychological insights. The drugs and the psychotherapy may be more sophisticated today than the methods used by Victorian and Edwardian alienists, but the underlying goal remains the same: to find the optimum union of neurological remedy and psychiatric comfort for each patient. Nor has contemporary psychiatry determined the role of heredity in the development of depression, a question always uppermost in nineteenth-century speculations. Despite accumulating evidence that inheritance does, in fact, play a considerable part in molding personality traits, mood disorders, and even specific forms of mental illness, the contributions of nature and nurture remain as controversial an issue as they were in Galton's day.

The line separating healthy from pathological is no sharper to psychiatrists now than it appeared to their Victorian forefathers, and political, ideological, or cultural biases are no less potent in defining normalcy and its opposite. The psychiatric profession is still highly vulnerable to charges of gender prejudice, and the always difficult area of doctor–patient relationships is no less troubling than in earlier decades. Comparing psychiatrists to other medical practitioners in the 1970s, Richard Hunter, president of the History of Medicine Section of the Royal Society of Medicine, observed accusingly that "no other specialty blames illness—and therapeutic failure—on patients."[56] All these reasons contribute to psychiatry's status in Great Britain, even today, as the poor relation among medical disciplines, the branch of healing most frequently derided by all the others. To point out the notable continuity between the problems, both theoretical and practical, which frustrated Victorian psychiatry and which harass its professional descendants a century later is not so much to discredit the latter as to lighten the burden of criticism that we level against the former. It is easy to dismiss nineteenth-century psychiatry as exasperatingly misguided in some of its assumptions and downright pernicious in certain of its practices. Yet alienists then faced the same daunting conceptual enigmas of mind's influence on body and body's impact on mind that psychiatrists struggle to address today. If those early psychiatrists reached a stalemate in their efforts to unravel the mystery, it is only fair to acknowledge not only that their tools were primitive, but that, in certain fundamental respects, today's neuropsychiatrists, working with the most advanced equipment, have not been able to improve on their predecessors' tentative answers.

In other respects, of course, there have been far-reaching and profound changes. Three of the most common neurotic diagnoses of the nineteenth century—hysteria, hypochondriasis, and neurasthenia—have either disappeared entirely from psychiatric nomenclature or have been utterly transformed by twentieth-century notions of psychosomatic illness. The explosion of knowledge about the brain in the last decade alone has filled, with minutely precise physiological detail, much that had hitherto remained blank in the picture of the mind. Extraordinarily complex technology has been marshaled to reveal the structure and workings of the cerebral neurons, to analyze the chemical codes that issue instructions to the brain, to monitor the brain's electrical activity, to examine the role of neurotransmitters and receptors in the brain, and to study how other bodily systems, such as the circulatory and endocrine, affect the nerves. Molecular geneticists are even trying to isolate the gene or genes responsible for manic-depression. In a sense, however, the wealth of information has brought medical and public attitudes toward depression right back to the perspective dominant in the early and middle years of the nineteenth century.

At the start of Victoria's reign, when the belief prevailed that functional nervous disorders had a definite somatic origin waiting to be discovered, nervous collapse carried with it no burden of shame. By the late nineteenth century, when those neuroses for which no organic cause had been identified were coming to be viewed as essentially psychological disorders, nervous breakdown was beginning to acquire the taint of dishonor that has clung to it almost to the present day. If the problem had its roots in the mind, it was widely considered more disgraceful to its victim than a purely somatic disability that did not fall under the province of the will. In 1913, Ernest Jones regretted the popular view that the neurotic patient could get better if he only tried, "that he wilfully refuses to take his mind away from himself and his symptoms, and [that] substantially he is suffering from either deliberate perversity or capricious failure to use the will-power and self-control at his command."[57] After the war, the interpretation of nervous breakdown centered almost exclusively on the concept of the will's dereliction, since nerve force no longer figured in psychiatric explanations, and such abdication of will inevitably indicated some humiliating weakness of character, a reluctance to face responsibilities, or a pathetic ploy for attention. Freudian explanations of psychoneurotic ailments further added to the embarrassment of families who sheltered a victim of nervous breakdown. Today the new emphasis on the evidence for depression's biochemical bases has brought the illness out of the shadows, for the brain's biochemical processes are unequivocally not the patient's own fault, apart, of course, from the ravages of substance abuse. Neurological and psychological troubles are merging together again, and, although politicians running for office in the United States are not supposed to suffer from depression, in anyone else the illness now evokes a degree of sympathy and stimulates reasonably candid discussion. The sympathy is always contingent on the patient remaining sane and nonviolent, and it is always compromised by the fundamental fear that healthy people experience when observing loss of self-control in others, but a notable public interest in the problem of depression nonetheless allows an open, wide-ranging literature on the subject to flourish.

Depression, furthermore, is the illness that has served to establish the limits of impersonal, bureaucratic medicine. It constantly forces doctors to remember that patients cannot simply be processed, like broken machines in a repair shop, and that no uniform therapy will serve the needs of all sufferers. Each depressed man, woman, and child needs treatment tailored to personal situations; the elements of medication and psychotherapy required to help will differ from one depressed patient to the next. Among all the medical specialists practicing today, psychiatrists are supposed to be most attuned to the subtle counterpoint of mind and body, of individual and society. Despite the constraints imposed by medical ignorance and by their own presuppositions, Victorian and Edwardian alienists never lost sight of those interactions. Because they could not locate a lesion or isolate a microbe to account for most of the maladies they confronted, they had to focus on the entire patient, not on one or another fragmented, malfunctioning part. They understood the extent to which illness can encompass the whole body. Even Maudsley, not noted for his sympathy toward human weakness, adopted a curative policy that focused on the unique quality of each case in all its aspects. "He required that treatment should be adapted to the particular patient—'always the rule of rules should be to treat an individual who is sick, not an abstract disease.'"[58] If virtually every aspect of medicine before World War I appears attuned to holistic concerns in comparison with medical practices today, psychiatry was particularly hostile to the separation of mind and body for therapeutic purposes.

The tragedy of British psychiatry in the nineteenth and early twentieth centuries was that the genuine desire of its practitioners to cure people who suffered from elusive neurotic ailments was nullified in large part by the doctors' own endeavors. They wanted their patients to be at once autonomous and connected by meaningful ties to the social community, but their intrusive morality defined both the autonomy and the social bonds in a narrow, restrictive manner. Freedom, in their vocabulary, tended to mean little more than self-control, while their vision of healthy social intercourse revealed the prejudices of their class and gender. Within Victorian culture, evangelical religion never ceased to exert a powerful influence, making the struggle for moral progress and the performance of duty inescapable imperatives for all who aspired to social authority or intellectual respectability. Doctors and patients alike were caught within the same inexorable system of values that set forth the proper forms of conduct and the appropriate responsibilities for men and women, as well as for society's privileged few and unfortunate many. This cultural framework restricted psychiatry's development in the nineteenth century fully as much as did the limited information about cerebral physiology.

Self-reliance, self-restraint, and emotional independence under reason's sway— these were the virtues that British psychiatrists, throughout the nineteenth century, extolled from their cultural prison, for these were the qualities that enabled the individual to become an instrument of progress, in the form both of personal advancement and of social betterment. A faith in such instrumentality was as central to Victorian psychiatric thought as it was to Victorian culture at large, and, needless to say, it always rested on a belief in the potency of the directing will. Self-help, whether in the artisan's Friendly Society or the invalid's sick room, depended on the exercise of individual volition. Even C. S. Myers, as late as 1918, reflected the longevity and vitality of this British psychiatric tradition when he claimed that, in treating certain cases of shell shock, the doctor had to compel "the patient to pull himself together and to resume control over himself."[59] Victorian and Edwardian alienists particularly valued nervous breakdown as an experience from which the sufferer could derive a valuable lesson, and from which wise patients could profit for their moral benefit. As the doctor busily commented and counseled, the invalid listened and learned, using medical guidance to gain insights into past mistakes and to plot future courses of action. However great the disappointment wrought by the failure of moral management in the asylums, psychiatrists before World War I never lost their confidence in morally managing neurotic men and women. That an appeal to the moral sense of these troubled people was ultimately not in vain remained a central tenet of their professional credo. That some patients were inspired by this message, while others found it oppressive, may be inferred from the accounts they left behind. What remains beyond doubt is that, as products of Victorian society, victims of nervous breakdown always bore a sense of personal accountability—whether to God or humanity—that admonished them even in the depths of their despair.

NOTES

The following abbreviations appear throughout the Notes:

BMJ   *British Medical Journal*
Bull Hist Med   *Bulletin of the History of Medicine*
DNB   *Dictionary of National Biography*
JMS   *Journal of Mental Science*
J Psych Med   *Journal of Psychological Medicine and Mental Pathology*
OED   *Oxford English Dictionary*
WRLAMR   *West Riding Lunatic Asylum Medical Reports*

Introduction

1. Arthur Christopher Benson, *Beside Still Waters* (New York and London: G. P. Putnam's, 1907), p. 48.
2. Symonds to Henry Sidgwick, 3 March 1868, in Herbert M. Schueller and Robert L. Peters, eds., *The Letters of John Addington Symonds,* 3 vols. (Detroit: Wayne State University Press, 1967–69), 1:795.
3. J. A. Symonds, *The Memoirs of John Addington Symonds,* ed. Phyllis Grosskurth (Chicago: University of Chicago Press, 1986), p. 133.
4. Gerald L. Klerman, "Depression and Related Disorders of Mood (Affective Disorders)," in Armand M. Nicholi, Jr., ed., *The New Harvard Guide to Psychiatry* (Cambridge, Mass. and London: Belknap Press of Harvard University Press, 1988), pp. 319–20.
5. Henry Maudsley, "Suicide in Simple Melancholy," *Medical Magazine* 1(1892–93):46.
6. John Charles Bucknill, "The Diagnosis of Insanity," *Asylum Journal of Mental Science* 3(1857):154–57, provides a typical example of Victorian efforts to classify melancholia. He uses Johnson as a case in point. For a detailed discussion of "Melancholia in the Nineteenth Century," see Stanley W. Jackson, *Melancholia and Depression: From Hippocratic Times to Modern Times* (New Haven and London: Yale University Press, 1986), ch. 8.
7. Daniel Noble, *Elements of Psychological Medicine: An Introduction to the Practical Study of Insanity* (London: Churchill, 1853), p. xii.
8. Maudsley, "Suicide in Simple Melancholy," p. 51; A. C. Benson, *Thy Rod and Thy Staff* (London: Smith, Elder, 1912), p. 1; Henry Bence Jones, *The Life and Letters of Faraday,* 2 vols. (London: Longmans, Green, 1870), 2:126.
9. Eric T. Carlson and Norman Dain, "The Meaning of Moral Insanity," *Bull Hist Med* 36(March–April 1962):130.
10. Margaret Oliphant, *A Memoir of the Life of John Tulloch, D.D., LL.D.,* 3d ed. (Edinburgh and London: William Blackwood, 1889), pp. 164–68. Also see Margaret Oliphant, *Autobiography and Letters of Mrs. Margaret Oliphant,* ed. Mrs. Harry Coghill (Leicester: Leicester University Press, 1974), pp. 89–90 (first published in 1899).
11. Francis Galton, *Memories of My Life* (New York: E. P. Dutton, 1909), p. 155.

12. See Richard Hunter and Ida Macalpine, eds., *Three Hundred Years of Psychiatry, 1535–1860: A History Presented in Selected English Texts* (London and New York: Oxford University Press, 1963; reprint ed., Hartsdale, N.Y.: Carlisle Publishing, 1982), pp. 473–75. Throughout this book, I employ *neurosis* and *neurotic* in their nineteenth-century guise, as synonymous with or pertaining to functional nervous disorders.

13. P. W. Latham, "Neuroses," in Richard Quain, ed., *A Dictionary of Medicine* (London: Longmans, Green, 1882), p. 1033; P. W. Latham, "Neuroses," in Richard Quain, ed., *A Dictionary of Medicine,* 2d ed. rev., 2 vols. (London: Longmans, Green, 1894), 2:219.

14. Alfred T. Schofield, *Functional Nerve Diseases* (London: Methuen, 1908), p. v.

15. Thomas Smethurst, *Hydrotherapia; or, The Water Cure* (London: John Snow, 1843), p. 223; T. Clifford Allbutt, "Nervous Diseases and Modern Life," *Contemporary Review* 67(1895):218.

16. Alfred T. Schofield, *Nerves in Disorder. A Plea for Rational Treatment* (London: Hodder & Stoughton, 1903), p. 156.

17. Stuart Sutherland, *Breakdown: A Personal Crisis and a Medical Dilemma,* rev. ed. (London: Weidenfeld & Nicolson, 1987), pp. 146, 62.

18. See W. F. Bynum, "The Nervous Patient in Eighteenth- and Nineteenth-Century Britain: The Psychiatric Origins of British Neurology," in W. F. Bynum, Roy Porter, and Michael Shepherd, eds., *The Anatomy of Madness: Essays in the History of Psychiatry,* 2 vols. (London and New York: Tavistock Publications, 1985), 1:89–90.

19. On French psychiatry, see Jan Goldstein, *Console and Classify: The French Psychiatric Profession in the Nineteenth Century* (Cambridge and New York: Cambridge University Press, 1987), and, on shifting French psychiatric ideologies in particular, Ian Dowbiggin, "French Psychiatry and the Search for a Professional Identity: The Société Médico-Psychologique, 1840–1870," *Bull Hist Med* 63 (Fall 1989):331–55.

20. Thomas Willis, *Cerebri Anatome* (1664), translated and quoted in Edwin Clarke and L. S. Jacyna, *Nineteenth-Century Origins of Neuroscientific Concepts* (Berkeley and Los Angeles: University of California Press, 1987), p. 4.

21. Robert Whytt, *Observations on the Nature, Causes, and Cure of those Disorders which have been Commonly Called Nervous, Hypochondriac, or Hysteric, . . .* (Edinburgh: J. Balfour, 1765), p. iii.

22. Edwin Lee, *A Treatise on Some Nervous Disorders,* 2d ed. enl. (London: Churchill, 1838), p. 15 (first published in 1833); George Cheyne, *The English Malady: or, a Treatise of Nervous Diseases of all kinds, as Spleen, Vapours, Lowness of Spirits, Hypochondriacal, and Hysterical Distempers, . . .* (1733; reprint ed., Delmar, N.Y.: Scholars' Facsimiles & Reprints, 1976), pp. i–ii.

23. William R. Gowers, "The Use of Drugs" (1895), in *Lectures on Diseases of the Nervous System,* 2d ser. (London: Churchill, 1904), p. 237.

Chapter 1

1. See p. 15, of this book, for Gowers's remark; Dr. Trevelyan appears in Arthur Conan Doyle's "The Resident Patient," *Memoirs of Sherlock Holmes;* T. Clifford Allbutt, "Nervous Diseases and Modern Life," *Contemporary Review* 67(1895):217.

2. Susan Wheeler, "What the Public Saw: Medicine in Caricature in the Eighteenth and Early Nineteenth Centuries" (Paper presented at the Mid-Atlantic Conference on British Studies, New Haven, Conn., October 1989).

3. M. Jeanne Peterson, *The Medical Profession in Mid-Victorian London* (Berkeley and Los

Angeles: University of California Press, 1978), pp. 6–9. Also see A. H. T. Robb-Smith, "Medical Education at Oxford and Cambridge Prior to 1850," in F. N. L. Poynter, ed., *The Evolution of Medical Education in Britain* (London: Pitman Medical Publishing Co., 1966), pp. 19–45.

4. On surgeons and apothecaries in the eighteenth century, see Peterson, *Medical Profession in Mid-Victorian London,* pp. 9–12. All three categories of medical men in Georgian England are also discussed in Ivan Waddington, *The Medical Profession in the Industrial Revolution* (Dublin: Gill and Macmillan; Atlantic Highlands, N.J.: Humanities Press, 1984).

5. Robb-Smith, "Medical Education at Oxford and Cambridge," p. 51.

6. This summary of the emergence of the general practitioners and consultants draws heavily on Peterson, *Medical Profession in Mid-Victorian London,* and Waddington, *Medical Profession in Industrial Revolution* (see p. 17 for his estimate that general practitioners provided 90% of the qualified medical services in England during the 1830s). Also important is Irvine Loudon, *Medical Care and the General Practitioner, 1750–1850* (Oxford: Clarendon, 1986).

7. See Appendix A, in Peterson, *Medical Profession in Mid-Victorian London,* pp. 289–90.

8. Ibid., pp. 17–18n, 233–34.

9. These criteria are discussed throughout W. J. Reader, *Professional Men: The Rise of the Professional Classes in Nineteenth-Century England* (London: Weidenfeld & Nicolson; New York: Basic Books, 1966). For the medical profession specifically, most of the recent literature acknowledges a debt to Eliot Freidson, *Profession of Medicine. A Study of the Sociology of Applied Knowledge* (New York: Dodd, Mead, 1970). Also see Noel Parry and José Parry, *The Rise of the Medical Profession: A Study of Collective Social Mobility* (London: Croom Helm, 1976), and Vern L. Bullough, *The Development of Medicine as a Profession* (New York: Hafner, 1966).

10. This, in an abridged form, is the argument propounded by N. D. Jewson, in "Medical Knowledge and the Patronage System in Eighteenth-Century England," *Sociology* 8(1974):369–85, and "The Disappearance of the Sick-Man from Medical Cosmology, 1770–1870," *Sociology* 10(1976):225–44. Although the theory has been widely adopted by medical historians, Loudon's picture of medical practice in *Medical Care and the General Practitioner* challenges it.

11. Among many others arguing along similar lines, see Frank Mort, *Dangerous Sexualities: Medico-Moral Politics in England since 1830* (London and New York: Routledge & Kegan Paul, 1987), pp. 66–67, 72.

12. On the evidence for overcrowding in the early Victorian medical profession and for the subsequent shortage of qualified practitioners, see Waddington, *Medical Profession in Industrial Revolution,* pp. 139–41, 148–50.

13. Peterson, *Medical Profession in Mid-Victorian London,* pp. 196 (for "occupational subservience"), 116.

14. As is well illustrated in the passages quoted by Myron F. Brightfield, "The Medical Profession in Early Victorian England, as Depicted in the Novels of the Period (1840–1870)," *Bull Hist Med* 35(1961):238–39.

15. William L. Parry-Jones, *The Trade in Lunacy: A Study of Private Madhouses in England in the Eighteenth and Nineteenth Centuries* (London: Routledge & Kegan Paul, 1972), is the leading work on this subject.

16. Andrew T. Scull, *Museums of Madness: The Social Organization of Insanity in Nineteenth-Century England* (New York: St. Martin's Press, 1979), p. 25; Michael Donnelly, *Managing the Mind: A Study of Medical Psychology in Early Nineteenth-Century Britain* (London and New York: Tavistock Publications, 1983), pp. 22–23.

17. Scull, *Museums of Madness,* pp. 51n, 89; Nicholas Hervey, "A Slavish Bowing Down: The Lunacy Commission and the Psychiatric Profession 1845–60," in W. F. Bynum, Roy Porter, and Michael Shepherd, eds., *The Anatomy of Madness: Essays in the History of Psychiatry,* 2 vols. (London and New York: Tavistock Publications, 1985), 2:98–102.

18. On Battie, Morison, Conolly, and the early teaching of psychiatry, see Richard Hunter and Ida Macalpine, eds., *Three Hundred Years of Psychiatry, 1535–1860: A History Presented in Selected English Texts* (London and New York: Oxford University Press, 1963; reprint ed., Hartsdale, N.Y.: Carlisle Publishing, 1982), pp. 402, 769–70. On Cullen, see Andrew T. Scull, "From Madness to Mental Illness: Medical Men as Moral Entrepreneurs," *Archives européennes de sociologie* 16(1975):224. Also Charles Newman, "The Rise of Specialism and Postgraduate Education," in Poynter, ed., *Evolution of Medical Education,* p. 171, on Battie at St. Luke's.

19. Andrew T. Scull, "Mad-doctors and Magistrates: English Psychiatry's Struggle for Professional Autonomy in the Nineteenth Century," *Archives européennes de sociologie* 17(1976):281–82; *DNB,* s.v. "Bucknill, Sir John Charles."

20. Scull, "Madness to Mental Illness," pp. 226–29, 234–37, 250, 255–56. On the founding of the York Retreat, see Anne Digby, *Madness, Morality and Medicine: A Study of the York Retreat, 1796–1914* (Cambridge and New York: Cambridge University Press, 1985), pp. 1–32. From the late eighteenth century, small private asylums, run by lay proprietors, often advertised their facilities explicitly in terms of gentle, kindly treatment and variegated, distracting activities for inmates. See Charlotte MacKenzie, "Women and Psychiatric Professionalization, 1780–1914," in London Feminist History Group, *The Sexual Dynamics of History: Men's Power, Women's Resistance* (London: Pluto Press, 1983), pp. 108, 110.

21. Two medical certificates, from different doctors, were needed to commit private patients, one plus a magistrate's detention order for pauper lunatics. See Donnelly, *Managing the Mind,* p. 26; Hervey, "Slavish Bowing Down," p. 101; Scull, "Madness to Mental Illness," pp. 250, 256–57, and "Mad-doctors and Magistrates," pp. 280, 288.

22. Scull, *Museums of Madness,* pp. 112–13, 163; Hervey, "Slavish Bowing Down," pp. 103–104; Digby, *Madness, Morality and Medicine,* pp. 112, 305 n31. The new Lunacy Commission included legal as well as medical authorities.

23. D. Hack Tuke, "Medico-Psychological Association of Great Britain and Ireland," in D. Hack Tuke, ed., *A Dictionary of Psychological Medicine,* 2 vols. (London: Churchill, 1892), 2:786, and "Presidential Address delivered at the Annual Meeting of the Medico-Psychological Association," *JMS* 27(Oct. 1881):307. Also see Scull, "Mad-doctors and Magistrates," p. 280.

24. *DNB,* s.v. "Winslow, Forbes Benignus."

25. Ibid., s.v. "Bucknill, Sir John Charles." There existed fifty-one county asylums in 1881, as Tuke commented in his "Presidential Address," pp. 310–11. Alienists who retired from service in public asylums sometimes owned and managed private ones, in addition to maintaining a consulting practice. Nonmedical control of private asylums declined steadily in the second half of the nineteenth century. The post of Lord Chancellor's Visitor in Lunacy is discussed in the next chapter.

26. S. T. Anning, "Provincial Medical Schools in the Nineteenth Century," in Poynter, ed., *Evolution of Medical Education,* p. 125; *Who Was Who, 1897–1916,* s.v. "Clouston, Sir Thomas Smith," and "Winslow, Lyttleton Stewart Forbes"; *Who Was Who, 1916–1928,* s.v. "Savage, Sir George Henry."

27. Andrew Scull, "A Brilliant Career? John Conolly and Victorian Psychiatry," *Victorian*

Studies 27(Winter 1984):228. Also see Michael Collie, *Henry Maudsley: A Victorian Psychiatrist. A Bibliographical Study* (Winchester, England: St. Paul's Bibliographies, 1988); Aubrey Lewis, "Henry Maudsley: His Work and Influence," *JMS* 97(April 1951):259–62, 268–69; *Who Was Who, 1916–1928,* s.v. "Maudsley, Henry."

28. Lewis, "Maudsley," p. 274.
29. Great Britain, *Parliamentary Papers,* vol. 13 (1877) (*Reports*), "Report of the Select Committee on the Operation of the Lunacy Law," question 1590.
30. Scull, "Mad-doctors and Magistrates," pp. 302, 292–93.
31. *OED,* s.v. "alienist," "psychiatry," "psychiatrics," "psychiater," and "psychiatrist." For "psychiatrician," see W. H. O. Sankey, "On Melancholia," *JMS* 9(1863):176. On French and German use of *psychiatrie,* see Jan Goldstein, *Console and Classify: The French Psychiatric Profession in the Nineteenth Century* (Cambridge and New York: Cambridge University Press, 1987), pp. 6–7.
32. Charles Mercier, *Conduct and Its Disorders Biologically Considered* (London: Macmillan, 1911), p. ix; T. S. Clouston, *Unsoundness of Mind* (London: Methuen, 1911), p. xiv.
33. Tuke, "Medico-Psychological Association," pp. 786–87.
34. *OED,* s.v. "neurologist" and "neurology"; Richard Hunter, "Psychiatry and Neurology: Psychosyndrome or Brain Disease," *Proceedings of the Royal Society of Medicine* 66(April 1973):362. For Willis's coinage of "neurologie," see W. F. Bynum, "The Nervous Patient in Eighteenth- and Nineteenth-Century Britain: The Psychiatric Origins of British Neurology," in Bynum, Porter, and Shepherd, eds., *Anatomy of Madness,* 1:91.
35. "Nervous Disorders Accounted for Philosophically," *Family Oracle of Health* 2(1825):291; Gordon Gordon-Taylor and E. W. Walls, *Sir Charles Bell: His Life and Times* (Edinburgh and London: Livingstone, 1958); *DNB,* s.v. "Mayo, Herbert." On the "reflex" researches of Hall and Laycock, see Edwin Clarke and L. S. Jacyna, *Nineteenth-Century Origins of Neuroscientific Concepts* (Berkeley and Los Angeles: University of California Press, 1987), pp. 114–24, 141–47.
36. Charlotte Hall, *Memoirs of Marshall Hall, M.D., F.R.S* (London: Richard Bentley, 1861), p. 142; William Hale-White, *Great Doctors of the Nineteenth Century* (London: Edward Arnold, 1935), pp. 85–105; *DNB,* s.v. "Hall, Marshall."
37. Thomas Laycock, "On the Naming and Classification of Mental Diseases and Defects," *JMS* 9(July 1863):153; T. S. Clouston, *The Hygiene of Mind* (London: Methuen, 1906), p. 66; *DNB,* s.v. "Laycock, Thomas."
38. Tuke, "Presidential Address," p. 340. The ophthalmoscope is an instrument for inspecting the retina; the sphygmograph reveals the pulse in a series of curves. Also see Hunter, "Psychiatry and Neurology," p. 362, and Bynum, "Nervous Patient," p. 96.
39. Bynum, "Nervous Patient," p. 96.
40. The officers, rules, and objects of the Neurological Society were published at the back of *Brain* 14(1891). A subsequent list of presidents appeared at the back of vol. 23(1900). On Tuke, see *DNB,* s.v. "Tuke, Daniel Hack."
41. Lewis, "Maudsley," p. 275.
42. These developments form the theme of Robert M. Young, *Mind, Brain and Adaptation in the Nineteenth Century: Cerebral Localization and its Biological Context from Gall to Ferrier* (Oxford: Clarendon, 1970).
43. Gordon Holmes, *The National Hospital, Queen Square, 1860–1948* (Edinburgh and London: Livingstone, 1954), pp. 7–11, 69–71; Bynum, "Nervous Patient," pp. 96–97.
44. George Savage, "Dr. Hughlings Jackson on Mental Disorders," *JMS* 63(July 1917):322–

23; E. Stengel, "Hughlings Jackson's Influence in Psychiatry," *British Journal of Psychiatry* 109(1963):351; H. Tristram Engelhardt, Jr., "John Hughlings Jackson and the Mind-Body Relation," *Bull Hist Med* 49(Summer 1975):147.

45. Stengel, "Jackson's Influence in Psychiatry," pp. 348, 352; James Sully, *My Life & Friends* (London: T. Fisher Unwin, 1918), p. 172.

46. Seymour J. Sharkey, "Hysteria and Neurasthenia," *Brain* 27(1904):2.

47. Stephen Trombley, *'All That Summer She Was Mad': Virginia Woolf and Her Doctors* (London: Junction Books, 1981), ch. 5 on Head; *DNB 1931–1940*, s.v. "Head, Sir Henry." Also see Quentin Bell, *Virginia Woolf, A Biography*, 2 vols. in 1 (New York: Harcourt Brace Jovanovich, 1972), 2:14–16.

48. Henry Harnett, "Observations on Insanity . . ." *Water Cure Journal and Hygienic Magazine* 2(1849):371.

49. W. S. Playfair, *The Systematic Treatment of Nerve Prostration and Hysteria* (London: Smith, Elder, 1883); *DNB 1901–1911*, s.v. "Playfair, Willliam Smoult."

50. Margaret Oliphant, *A Memoir of the Life of John Tulloch, D.D., LL.D.*, 3d ed. (Edinburgh and London: William Blackwood, 1889), pp. 244–45; J. A. Symonds, *The Memoirs of John Addington Symonds*, ed. Phyllis Grosskurth (Chicago: University of Chicago Press, 1986), pp. 134–35, 151–52. On Wells's career, see John A. Shepherd, *Spencer Wells: The Life and Work of a Victorian Surgeon* (Edinburgh and London: Livingstone, 1965), and *DNB*, s.v. "Wells, Sir Thomas Spencer."

51. Great Britain, *Parliamentary Papers* (Commons), vol. 61 (1884) (*Accounts and Papers*, vol. 15), "Elementary Schools (Dr. Crichton-Browne's Report)," p. 20 [of the report]; *DNB Supplement*, s.v. "Quain, Sir Richard"; and "Obituary. Sir Richard Quain, Bart.," *BMJ*, 19 March 1898, pp. 793–95.

52. *DNB Supplement*, vol. 2, s.v. "Clark, Sir Andrew." Also see "Obituary. Sir Andrew Clark, Bart.," *Lancet*, 11 Nov. 1893, pp. 1222–25, and "Obituary. Sir Andrew Clark, Bart.," *BMJ*, 11 Nov. 1893, pp. 1055–62. On Clark and Spencer, see Walter Troughton, "Typescript Account of H. Spencer's Life, 1888–1903," Herbert Spencer Papers, MS 791/355/3, University of London Library, Senate House, London, p. 5. Ralph Colp, Jr., *To Be an Invalid: The Illness of Charles Darwin* (Chicago: University of Chicago Press, 1977), pp. 88–90, discusses Clark's prescriptions for Darwin in the 1870s. On Clark and Tulloch, see Oliphant, *Tulloch*, p. 375. The casebooks of Frederick Parkes Weber in the Contemporary Medical Archives Centre of the Wellcome Institute for the History of Medicine, London, suggest the degree to which indefinite nervous complaints figured in the practice of a Harley St. consultant between about 1890 and World War I.

53. David Drummond, "Neurasthenia: Its Nature and Treatment," *BMJ*, 7 July 1906, p. 11.

54. Todd is frequently mentioned in David Newsome, *On the Edge of Paradise: A. C. Benson: The Diarist* (London: John Murray, 1980). For Margaret Benson's breakdown in 1907, see pp. 219–20.

55. Alfred T. Schofield, *The Management of a Nerve Patient* (London: Churchill, 1906), pp. 240–41. Information on Dowse was gleaned from the title pages of his books. For Schofield, I also used his singularly uninformative entry in *Who Was Who, 1929–1940*.

56. Erwin H. Ackerknecht, *A Short History of Medicine*, rev. ed. (Baltimore: Johns Hopkins University Press, 1982), p. 163.

57. Tuke, "Presidential Address," p. 326.

58. See Scull, "From Madness to Mental Illness," pp. 251–52 n132, for a mass of quotations to that effect, taken from the first half of the nineteenth century.

59. Tuke, "Presidential Address," pp. 326–27, 330.

60. Sankey, "On Melancholia," p. 175; Tuke, "Presidential Address," pp. 326, 330; T. S.

Clouston, "The Prodromata of the Psychoses, and Their Meaning," *Review of Neurology and Psychiatry* 1(1903):789–90.

61. "Desk Diseases," *Family Oracle of Health* 1(1824):417–19, and "October Diseases, and the Means of Escaping Them," *Family Oracle of Health* 2(1825):85, among numerous examples; Benjamin Collins Brodie, *Autobiography of the Late Sir Benjamin C. Brodie, Bart.* (London: Longman, Green, Longman, Roberts, & Green, 1865), pp. 112–13; Clouston, *Hygiene of Mind*, p. 34.

62. Scull, "From Madness to Mental Illness," p. 251.

63. For examples of "functional lesion" spanning the Victorian and Edwardian decades, see John Conolly, "Hysteria," in John Forbes, Alexander Tweedie, and John Conolly, eds., *The Cyclopædia of Practical Medicine*, 4 vols. (London: Sherwood, Gilbert, Piper, Baldwin, and Cradock, 1833–35), 2:567, and A. T. Schofield, *Functional Nerve Diseases* (London: Methuen, 1908), p. 60.

64. Tuke, "Presidential Address," pp. 326–29.

65. See Scull, "Mad-doctors and Magistrates," pp. 285–86, 301.

66. Tuke, "Presidential Address," pp. 324–25.

67. Charlotte MacKenzie, "Social Factors in the Admission, Discharge, and Continuing Stay of Patients at Ticehurst Asylum, 1845–1917," in Bynum, Porter, and Shepherd, eds., *Anatomy of Madness*, 2:169.

68. This paragraph is heavily indebted to Christopher Lawrence, "Incommunicable Knowledge: Science, Technology and the Clinical Art in Britain 1850–1914," *Journal of Contemporary History* 20(October 1985):503–20. Also see Peterson, *Medical Profession in Mid-Victorian London*, pp. 152–57.

69. *DNB*, s.v. "Holland, Sir Henry." Colp, *To Be an Invalid*, makes frequent reference to Holland, who was Darwin's second cousin, as well as sometime medical attendant.

70. Zuzanna Shonfield, *The Precariously Privileged: A Professional Family in Victorian London* (Oxford and New York: Oxford University Press, 1987), p. 137.

71. "Obituary. Sir Andrew Clark," *Lancet*, 11 Nov. 1893, p. 1224; C. Hall, *Memoirs of Marshall Hall*, pp. 121–22.

72. See Hervey, "Slavish Bowing Down," pp. 115, 126 n112, 128–29; Peterson, *Medical Profession in Mid-Victorian London*, p. 156; *DNB*, s.v. "Morison, Sir Alexander," and "Southey, Henry Herbert."

73. Elaine Showalter, *The Female Malady: Women, Madness, and English Culture, 1830–1980* (New York: Pantheon Books, 1985), p. 117, discusses the sporting passions of late Victorian alienists. Also see *Who Was Who, 1916–1928*, s.v. "Savage, Sir George."

74. Peterson, *Medical Profession in Mid-Victorian London*, pp. 204, 344 n28; Richard A. Hunter and H. Phillip Greenberg, "Sir William Gull and Psychiatry," *Guy's Hospital Reports* 105(1956):372–73; *DNB*, s.v. "Gull, Sir William Withey," and *DNB 1901–1911*, s.v. "Wilks, Sir Samuel." Wilks's *Lectures on Diseases of the Nervous System* first appeared in 1878, with a second edition in 1883.

75. Hunter and Macalpine, *Three Hundred Years of Psychiatry*, p. 870.

76. *DNB 1922–1930*, s.v. "Allbutt, Sir Thomas Clifford," and *Who Was Who, 1897–1916*, s.v. "Clouston, Sir Thomas Smith."

77. Mort, *Dangerous Sexualities*, explores this theme in great detail.

78. David Skae, "A Rational and Practical Classification of Insanity," *JMS* 9(Oct. 1863):314; for a sample of Maudsley's statements on this topic, see his *Body and Mind: An Inquiry into their Connection and Mutual Influence* (London: Macmillan, 1870), p. 108; *The Pathology of Mind* (London: Macmillan, 1879), p. 68; *Natural Causes and Supernatural Seemings*, 2d ed. (London: Kegan Paul, Trench, 1887), p. 191.

79. N. D. Jewson's work has been particularly influential in establishing this interpretation. See Jewson, "Disappearance of Sick-Man," pp. 228–29, 233, 235–37 (p. 229 for the quotation). Eric T. Carlson and Norman Dain discuss the "psychosomatic orientation" of eighteenth- and early nineteenth-century medicine, and its decline later in the Victorian period, in "The Meaning of Moral Insanity," *Bull Hist Med* 36(March–April 1962):134, 137. Also see Charles E. Rosenberg, "Body and Mind in Nineteenth-Century Medicine: Some Clinical Origins of the Neurosis Construct," *Bull Hist Med* 63(Summer 1989): 185–97.

80. Benjamin Ward Richardson, *The Field of Disease: A Book of Preventive Medicine* (London: Macmillan, 1883), p. 618.

81. Bruce Haley, *The Healthy Body and Victorian Culture* (Cambridge, Mass: Harvard University Press, 1978), p. 45; Clouston, *Hygiene of Mind,* pp. 93–100.

82. See Michael J. Clark, "The Rejection of Psychological Approaches to Mental Disorder in Late Nineteenth-Century British Psychiatry," in Andrew Scull, ed., *Madhouses, Mad-Doctors, and Madmen: The Social History of Psychiatry in the Victorian Era* (London: Athlone Press; Philadelphia: University of Pennsylvania Press, 1981), pp. 274–76, for a summary of the Victorian psychiatric theory of the will; also Haley, *Healthy Body,* pp. 40–45.

83. J. D. Morell, "Modern English Psychology," *British and Foreign Medico-Chirurgical Review,* n.s. 17 (1856):351.

84. Th. Ribot, "Disorders of Will," in Tuke, ed., *Dictionary of Psychological Medicine,* 2:1366–68.

85. Lewis, "Maudsley," p. 270. Also see L. S. Jacyna, "The Physiology of Mind, the Unity of Nature, and the Moral Order in Victorian Thought," *British Journal for the History of Science* 14(July 1981):114–15.

86. Henry Holland, *Chapters on Mental Physiology,* 2d ed., rev. and enl. (London: Longman, Brown, Green, Longmans, & Roberts, 1858), p. 95; Richardson, *Field of Disease,* p. 629; and Henry Maudsley, "Suicide in Simple Melancholy," *Medical Magazine* 1(1892–93):48.

87. J. C. Bucknill, "The President's Address to the Association," *JMS* 7(Oct. 1860):7.

88. Charles Darwin, *The Autobiography of Charles Darwin 1809–1882,* ed. Nora Barlow (New York: Norton, 1969), pp. 31–32.

89. Clark, "Rejection of Psychological Approaches," pp. 292–300, offers a penetrating discussion of these moral-pastoral responsibilities, especially with regard to psychiatrists.

90. The story, from Samuel Wilks, *Lectures on Diseases of the Nervous System,* 2d ed. (1883), is told in Hunter and Greenberg, "Gull and Psychiatry," p. 374.

91. Leonard G. Guthrie, *Functional Nervous Disorders in Childhood* (London: Oxford University Press, 1907), pp. 4, 23. For reservations about the place of "the confessional" in psychiatry, see Joseph A. Ormerod, "Hysteria," in Clifford Allbutt and Humphry Davy Rolleston, eds., *A System of Medicine,* 2d ed. rev., 9 vols. (London: Macmillan, 1905–1911), 8:693.

92. Goldstein, *Console and Classify,* p. 5. Also see Ruth Harris, "Murder under Hypnosis in the Case of Gabrielle Bompard: Psychiatry in the Courtroom in Belle Epoque Paris," in Bynum, Porter, and Shepherd, eds., *Anatomy of Madness,* 2:221.

93. See Mort, *Dangerous Sexualities,* pt. 1, for a lengthy discussion of this alliance.

94. Daniel Noble, *Elements of Psychological Medicine. An Introduction to the Practical Study of Insanity* (London: Churchill, 1853), pp. 82–83.

95. Thomas Stretch Dowse, *On Brain and Nerve Exhaustion: 'Neurasthenia'. Its Nature and Curative Treatment* (London: Baillière, Tindall, & Cox, 1880), p. 35. Also see William F. Bynum, Jr., "Rationales for Therapy in British Psychiatry, 1780–1835," in Scull, ed.,

Madhouses, pp. 38–40, 49; Clark, "Rejection of Psychological Approaches," p. 285; Scull, *Museums of Madness,* pp. 159–60.

96. As Jacyna observes, in "Physiology of Mind," p. 117. Although I disagree with some of Jacyna's conclusions, my ideas in the paragraph were aroused by his invaluable article.

97. Tuke, "Medico-Psychological Association," p. 786; Hervey, "Slavish Bowing Down," pp. 128–29; *DNB,* s.v. "Prichard, James Cowles."

98. James Cowles Prichard, *A Treatise on Insanity and Other Disorders Affecting the Mind* (London: Sherwood, Gilbert, and Piper, 1835), p. 19; George H. Savage, "Moral Insanity," *JMS* 27(July 1881):148. Also see Carlson and Dain, "Meaning of Moral Insanity," pp. 130–40; and Denis Leigh, *The Historical Development of British Psychiatry,* vol. 1 (Oxford: Pergamon Press, 1961), pp. 186–89, for a useful summary of the problems implicit in Prichard's concept.

99. Prichard, *Treatise on Insanity,* p. 18; Savage, "Moral Insanity," p. 154.

100. The diagnosis of moral insanity was not applied constantly after 1835, but enjoyed spurts of popularity during the rest of Victoria's reign. When applied in cases of suicide, or in criminal trials, it represented an effort to liberalize the law in the name of humane reform rather than an exercise in labeling deviancy. See Olive Anderson, *Suicide in Victorian and Edwardian England* (Oxford: Clarendon, 1987), pp. 229–30.

101. Michel Foucault, *Madness and Civilization: A History of Insanity in the Age of Reason,* trans. Richard Howard (New York: Pantheon, 1965)—first published in Paris in 1961. Andrew Scull has played a leading role in coloring the study of Victorian psychiatry in the tones of social control theory. In addition to Scull's *Museums of Madness,* see "From Madness to Mental Illness," p. 219, and "Was Insanity Increasing? A Response to Edward Hare," *British Journal of Psychiatry* 144(1984):432–36, for examples of the social control assumptions dominating his work. Roger Smith shares this viewpoint in *Trial by Medicine: Insanity and Responsibility in Victorian Trials* (Edinburgh: Edinburgh University Press, 1981), and so does Richard Russell, "Mental Physicians and Their Patients: Psychological Medicine in the English Pauper Lunatic Asylums of the Later Nineteenth Century" (Ph.D. diss., University of Sheffield, 1983). It is impossible to list here all the books, articles, and theses that embrace this perspective. It often appears as a simple statement of fact, as, for example, in Trombley, *'All That Summer She Was Mad,'* p. 2. For an overview of the subject, beyond the field of medical history, see A. P. Donajgrodzki, ed., *Social Control in Nineteenth Century Britain* (London: Croom Helm; Totowa, N.J.: Rowman & Littlefield, 1977); and F. M. L. Thompson's thoughtful critique of the concept, "Social Control in Victorian Britain," *Economic History Review,* 2d ser., 34(May 1981):189–208.

102. MacKenzie, "Patients at Ticehurst," p. 151. For challenges to, or modifications of, the social control hypothesis with regard to Victorian psychiatry, also see J. K. Walton, "Casting Out and Bringing Back in Victorian England: Pauper Lunatics, 1840–70," in Bynum, Porter, and Shepherd, eds., *Anatomy of Madness,* 2:132–46; in the same volume, Anne Digby, "Moral Treatment at the Retreat, 1796–1846," pp. 52–72 (as well as her book, *Madness, Morality and Medicine*); and Henry Gilbert Orme and William H. Brock, *Leicestershire's Lunatics: The Institutional Care of Leicestershire's Lunatics during the Nineteenth Century* (Leicester, England: Leicestershire Museum Publications, 1987).

103. Thompson, "Social Control in Victorian Britain," p. 189.

104. Tuke, "Presidential Address," pp. 340–41.

105. Walton, "Casting Out and Bringing Back," p. 135.

106. Karl Figlio, for example, offers such an argument in "Chlorosis and Chronic Disease in

Nineteenth-Century Britain: The Social Constitution of Somatic Illness in a Capitalist Society,'' *Social History* 3(May 1978):176, 179. Many of the points raised in this paragraph also apply to the treatment of affluent insane patients in private asylums.

107. The relevance of the psychiatric theory of the will for notions of social order and governing hierarchy is explored in Elizabeth Fee, ''Psychology, Sexuality, and Social Control in Victorian England,'' *Social Science Quarterly* 58(March 1978):632–42, and Jacyna, ''Physiology of Mind,'' where the argument is extended to concepts of universal order and divine will, which did not invariably figure in the man-centered concerns of Victorian alienists. Thompson, ''Social Control in Victorian Britain,'' p. 206, also sparked some of the ideas in this paragraph. One important criticism of the social control hypothesis, not directly pertinent to my discussion, centers on the richness, strength, and diversity of working-class culture, which was far less amenable to molding from above than is often assumed.

Chapter 2

1. Throughout this volume, I hyphenate ''Crichton-Browne,'' although Sir James himself did not begin to do so until the late 1870s, and not even consistently thereafter. Most indexes and bibliographies today, however, alphabetize him under ''C.'' The *DNB 1931–1940* is a notable exception.

2. James Crichton-Browne, Foreword (dated 1936) to *The Chronicle of Crichton Royal (1833–1936)*, by Charles Cromhall Easterbrook (Dumfries: Courier Press, 1940), p. 1; ''Obituary. Sir James Crichton–Browne,'' *Times* (London), 1 Feb. 1938, p. 16; G. M. Holmes, ''Sir James Crichton-Browne,'' *Obituary Notices of Fellows of the Royal Society* 2(1936–38):520; ''Obituary. Sir James Crichton-Browne,'' *BMJ,* 5 Feb. 1938, pp. 311–12; ''Obituary. Sir James Crichton-Browne,'' *Lancet,* 12 Feb. 1938, pp. 406–407.

3. D. Hack Tuke, ''Presidential Address delivered at the Annual Meeting of the Medico-Psychological Association,'' *JMS* 27(Oct. 1881):311, and ''Medico-Psychological Association of Great Britain and Ireland,'' in D. Hack Tuke, ed., *A Dictionary of Psychological Medicine,* 2 vols. (London: Churchill, 1892), 2:786; James Harper, ''Dr. W. A. F. Browne,'' *Proceedings of the Royal Society of Medicine* 48(1955):590–93; Easterbrook, *Crichton Royal,* pp. ix, 1–3; Richard Hunter and Ida Macalpine, eds., *Three Hundred Years of Psychiatry, 1535–1860: A History Presented in Selected English Texts* (London and New York: Oxford University Press, 1963; reprint ed., Hartsdale, N.Y.: Carlisle Publishing, 1982), pp. 865–66.

4. W. A. F. Browne, ''The Moral Treatment of the Insane,'' *JMS* 10(Oct. 1864):311. Andrew T. Scull, *Museums of Madness: The Social Organization of Insanity in Nineteenth-Century England* (New York: St. Martin's Press, 1979), p. 160, discusses ''the ultimately theological grounds'' for Browne's ''somatic ideology,'' which were apparent in *What Asylums Were, Are, and Ought to Be: Being the Substance of Five Lectures Delivered Before the Managers of the Montrose Royal Lunatic Asylum* (Edinburgh: Adam & Charles Black, 1837).

5. Lional John Beale, *The Senses, the Brain, and the Mind; Their Connections and Relations* (London: Harrison, 1860), p. 22. See Janet Oppenheim, *The Other World: Spiritualism and Psychical Research in England, 1850–1914* (Cambridge and New York: Cambridge University Press, 1985), pp. 208–10, for the spiritual strain lurking beneath phrenology's materialist veneer.

6. William F. Bynum, Jr., ''Rationales for Therapy in British Psychiatry, 1780–1835,'' in Andrew Scull, ed., *Madhouses, Mad-Doctors, and Madmen: The Social History of*

Psychiatry in the Victorian Era (London: Athlone Press; Philadelphia: University of Pennsylvania Press, 1981), pp. 50–52.

7. Jan Goldstein, *Console and Classify: The French Psychiatric Profession in the Nineteenth Century* (Cambridge and New York: Cambridge University Press, 1987), pp 155–56. See Chapters 3 and 5 of this invaluable study for a detailed discussion of Pinel's contribution to the theory and practice of moral management, and Esquirol's concept of monomania.

8. Anne Digby, *Madness, Morality and Medicine: A Study of the York Retreat, 1796–1914* (Cambridge and New York: Cambridge University Press, 1985), pp. 244–45, and "Moral Treatment at the Retreat, 1796–1846," in W. F. Bynum, Roy Porter, and Michael Shepherd, eds., *The Anatomy of Madness: Essays in the History of Psychiatry*, 2 vols. (London and New York: Tavistock Publications, 1985), 2:63; Andrew Scull, "A Victorian Alienist: John Conolly, FRCP, DCL (1794–1866)," in *Anatomy of Madness*, 1:123–25; Bynum, "Rationales for Therapy," pp. 51–52; on the Ellises at Hanwell, see Charlotte MacKenzie, "Women and Psychiatric Professionalization, 1780–1914," in London Feminist History Group, *The Sexual Dynamics of History: Men's Power, Women's Resistance* (London: Pluto Press, 1983), pp. 111–12.

9. Harper, "Dr. W. A. F. Browne," p. 592. All the information concerning Browne's activities at Crichton Royal comes from Harper's article and from Easterbrook, *Chronicle of Crichton Royal*, p. 4. Crichton-Browne reminisced about his father's work in *What the Doctor Thought* (London: Ernest Benn, 1930), pp. 41–42, and *Stray Leaves from a Physician's Portfolio* (London: Hodder & Stoughton, [1927]), p. 350.

10. Harper, "Dr. W. A. F. Browne," passim.

11. Quoted in Ibid., pp. 592, 591.

12. "Obituary. Sir James Crichton-Browne," *Times* (London), 1 Feb. 1938, p. 16; James Crichton-Browne, *Victorian Jottings from an Old Commonplace Book* (London: Etchells & MacDonald, 1926), pp. 15–16; *DNB*, s.v. "Riddell, Henry Scott," where Riddell's asylum confinement is dated 1841–44.

13. Browne's 1864 lecture, "The Moral Treatment of the Insane," reveals a heavy stress on the physiological side of mental illness. Andrew T. Scull, "From Madness to Mental Illness: Medical Men as Moral Entrepreneurs," *Archives européennes de sociologie* 16(1975):252–53, 255, comments on the moral *and* somatic emphases in Browne's work.

14. Crichton-Browne, *Victorian Jottings*, pp. 1–7, 28; Easterbrook, *Chronicle of Crichton Royal*, p. 4; *DNB*, s.v. "Balfour, John Hutton."

15. John Dixon Comrie, *History of Scottish Medicine*, 2d ed., 2 vols. (London: Baillière, Tindall & Cox, for the Wellcome Historical Medical Museum, 1932), 1:303, 340, 365, 2:715; H. P. Tait, "Medical Education at the Scottish Universities to the Close of the Eighteenth Century," in F. N. L. Poynter, ed., *The Evolution of Medical Education in Britain* (London: Pitman Medical Publishing Co., 1966), pp. 53–68; Vern and Bonnie Bullough, "The Causes of the Scottish Medical Renaissance of the Eighteenth Century," *Bull Hist Med* 45(Jan.–Feb. 1971):13–28; Christopher Lawrence, "Ornate Physicians and Learned Artisans: Edinburgh Medical Men, 1726–1776," in W. F. Bynum and Roy Porter, eds., *William Hunter and the Eighteenth-Century Medical World* (Cambridge: Cambridge University Press, 1985), pp. 153–76.

16. A. J. Youngson, *The Scientific Revolution in Victorian Medicine* (London: Croom Helm, 1979), p. 57. Also see A. H. T. Robb-Smith, "Medical Education at Oxford and Cambridge Prior to 1850," in Poynter, ed., *Evolution of Medical Education*, pp. 19–52.

17. Forbes Winslow, *On the Preservation of the Health of Body and Mind* (London: Henry Renshaw, 1842), p. 139.

18. *DNB 1931–1940*, s.v. "Browne, Sir James Crichton-," gives a list of his professors at Edinburgh. Crichton-Browne wrote about some of his teachers in *What the Doctor*

Thought, p. 202, and *From the Doctor's Notebook* (London: Duckworth, 1937), pp. 32, 59–60. See individual entries in the *DNB* for biographical information about these men.

19. Crichton-Browne, *Victorian Jottings,* p. 36.

20. J. Crichton-Browne, "The History and Progress of Psychological Medicine," *JMS* 7(April 1861):19, 23–26, 30. On the Royal Medical Society, see Tait, "Medical Education at the Scottish Universities," p. 67, and Charlotte Hall, *Memoirs of Marshall Hall, M.D., F.R.S.* (London: Richard Bentley, 1861), pp. 13–14. The title page of W. A. F. Browne's *What Asylums Were, Are, and Ought to Be* describes him as a former president of the society.

21. J. Crichton-Browne, "Psychical Diseases of Early Life," *JMS* 6(April 1860):299–301, 320. Harper, "Dr. W. A. F. Browne," p. 592, comments that William Browne noted the significance of behavior disorders in children, but it was not a major concern in his work. Crichton-Browne's views on childhood nervousness are discussed further in Chapter 7 of this book.

22. Crichton-Browne, *Victorian Jottings,* pp. 239–40, and *The Doctor's Second Thoughts* (London: Ernest Benn, 1931), p. 14.

23. See Ian Dowbiggin, "Degeneration and Hereditarianism in French Mental Medicine 1840–90: Psychiatric Theory as Ideological Adaptation," in Bynum, Porter, and Shepherd, eds., *Anatomy of Madness,* 1:188–232. Degeneration theory is explored in Chapter 8 of this book.

24. J. Crichton-Browne, "Personal Identity, and its Morbid Modifications," *JMS* 8(Oct. 1862):385. Other information in the paragraph is from Crichton-Browne's entry in the *DNB 1931–1940* and his obituary in the *Times.* He and his wife had two children: a son, Harold, born in 1866, and a daughter Florence, in 1878.

25. For the inmate–attendant ratio at Wakefield, see Digby, *Madness, Morality and Medicine,* p. 146. Crichton-Browne discussed conditions at the Wakefield asylum in his testimony to the Select Committee on the Lunacy Law. See Great Britain, *Parliamentary Papers,* vol. 13 (1877) (*Reports*), "Report of the Select Committee on the Operation of the Lunacy Law," questions 1590, 1611, 1701. On Colney Hatch asylum as a symbol of modernity, see Elaine Showalter, *The Female Malady: Women, Madness, and English Culture, 1830–1980* (New York: Pantheon, 1985), pp. 23–24.

26. Case notes incorporated into J. Crichton-Browne, "Notes on the Pathology of General Paralysis of the Insane," *WRLAMR* 6(1876):205, 208. For the new water filter-beds at Wakefield, see Richard Russell, "Mental Physicians and Their Patients: Psychological Medicine in the English Pauper Lunatic Asylums of the Later Nineteenth Century" (Ph.D. diss., University of Sheffield, 1983), pp. 220–23.

27. Crichton-Browne's report from the West Riding Lunatic Asylum was quoted in a section on "Female Nursing in Asylums," under "Occasional Notes of the Quarter," *JMS* 14(July 1868):203–204.

28. See Roger Smith, *Trial by Medicine: Insanity and Responsibility in Victorian Trials* (Edinburgh: Edinburgh University Press, 1981), pp. 5–6; Scull, *Museums of Madness,* pp. 221–53; Edward Hare, "Was Insanity on the Increase?" *British Journal of Psychiatry* 142(1983):439–55; Andrew Scull, "Was Insanity Increasing? A Response to Edward Hare," *British Journal of Psychiatry* 144(1984):432–36.

29. J. K. Walton, "Casting Out and Bringing Back in Victorian England: Pauper Lunatics, 1840–70," in Bynum, Porter, and Shepherd, eds., *Anatomy of Madness,* 2:142. These figures do not, of course, include lunatics in other institutions, such as workhouses or private asylums.

30. Tuke, "Presidential Address," pp. 318–19. Also see Nicholas Hervey, "A Slavish Bowing Down: The Lunacy Commission and the Psychiatric Profession 1845–60," in

Bynum, Porter, and Shepherd, eds., *Anatomy of Madness*, 2:119; Scull, *Museums of Madness*, p. 176, and "Mad-doctors and Magistrates: English Psychiatry's Struggle for Professional Autonomy in the Nineteenth Century," *Archives européennes de sociologie* 17(1976):282, 292–93, 301.

31. Sander L. Gilman, "Darwin Sees the Insane," *Journal of the History of the Behavioral Sciences* 15(1979):253–62, revised as "Darwin's Influence on Seeing the Insane," in Gilman, *Seeing the Insane* (New York: John Wiley/Brunner, Mazel, 1982); Janet Browne, "Darwin and the Face of Madness," in Bynum, Porter, and Shepherd, eds., *Anatomy of Madness*, 1:151–65.

32. Crichton-Browne to Charles Darwin, 1 June 1869, in Cambridge University Library, Darwin Correspondence, DAR 161³, a folder marked "Letters and Memoranda from James Crichton-Browne," and containing Crichton-Browne's original letters. Copies of Darwin's letters to Crichton-Browne are in DAR 143, alphabetized under "B." All subsequent quotations from Crichton-Browne's and Darwin's letters to each other are from this material in the Cambridge University Library.

33. Darwin to Crichton-Browne, 31 January [1870]; Crichton-Browne to Darwin, 15 March and 6 June 1870. Crichton-Browne alluded to family sorrows on black-bordered stationery. I have not been able to ascertain which member of his family died, but I suspect that he and his wife lost a young child sometime in late 1869 or early 1870. His son was twelve years older than his daughter, a gap that suggests the brief life of at least one other sibling.

34. Darwin to Crichton-Browne, 8 Feb. 1871, and Crichton-Browne to Darwin, 16 Feb. 1871.

35. Crichton-Browne to Darwin, 2 March 1873.

36. Darwin to Crichton-Browne, 20 Feb. [1871]; also see Darwin to Crichton-Browne, 7 April [1871], and 28 Feb. [1873], for similar expressions of concern.

37. Darwin to Crichton-Browne, 26 March [1872?] and 30 Dec. 1873.

38. James Crichton-Browne, "The First Maudsley Lecture," *JMS* 66(July 1920):202.

39. James Crichton-Browne, Editor's Preface to *WRLAMR* 1(1871):iii.

40. "Obituary. Sir James Crichton-Browne," *BMJ*, 5 Feb. 1938, p. 311; "Obituary. Sir James Crichton-Browne," *Times* (London), 1 Feb. 1938, p. 16.

41. Charles Mercier, *Psychology Normal and Morbid* (London: Swan Sonnenschein; New York: Macmillan, 1901), dedication page. Allbutt's tribute is quoted in Henry R. Viets, "West Riding, 1871–76," *Bulletin of the Institute of the History of Medicine* 6(1938):479. Also see Christopher Lawrence, "Incommunicable Knowledge: Science, Technology and the Clinical Art in Britain 1850–1914," *Journal of Contemporary History* 20(Oct. 1985):508, 514, 516, on Allbutt. For Crichton-Browne's clinical clerkships at Wakefield, see "Report of the Select Committee on the Lunacy Law," question 1590. W. F. Bynum, "The Nervous Patient in Eighteenth- and Nineteenth-Century Britain: The Psychiatric Origins of British Neurology," in Bynum, Porter, and Shepherd, eds., *Anatomy of Madness*, 1:96, discusses Crichton-Browne's work to stimulate research at Wakefield.

42. "Report of Select Committee on the Lunacy Law," questions 1637–42; Viets, "West Riding," pp. 478–79. The larger issue is discussed in Ruth Richardson, *Death, Dissection and the Destitute* (London: Routledge & Kegan Paul, 1987).

43. *DNB 1922–1930*, s.v. "Ferrier, Sir David." See David Ferrier, "Experimental Researches in Cerebral Physiology and Pathology," *WRLAMR* 3(1873):30–96, and "Pathological Illustrations of Brain Function," *WRLAMR* 4(1874):30–62; William B. Carpenter, "On the Physiological Import of Dr. Ferrier's Experimental Investigations into the Functions of the Brain," *WRLAMR* 4(1874):1–23; Viets, "West Riding," pp. 481–82.

44. Crichton-Browne to Darwin, 16 April 1873; Darwin to Crichton-Browne, 7 Sept. [1873].

45. Bernard Hollander, *In Search of the Soul, and the Mechanism of Thought, Emotion, and*

Conduct, 2 vols. (London: Kegan Paul, Trench, Trubner; New York: E. P. Dutton, [1921]) 1:407. Robert M. Young, *Mind, Brain and Adaptation in the Nineteenth Century: Cerebral Localization and its Biological Context from Gall to Ferrier* (Oxford: Clarendon, 1970), p. 238 n4, evaluates Hollander's assertion.

46. J. Crichton-Browne, "Notes on Homicidal Insanity," *JMS* 9(July 1863):210 (for the quotation); also, 199–200, 203, 205, 206, 208; *The Story of the Brain* (Edinburgh and London: Oliver & Boyd, 1924), pp. 1–4, 8–9. For another endorsement of phrenology's basic truths, see Crichton-Browne's "Presidential Address to the Medico-Psychological Association," *JMS* 24(Oct. 1878):346.

47. J. Crichton-Browne, "Cranial Injuries and Mental Diseases," *WRLAMR* 1(1871):2, and *WRLAMR* 2(1872):97–136; "Nitrite of Amyl in Epilepsy," *WRLAMR* 3(1873):153–74; "Notes on Epilepsy, and its Pathological Consequences," *JMS* 19(April 1873):21; "Acute Dementia," *WRLAMR* 4(1874):265–90; "The Functions of the Thalami Optici" and "Note on Chronic Mania," *WRLAMR* 5(1875):227–56, and 284–92.

48. Crichton-Browne, "Notes on the Pathology of General Paralysis of the Insane," p. 226. Also see Browne, "Darwin and the Face of Madness," p. 165 n29, and Showalter, *Female Malady,* pp. 110–12.

49. Crichton-Browne's contribution to the discussion following Robert Boyd's paper on general paralysis of the insane, read at a quarterly meeting of the Medico-Psychological Association in London, in "Notes and News," *JMS* 17(April 1871):147–49.

50. Crichton-Browne to Darwin, 27 Dec. 1873.

51. Crichton-Browne, "Notes on the Pathology of General Paralysis of the Insane," pp. 186, 182, 203, 181, 200, 218, 171.

52. In addition to the table of contents of the six volumes of *WRLAMR,* see Bynum, "Nervous Patient," p. 96, and Viets, "West Riding," pp. 483–87.

53. "Notes and News: Appointments," *JMS* 21(Jan. 1876):633–34.

54. Crichton-Browne, *Victorian Jottings,* p. 154.

55. Crichton-Browne's responses, in "Report of Select Committee on the Lunacy Law," questions 1253, 1276, 1342–47, 1353, 1458–63.

56. Ibid., questions 1259, 1283, 1446–48, 1585–87 (on wrongful confinement); 1583–84, 1589–90 (on education in "cerebral disease"), and 1313, 1315, 1262 (optimism about insanity); Crichton-Browne, Preface to *WRLAMR* 5(1875):vi.

57. Crichton-Browne, "Nitrite of Amyl in Epilepsy," p. 153.

58. Quotations from Tulloch's diaries and letters, in Margaret Oliphant, *A Memoir of the Life of John Tulloch, D.D., LL.D.,* 3d ed. (Edinburgh and London: William Blackwood, 1889), pp. 374–76, 379–80, 470, and Oliphant's comments, pp. 471–72. Crichton-Browne briefly discussed Tulloch's case in *What the Doctor Thought,* pp. 73–75.

59. On Eliot, Crichton-Browne, *Doctor's Second Thoughts,* pp. 286–89, and *DNB 1931–1940,* s.v. "Eliot, Sir Charles Norton Edgecumbe." On Jones, James Crichton-Browne, *The Doctor's After Thoughts* (London: Ernest Benn, 1932), p. 269.

60. J. Crichton-Browne, "On the Weight of the Brain and Its Component Parts in the Insane," *Brain* 1(1878–79):504–505, and 2(1879–80):60–61, 63, 66; also "A Plea for the Minute Study of Mania," *Brain* 3(1880–81):347–62, and "The Pulmonary Pathology of General Paralysis," *Brain* 6(1883–84):317–41—based on his research at Wakefield.

61. Volume 14 of *Brain* (1891) was the first to contain information about the Neurological Society at the end of the journal. Crichton-Browne figures on the membership list in that volume, with a notice about his status as a founding member and about the offices that he held in the society. The next membership list appears at the back of vol. 17 (1894), by which time his name was no longer included.

62. Bynum, "Nervous Patient," pp. 96–97.

63. James Crichton-Browne, comments on H. Charlton Bastian, "The 'Muscular Sense': Its Nature, and Cortical Localisation," *Brain* 10(1887–88):105.

64. Crichton-Browne, *Story of Brain,* pp. 21–22. For an early (1863) expression of Crichton-Browne's belief in the will's central significance to psychiatric theory, see his "Homicidal Insanity," p. 203.

65. See Chapter 8 of this book for Crichton-Browne's work as a moral hygienist. Many of his speeches were published as separate pamphlets or appeared in the medical press.

66. Crichton-Browne, "Presidential Address," pp. 353, 372.

67. Crichton-Browne, "First Maudsley Lecture," p. 200.

68. Crichton-Browne, *Doctor's Second Thoughts,* pp. 58–64; Oppenheim, *Other World,* pp. 285–86.

69. Crichton-Browne, "Presidential Address," p. 370.

70. Crichton-Browne, "Notes on the Pathology of General Paralysis of the Insane," p. 189; J. Milner Fothergill, *The Maintenance of Health: A Medical Work for Lay Readers* (London: Smith, Elder, 1874), p. 262.

71. James Crichton-Browne to Sir Edward Sharpey-Schafer, 22 Feb. 1931, document ESS/ B.26/16, in the Sharpey-Schafer Correspondence, Contemporary Medical Archives Centre, The Wellcome Institute for the History of Medicine, London. Crichton-Browne's letters of 26 Feb. and 14 April 1931 (ESS/B.26/17, 18) continue to discuss the subject with Sharpey-Schafer.

Chapter 3

1. James Manby Gully, *An Exposition of the Symptoms, Essential Nature, and Treatment of Neuropathy, or Nervousness* (London: Churchill, 1837), p. vii.

2. Eric T. Carlson and Meribeth M. Simpson, "Models of the Nervous System in Eighteenth Century Psychiatry," *Bull Hist Med* 43(March–April 1969):103–106 (quoted phrase on p. 106).

3. John Cooke, *A Treatise on Nervous Diseases,* 2 vols. (London: Longman, Hurst, Rees, Orme, & Brown, 1820–23), 1:115. For detailed discussions of the points touched on in the previous paragraphs, see Carlson and Simpson, "Models of the Nervous System," pp. 101–15; Edwin Clarke and L. S. Jacyna, *Nineteenth-Century Origins of Neuroscientific Concepts* (Berkeley and Los Angeles: University of California Press, 1987), ch. 5; Stanley W. Jackson, "Force and Kindred Notions in Eighteenth-Century Neurophysiology and Medical Psychology," *Bull Hist Med* 44(Nov.–Dec. 1970):397–410, 539–54; Roderick W. Home, "Electricity and the Nervous Fluid," *Journal of the History of Biology* 3(1970):235–51; Roger Smith, "The Background of Physiological Psychology in Natural Philosophy," *History of Science* 11(1973):80–88.

4. Forbes Winslow, *On the Preservation of the Health of Body and Mind* (London: Henry Renshaw, 1842), p. 152n.

5. Henry Holland, *Chapters on Mental Physiology,* 2d ed., rev. and enl. (London: Longman, Brown, Green, Longmans, & Roberts, 1858), pp. 314–15 (first published 1852).

6. Thomas Dixon Savill, *Clinical Lectures on Neurasthenia,* 3d ed., rev. and enl. (London: H. J. Glaisher, 1906), p.93 (first published 1899).

7. Holland, *Chapters on Mental Physiology,* p. 303n.

8. Clark quoted in F. B. Smith, *Florence Nightingale: Reputation and Power* (London and Canberra: Croom Helm, 1982), p. 92.

9. Arthur Christopher Benson, *Beside Still Waters* (New York and London: G. P. Putnam's, 1907), pp. 47, 339–40, for example; Herbert Spencer, *An Autobiography,* 2 vols.

(London: Williams & Norgate, 1904), 1:487–88; Beatrice Webb, *The Diary of Beatrice Webb*, vol. 1: *1873–1892: "Glitter Around and Darkness Within,"* ed. Norman Mac-Kenzie and Jeanne MacKenzie (Cambridge, Mass.: Harvard University Press, 1982), p. 214 (29 Aug. 1887).

10. Alfred T. Schofield, *Nerves in Order or the Maintenance of Health* (London: Hodder & Stoughton, 1905), p. 207; Carlson and Simpson, "Models of the Nervous System," pp. 106, 111, trace these ideas, for example, in the work of Boerhaave and Cullen.

11. For the applicability of nervous reflex theory to nervous exhaustion, see Charles E. Rosenberg, "George M. Beard and American Nervousness," in his collection of essays, *No Other Gods: On Science and American Social Thought* (Baltimore: Johns Hopkins University Press, paperback ed., 1978), pp. 102–103—first published as "The Place of George M. Beard in Nineteenth-Century Psychiatry," *Bull Hist Med* 36(May–June 1962):245–59; Barbara A. Sicherman, "The Uses of a Diagnosis: Doctors, Patients, and Neurasthenia," in Judith Walzer Leavitt and Ronald L. Numbers, eds., *Sickness and Health in America: Readings in the History of Medicine and Public Health* (Madison, Wisc.: University of Wisconsin Press, 1978), p. 25.

12. Henry Maudsley, "Sex in Mind and in Education," *Fortnightly Review*, n.s., 15 (1874):467.

13. On this subject, see the collection of essays in James Paradis and Thomas Postlewait, eds., *Victorian Science and Victorian Values: Literary Perspectives* (New Brunswick, N.J.: Rutgers University Press, 1985).

14. As Owsei Temkin argued in "Metaphors of Human Biology," in Robert C. Stauffer, ed., *Science and Civilization* (Madison, Wisc.: University of Wisconsin Press, 1949), pp. 169–94. Also see Jackson, "Force and Kindred Notions," pp. 550–52, and Charles E. Rosenberg, "Medicine and Community in Victorian Britain," *Journal of Interdisciplinary History* 11(Spring 1981):680–81, 683. Susan Sontag explores the metaphorical exploitation of disease, particularly tuberculosis and cancer, in *Illness as Metaphor* (New York: Farrar, Straus, and Giroux, paperback ed., 1988).

15. Henry Holland, *Recollections of Past Life* (London: Longmans, Green, 1872), p. 333.

16. Savill, *Clinical Lectures on Neurasthenia*, pp. 12–13.

17. T. Clifford Allbutt, *On Visceral Neuroses* (London: Churchill, 1884), p. 95; J. Crichton-Browne, "Notes on the Pathology of General Paralysis of the Insane," *WRLAMR* 6(1876):195; "Cases Illustrative of the Powers of the Water System in the Cure of Various Diseases," *Water Cure Journal and Hygienic Magazine* 1(1847–48):507.

18. J. Milner Fothergill, *The Maintenance of Health: A Medical Work for Lay Readers* (London: Smith, Elder, 1874), p. 244; J. A. Symonds, *The Memoirs of John Addington Symonds*, ed. Phyllis Grosskurth (Chicago: University of Chicago Press, 1986), pp. 234, 236.

19. Alfred T. Schofield, *Nerves in Disorder: A Plea for Rational Treatment* (London: Hodder & Stoughton, 1903), p. 4. The similar concept of a "spermatic economy" is discussed in Chapter 5 of this book.

20. Karl Figlio, "Chlorosis and Chronic Disease in Nineteenth-Century Britain: The Social Constitution of Somatic Illness in a Capitalist Society," *Social History* 3(May 1978):170.

21. Fothergill, *Maintenance of Health*, pp. 249–50.

22. Gerald L. Klerman, "Depression and Related Disorders of Mood (Affective Disorders)," in Armand M. Nicholi, Jr., ed., *The New Harvard Guide to Psychiatry* (Cambridge, Mass. and London: Belknap Press of Harvard University Press, 1988), p. 309.

23. Ralph Browne, *Neurasthenia and Its Treatment by Hypodermic Transfusions* (London: Churchill, 1894), p. 33.

24. William Thorburn, "The Traumatic Neuroses," *Proceedings of the Royal Society of Medicine* 7(1913–14), pt. 2 (Neurological Section): 4.
25. William George Willoughby, "Temperament," in D. Hack Tuke, ed., *A Dictionary of Psychological Medicine*, 2 vols. (London: Churchill, 1892), 2:1276.
26. J. Crichton-Browne, "Cranial Injuries and Mental Diseases," *WRLAMR* 1(1871):15; Patrick Nicol, "The Mental Symptoms of Ordinary Disease," *WRLAMR* 2(1872):202; T. S. Clouston, *Clinical Lectures on Mental Diseases*, 2d ed. (London: Churchill, 1887), p. 33; Willoughby, "Temperament," p. 1277; Herbert Mayo, *The Philosophy of Living* (London: John W. Parker, 1837), p. 13.
27. A. Clark, "Some Observations Concerning What is Called Neurasthenia," *Lancet*, 2 January 1886, pp. 1–2.
28. Alfred T. Schofield, *Functional Nerve Diseases* (London: Methuen, 1908), p. 62; John James Graham Brown, *The Treatment of Nervous Disease* (Edinburgh and London: William Green, 1905), p. 368.
29. Symonds, *Memoirs*, pp. 38, 64, 55; Spencer, *Autobiography*, 1:66–67, 413–15; Webb, *Diary*, 1:96–97, 214–15; Benson, *Beside Still Waters*, pp. 4, 258-59.
30. Symonds, *Memoirs*, p. 64; Leonard G. Guthrie, *Functional Nervous Disorders in Childhood* (London: Oxford Medical Publications, Oxford University Press, 1907), p. 22; T. Clifford Allbutt, "Nervous Diseases and Modern Life," *Contemporary Review* 67(1895):221.
31. Arnold Toynbee to Robert Darbishire, 13 June 1913, quoted in William H. McNeill, *Arnold J. Toynbee, A Life* (New York and Oxford: Oxford University Press, 1989), p. 51.
32. H. Charlton Bastian, "Nervous" in Richard Quain, ed., *A Dictionary of Medicine* (London: Longmans, Green, 1882), p. 1025.
33. Alfred T. Schofield, *Manual of Personal and Domestic Hygiene*, in 2 parts (London: Allman, [1890]), pt. 2, p. 140.
34. Charles Kingsley, *The Water-Babies: A Fairy Tale for a Land-Baby* (1863), ch. 1.
35. Allbutt, "Nervous Diseases and Modern Life," p. 220.
36. Rosenberg, "Beard and American Nervousness," pp. 99–100, 105, 236–37 ns 9, 21; Sicherman, "Uses of a Diagnosis," p. 30; and, for earlier English-language uses of neurasthenia, Francis Schiller, "Spinal Irritation and Osteopathy," *Bull Hist Med* 45(May–June 1971):258.
37. Beard's first book-length treatment of neurasthenia—*A Practical Treatise on Nervous Exhaustion (Neurasthenia), Its Symptoms, Nature, Sequences, Treatment* (New York: W. Wood, 1880–dealt with the myriad manifestations of the disorder. A summary of Beard's list of symptoms was offered to British medical men in the review of the *Practical Treatise* published in *J Psych Med*, pt. 1, n.s., 7(1881):97–117. Also see Rosenberg, "Beard and American Nervousness," pp. 100–101, and Sicherman, "Uses of a Diagnosis," p. 25.
38. Rosenberg, "Beard and American Nervousness," pp. 105–107, discusses the nationalism implicit in Beard's understanding of neurasthenia, as Beard argued in *American Nervousness, Its Causes and Consequences* (New York: G. P. Putnam's, 1881).
39. See, for example, the review of Beard's *Practical Treatise*, in *J Psych Med*, pt. 1, n.s., 7(1881):118.
40. Stanley W. Jackson, *Melancholia and Depression, From Hippocratic Times to Modern Times* (New Haven and London: Yale University Press, 1986), p. 183, and "Force and Kindred Notions," p. 542; also Erwin H. Ackerknecht, *A Short History of Medicine*, rev. ed. (Baltimore: Johns Hopkins University Press, paperback ed., 1982), p. 129.
41. Schiller, "Spinal Irritation," pp. 251–57.

42. For example, James Ross, *Handbook of the Diseases of the Nervous System* (London: Churchill, 1885), pp. 578–79.

43. Oliver Sacks, *Migraine: Understanding a Common Disorder,* rev. and enl. ed. (Berkeley and Los Angeles: University of California Press, paperback ed., 1986), p. 3; Rosenberg, "Beard and American Nervousness," pp. 102–103.

44. Clark, "Some Observations Concerning Neurasthenia," p. 1; Guthrie, *Functional Nervous Disorders in Childhood,* p. 17; Rudolf Arndt, "Neurasthenia," in Tuke, ed., *Dictionary of Psychological Medicine,* 2:840–41, and W. S. Playfair, "Neuroses, Functional, The Systematic Treatment of," in the same volume, p. 851.

45. J. Strahan, "Puzzling Conditions of the Heart and Other Organs Dependent on Neurasthenia," *BMJ,* 5 Sept. 1885, p. 435; W. S. Playfair, "Some Observations Concerning What is Called Neurasthenia," *BMJ,* 6 Nov. 1886, p. 854; William R. Gowers, *A Manual of Diseases of the Nervous System,* 2 vols. (London: Churchill, 1886–88), 2:959.

46. Savill, *Clinical Lectures on Neurasthenia,* pp. 48–49.

47. Seymour J. Sharkey, "Hysteria and Neurasthenia," *Brain* 27 (Spring 1904):18. No wonder some American doctors spoke of "hystero-neurasthenia." See Francis G. Gosling, "Neurasthenia in Pennsylvania: A Perspective on the Origins of American Psychotherapy, 1870–1910," *Journal of the History of Medicine and Allied Sciences* 40(April 1985):193.

48. George H. Savage's contribution to "Discussion on Neurasthenia and its Treatment," at the 1894 annual meeting of the British Medical Association, reported in *BMJ,* 8 Sept. 1894, p. 522.

49. Sicherman, "Uses of a Diagnosis," p. 28. Also see Rosenberg, "Beard and American Nervousness," pp. 100, 104.

50. Herbert W. Page, "On the Abuse of Bromide of Potassium in the Treatment of Traumatic Neurasthenia," *Medical Times and Gazette,* 4 April 1885, pp. 439, 438. On the international belief that railroads were a potent source of neurotic illness, with specific reference to Page, see George Frederick Drinka, *The Birth of Neurosis: Myth, Malady, and the Victorians* (New York: Simon & Schuster, 1984), pp. 108–22.

51. Guthrie, *Functional Nervous Disorders in Childhood,* p. 17; Herbert W. Page, *Injuries of the Spine and Spinal Cord without Apparent Mechanical Lesion, and Nervous Shock, in the Surgical and Medico-Legal Aspects* (London: Churchill, 1883), and *Railway Injuries: With Special Reference to those of the Back and Nervous System, in their Medico-Legal and Clinical Aspects* (London: C. Griffin, 1891). Also see Thorburn, "Traumatic Neuroses," pp. 1–14.

52. Savill, *Clinical Lectures on Neurasthenia,* p. 122. See Alfred T. Schofield, *The Force of Mind or the Mental Factor in Medicine* (London: Churchill, 1902), p. 105, for the "many varieties of neurasthenia." The proliferation of neurasthenic categories only underscores, needless to say, the inadequacy of neurasthenia as a unified disease construct.

53. Strahan, "Puzzling Conditions," p. 435; Flora Thompson, *Lark Rise to Candleford* (London: Reprint Society, 1948), pp. 127, 212; "Pathology of the Nerves and Nervous Maladies," *J Psych Med* 2(Jan. 1849):114.

54. Savill, *Clinical Lectures on Neurasthenia,* p. 188.

55. George Cheyne, *The English Malady: or, a Treatise of Nervous Diseases of all kinds, as Spleen, Vapours, Lowness of Spirits, Hypochondriacal, and Hysterical Distempers,* . . . (1733; reprint ed., Delmar, N.Y.: Scholars' Facsimiles & Reprints, 1976), pp. i, ii, 10, 34–36, 38–39. Also see Oswald Doughty, "The English Malady of the Eighteenth Century," *Review of English Studies* 2(July 1926):257–69; Vieda Skultans, *English Madness: Ideas on Insanity, 1580–1890* (London: Routledge & Kegan Paul, 1979), ch.3.

56. The *OED* traces the shifting meanings of *nervous.* Also see W. F. Bynum, "The Nervous

Patient in Eighteenth- and Nineteenth-Century Britain: The Psychiatric Origins of British Neurology," in W. F. Bynum, Roy Porter, and Michael Shepherd, eds., *The Anatomy of Madness: Essays in the History of Psychiatry,* 2 vols. (London and New York: Tavistock Publications, 1985), 1:91.

57. Thomas Stretch Dowse, *On Brain and Nerve Exhaustion. 'Neurasthenia.' Its Nature and Curative Treatment* (London: Baillière, Tindall, & Cox, 1880), p. 40; "Pathology of the Nerves and Nervous Maladies," pp. 111–12; Frederick MacCabe, "On Mental Strain and Overwork," *JMS* 21(Oct. 1875):398.

58. Great Britain, *Parliamentary Papers* (Commons), vol. 61 (1884), (*Accounts and Papers,* vol. 15), "Elementary Schools (Dr. Crichton-Browne's Report)," p. 17 [of the report]. Also see his "Presidential Address to the Medico-Psychological Association," *JMS* 24(Oct. 1878):359.

59. J. C. Bucknill, "President's Address to the Association of Medical Officers of Asylums and Hospitals for the Insane," *JMS* 7(Oct. 1860):2; Maudsley discussed insanity's various causes, predisposing and proximate, in *The Physiology and Pathology of Mind* (London: Macmillan, 1867), pp. 197–258; Daniel H. Tuke, "Does Civilization Favour the Generation of Mental Disease?" *Asylum Journal of Mental Science* 4(Oct. 1857):104–109.

60. Marshall Hall, quoted in Charlotte Hall, *Memoirs of Marshall Hall, M.D., F.R.S.* (London: Richard Bentley, 1861), pp. 275–76. On urban–rural mortality statistics in Victorian England, see Robert Woods and P. R. Andrew Hinde, "Mortality in Victorian England: Models and Patterns," *Journal of Interdisciplinary History* 18(Summer 1987): 48–52.

61. Olive Anderson, *Suicide in Victorian and Edwardian England* (Oxford: Clarendon, 1987), pp. 84, 89–93, 345.

62. James Crichton-Browne, "On the Weight of the Brain and Its Component Parts in the Insane," *Brain* 1(1878–79):511, and *The Prevention of Senility and A Sanitary Outlook* (London: Macmillan, 1905), p. 106.

63. Ivan Waddington, *The Medical Profession in the Industrial Revolution* (Dublin: Gill and Macmillan; Atlantic Highlands, N.J.: Humanities Press, 1984), pp. 196–98, discusses how these trends influenced the Victorian medical profession in general.

64. As, for example, T. Clifford Allbutt, "Neurasthenia," in T. C. Allbutt and Humphry Davy Rolleston, eds., *A System of Medicine,* 2d ed. rev., 9 vols. (London: Macmillan, 1905–11), 8:738.

65. See Figlio, "Chlorosis and Chronic Disease," pp. 186–87, for a heavily ideological discussion of the broader issues sketched in this paragraph.

66. Tuke, "Does Civilization Favour the Generation of Mental Disease?" p. 96.

67. Edwin Lee, *A Treatise on Some Nervous Disorders,* 2d. ed. enl. (London: Churchill, 1838), p. 14 (first published 1833). Lee, a medical writer and practitioner, subsequently advocated hydropathy and spent much of his time on the continent. Edward J. Tilt, *On the Preservation of the Health of Women at the Critical Periods of Life* (London: Churchill, 1851), pp. 36, 40, differentiated wealthy from poor women precisely in terms of nervous development.

68. Playfair, "Some Observations Concerning Neurasthenia," p. 854. Also see Sicherman, "Uses of a Diagnosis," p. 30.

69. Thomas Trotter, *A View of the Nervous Temperament* (London: Longman, Hurst, Rees, & Orme, 1807); Daniel Noble, *Facts and Observations Relative to the Influence of Manufactures Upon Health and Life* (London: Churchill, 1843), p. 20.

70. James Phillips Kay, *The Moral and Physical Condition of the Working Classes Employed in the Cotton Manufacture in Manchester* (London: Ridgeway, 1832), excerpted in Philip

A. M. Taylor, *The Industrial Revolution in Britain: Triumph or Disaster?*, rev. ed. (Lexington, Mass.: D. C. Heath, 1970), p. 8. Anderson discusses many such cases throughout *Suicide in Victorian and Edwardian England*. Chapter 9 is entitled "Good Samaritans."

71. J. Milner Fothergill, "Notes on the Therapeutics of Some Affections of the Nervous System," *WRLAMR* 6(1876):254–56; Charles Henry Mayhew, "Acute Delirious Melancholia," *WRLAMR* 1(1871):257.

72. This important shift is discussed in Chapter 5 of this book.

73. Thomas Stretch Dowse, *The Brain and the Nerves: Their Ailments and Their Exhaustion* (London: Baillière, Tindall, & Cox, [1884]), p. 121.

74. Guthrie, *Functional Nervous Disorders in Childhood*, p. 17; Savill, *Clinical Lectures on Neurasthenia*, pp. 27–30.

75. Gosling, "Neurasthenia in Pennsylvania," p. 195; anonymous review of Levillain's volume, in *JMS* 37(Oct. 1891):587–88; Allbutt, "Neurasthenia," p. 738. For an extended discussion of this process in the American context, see F. G. Gosling, *Before Freud: Neurasthenia and the American Medical Community, 1870–1910* (Urbana and Chicago: University of Illinois Press, 1987).

76. "The Nature and Causes of Depression—Part II," *Harvard Medical School Mental Health Letter* 4(Feb. 1988):3.

77. Allbutt, "Neurasthenia," p. 741.

78. J. C. Prichard, "Hypochondriasis," in John Forbes, Alexander Tweedie, and John Conolly, eds., *The Cyclopædia of Practical Medicine*, 4 vols. (London: Sherwood, Gilbert, Piper, Baldwin, & Cradock, 1833–35), 2:553.

79. Anderson, *Suicide in Victorian and Edwardian England*, pp. 386–87.

80. Quentin Bell, *Virginia Woolf, A Biography*, 2 vols. in 1 (New York: Harcourt Brace Jovanovich, 1972), 1:89–90; Stephen Trombley, *'All That Summer She Was Mad': Virginia Woolf and Her Doctors* (London: Junction Books, 1981), p. 3; Elaine Showalter, *The Female Malady: Women, Madness, and English Culture, 1830–1980* (New York: Pantheon, 1985), pp. 143–44; Virginia Stephen to Violet Dickinson, 30 Oct. [1904], in Nigel Nicolson and Joanne Trautmann, eds., *The Letters of Virginia Woolf*, vol. 1: *1888–1912 (Virginia Stephen)* (New York and London: Harcourt Brace Jovanovich, 1975), p. 147. Sicherman, "Uses of a Diagnosis," p. 30, mentions the social implications of Virginia Stephen's medical treatment.

81. See, for example, the case depicted by Anderson, *Suicide in Victorian and Edwardian England*, pp. 333–34.

82. For a fascinating discussion of several hundred working-class autobiographies and the interpretative questions they raise, see Regenia Gagnier, "Social Atoms: Working-Class Autobiography, Subjectivity, and Gender," *Victorian Studies* 30(Spring 1987):335–63.

83. Ben Tillett, *Memories and Reflections* (London: John Long, 1931), pp. 180–81, 196; Jonathan Schneer, *Ben Tillett: Portrait of a Labour Leader* (London and Canberra: Croom Helm, 1982), pp. 112–15, 210.

84. Savage, "Discussion on Neurasthenia and its Treatment," p. 523; Allbutt, "Neurasthenia," p. 728. On the demise of neurasthenia, also see Sicherman, "Uses of a Diagnosis," p. 26.

Chapter 4

1. A. C. Wootton, *Chronicles of Pharmacy*, 2 vols. (London: Macmillan, 1910), 2:243–48, 256–73; Michael W. Perrin, "The Influence of the Pharmaceutical Industry on the

Evolution of British Medical Practice,'' in F. N. L. Poynter, ed., *The Evolution of Medical Practice in Britain* (London: Pitman Medical Publishing Co., 1961), pp. 97–107.

2. Francis Galton, *Memories of My Life* (New York: E. P. Dutton, 1909), pp. 26–28; Wootton, *Chronicles of Pharmacy,* 2:61–69; *Monthly Gazette of Health* 1(1816):234, and 2(1816–17):720; Charles Dickens, *The Posthumous Papers of the Pickwick Club* (1836–37), ch. 48.

3. Erwin H. Ackerknecht, *A Short History of Medicine,* rev. ed. (Baltimore: Johns Hopkins University Press, paperback ed., 1982), p. 45; Wootton, *Chronicles of Pharmacy,* 1:399.

4. J. Crichton-Browne, "Psychical Diseases of Early Life," *JMS* 6 (April 1860):317.

5. Rudolf Arndt, "Neurasthenia," in D. Hack Tuke, ed., *A Dictionary of Psychological Medicine,* 2 vols. (London: Churchill, 1892), 2:849; Thomas Stretch Dowse, *The Brain and the Nerves: Their Ailments and Their Exhaustion* (London: Baillière, Tindall, & Cox, [1884]), p. 106.

6. Charlotte Hall, *Memoirs of Marshall Hall, M.D., F.R.S.* (London: Richard Bentley, 1861), p. 126; Alfred T. Schofield, *The Management of a Nerve Patient* (London: Churchill, 1906), p. 170; Bruce Haley, *The Healthy Body and Victorian Culture* (Cambridge, Mass.: Harvard University Press, 1978), p. 29 (on Huxley); T. C. Allbutt, "Nervous Diseases and Modern Life," *Contemporary Review* 67(Jan.–June 1895):217.

7. Wootton, *Chronicles of Pharmacy,* 2:67, 133–35; Thomas Stretch Dowse, *On Brain and Nerve Exhaustion. 'Neurasthenia.' Its Nature and Curative Treatment* (London: Baillière, Tindall, & Cox, 1880), pp. 51–52; H. B. Donkin, "Hysteria," and Charles Mercier, "Melancholia," in Tuke, ed., *Dictionary of Psychological Medicine,* 1:627, 640, 2:794; Ralph Colp, Jr., *To Be an Invalid: The Illness of Charles Darwin* (Chicago: University of Chicago Press, 1977), pp. 132–39, discusses and dismisses the argument for Darwin's arsenic poisoning, proposed by John H. Winslow in *Darwin's Victorian Malady: Evidence for its Medically Induced Origin* (Philadelphia: American Philosophical Society, 1971). Also see Lawrence A. Kohn, "Charles Darwin's Chronic Ill Health," *Bull Hist Med* 37(May–June 1963):240, 252.

8. Benjamin Rush, *Medical Inquiries and Observations, upon the Diseases of the Mind* (1812; facsimile ed., New York: Hafner Publishing Co., 1962), p. 105; Wootton, *Chronicles of Pharmacy,* 1:408–18; K. D. Keele, "The Influence of Clinical Research on the Evolution of Medical Practice in Britain," in Poynter, ed., *Evolution of Medical Practice,* pp. 92–93.

9. Henry Holland, *Medical Notes and Reflections,* 3d ed. (London: Longman, Brown, Green, & Longmans, 1855), pp. 417–18, 541–42; Peter Mere Latham, *The Collected Works of Dr. P. M. Latham, with Memoir by Sir Thomas Watson, Bart., M.D.,* 2 vols. (London: New Sydenham Society, 1876), 1:171; J. Crichton-Browne, "Notes on the Pathology of General Paralysis of the Insane," *WRLAMR* 6(1876):174–75; T. S. Clouston, "The Prodromata of the Psychoses, and Their Meaning," *Review of Neurology and Psychiatry* 1(1903):789; William Allingham, *A Diary, 1824–1889,* ed. H. Allingham and D. Radford (Harmondsworth: Penguin Books, 1985), p. 218 (first published in 1907).

10. Richard Reece, *The Medical Guide,* 12th ed. (London: Longman, Hurst, Rees, Orme, & Brown, 1817), p. 35; James Walvin, *A Child's World: A Social History of English Childhood 1800–1914* (Harmondsworth: Penguin Books, 1982), p. 26.

11. Terry M. Parssinen, *Secret Passions, Secret Remedies: Narcotic Drugs in British Society 1820–1930* (Philadelphia: Institute for the Study of Human Issues, 1983), pp. 79, 99. The discussion here is also indebted to Virginia Berridge and Griffith Edwards, *Opium and the People: Opiate Use in Nineteenth-Century England* (New Haven and London: Yale University Press, paperback ed., 1987) (first published in 1981).

12. Rachel Grant-Smith, *The Experiences of an Asylum Patient* (London: George Allen &

Unwin, 1922), pp. 51–52; Parssinen, *Secret Passions*, pp. 84, 94, 100–101; Berridge and Edwards, *Opium and the People*, pp. 68, 228.

13. Berridge and Edwards, *Opium and the People*, p. 65; Margaret Oliphant, *Autobiography and Letters of Mrs. Margaret Oliphant*, ed. Mrs. Harry Coghill (Leicester: Leicester University Press, 1974), p. 63 (first published in 1899).

14. Margaret Oliphant, *A Memoir of the Life of John Tulloch, D.D., LL.D.*, 3d ed. (Edinburgh and London: William Blackwood, 1889), p. 244; E. Mazière Courtenay, "The Use of Opium in the Treatment of Melancholia," *WRLAMR* 2(1872):256–58; Dowse, *Brain and Nerve Exhaustion*, pp. 51–52.

15. Benjamin Wood Richardson, *Diseases of Modern Life* (London: Macmillan, 1876), p. 330.

16. J. Strahan, "Puzzling Conditions of the Heart and Other Organs Dependent on Neurasthenia," *BMJ*, 5 Sept. 1885, p. 436; W. S. Playfair, "The Systematic Treatment of Functional Neuroses," in Tuke, ed., *Dictionary of Psychological Medicine*, 2:852; Donkin, "Hysteria," p. 625. The phrase "therapeutic nihilism" is Barbara Sicherman's in "The Uses of a Diagnosis: Doctors, Patients, and Neurasthenia," in Judith Walzer Leavitt and Ronald L. Numbers, eds., *Sickness and Health in America: Readings in the History of Medicine and Public Health* (Madison, Wisc.: University of Wisconsin Press, 1978), p. 27.

17. Charlotte Brontë, *Villette*, chs. 15, 17.

18. Dowse, *Brain and Nerves*, p. 116; Ackerknecht, *Short History of Medicine*, pp. 163–64, on "the introduction of a new scientific dietetics into medicine."

19. Richard A. Hunter and H. Phillip Greenberg, "Sir William Gull and Psychiatry," *Guy's Hospital Reports* 105(1956):361, 370; William Withey Gull, "Anorexia Nervosa (Apepsia Hysterica, Anorexia Hysterica)," *Transactions of the Clinical Society of London* 7(1874):24, 26–27; Leonard Woolf, *Beginning Again: An Autobiography of the Years 1911 to 1918* (New York: Harcourt Brace & World, 1964), p. 79.

20. Oliphant, *Tulloch*, pp. 374–76; Beatrice Webb, *My Apprenticeship* (London: Longmans, Green, 1926), p. 219. For Mary Booth's comments on her husband's health, see T. S. Simey and M. B. Simey, *Charles Booth, Social Scientist* (London: Oxford University Press, 1960), pp. 51–61; Belinda Norman-Butler describes her grandfather's breakdown in *Victorian Aspirations: The Life and Labour of Charles and Mary Booth* (London: George Allen & Unwin, 1972), pp. 44–46.

21. Audrey C. Peterson, "Brain Fever in Nineteenth-Century Literature: Fact and Fiction," *Victorian Studies* 19(June 1976):447, 449, 450, 460; Olive Anderson, *Suicide in Victorian and Edwardian England* (Oxford: Clarendon, 1987), pp. 159–60, 185, 408.

22. "November Diseases and the Means of Escaping Them," *Family Oracle of Health* 1(1824):127; Herbert Mayo, *The Philosophy of Living* (London: John W. Parker, 1837), pp. 15–16.

23. Anne Digby, "Moral Treatment at the Retreat, 1796–1846," in W. F. Bynum, Roy Porter, and Michael Shepherd, eds., *The Anatomy of Madness: Essays in the History of Psychiatry*, 2 vols. (London and New York: Tavistock Publications, 1985), 2:66.

24. William R. Gowers, *A Manual of Diseases of the Nervous System*, 2 vols. (London: Churchill, 1886–88), 2:938.

25. Eric T. Carlson and Meribeth M. Simpson, "Models of the Nervous System in Eighteenth Century Psychiatry," *Bull Hist Med* 43(March–April 1969):112; also see Roy Porter, "Being Mad in Georgian England," *History Today* 31(Dec. 1981):44.

26. John Conolly, "Hysteria," in John Forbes, Alexander Tweedie, and John Conolly, eds., *The Cyclopædia of Practical Medicine*, 4 vols. (London: Sherwood, Gilbert, Piper, Baldwin, & Cradock, 1833–35), 2:584; James Manby Gully, *An Exposition of the*

Symptoms, Essential Nature, and Treatment of Neuropathy, or Nervousness (London: Churchill, 1837), p. 190; Dickens, *Pickwick Papers*, ch. 48.

27. J. Crichton-Browne, "Cranial Injuries and Mental Diseases," *WRLAMR* 2(1872):122; Barbara Sicherman, "The Paradox of Prudence: Mental Health in the Gilded Age," in Andrew Scull, ed., *Madhouses, Mad-Doctors, and Madmen: The Social History of Psychiatry in the Victorian Era* (London: Athlone Press; Philadelphia: University of Pennsylvania Press, 1981), p. 226; W. S. Playfair, *The Systematic Treatment of Nerve Prostration and Hysteria* (London: Smith, Elder, 1883), pp. 19–20.

28. Thomas Dixon Savill, *Clinical Lectures on Neurasthenia*, 3d ed., rev. and enl. (London: Henry Glaisher, 1906), p. 120; J. J. Graham Brown, *The Treatment of Nervous Disease* (Edinburgh and London: William Green, 1905), p. 398; Dowse, *Brain and Nerves*, p. 121; Alfred T. Schofield, *Nerves in Disorder. A Plea for Rational Treatment* (London: Hodder & Stoughton, 1903), p. 158; J. Michell Clarke, *Hysteria & Neurasthenia* (London: The Bodley Head, 1905), p. 281 (on electrical baths.)

29. Gordon Holmes, *The National Hospital, Queen Square, 1860–1948* (Edinburgh and London: Livingstone, 1954), pp. 14, 17, 20–21; Alfred T. Schofield, *Manual of Personal and Domestic Hygiene*, in 2 parts (London: Allman, [1890]), pt. 2, p. 144, and *Nerves in Disorder*, p. 168.

30. Ralph Browne, *Neurasthenia and Its Treatment by Hypodermic Transfusions* (London: Churchill, 1894), p. 28 (italics in original); Maurice Craig, *Psychological Medicine: A Manual on Mental Diseases for Practitioners and Students* (London: Churchill, 1905), p. 247; W. H. B. Stoddart, *Mind and Its Disorders: A Text-Book for Students and Practitioners* (London: H. K. Lewis, 1908), pp. 366–67.

31. Hall, *Memoirs of Marshall Hall*, p. 195; T. S. Clouston, *The Hygiene of Mind* (London: Methuen, 1906), pp. 35, 115, 228.

32. Jane Austen, *Sanditon, The Watsons, Lady Susan, and Other Miscellanea* (London: Dent, Everyman's Library, 1978), p. 65; Dr. Armstrong, "Abstract of Lectures on Chronic Affections of the Brain and Nervous System," *Lancet*, 23 July 1825, pp. 71–72, and Dr. Clutterbuck, "Lectures on the Diseases of the Nervous System," *Lancet*, 7 July 1827, p. 419; Colp, *To Be an Invalid*, p. 86; Leonard Huxley, *Life and Letters of Thomas Henry Huxley*, 2 vols. (New York: D. Appleton, 1900), 1:154–55.

33. James Crichton-Browne, *Stray Leaves from a Physician's Portfolio* (London: Hodder & Stoughton, [1927]), p. 140.

34. John Bright, *The Diaries of John Bright*, ed. R. A. J. Walling (London: Cassell: 1930), pp. 204–205, 229, 345–46; George M. Trevelyan, *The Life of John Bright* (London: Constable, 1913), pp. 254–55; Herman Ausubel, *John Bright, Victorian Reformer* (New York and London: John Wiley, 1966), pp. 80–81 (for Cobden's advice).

35. Walter Troughton, "Typescript Account of H. Spencer's Life, 1888–1903," Herbert Spencer Papers, MS 791/355/3, University of London Library, Senate House, London, pp. 10, 2; Richard Ormond, *Sir Edwin Landseer* (London: The Tate Gallery; Philadelphia: Philadelphia Museum of Art, 1981), p. 10.

36. Digby, "Moral Treatment at the Retreat," p. 65; J. Crichton-Browne, "Acute Dementia," *WRLAMR* 4(1874):285, 287–88; Anderson, *Suicide in Victorian and Edwardian England*, pp. 346, 348–50 (on Farr); John P. Wright, "Hysteria and Mechanical Man," *Journal of the History of Ideas* 41(April–June 1980):242 (on Sydenham).

37. Kitty Muggeridge and Ruth Adam, *Beatrice Webb: A Life, 1858–1943* (London: Secker & Warburg, 1967), pp. 135–36.

38. Galton, *Memories of My Life*, p. 44; Allbutt, "Nervous Diseases and Modern Life," p. 224. See John Pemble, *The Mediterranean Passion: Victorians and Edwardians in the South* (Oxford: Clarendon, 1987), pp. 91–92 (for "the object of nature-therapy").

39. Brontë, *Villette,* ch. 17.

40. Craig, *Psychological Medicine,* pp. 247–48; Frances Kingsley, ed., *Charles Kingsley, His Letters and Memories of His Life,* abr. ed. (New York: Charles Scribner's, 1877), pp. 111, 118–19; Susan Chitty, *The Beast and the Monk: A Life of Charles Kingsley* (New York: Mason/Charter, 1975), pp. 116–19, 123–26 (p. 118 for "poor addle brain.")

41. Savill, *Clinical Lectures on Neurasthenia,* p. 160.

42. David Newsome, *On the Edge of Paradise. A. C. Benson: The Diarist* (London: John Murray, 1980), pp. 224–27, 230.

43. James Crichton-Browne, *What the Doctor Thought* (London: Ernest Benn, 1930), p. 211; T. Clifford Allbutt, *On Visceral Neuroses* (London: Churchill, 1884), p. 98; Brown, *Treatment of Nervous Disease,* pp. 405–406.

44. Thomas Hughes, *Tom Brown's Schooldays,* ch. 1; Kingsley, ed., *Charles Kingsley,* pp. 346–47. The third and fourth editions of Clark's book, published in 1841 and 1846, were entitled *The Sanative Influence of Climate.* He was the physician who tragically misdiagnosed Lady Flora Hasting's tumor as pregnancy, thereby rocking Queen Victoria's court in 1839.

45. Austen, *Sanditon,* p. 19.

46. Benjamin Collins Brodie, *Autobiography of the Late Sir Benjamin C. Brodie, Bart.* (London: Longman, Green, Longmans, Roberts, & Green, 1865), pp. 112–13; Keith Robbins, *John Bright* (London and Boston: Routledge & Kegan Paul, 1979), p. 210; John Tyndall, *Faraday as a Discoverer* (London: Longmans, Green, 1868), p. 76. Also see L. Pearce Williams, *Michael Faraday: A Biography* (New York: Basic Books, 1965), pp. 358–59, and Edward Hare, "Michael Faraday's Loss of Memory," *Proceedings of the Royal Institution of Great Britain* 49 (1976):33–35.

47. Jo Manton, *Mary Carpenter and the Children of the Streets* (London: Heinemann Educational Books, 1976), p. 55; Grant-Smith, *Experiences of an Asylum Patient,* p. 54; Herbert Spencer, *An Autobiography,* 2 vols. (London: Williams & Norgate, 1904), 1:466–68, 482–83, 2:411.

48. Henry Maudsley, "Suicide in Simple Melancholy," *Medical Magazine* 1(1892–93):49.

49. Newsome, *Edge of Paradise,* p. 225; also see A. C. Benson, *The Diary of Arthur Christopher Benson,* ed. Percy Lubbock (New York: Longmans, Green, 1926), p. 155; Henry Bence Jones, *The Life and Letters of Faraday,* 2 vols. (London: Longmans, Green, 1870), 2:126–27, 151–54, and *DNB,* s.v. "Faraday, Michael," by John Tyndall.

50. J. Crichton-Browne, "Education and the Nervous System," in Malcolm Morris, ed., *The Book of Health* (London: Cassell, 1883), pp. 318–19; on Eliot, see Chapter 2, p. 73, of this book; Oliphant, *Tulloch,* p. 172; Norman-Butler, *Victorian Aspirations,* pp. 45–46 (on Booth); Manton, *Mary Carpenter,* pp. 32, 55–57; Ben Tillett, *Memories and Reflections* (London: John Long, 1931), p. 196, and Jonathan Schneer, *Ben Tillett: Portrait of a Labour Leader* (London and Canberra: Croom Helm, 1982), p. 131 (on Bottomley).

51. This paragraph is indebted to Pemble, *Mediterranean Passion.*

52. Ibid., p. 86; Bright, *Diaries,* pp. 205–30; Spencer, *Autobiography,* 2:320–22, 333–47, and David Duncan, *The Life and Letters of Herbert Spencer* (London: Methuen, 1908), pp. 196–97, 204–206; James Sully, *My Life and Friends: A Psychologist's Memories* (London: T. Fisher Unwin, 1918), pp. 149–61; Edward Lyttelton, *Alfred Lyttelton: His Home-Training and Earlier Life* (Privately printed, [1916?]), pp. 42–43 (Edward and Alfred were Lord Lyttelton's sons).

53. Dowse, *Brain and Nerve Exhaustion,* pp. 57–58. For some other examples of Alpine therapy applied to depressed and nervous patients, see J. A. Symonds, *The Memoirs of John Addington Symonds,* ed. Phyllis Grosskurth (Chicago: University of Chicago Press, 1986), p. 137; Norman-Butler, *Victorian Aspirations,* pp. 44–45, and Simey and Simey,

Charles Booth, pp. 51–53; Sully, *My Life and Friends,* p. 172; Huxley, *Life and Letters of T. H. Huxley,* 1:155.

54. Galton, *Memories of My Life,* p. 79; Edwin Landseer to Miss Potts and Jessica Landseer, 28 August 1840, Landseer Correspondence, Eng MS, 86 RR, vol. 3, no. 186, Victoria and Albert Museum Library, London; and Ormond, *Landseer,* p. 10.

55. D. H. Lawrence, *Lady Chatterley's Lover,* ch. 7.

56. "Desk Diseases, as Contracted in Counting-Houses, Libraries, and Public Offices," *Family Oracle of Health* 1(1824):420–21; on the eighteenth-century background, see Richard Metcalfe, *The Rise and Progress of Hydropathy in England and Scotland* (London: Simpkin, Marshall, Hamilton, Kent, 1906), pp. 6–19.

57. R. T. Claridge, *Hydropathy; or, The Cold Water Cure, as Practised by Vincent Priessnitz, at Graefenberg, Silesia, Austria* (London: James Madden, 1842); Metcalfe, *Rise and Progress of Hydropathy,* pp. 31–41, 58; Marshall Scott Legan, "Hydropathy in America: A Nineteenth Century Panacea," *Bull Hist Med* 45(May–June 1971):268–71.

58. Metcalfe, *Rise and Progress of Hydropathy,* pp. 48–49, 50–53.

59. The prospectus for Metcalfe's hydros is printed in Richard Metcalfe, ed., *Testimonies to the Efficacy of Hydropathy in the Cure of Disease* (London: W. Tweedie, [1878]), pp. 6–10.

60. Gully, *Neuropathy,* p. 106; *A Prospectus of the Water Cure Establishment at Malvern, under the Professional Management of James Wilson, M.D., and James M. Gully, M.D.* (London: Cunningham & Mortimer, 1843), pp. 2–11; Metcalfe, *Rise and Progress of Hydropathy,* pp. 58–74.

61. Metcalfe, *Rise and Progress of Hydropathy,* pp. 99–106, on McLeod, whose name Metcalfe incorrectly spells as "Macleod." Gully's hydropathic works include *The Water Cure in Chronic Disease* (London: Churchill; Malvern: Henry Lamb, 1846); *A Guide to Domestic Hydrotherapeia: The Water Cure in Acute Disease* (London: Simpkin, 1863); and *A Monograph on Fever and Its Treatment by Hydro-therapeutic Means* (London: Simpkin, Marshall, 1885).

62. James Freeman, *Medical Reflections on the Water Cure* (London: Saunders & Otley, 1842), pp. 22–23.

63. Edward Johnson, *Hydropathy. The Theory, Principles, and Practice of the Water Cure Shewn to Be in Accordance with Medical Science and the Teachings of Common Sense* (London: Simpkin, Marshall; Ipswich: Burton, 1843), pp. xiv–xv.

64. Gully, *Water Cure in Chronic Disease,* pp. 281n, 277.

65. Ibid., p. 279; Thomas J. Graham, *The Cold-Water System,* 2d ed. (London: Simpkin, Marshall, and Hatchards, 1843), p. 128.

66. For a sympathetic account of Gully as a psychotherapist, particularly skilled in treating troubled women, see Mary S. Hartman, *Victorian Murderesses: A True History of Thirteen Respectable French and English Women Accused of Unspeakable Crimes* (New York: Schocken Books, 1977), ch. 4.

67. Gully, *Neuropathy,* p. 106; James Wilson and James M. Gully, *The Dangers of the Water Cure and Its Efficacy Examined and Compared with Those of the Drug Treatment of Diseases* (London: Cunningham & Mortimer, 1843), pp. 41–42; Henry Harnett, "Observations on Insanity. . ." *Water Cure Journal and Hygienic Magazine* 2(1849):375. Homeopathy, another unorthodox medical response to promiscuous drugging in the first half of the nineteenth century, was not much used for cases of nervous exhaustion.

68. Haley, *Healthy Body and Victorian Culture,* pp. 16, 34.

69. Elizabeth Jenkins, *Tennyson and Dr. Gully* (Lincoln: The Tennyson Society, Tennyson Research Centre, 1974), pp. 4, 9–10; Carlyle quoted in James Crichton-Browne, *The Doctor's Second Thoughts* (London: Ernest Benn, 1931), pp. 254–55; Metcalfe, *Rise and*

Progress of Hydropathy, p. 74 (giving the correct date of Carlyle's visit to Malvern, which Crichton-Browne erroneously stated as 1831); Colp, *To Be an Invalid*, pp. 40–43, 45, 57–69, 75–76; Kohn, ''Darwin's Chronic Ill Health,'' pp. 244–46.

70. Spencer, *Autobiography*, 1:413–14, 448–50, 480; Bright, *Diaries*, p. 204; Metcalfe, *Rise and Progress of Hydropathy*, p. 106, reported that the large hydros in their heyday accommodated 150 to 200 patients at a time.

71. Oliphant, *Tulloch*, pp. 169–70; Jenkins, *Tennyson and Gully*, p. 10 (on Nightingale); Samuel Greg, *A Layman's Legacy in Prose and Verse* (London: Macmillan, 1877), pp. 21–23; Sully, *My Life and Friends*, p. 183 (on Bain).

72. F. B. Smith, *The People's Health, 1830–1910* (London: Croom Helm, 1979), p. 342.

73. No one was ever found guilty of the murder, although the jury refused to call Charles Bravo's death a suicide. See Hartman, *Victorian Murderesses*, ch. 4.

74. Ernest Jones, ''The Treatment of the Neuroses, Including the Psychoneuroses,'' in William A. White and Smith Ely Jelliffe, eds., *The Modern Treatment of Nervous and Mental Diseases*, vol. 1 (London: Henry Kimpton; Glasgow: Alexander Stenhouse, 1913), p. 349.

75. James Johnson, *An Essay on Morbid Sensibility of the Stomach and Bowels, as the Proximate Cause, or Characteristic Condition of Indigestion, Nervous Irritability, Mental Despondency, Hypochondriasis . . .* (London: Underwood, 1827), p. 118.

76. Dowse, *Brain and Nerve Exhaustion*, p. 61; Allbutt, *Visceral Neuroses*, p. 98; Amy Levy, *Reuben Sachs, A Sketch* (London: Macmillan, 1888), pp. 3, 5; W. Clark, ''Hydropathic Institution for Working Classes,'' *Water Cure Journal* 1(1847):180–82; also ''Correspondence and Remarks,'' *Water Cure Journal* 1(1847):147–49; Metcalfe, *Rise and Progress of Hydropathy*, pp. 56, 105.

77. Daniel Noble, *Facts and Observations Relative to the Influence of Manufactures upon Health and Life* (London: Churchill, 1843), p. 81; J. Michell Clarke, *Hysteria & Neurasthenia* (London: The Bodley Head, 1905), p. 262.

78. Alfred T. Schofield, *Unconscious Therapeutics; or, The Personality of the Physician* (London: Churchill, 1904), p. 107. Also see Sara Coleridge's comments to a similar effect in her dialogue on ''Nervousness'' (1834), reprinted in Bradford Keyes Mudge, *Sara Coleridge, A Victorian Daughter* (New Haven and London: Yale University Press, 1989), pp. 207–208.

79. Ian Dowbiggin, ''Degeneration and Hereditarianism in French Mental Medicine 1840–90: Psychiatric Theory as Ideological Adaptation,'' in Bynum, Porter, and Shepherd, eds., *Anatomy of Madness*, 1:200. ''Therapeutic eclecticism'' is also Dowbiggin's phrase, translating from the French of Jean-Pierre Falret, a nineteenth-century psychiatrist.

80. See the ''Introduction,'' in Bynum, Porter, and Shepherd, eds., *Anatomy of Madness*, 1:16.

81. Stuart Sutherland, *Breakdown: A Personal Crisis and a Medical Dilemma*, rev. ed. (London: Weidenfeld & Nicolson, 1987), p. 215; also see pp. 62, 94, 204.

82. Alexander Bain, *John Stuart Mill, A Criticism, with Personal Recollections* (London: Longmans, Green, 1882), p. 91.

Chapter 5

1. Arthur Christopher Benson, *The Life of Edward White Benson, Sometime Archbishop of Canterbury*, new ed., abr. (London: Macmillan, 1901), p. 240; Margaret Oliphant, *Autobiography and Letters of Mrs. Margaret Oliphant*, ed. Mrs. Harry Coghill (1899; Leicester: Leicester University Press, 1974), pp. 120, 123–24; Regenia Gagnier, ''Social Atoms: Working-Class Autobiography, Subjectivity, and Gender,'' *Victorian Studies* 30(Spring 1987):361.

2. Daniel H. Tuke, "On the Various Forms of Mental Disorder," *Asylum Journal of Mental Science* 3(1857):230; Alfred T. Schofield, *The Force of Mind or the Mental Factor in Medicine* (London: Churchill, 1902), p. 105. For the transition from melancholy to hypochondriasis, and thence to neurasthenia, see Esther Fischer-Homberger, "Hypochondriasis of the Eighteenth Century—Neurosis of the Present Century," *Bull Hist Med* 46(July–Aug. 1972):391–97, and, at much greater length, *Hypochondrie. Melancholie bis Neurose: Krankheiten und Zustandbilder* (Bern: Hans Huber, 1970). Also see Ilza Veith, "On Hysterical and Hypochondriacal Afflictions," *Bull Hist Med* 30(May–June 1956):234–39, and Susan Baur, *Hypochondria: Woeful Imaginings* (Berkeley and Los Angeles: University of California Press, 1988), pp. 21–28. Stanley W. Jackson traces the relationships among the changing names for depressive symptoms throughout *Melancholia and Depression: From Hippocratic Times to Modern Times* (New Haven and London: Yale University Press, 1986).

3. Benjamin Rush, *Medical Inquiries and Observations, upon the Diseases of the Mind* (1812; facsimile ed., New York: Hafner Publishing Co., 1962), p. 77; J. C. Prichard, "Hypochondriasis," in John Forbes, Alexander Tweedie, and John Conolly, eds., *The Cyclopædia of Practical Medicine,* 4 vols. (London: Sherwood, Gilbert, Piper, Baldwin, & Cradock, 1833–35), 2:552; John Charles Bucknill and Daniel H. Tuke, *A Manual of Psychological Medicine* (London: Churchill, 1858), p. 168. On the enfeeblement of the will in hypochondriasis, see James Manby Gully, *The Water Cure in Chronic Disease* (London: Churchill; Malvern: Henry Lamb, 1846), p. 280, and Henry Holland, *Medical Notes and Reflections,* 3d ed. (London: Longman, Brown, Green, and Longmans, 1855), p. 419.

4. John Conolly, "Hysteria," in Forbes, Tweedie, and Conolly, eds., *Cyclopædia of Practical Medicine,* 2:565.

5. Thomas Laycock, *A Treatise on the Nervous Diseases of Women* (London: Longman, Orme, Brown, Green, and Longmans, 1840), pp. 8, 82; C. H. F. Routh, *On Overwork and Premature Mental Decay: Its Treatment* (London: Baillière, Tindall, & Cox, 1876), p. 19; "The Systematic Treatment of Nerve Prostration," *Medical Times and Gazette,* 7 Feb. 1885, pp. 188–89.

6. Mark S. Micale, "Diagnostic Discriminations: Jean-Martin Charcot and the Nineteenth-Century Idea of Masculine Hysterical Neurosis," unpublished paper, presented to the Wellcome Institute for the History of Medicine, London, 20 Oct. 1987, pp. 22–23 (I am very grateful to Dr. Micale for sending me his paper); Thomas Stretch Dowse, *Lectures on Massage & Electricity in the Treatment of Disease* (London: Hamilton, Adams; Bristol: John Wright, [1889]), p. 197; H. B. Donkin, "Hysteria," in D. Hack Tuke, ed., *A Dictionary of Psychological Medicine,* 2 vols. (London: Churchill, 1892), 1:624. Also see, in the same volume, J. M. Charcot and Pierre Marie, "Hysteria, Mainly Hystero-Epilepsy," pp. 627–41.

7. Donkin, "Hysteria," p. 625.

8. J. Michell Clarke, "Hysteria and Neurasthenia," *Brain* 17(1894):122 (on sturdy and delicate neurasthenics); Schofield, *Force of Mind,* p. 101.

9. James Johnson, *Change of Air, or the Pursuit of Health* (London: S. Highley and T. G. Underwood, 1831), p. 3.

10. Two recent books on Victorian suicide point out that British romanticism was not, generally speaking, sympathetic to the cult of Goethe's young Werther, which engulfed continental Europe in the late eighteenth and early nineteenth centuries: Olive Anderson, *Suicide in Victorian and Edwardian England* (Oxford: Clarendon, 1987), pp. 213, 249, and Barbara T. Gates, *Victorian Suicide: Mad Crimes and Sad Histories* (Princeton: Princeton University Press, 1988), pp. 24–25.

11. All discussions of early Victorian ideals of manliness owe a debt of gratitude to David Newsome, *Godliness and Good Learning: Four Studies on a Victorian Ideal* (London: John Murray, 1961). For the ideas summarized in this paragraph, see pp. 25, 34, 83–91, 195–97. Jeffrey Richards, "'Passing the Love of Women': Manly Love and Victorian Society," in James A. Mangan and James Walvin, eds., *Manliness and Morality: Middle-Class Masculinity in Britain and America, 1800–1940* (Manchester: Manchester University Press; New York: St. Martin's Press, 1987), pp. 92–122, provides a valuable discussion of the subject and breaks down the Victorian concept of manliness into the three periods roughly adopted here.

12. For the rich variety in early nineteenth-century British views of manliness, see Norman Vance, *The Sinews of the Spirit: The Ideal of Christian Manliness in Victorian Literature and Religious Thought* (Cambridge and New York: Cambridge University Press, 1985), ch. 1.

13. Leonore Davidoff and Catherine Hall, *Family Fortunes: Men and Women of the English Middle Class, 1780–1850* (Chicago: University of Chicago Press, 1987), persuasively portray the construction of this domesticated middle-class ideal of manliness under the influence of evangelicalism.

14. For some of the ideas discussed in this paragraph, see Charles E. Rosenberg, "Body and Mind in Nineteenth-Century Medicine: Some Clinical Origins of the Neurosis Construct," *Bull Hist Med* 63(Summer 1989):187, 191–92, and Vieda Skultans, *English Madness: Ideas on Insanity, 1580–1890* (London: Routledge & Kegan Paul, 1979), p. 86.

15. As Vance argues throughout *Sinews of the Spirit*.

16. Frances Kingsley, ed., *Charles Kingsley, His Letters and Memories of His Life*, abr. ed. (New York: Charles Scribner's, 1877), p. 113. Also see Bruce Haley, *The Healthy Body and Victorian Culture* (Cambridge, Mass.: Harvard University Press, 1978), p. 109, and Allen Warren, "Popular Manliness: Baden-Powell, Scouting, and the Development of Manly Character," in Mangan and Walvin, eds., *Manliness and Morality*, p. 199.

17. Henry Maudsley, "Memoir of the Late John Conolly," *JMS* 12(July 1866):160–61, 173.

18. Wilkie Collins, *The Woman in White*, ed. Julian Symons (Harmondsworth: Penguin, 1974), pp. 61, 66, 370. For a fascinating, if overwrought, discussion of Fairlie and gender surprises in this novel, see D. A. Miller, "*Cage aux Folles:* Sensation and Gender in Wilkie Collins's *The Woman in White*," *Representations*, no. 14(Spring 1986):107–36.

19. "Mr. Bright's Retirement," *Economist*, 24 Dec. 1870, p. 1545—attributed to Bagehot by Keith Robbins, *John Bright* (London: Routledge & Kegan Paul, 1979), p. 210; J. Milner Fothergill, *The Maintenance of Health: A Medical Work for Lay Readers* (London: Smith, Elder, 1874), pp. 260–61.

20. This is the crux of the argument in J. A. Mangan, "Social Darwinism and Upper-Class Education in Late Victorian and Edwardian England," in Mangan and Walvin, eds., *Manliness and Morality*, pp. 135–59.

21. See J. A. Mangan and James Walvin, "Introduction," in Mangan and Walvin, eds., *Manliness and Morality*, p. 1. Mangan has explored the themes discussed here in great detail in *Athleticism in the Victorian and Edwardian Public School: The Emergence and Consolidation of an Educational Ideology* (Cambridge and New York: Cambridge University Press, 1981) and *The Games Ethic and Imperialism: Aspects of the Diffusion of an Ideal* (Harmondsworth and New York: Viking, 1986).

22. John Springhall, "Building Character in the British Boy: The Attempt to Extend Christian Manliness to Working-Class Adolescents, 1880–1914," in Mangan and Walvin, eds., *Manliness and Morality*, pp. 52–74, explores the degree to which working-class boys accepted the middle- and upper-class ideals of manliness, and the extent to which they

clung to their own ethos, "which placed a heavy emphasis on drinking and fighting" (p. 69). In the same volume, also see John M. MacKenzie, "The Imperial Pioneer and Hunter and the British Masculine Stereotype in Late Victorian and Edwardian Times," pp. 176–80, and Warren, "Popular Manliness," pp. 200–202.

23. Benjamin Ward Richardson, *The Field of Disease. A Book of Preventive Medicine* (London: Macmillan, 1883), pp. 627–28.

24. Charles Mercier, "Melancholia," in Tuke, ed., *Dictionary of Psychological Medicine*, 2:788; Jules Verne, *Around the World in Eighty Days* (1873), ch. 18.

25. Mangan, "Social Darwinism and Upper-Class Education," pp. 140–43, 152.

26. Henry Maudsley, "Suicide in Simple Melancholy," *Medical Magazine* 1(1892–93):48, 47.

27. Thomas Smith Clouston, *The Hygiene of Mind* (London: Methuen, 1906), p. 36; W. S. Hedley, "The Insomnia of Neurasthenia," *Lancet,* 10 June 1893, p. 1381.

28. See Martin Stone, "Shellshock and the Psychologists," in W. F. Bynum, Roy Porter, and Michael Shepherd, eds., *The Anatomy of Madness: Essays in the History of Psychiatry,* 2 vols. (London and New York: Tavistock Publications, 1985), 2:242–71.

29. "The Nature and Causes of Depression—Part III," *Harvard Medical School Mental Health Letter* 4(March 1988):3–4.

30. See Chapter 6 of this book for a discussion of the way nerves and gender stereotypes figured in evolutionary theory.

31. As G. J. Barker-Benfield points out, in "Mary Wollstonecraft's Depression and Diagnosis: The Relation Between Sensibility and Women's Susceptibility to Nervous Disorders," *Psychohistory Review* 13(1985):21.

32. Edwin Lee, *A Treatise on Some Nervous Disorders,* 2d ed. enl. (London: Churchill, 1838), p. 16.

33. Routh, *On Overwork,* p. 15; James Crichton-Browne, "An Oration on Sex in Education," *Lancet,* 7 May 1892, p. 1017; Seymour J. Sharkey, "Hysteria and Neurasthenia," *Brain* 27(Spring 1904):18–19; Arthur Conan Doyle, "The Adventure of the Devil's Foot," *His Last Bow.*

34. J. C. Bucknill, "The President's Address," *JMS* 7(Oct. 1860):7–8; J. Strahan, "Puzzling Conditions of the Heart and Other Organs Dependent on Neurasthenia," *BMJ,* 5 Sept. 1885, p. 435; Thomas Stretch Dowse, *The Brain and the Nerves: Their Ailments and Their Exhaustion* (London: Baillière, Tindall, & Cox, [1884]), p. 131; T. Wemyss Reid, ed., *A Memoir of John Deakin Heaton, M.D., of Leeds* (London: Longmans, Green, 1883), pp. 248–49; Anderson, *Suicide in Victorian and Edwardian England,* pp. 70, 94–95.

35. Benjamin Ward Richardson, *Diseases of Modern Life* (London: Macmillan, 1876), p. 123—a volume that incorporated an earlier series of Richardson's articles on the diseases of overworked men; Frederick MacCabe, "On Mental Strain and Overwork," *JMS* 21(Oct. 1875):394–401; Thomas Stretch Dowse, *On Brain and Nerve Exhaustion. 'Neurasthenia.' Its Nature and Curative Treatment* (London: Baillière, Tindall, & Cox, 1880), p. 42.

36. J. J. Graham Brown, *The Treatment of Nervous Disease* (Edinburgh and London: William Green, 1905), pp. 373–74.

37. Johnson, *Change of Air,* pp. 2–3.

38. C. Mercier, "Delusion," in Tuke, ed., *Dictionary of Psychological Medicine,* 1:346. Among innumerable other examples, see Andrew Wynter, *The Borderlands of Insanity and Other Allied Papers* (London: Robert Hardwicke, 1875), p. 13, and John Michell Clarke, *Hysteria & Neurasthenia* (London: The Bodley Head, 1905), p. 180.

39. Arthur Conan Doyle, *The Hound of the Baskervilles* (1902), ch. 14. A trip around the world set Sir Henry right.

40. G. M. Trevelyan, *The Life of John Bright* (London: Constable, 1913), p. 254. Also see George Barnett Smith, *The Life and Speeches of the Right Hon. John Bright, M.P.*, 2 vols. (London: Hodder & Stoughton, 1881), 1:423; William Robertson, *Life and Times of the Right Hon. John Bright* (London: Cassell, 1883), p. 322; Francis Watt, *The Life and Opinions of the Right Hon. John Bright* (London: James Sangster, [1886]), p. 151.

41. James A. Manson, *Sir Edwin Landseer, R.A.* (London: Walter Scott, and New York: Scribner's 1902), pp. 100–101, 108–112; Alexander Bain, *John Stuart Mill, A Criticism, with Personal Recollections* (London: Longmans, Green, 1882), pp. 37–38; Henry Bence Jones, *The Life and Letters of Faraday*, 2 vols. (London: Longmans, Green, 1870), 2:126; J. H. Gladstone, *Michael Faraday* (London: Macmillan, 1872), p. 38.

42. James Sully, *My Life and Friends: A Psychologist's Memories* (London: T. Fisher Unwin, 1918), p. 149; Francis Galton, *Memories of My Life* (New York: E. P. Dutton, 1909), pp. 78–79; Sarah Austin quoted in Lotte Hamburger and Joseph Hamburger, *Troubled Lives: John and Sarah Austin* (Toronto: University of Toronto Press, 1985), p. 152.

43. Herbert Spencer, *An Autobiography*, 2 vols. (London: Williams & Norgate, 1904), 1:495, 466, 464. See Lee Krenis's astute comment on Spencer's "intellectual hubris," in "Authority and Rebellion in Victorian Autobiography," *Journal of British Studies* 18(Fall 1978):126. Doctors considered unusual head pains to signify suicidal tendencies, according to Anderson, *Suicide in Victorian and Edwardian England*, pp. 385–86.

44. Lionel John Beale, *The Laws of Health, in Relation to Mind and Body* (London: Churchill, 1851), p. 214.

45. Beatrice Webb, *Our Partnership*, ed. Barbara Drake and Margaret I. Cole (London: Longmans, Green, 1948), p. 348. Also see Kitty Muggeridge and Ruth Adam, *Beatrice Webb, A Life 1858–1943* (London: Secker & Warburg, 1967), p. 182.

46. Arthur Christopher Benson, *Beside Still Waters* (New York and London: G. P. Putnam's, 1907), p. 257.

47. "Woman in Her Psychological Relations," *J Psych Med* 4(Jan. 1851):46; Forbes Winslow, *On Softening of the Brain Arising from Anxiety & Undue Mental Exercise and Resulting in Impairment of Mind* (London: Churchill, 1849), p. 13. See E. H. Hare, "Masturbatory Insanity: The History of an Idea," *JMS* 108(Jan. 1962):1–25.

48. J. Crichton-Browne, "Acute Dementia," *WRLAMR* 4(1874):270–71.

49. Among extensive writings of these topics, see H. Tristram Engelhardt, Jr., "The Disease of Masturbation: Values and the Concept of Disease," *Bull Hist Med* 48(1974):234–48; Arthur N. Gilbert, "Doctor, Patient, and Onanist Diseases in the Nineteenth Century," *Journal of the History of Medicine and Allied Sciences* 30(July 1975):217–34, and "Masturbation and Insanity: Henry Maudsley and the Ideology of Sexual Repression," *Albion* 12(Fall 1980):268–82; Robert H. MacDonald, "The Frightful Consequences of Onanism: Notes on the History of a Delusion," *Journal of the History of Ideas* 28(1967):423–31; Skultans, *English Madness*, pp. 69–76. For a historical overview, see Jean Stengers and Anne Van Neck, *Histoire d'une Grande Peur: La Masturbation* (Brussels: Editions de l'Université de Bruxelles, 1984).

50. Peter T. Cominos drew attention to the presumed links between sexual continence and capitalist accumulation in "Late-Victorian Sexual Respectability and the Social System," *International Review of Social History* 8(1963):18–48, 216–50, and G. J. Barker-Benfield elaborated on the idea in "The Spermatic Economy: A Nineteenth Century View of Sexuality," *Feminist Studies* 1(1973):45–74.

51. MacDonald, "Frightful Consequences of Onanism," p. 431.

52. Anderson, *Suicide in Victorian and Edwardian England*, pp. 187–88; Gilbert, "Doctor, Patient, and Onanist Diseases," pp. 225–28, 233; Engelhardt, "Disease of Masturbation," pp. 244–45; MacDonald, "Frightful Consequences of Onanism," p. 429.

53. As Gilbert argues, in "Doctor, Patient, and Onanist Diseases," pp. 222–23, 225–28, 231–33.

54. See Hare, "Masturbatory Insanity," pp. 11–12.

55. R. P. Neuman, "Masturbation, Madness, and the Modern Concepts of Childhood and Adolescence," *Journal of Social History* 8(Spring 1975):6.

56. F. B. Smith, *The People's Health, 1830–1910* (London: Croom Helm, 1979), pp. 295–96.

57. James Paget, *Clinical Lectures and Essays,* ed. Howard Marsh (London: Longmans, Green, 1875), pp. 277, and 268–91 passim; E. Stengel, "Hughlings Jackson's Influence in Psychiatry," *British Journal of Psychiatry* 109(1963):353; Alfred T. Schofield, *Functional Nerve Diseases* (London: Methuen, 1908), p. 67. On Paget, also see M. Jeanne Peterson, "Dr. Acton's Enemy: Medicine, Sex, and Society in Victorian England," *Victorian Studies* 29(Summer 1986):569–90.

58. Engelhardt, "Disease of Masturbation," p. 234.

59. See Frank Mort, *Dangerous Sexualities: Medico-Moral Politics in England since 1830* (London and New York: Routledge & Kegan Paul, 1987), pp. 77–79. Medical opinion in the late nineteenth century also debated whether sexual feeling was located in the genitals, as traditionally believed, or was a product of the mind, as some modern writers contended.

60. James Ross, *Handbook of the Diseases of the Nervous System* (London: Churchill, 1885), p. 579; Strahan, "Puzzling Conditions," p. 436; Maurice Craig, *Psychological Medicine. A Manual on Mental Diseases for Practitioners and Students* (London: Churchill, 1905), p. 245.

61. See Peterson, "Dr. Acton's Enemy," pp. 569–71, for a helpful summary of the recent debate over Victorian attitudes toward sexuality.

62. For example, Conolly, "Hysteria," p. 565; Donkin, "Hysteria," p. 625; Robert Brudenell Carter, *On the Pathology and Treatment of Hysteria* (London: Churchill, 1853), p. 33.

63. J. A. Symonds, *The Memoirs of John Addington Symonds,* ed. Phyllis Grosskurth (Chicago: University of Chicago Press, 1986), pp. 151–52, and Phyllis Grosskurth, *John Addington Symonds, A Biography* (London: Longmans, 1964), p. 85. Also see Schofield, *Functional Nerve Diseases,* p. 127, and Clifford Allbutt, "Neurasthenia," in Clifford Allbutt and Humphry Davy Rolleston, eds., *A System of Medicine,* 2d ed. rev., 9 vols. (London: Macmillan, 1905–11), 8:761.

64. Blackwell quoted in Jeffrey Weeks, "'Sins and Diseases': Some Notes on Homosexuality in the Nineteenth Century," *History Workshop,* issue 1(Spring 1976):214; Symonds, *Memoirs,* p. 152; Clouston, *Hygiene of Mind,* p. 245.

65. For the Kingsley-Grenfell letters, see Susan Chitty, *The Beast and the Monk: A Life of Charles Kingsley* (New York: Mason/Charter, 1975), pp. 79–88; Spencer, *Autobiography,* 1:478, 493.

66. Spencer, *Autobiography,* 1:478–79, 497; on the Cripps children's visit, see Walter Troughton, "Typescript Account of H. Spencer's Life, 1888–1903," Herbert Spencer Papers, MS 791/355/3, University of London Library, Senate House, London, pp. 14–15.

67. Since there is no complete agreement concerning the terminal date of adolescence, I am using eighteen years old as the beginning of adulthood and discussing these cases in this chapter, rather than in Chapter 7, all the more so since most of the men discussed here continued to suffer from intermittent bouts of depression throughout their adult lives.

68. Frank Podmore, *Modern Spiritualism: A History and a Criticism,* 2 vols. (London: Methuen, 1902), 2:275; Spencer, *Autobiography,* 1:475.

69. William Withey Gull, "Anorexia Nervosa (Apepsia Hysterica, Anorexia Hysterica)," *Transactions of the Clinical Society of London* 7(1874):22; Elizabeth Garrett Anderson,

"Sex in Mind and Education: A Reply," *Fortnightly Review,* n.s., 15(1874):589; W. H. B. Stoddart, *Mind and Its Disorders. A Text-Book for Students and Practitioners* (London: H. K. Lewis, 1908), p. 362. Also see Thomas Dixon Savill, *Clinical Lectures on Neurasthenia,* 3d ed., rev. and enl. (London: Henry Glaisher, 1906), p. 48.

70. On Galton's exams, see Daniel J. Kevles, *In the Name of Eugenics: Genetics and the Uses of Human Heredity* (Berkeley and Los Angeles: University of California Press, paperback ed., 1986), p. 9; Galton, *Memories of My Life,* pp. 78–81; Toynbee quoted in William H. McNeill, *Arnold J. Toynbee, A Life* (Oxford and New York: Oxford University Press, 1989), p. 34.

71. For his parents' interpretation of Ruskin's breakdown, see Van Akin Burd, Introduction to *John Ruskin and Rose La Touche: Her Unpublished Diaries of 1861 and 1867* (Oxford: Clarendon, 1979), p. 64. A persuasively argued example of recent studies that focus on the relationships within the Ruskin family is Michael Brooks's essay, "Love and Possession in a Victorian Household: The Example of the Ruskins," in Anthony S. Wohl, ed., *The Victorian Family: Structure and Stresses* (New York: St. Martin's Press, 1978), pp. 82–100. Ruskin's case was complicated by the fact that he was suffering from tuberculosis at the time.

72. This is the main thread of argument in Krenis, "Authority and Rebellion," pp. 107–30. A far less balanced assessment is provided by Stephen Kern, in "Explosive Intimacy: Psychodynamics of the Victorian Family," *History of Childhood Quarterly* 1(1973–74):437–61, which, in any case, draws far more heavily on German than British sources to present a picture of the conflict-laden Victorian family.

73. Summary drawn from the first six chapters of Sully, *My Life and Friends.* The "depressing reaction" of 1866–67 appears on p. 77.

74. Jeannette Marshall's diaries quoted in Zuzanna Shonfield, *The Precariously Privileged: A Professional Family in Victorian London* (Oxford and New York: Oxford University Press, 1987), pp. 104–105, 122–32.

75. Oscar Browning, "Personal Recollection of Sir John Seeley and Lord Acton," *Albany Review* 2(Feb. 1908):550; Roy Jenkins, *Sir Charles Dilke, A Victorian Tragedy* (London: Collins, 1958), pp. 89–91.

76. Edward Hare, "Michael Faraday's Loss of Memory," *Proceedings of the Royal Institution of Great Britain* 49(1976):43–45; Lister's father quoted in Rickman John Godlee, *Lord Lister* (London: Macmillan, 1917), pp. 15–16. On influenza and depression, see Anderson, *Suicide in Victorian and Edwardian England,* p. 169.

77. Charlotte Brontë, *Villette* (1853), ch. 1; Margaret Oliphant, *A Memoir of the Life of John Tulloch, D.D., LL.D.,* 3d ed. (Edinburgh and London: William Blackwood, 1889), pp. 166–67.

78. W. L. Courtney, *Life of John Stuart Mill* (London: Walter Scott, 1889), p. 56.

79. Arthur Christopher Benson, *The House of Quiet, An Autobiography* (New York: E. P. Dutton, 1906), pp. 56–60, and David Newsome, *On the Edge of Paradise. A. C. Benson: The Diarist* (London: John Murray, 1980), pp. 37–43; Arthur Christopher Benson, *Ruskin, a Study in Personality* (London: Smith, Elder, 1911), pp. 18, 20; E. T. Cook, *The Life of John Ruskin,* 2 vols. (New York: Macmillan; London: George Allen, 1911), 1:96.

80. E. M. Forster, *A Room With a View* (1908), ch. 14.

81. Mill's disappointingly uninformative letters from this period are found in Francis E. Mineka, ed., *The Earlier Letters of John Stuart Mill, 1812–1848,* vol. 12 of *The Collected Works of John Stuart Mill* (Toronto: University of Toronto Press, and London: Routledge & Kegan Paul, 1963), pp. 16–25 (with no letters from 1826 itself.) For a full-blown psychoanalytic treatment, complete with Oedipal crisis, see Bruce Mazlish, *James and*

John Stuart Mill: Father and Son in the Nineteenth Century (New York: Basic Books, 1975), pp. 205–30.

82. J. S. Mill, *Autobiography* (London: Longmans, Green, Reader, & Dyer, 1873), pp. 133–38, 140–41, 143.

83. Michael St. John Packe, *The Life of John Stuart Mill* (London: Secker & Warburg, 1954), p. 80; Gagnier, "Social Atoms," p. 344, on the format of spiritual autobiography. Janice Carlisle, "J. S. Mill's *Autobiography:* The Life of a 'Bookish Man','' *Victorian Studies* 33(Autumn 1989):134–39, reads Mill's crisis in terms of his vocational aspirations, which James Mill threatened by obtaining a clerical post for his son at the East India Company.

84. Bain, *Mill,* pp. 42–44, 77–78, 90–91, 95; on "change of scene," see Mill to Alexis de Tocqueville, 15 June 1836, in Mineka, ed., *Earlier Letters,* p. 306. Also see Gertrude Himmelfarb, *Victorian Minds* (New York: Harper & Row, Harper Torchbooks ed., 1970), p. 125, and Gates, *Victorian Suicide,* p. 32.

85. Betty Balfour, ed., *Personal and Literary Letters of Robert, First Earl of Lytton,* 2 vols. (London: Longmans, Green, 1906), 1:226.

86. Grosskurth, Foreword and Introduction to Symonds, *Memoirs,* pp. 9–11, 15.

87. Louis Crompton, *Byron and Greek Love: Homophobia in 19th-Century England* (Berkeley and Los Angeles: University of California Press, 1985), pp. 14, 21–22, 37–38; Jeffrey Weeks, *Sex, Politics and Society: The Regulation of Sexuality Since 1800* (London and New York: Longman, 1981), pp. 99–100, 118–19 n12.

88. See J. R. de S. Honey, *Tom Brown's Universe: The Development of the English Public School in the Nineteenth Century* (New York: Quadrangle/The New York Times Book Co., 1977), pp. 185–94.

89. Weeks, *Sex, Politics and Society,* pp. 102–103; Mort, *Dangerous Sexualities,* pp. 113–14.

90. For a summary of this literature, see Weeks, *Sex, Politics and Society,* pp. 104–105; Grosskurth, Introduction to Symonds, *Memoirs,* pp. 19–20; Jane Caplan, "Sexuality and Homosexuality," in Cambridge Women's Studies Group, ed., *Women in Society: Interdisciplinary Essays* (London: Virago, 1981), pp. 153–55 (on Krafft-Ebing). The theory of degenerate inheritance is examined in Chapter 8 of this book.

91. Morison's discussion appeared in *The Physiognomy of Mental Diseases* (1838), excerpted in Richard Hunter and Ida Macalpine, eds., *Three Hundred Years of Psychiatry, 1535–1860: A History Presented in Selected English Texts* (London and New York: Oxford University Press, 1963; reprint ed., Hartsdale, N.Y.: Carlisle Publishing, 1982), p. 773; Grosskurth, *Symonds, A Biography,* pp. 272, 281.

92. Grosskurth, *Symonds, A Biography,* pp. 286–92. On the origin of the word *homosexuality,* see Weeks, "Sins and Diseases," p. 213, and Michael Lynch, "'Here is Adhesiveness': From Friendship to Homosexuality," *Victorian Studies* 29(Autumn 1985):88.

93. Weeks, *Sex, Politics and Society,* pp. 112–13. Also see Samuel Hynes, *The Edwardian Turn of Mind* (Princeton: Princeton University Press, 1968), p. 153.

94. Symonds, *Memoirs,* pp. 166, 128, 224, 230, 125, 134–35, 174, 282; Symonds's letter about his "stripped" nerves is quoted in Grosskurth, *Symonds, A Biography,* p. 84.

95. Symonds, *Memoirs,* pp. 234–35, 252.

96. Ibid., p. 283.

97. Havelock Ellis, *Studies in the Psychology of Sex,* vol. 1: *Sexual Inversion* (London: The University Press, 1897), pp. 59–63 (also reprinted as Appendix I in Symonds, *Memoirs,* pp. 284–88). On classical stipulations concerning homosexual relations, see Richards, "Passing the Love of Women," p. 95.

352 *Notes*

98. Grant Allen, "Plain Words on the Woman Question," *Fortnightly Review*, n.s., 46(Oct. 1889):448–58; Mary Paley Marshall, *What I Remember* (Cambridge: The University Press, 1947), p. 24.
99. Benson, *Beside Still Waters*, pp. 186, 353, 356–57.
100. A. C. Benson, *The Diary of Arthur Christopher Benson*, ed. Percy Lubbock (New York: Longmans, Green, 1926), p. 133 (editor's comment).
101. Samuel Greg, *A Layman's Legacy in Prose and Verse* (London: Macmillan, 1877), pp. 22–23, vii, 54.

Chapter 6

1. Joan Perkin, *Women and Marriage in Nineteenth-Century England* (London: Routledge; Chicago: Lyceum Books, 1989), p. 28.
2. "Woman in Her Psychological Relations," *J Psych Med* 4(Jan. 1851):30.
3. Charles Darwin, *The Descent of Man, and Selection in Relation to Sex*, 2 vols. (London: John Murray, 1871), 2:329, 326–27.
4. In recent years, there has been a veritable explosion of studies that explore the misogynist thread in Victorian biology and anthropology. Among the most helpful and provocative are Flavia Alaya, "Victorian Science and the 'Genius' of Woman," *Journal of the History of Ideas* 38(1977):261–80; Susan Sleeth Mosedale, "Science Corrupted: Victorian Biologists Consider 'The Woman Question'," *Journal of the History of Biology* 11 (Spring 1978):1–55; Rosalind Rosenberg, "In Search of Woman's Nature, 1850–1920," *Feminist Studies* 3(1975–76):141–54; Jill Conway, "Stereotypes of Femininity in a Theory of Sexual Evolution," *Victorian Studies* 14(Sept. 1970):47–62; Lorna Duffin, "Prisoners of Progress: Women and Evolution," in Sara Delamont and Lorna Duffin, eds., *The Nineteenth-Century Woman: Her Cultural and Physical World* (London: Croom Helm; New York: Barnes & Noble, 1978), pp. 57–91; Elizabeth Fee, "The Sexual Politics of Victorian Anthropology," in Mary S. Hartman and Lois Banner, eds., *Clio's Consciousness Raised: New Perspectives of the History of Women* (New York: Harper & Row, Harper Torchbooks, ed., 1974), pp. 86–102; Cynthia Eagle Russett, *Sexual Science: The Victorian Construction of Womanhood* (Cambridge, Mass.: Harvard University Press, 1989); and Ludmilla Jordanova, *Sexual Visions:Images of Gender in Science and Medicine Between the Eighteenth and Twentieth Centuries* (Madison, Wisc.: University of Wisconsin Press, 1989).
5. Harry Campbell, *Differences in the Nervous Organisation of Man and Woman: Physiological and Pathological* (London: H. K. Lewis, 1891), p. 155.
6. J. Crichton-Browne, "Education and the Nervous System," in Malcolm Morris, ed., *The Book of Health* (London: Cassell, 1883), p. 342; George J. Romanes, "Mental Differences Between Men and Women," *Nineteenth Century* 21(May 1887):659; Rudyard Kipling, *Stalky & Co.* (1899), ch. 7.
7. Elizabeth Fee "Nineteenth-Century Craniology: The Study of the Female Skull," *Bull Hist Med* 53(1979):419.
8. Ibid., pp. 415–17, 419, 420–22, 426–27, 429–32; Mosedale, "Science Corrupted," p. 18; Rosenberg, "In Search of Woman's Nature," pp. 147–49.
9. J. Crichton-Browne, "On the Weight of the Brain and its Component Parts in the Insane," *Brain* 1(1878–79):504–505, 510–11, 513, 515.
10. See, for example, the following works by Crichton-Browne: "On the Weight of the Brain and its Component Parts in the Insane," con't., *Brain* 2(1879–80):62–63; "An Oration on Sex in Education," *Lancet*, 7 May 1892, pp. 1011–12; and *The Story of the Brain*

(Edinburgh and London: Oliver & Boyd, 1924), pp. 10–11. Also see Romanes, "Mental Differences Between Men and Women," pp. 654–55, 666.

11. Campbell, *Differences in the Nervous Organisation of Man and Woman,* pp. 162, 155. On the "infantile characteristics" of the female skull, see Fee, "Nineteenth-Century Craniology," pp. 422–24. The fact that many gynecologists/obstetricians held the post of "physician for the diseases of women and children" at diverse hospitals is telling.

12. Nancy Stepan, *The Idea of Race in Science: Great Britain 1800–1960* (London: Macmillan; Hamden, Conn.: Archon Books, 1982), pp. xv, xviii. Stepan's comments here about the construction of racist thought apply with equal validity to the construction of gender stereotypes.

13. As Perkin amply illustrates in *Women and Marriage,* pp. 76–101. For the impact of evangelical religion on the emergence of the ideology of separate spheres, see Leonore Davidoff and Catherine Hall, *Family Fortunes: Men and Women of the English Middle Class, 1780–1850* (Chicago: University of Chicago Press, 1987).

14. Thomas Laycock, *Mind and Brain* 2d ed., 2 vols. (London: Simpkin, Marshall, 1869), 2:317; H. Charlton Bastian, "Nervous," in Richard Quain, ed., *A Dictionary of Medicine* (London: Longmans, Green, 1882), p. 1025.

15. Thomas Addison, *Observations on the Disorders of Females Connected with Uterine Irritation* (London: S. Highley, 1830), pp. 10–12, 14–15; Samuel Ashwell, *A Practical Treatise on the Diseases Peculiar to Women* (London: S. Highley, 1844), pp. 240, 242.

16. Edward John Tilt, *On Diseases of Women and Ovarian Inflammation, in Relation to Morbid Menstruation, Sterility, Pelvic Tumours, & Affections of the Womb,* 2d ed. (London: Churchill, 1853), p. 85.

17. W. Tyler Smith, "The Climacteric Disease in Women," *London Journal of Medicine* 2(July 1849):601.

18. Charles Mercier, "Melancholia," in D. Hack Tuke, ed., *A Dictionary of Psychological Medicine,* 2 vols. (London: Churchill, 1892), 2:792; Olive Anderson, *Suicide in Victorian and Edwardian England* (Oxford: Clarendon, 1987), pp. 224, 226. The crises of puberty are further discussed in Chapter 7 of this book.

19. For one among many such assertions, see Henry Sutherland, "Menstrual Irregularities and Insanity," *WRLAMR* 2(1872):53–72. Anne Digby, "Women's Biological Straitjacket," in Susan Mendus and Jane Rendall, eds., *Sexuality and Subordination: Interdisciplinary Studies of Gender in the Nineteenth Century* (London and New York: Routledge, 1989), pp. 192–220, provides a helpful discussion of the links between female insanity and the reproductive cycle in Victorian psychiatric literature. A useful collection of documents, largely reflecting medical opinion about the female life cycle but with some comments from women themselves, is found in Pat Jalland and John Hooper, eds., *Women from Birth to Death: The Female Life Cycle in Britain 1830–1914* (Brighton: Harvester Press; Atlantic Highlands, N. J.: Humanities Press, 1986).

20. James Crichton-Browne, Introduction to *New Letters and Memorials of Jane Welsh Carlyle,* ed. Alexander Carlyle, 2 vols. (London: John Lane, The Bodley Head, 1903), 1:lvii.

21. E. J. Tilt, *On the Preservation of the Health of Women at the Critical Periods of Life* (London: Churchill, 1851), pp. 18, 24 (italics in original).

22. See Vern Bullough and Martha Voght, "Women, Menstruation, and Nineteenth-Century Medicine," *Bull Hist Med* 47(1973):66–82; Elaine Showalter and English Showalter, "Victorian Women and Menstruation," in Martha Vicinus, ed., *Suffer and Be Still: Women in the Victorian Age* (Bloomington, Ind.: Indiana University Press, 1972), pp. 38–44; Thomas Laqueur, "Orgasm, Generation, and the Politics of Reproductive Biology," *Representations,* no. 14(Spring 1986):3, 25–31.

23. Henry Maudsley, "Sex in Mind and in Education," *Fortnightly Review*, n.s., 15 (1874):479–80; Mary Wollstonecraft, *Vindication of the Rights of Woman* (1792), ch. 3. Less negative interpretations of menstruation, expressed in classical and Renaissance texts, are discussed in Laqueur, "Orgasm, Generation, and the Politics of Reproductive Biology." For seventeenth-century ambivalence about the healthiness of menstruation, see Patricia Crawford, "Attitudes to Menstruation in Seventeenth-Century England," *Past & Present*, no. 91 (May 1981):47–73.

24. Thomas Laycock, "On the Naming and Classification of Mental Diseases and Defects," *JMS* 9(July 1863):160; Smith, "Climacteric Disease in Women," for example. Many of the themes discussed here are explored in Lorna Duffin, "The Conspicuous Consumptive: Woman as an Invalid," in Delamont and Duffin, eds., *The Nineteenth-Century Woman*, pp. 26–56.

25. W. S. Playfair, "Remarks on the Systematic Treatment of Aggravated Hysteria and Certain Allied Forms of Neurasthenic Disease," *BMJ*, 19 Aug. 1882, p. 309; Thomas Stretch Dowse, *The Brain and the Nerves: Their Ailments and Their Exhaustion* (London: Baillière, Tindall, & Cox, [1884]), pp. 57–58; T. Clifford Allbutt, *On Visceral Neuroses* (London: Churchill, 1884), pp. 15, 17.

26. James Manby Gully, *An Exposition of the Symptoms, Essential Nature, and Treatment of Neuropathy, or Nervousness* (London: Churchill, 1837), pp. 27–73, for the cases, and p. 76, for the general conclusion from them; J. Crichton-Browne, "Cranial Injuries and Mental Diseases," *WRLAMR* 1(1871):8–10; Romanes, "Mental Differences Between Men and Women," pp. 656–57; Campbell, *Differences in the Nervous Organisation of Man and Woman*, pp. 171–72. Mosedale, "Science Corrupted," pp. 19–24, subjects Romanes's inconsistencies to a withering analysis.

27. James E. Pollock, "The Influence of Our Surroundings on Health," in Morris, ed., *Book of Health*, p. 553; Great Britain, *Parliamentary Papers* (Commons), vol. 61 (1884), (*Accounts and Papers*, vol. 15), "Elementary Schools (Dr. Crichton-Browne's Report)," p. 24 [of the report]; Romanes, "Mental Differences Between Men and Women," pp. 656, 660; Thomas S. Clouston, *The Hygiene of Mind* (London: Methuen, 1906), pp. 208–209. Also see Mosedale, "Science Corrupted," p. 18.

28. See Joan N. Burstyn, *Victorian Education and the Ideal of Womanhood* (London: Croom Helm; Totowa, N.J.: Barnes & Noble, 1980), p. 85; Bullough and Voght, "Women, Menstruation, and Nineteenth-Century Medicine," p. 69; Brian Harrison, "Women's Health and the Women's Movement in Britain: 1840–1940," in Charles Webster, ed., *Biology, Medicine and Society 1840–1940* (Cambridge: Cambridge University Press, 1981), pp. 31–32.

29. Thomas Stretch Dowse, *On Brain and Nerve Exhaustion. 'Neurasthenia.' Its Nature and Curative Treatment* (London: Baillière, Tindall, & Cox, 1880), p. 14.

30. Thomas Smith Clouston, *Female Education from a Medical Point of View* (Edinburgh: Macniven & Wallace, 1882), p. 20.

31. Romanes, "Mental Differences Between Men and Women," p. 668; Crichton-Browne, "Sex in Education," p. 1018.

32. T. S. Clouston, *Clinical Lectures on Mental Diseases*, 2d ed. (London: Churchill, 1887), pp. 40–42, and *Female Education*, p. 43.

33. James Crichton-Browne, *What the Doctor Thought* (London: Ernest Benn, 1930), pp. 52–53; also see *The Doctor's Second Thoughts* (London: Ernest Benn, 1931), pp. 30, 104–105, 117–18; *The Doctor's After Thoughts* (London: Ernest Benn, 1932), pp. 152, 235–38; *From the Doctor's Notebook* (London: Duckworth, 1937), p. 220.

34. J. Crichton-Browne, Introduction to Niels T. A. Hertel, *Overpressure in High Schools in Denmark* (London: Macmillan, 1885), pp. xxix–xxx, xxxiii–xxxv.

35. See Carol Dyhouse, "Mothers and Daughters in the Middle-Class Home, c. 1870–1914," in Jane Lewis, ed., *Labour and Love: Women's Experience of Home and Family, 1850–1940* (Oxford and New York: Basil Blackwell, 1986), pp. 35–36; and Deborah Gorham, *The Victorian Girl and the Feminine Ideal* (London and Canberra: Croom Helm, 1982), p. 85.

36. Quoted in Louisa Garrett Anderson, *Elizabeth Garrett Anderson 1836–1917* (London: Faber & Faber, 1939), p. 58.

37. Elizabeth Garrett Anderson, "Sex in Mind and Education: A Reply," *Fortnightly Review*, n.s., 15(1874):585, 590, 594. For Maudsley's article, see "Sex in Mind and in Education," 15(1874):466–83. Both Maudsley and Anderson were writing in response— approving and disapproving, respectively—to *Sex in Education*, a book published the previous year by Edward Clarke of Harvard, who maintained that university education was making American women unfit to bear children.

38. Romanes, "Mental Differences Between Men and Women," p. 670. For a summary of the Sidgwick study, see Richard Allen Soloway, *Birth Control and the Population Question in England, 1877–1930* (Chapel Hill, N.C.: University of North Carolina Press, 1982), pp. 140–42. Also see Burstyn, *Victorian Education and the Ideal of Womanhood*, pp. 150–51; Bullough and Voght, "Women, Menstruation, and Nineteenth-Century Medicine," pp. 72, 76; Kathleen E. McCrone, "Play Up! Play Up! And Play the Game! Sport at the Late Victorian Girls' Public School," *Journal of British Studies* 23(Spring 1984):115 n39.

39. Arabella Kenealy, "Woman as an Athlete," *Nineteenth Century* 45(April 1899):637, 642–43; Mary Scharlieb, "Adolescent Girlhood under Modern Conditions, with Special Reference to Motherhood," *Eugenics Review* 1(1909–10):178–79. It comes as no surprise to learn that Kenealy, much given to hyperbole, was subsequently the author of *Feminism and Sex-Extinction* (1920).

40. Harrison, "Women's Health and Women's Movement," pp. 56–57. Little has been written about the status of women specifically in the psychiatric branch of the medical profession by the late nineteenth century. For an initial exploration of the subject, see Charlotte MacKenzie, "Women and Psychiatric Professionalization, 1780–1914," in London Feminist History Group, *The Sexual Dynamics of History: Men's Power, Women's Resistance* (London: Pluto Press, 1983), pp. 116–19.

41. Margaret Oliphant, *The Autobiography and Letters of Mrs. Margaret Oliphant*, ed. Mrs. Harry Coghill (1899; Leicester: Leicester University Press, 1974), p. 36; E. Lynn Linton, "The Higher Education of Woman," *Fortnightly Review*, n.s., 40(Oct. 1886):504. See Nancy Fix Anderson, *Woman Against Women in Victorian England: A Life of Eliza Lynn Linton* (Bloomington, Ind.: Indiana University Press, 1987), for an attempt to explain E. Lynn Linton's attitudes in psychoanalytic terms.

42. For some examples, see Gorham, *Victorian Girl and Feminine Ideal*, pp. 164, 172–76.

43. From *Democracy and Liberty*, quoted in Harrison, "Women's Health and Women's Movement," p. 41; also see pp. 38–40, for the feminist campaign against female invalidism. Kathleen E. McCrone explores these themes at length in *Playing the Game: Sport and the Physical Emancipation of English Women, 1870–1914* (Lexington, Ky.: University Press of Kentucky, 1988).

44. Kenealy, "Woman as an Athlete," pp. 641, 643–44; McCrone, "Play Up!" pp. 114, 129; Paul Atkinson, "Fitness, Feminism and Schooling," in Delamont and Duffin, eds., *Nineteenth-Century Woman*, pp. 92–133.

45. John Stuart Mill, *On the Subjection of Women* (1869), ch. 3.

46. "Nervous Disorders of Ladies," *Family Oracle of Health* 3(1826):96; J. Conolly, "Hysteria," in John Forbes, Alexander Tweedie, and John Conolly, eds., *The Cyclo-*

pædia of Practical Medicine, 4 vols. (London: Sherwood, Gilbert, Piper, Baldwin, & Cradock, 1833–35), 2:573; Tilt, *Preservation of Health of Women,* p. 37.

47. Lionel John Beale, *The Laws of Health, in Relation to Mind and Body* (London: Churchill, 1851), pp. 199–200; Hall's advice quoted in Charlotte Hall, *Memoirs of Marshall Hall, M.D., F.R.S.* (London: Richard Bentley, 1861), pp. 137–38.

48. Crichton-Browne, "Education and the Nervous System," p. 312.

49. Romanes, "Mental Differences Between Men and Women," p. 671.

50. William Acton, *The Functions and Disorders of the Reproductive Organs in Childhood, Youth, Adult Age, and Advanced Life; considered in Their Physiological, Social and Moral Relations* (1857), excerpted, from a subsequent edition, in Sheila Jeffreys, ed., *The Sexuality Debates* (London and New York: Routledge & Kegan Paul, 1987), p. 61. M. Jeanne Peterson, "Dr. Acton's Enemy: Medicine, Sex, and Society in Victorian England," *Victorian Studies* 29(Summer 1986):570 n5, points out that Acton never earned the M.D. degree.

51. F. Barry Smith, "Sexuality in Britain, 1800–1900: Some Suggested Revisions," in Martha Vicinus, ed., *A Widening Sphere: Changing Roles of Victorian Women* (Bloomington, Ind.: Indiana University Press, 1977), pp. 185–86, and Peterson, "Acton's Enemy," challenge the validity of using Acton as a spokesman for mid-Victorian medical attitudes about sexuality. Both trace the tendency of Victorianists today to treat him as such to the influence of Steven Marcus's book, *The Other Victorians: A Study of Sexuality and Pornography in Mid-Nineteenth-Century England* (New York: Basic Books, 1966).

52. Sheila Jeffreys, Introduction, in Jeffreys, eds., *Sexuality Debates,* pp. 2–5. Also see Peter T. Cominos, "Innocent Femina Sensualis in Unconscious Conflict," in Vicinus, ed., *Suffer and Be Still,* pp. 156–63—an argument marred by reliance on Acton as typical of Victorian medical views of female sexuality—and Frank Mort, *Dangerous Sexualities: Medico-Moral Politics in England since 1830* (London and New York: Routledge & Kegan Paul, 1987), pp. 94–95, 98, 138.

53. See Cominos, "Innocent Femina Sensualis," pp. 156, 158, 162, 167, 171, and Carol Christ, "Victorian Masculinity and the Angel in the House," in Vicinus, ed., *Widening Sphere,* p. 152.

54. For remarks on the lack of a Georgian Acton, see Roy Porter, "Mixed Feelings: The Enlightenment and Sexuality in Eighteenth-Century Britain," in Paul-Gabriel Boucé, ed., *Sexuality in Eighteenth-Century Britain* (Manchester: Manchester University Press; Totowa, N.J.: Barnes & Noble, 1982), p. 15; on Pamela, see Vieda Skultans, *English Madness: Ideas on Insanity, 1580–1890* (London: Routledge & Kegan Paul, 1979), p. 78.

55. Peterson, "Acton's Enemy," pp. 575–76, 580.

56. Elizabeth Blackwell, *The Human Element in Sex* (1884), quoted in Jane Lewis, *Women in England 1870–1950: Sexual Divisions and Social Change* (Sussex: Wheatsheaf Books; Bloomington, Ind.: Indiana University Press, 1984), p. 128; on opposition to ovariotomies, see F. B. Smith, *The People's Health 1830–1910* (London: Croom Helm, 1979), p. 296; Aubrey Lewis, "Henry Maudsley: His Work and Influence," *JMS* 97(April 1951):271; on Dr. Solomon, see Smith, "Sexuality in Britain," pp. 194–95.

57. I'm arguing here against Mort's analysis in *Dangerous Sexualities,* pp. 80–83.

58. Stanley Weintraub, *Victoria, An Intimate Biography* (New York: E. P. Dutton, 1987), pp. 238–39.

59. Lucy Bland, "Marriage Laid Bare: Middle-Class Women and Marital Sex 1880s–1914," in Lewis, ed., *Labour and Love,* pp. 128–31. Also see Judith R. Walkowitz, "Science, Feminism and Romance: The Men and Women's Club 1885–1889," *History Workshop,* issue 21(Spring 1986):37–59, and Smith, "Sexuality in Britain," pp. 188–90, for neo-Malthusian views on human sexuality.

60. Thomas Laycock, *A Treatise on the Nervous Diseases of Women* (London: Longman, Orme, Brown, Green, & Longmans, 1840), p. 83 (also pp. 128, 142, 177, 212–13); Conolly, "Hysteria," p. 585. Also see Robert Brudenell Carter, *On the Pathology and Treatment of Hysteria* (London: Churchill, 1853), pp. 21–22; Alfred T. Schofield, *The Force of Mind or the Mental Factor in Medicine* (London: Churchill, 1902), pp. 254–55; and Mark S. Micale, "Diagnostic Discriminations: Jean-Martin Charcot and the Nineteenth-Century Idea of Masculine Hysterical Neurosis," unpublished paper, presented to the Wellcome Institute for the History of Medicine, London, 20 Oct. 1987, pp. 1, 21–23.

61. T. S. Clouston, *The Hygiene of Mind* (London: Methuen, 1906), p. 209; Alfred T. Schofield, *Functional Nerve Diseases* (London: Methuen, 1908), p. 68.

62. Jeffrey Weeks, in *Sex, Politics and Society: The Regulation of Sexuality since 1800* (London and New York: Longman, 1981), pp. 105–106, 115–17, and "'Sins and Diseases': Some Notes on Homosexuality in the Nineteenth Century," *History Workshop,* issue 1(Spring 1976):215, offers valuable comments about late Victorian and Edwardian attitudes toward lesbianism. On the implications of the Incest Act of 1908, see Anthony S. Wohl, "Sex and the Single Room: Incest among the Victorian Working Classes," in Anthony S. Wohl, ed., *The Victorian Family: Structure and Stresses* (New York: St. Martin's Press, 1978), p. 210.

63. William Campbell, *Introduction to the Study and Practice of Midwifery, and the Diseases of Women and Children* (Edinburgh: Adam & Charles Black; London: Longman, Rees, Orme, Brown, Green, & Longman, 1833), p. 443.

64. James Cowles Prichard, *A Treatise on Insanity and Other Disorders Affecting the Mind* (London: Sherwood, Gilbert, & Piper, 1835), p. 19.

65. See Leonore Davidoff, "Class and Gender in Victorian England: The Diaries of Arthur J. Munby and Hannah Cullwick," *Feminist Studies* 5(Spring 1979):90, 113.

66. Kate Millett, "The Debate over Women: Ruskin vs. Mill," in Vicinus, ed., *Suffer and Be Still,* p. 121.

67. Katharine Moore, *Victorian Wives* (London and New York: Allison and Busby, paperback ed., 1985), p. 119.

68. Wollstonecraft, *Vindication,* "Author's Introduction," in particular; on Tennyson and Patmore, see Christ, "Victorian Masculinity and the Angel in the House," pp. 148, 155; Oliphant, *Autobiography and Letters,* p. 82.

69. Forbes B. Winslow, *Anatomy of Suicide* (London: Henry Renshaw, 1840), p. 56; Crichton-Browne, *What the Doctor Thought,* p. 279. Sandra M. Gilbert and Susan Gubar offer a fascinating exploration of the implications of female selflessness in Victorian literature, in *The Madwoman in the Attic: The Woman Writer and the Nineteenth-Century Literary Imagination* (New Haven: Yale University Press, 1979), pp. 21–27.

70. See Duffin, "Prisoners of Progress," pp. 70–74, on woman's "moral constitution."

71. So many of the recent studies of Victorian gender stereotyping discuss the fundamental contradiction between fragility and strength in the nineteenth-century models of womanhood that it would be impossible to cite them all. Suffice it to say that it is an underlying theme in Davidoff and Hall, *Family Fortunes,* and Gorham, *Victorian Girl and Feminine Ideal.* Also see Patricia Branca, "Image and Reality: The Myth of the Idle Victorian Woman," in Hartman and Banner, eds., *Clio's Consciousness Raised,* pp. 179–91.

72. Romanes, "Mental Differences Between Men and Women," p. 663.

73. 13 Oct. 1836, William Baly MSS 715/209, Royal College of Physicians of London (italics in original): Crichton-Browne, *What the Doctor Thought,* p. 37.

74. Jane Austen, *Pride and Prejudice,* ch. 1; Charles Dickens, *Nicholas Nickleby* (1838–39),

ch. 28; on Queen Victoria, see E. F. Benson, *As We Were: A Victorian Peep-Show* (1930; London: Hogarth Press, 1985), p. 38.

75. See Gilbert and Gubar, *Madwoman in Attic*, pp. 27–36, on woman as monster. Bram Dijkstra, *Idols of Perversity: Fantasies of Feminine Evil in Fin-de-Siècle Culture* (New York and Oxford: Oxford University Press, 1986), explores these images in western art and literature at the turn of the century.

76. Romanes, "Mental Differences Between Men and Women," p. 657; J. Michell Clarke, "Hysteria and Neurasthenia," *Brain* 17(1894):140; Seymour J. Sharkey, "Hysteria and Neurasthenia," *Brain* 27(1904):5.

77. Conolly, "Hysteria," p. 563; Daniel Hack Tuke, *Illustrations of the Influence of the Mind upon the Body in Health and Disease Designed to Elucidate the Action of the Imagination* (London: Churchill, 1872), p. 386; Clifford Allbutt, "Neurasthenia," in Clifford Allbutt and Humphry Davy Rolleston, eds., *A System of Medicine*, 2d ed. rev., 9 vols. (London: Macmillan, 1905 11), 8:789. Also see Carroll Smith-Rosenberg, "The Hysterical Woman: Sex Roles and Role Conflict in 19th-Century America," *Social Research* 39(Winter 1972):675, and Michael J. Clark, "The Rejection of Psychological Approaches to Mental Disorder in Late Nineteenth-Century British Psychiatry," in Andrew Scull, ed., *Madhouses, Mad-Doctors, and Madmen: The Social History of Psychiatry in the Victorian Era* (London: Athlone Press; Philadelphia: University of Pennsylvania Press, 1981), pp. 293–94. Barbara T. Gates, *Victorian Suicide: Mad Crimes and Sad Histories* (Princeton: Princeton University Press, 1988), pp. 128–31, discusses the Victorian debate over will-less or willful women, in the context of opinions about female suicide.

78. For a summary of attitudes toward self-starvation prior to the second half of the nineteenth century, see Joan Jacobs Brumberg, *Fasting Girls: The Emergence of Anorexia Nervosa as a Modern Disease* (Cambridge, Mass.: Harvard University Press, 1988), chs. 2, 3.

79. William Withey Gull, "Anorexia Nervosa (Apepsia Hysterica, Anorexia Hysterica)," *Transactions of the Clinical Society of London* 7(1874):25–26, 22; Richard A. Hunter and H. Phillip Greenberg, "Sir William Gull and Psychiatry," *Guy's Hospital Reports* 105(1956):373; Brumberg, *Fasting Girls*, pp. 101, 111–21.

80. Gull, "Anorexia Nervosa" (1874), pp. 26, 28, and "Anorexia Nervosa," *Lancet*, 17 March 1888, p. 517; Brumberg, *Fasting Girls*, pp. 102–10.

81. In Tuke's *Dictionary of Psychological Medicine*, see Donkin, "Hysteria," 1:624, and the definition of "Anorexia Hysterica," 1:94; Brumberg, *Fasting Girls*, pp. 127, 149–50.

82. Playfair, "Systematic Treatment of Aggravated Hysteria," p. 310.

83. Gull, "Anorexia Nervosa" (1874), p. 26; Hunter and Greenberg, "Gull and Psychiatry," p. 361. I shall resist the temptation, in this context, to discuss the literature that speculatively identifies Gull as Jack the Ripper.

84. Gull, "Anorexia Nervosa" (1874), p. 24; W. S. Playfair, "Neuroses, Functional, The Systematic Treatment of," in Tuke, ed., *Dictionary of Psychological Medicine*, 2:852.

85. Suzanne Poirier, "The Weir Mitchell Rest Cure: Doctor and Patients," *Women's Studies* 10(1983):20–23, 30; also see Barbara Sicherman, "The Uses of a Diagnosis: Doctors, Patients, and Neurasthenia," in Judith Walzer Leavitt and Ronald L. Numbers, eds., *Sickness and Health in America: Readings in the History of Medicine and Public Health* (Madison, Wisc.: University of Wisconsin Press, 1978), p. 33. Virtually every recent book and article on Victorian women's health discusses the Weir Mitchell treatment, in passing or in detail.

86. See, for example, "Woman in Her Psychological Relations," p. 34, and Donkin, "Hysteria," p. 624.

87. W. S. Playfair, *The Systematic Treatment of Nerve Prostration and Hysteria* (London:

Smith, Elder, 1883), pp. 8–9; Donkin, "Hysteria," p. 624; Allbutt, "Neurasthenia," p. 779; W. R. Gowers, *A Manual of Diseases of the Nervous System*, 2 vols. (London: Churchill, 1886–88), 2:938.

88. *Fat and Blood* was the title of his best-selling book, first published in 1877 and going through eight editions by 1911. See Poirier, "Weir Mitchell Rest Cure," pp. 17, 20.

89. Playfair, *Systematic Treatment of Nerve Prostration*, pp. 15–16, and "Neuroses, Functional," p. 853. Also see J. J. Graham Brown, *The Treatment of Nervous Disease* (Edinburgh and London: William Green, 1905), pp. 418–19, and Dowse, *Brain and Nerves*, p. 58. Brumberg, *Fasting Girls*, pp. 126–40, 156–63, examines Lasègue's work and faults British doctors for betraying no similar interest in the psychological impulses behind self-starvation in young women.

90. Poirier, "Weir Mitchell Rest Cure," p. 27.

91. Beatrice Webb, *The Diary of Beatrice Webb*, vol. 1: *1873–1892*, *"Glitter Around and Darkness Within,"* ed. Norman MacKenzie and Jeanne MacKenzie (Cambridge, Mass.: Harvard University Press, 1982), pp. 275 (7 March 1889), 157 (15 March 1886).

92. "An Appeal Against Female Suffrage," *Nineteenth Century* 25(June 1889):782 (Miss Beatrice Potter's name appears on p. 786); Beatrice Webb, *My Apprenticeship* (London: Longmans, Green, 1926), pp. 353–55, and *Our Partnership*, ed. Barbara Drake and Margaret I. Cole (London: Longmans, Green, 1948), pp. 360–63. Also see Barbara Caine, "Beatrice Webb and the 'Woman Question'," *History Workshop*, issue 14(Autumn 1982):33–35.

93. Webb, *Diary*, 1:45 (12 Sept. 1881). For examples of her denigration of female intelligence, see Ibid., pp. 63 (25 Nov. 1882), 77 (1 March 1883), 328 (29 March 1890), 359 (7 July 1891).

94. Ibid., 1:19 (11 Dec. 1874), 157 (21 March 1886), 250 (5 May 1888), 284 (4 June 1889) (italics in original), 357 (20 June 1891); and Caine, "Beatrice Webb," pp. 37–38.

95. Webb, *Diary*, 1:188–89 (10 Dec. 1886).

96. Ibid., 1:117–18 (9 May 1884), 126 (26 Nov. 1884) (italics in original), 264 (7 Nov. 1888), 267 (24 Nov. 1888), 276 (10 March 1889).

97. Webb, *My Apprenticeship*, p. 324; Webb, *Diary*, 1:252 (28 May 1888), 259 (28 Aug. 1888).

98. Webb, *Our Partnership*, pp. 392–94. She showed the commissioners all the letters from medical officers that supported her own viewpoint and withheld most of those that did not.

99. Kitty Muggeridge and Ruth Adam, *Beatrice Webb, A Life 1858–1943* (London: Secker & Warburg, 1967), pp. 163–66. Webb dedicated *My Apprenticeship* to "The Other One" and began *Our Partnership* with an introductory chapter on "The Other One."

100. Webb, *Diary*, 1:359 (7 July 1891).

101. Havelock Ellis, *My Life* (Boston: Houghton, Mifflin, 1939), p. 230; Ruth First and Ann Scott, *Olive Schreiner* (London: Andre Deutsch, 1980), p. 150, for Schreiner and Donkin in the Men and Women's Club. My views of Schreiner are indebted to the interpretation put forward throughout the splendid biography by First and Scott.

102. First and Scott, *Schreiner*, pp. 166–67, 116; Phyllis Grosskurth, *Havelock Ellis, A Biography* (London: Allen Lane; New York: Alfred A. Knopf, 1980), p. 80.

103. S. C. Cronwright-Schreiner, ed., *The Letters of Olive Schreiner 1876–1920* (London: T. Fisher Unwin, 1924), pp. 22 (16 June 1884), 23 (29 June 1884), 40 (5 Sept. 1884), 56 (12 Jan. 1885), 57 (28 Jan. 1885).

104. First and Scott, *Schreiner*, p. 137; Cronwright-Schreiner, ed., *Letters of Olive Schreiner*, p. 41 (13 Oct. 1884), 56 (17 Jan. 1885).

105. Maria Sharpe, "Autobiographical Notes on 'Men & Women's Club'," Karl Pearson

Papers 10/1, The Library, University College London, pp. 63–64, 23.

106. Ibid., pp. 54–55.

107. Ibid., pp. 5–6.

108. Ibid., pp. 18–19, 64–65, 82, 72, 73, 78.

109. Ibid., pp. 84, 20. See Walkowitz, "Science, Feminism and Romance," pp. 51–53, for an account of the Sharpe–Pearson relationship; also Daniel J. Kevles, *In the Name of Eugenics: Genetics and the Uses of Human Heredity* (Berkeley and Los Angeles: University of California Press, paperback ed., 1986), pp. 25–26. Schreiner did give birth to a daughter in 1895, but the baby died within twenty-four hours.

110. Eleanor Marx to Jenny Marx Longuet, 8 Jan. 1882, in *The Daughters of Karl Marx: Family Correspondence 1866–1898,* trans. Faith Evans, with notes by Olga Meier (Harmondsworth: Penguin, 1984), pp. 145–46 (italics in original). For Karl Marx's hint about Eleanor's sexual frustration, see Yvonne Kapp, *Eleanor Marx,* 2 vols. (London: Virago, 1979), 1:229.

111. Eleanor Marx to Jenny Longuet, 15 Jan. 1882, in *Daughters of Karl Marx,* p. 148, and Kapp, *Eleanor Marx,* 1:143–61, 227–28.

112. Kapp, *Eleanor Marx,* 2:259–60; Amy Levy, *Reuben Sachs, A Sketch* (London and New York: Macmillan, 1888), p. 230; Levy's letter to Schreiner is quoted in First and Scott, *Schreiner,* p. 187.

113. Martha Vicinus, *Independent Women: Work and Community for Single Women, 1850–1920* (Chicago: University of Chicago Press; London: Virago, 1985), p. 138, and Edyth M. Lloyd, ed., *Anna Lloyd (1837–1925): A Memoir, with Extracts from her Letters* (London: Cayme Press, 1928), pp. 58–59, 71–72, 38.

114. It may seem odd that I have hitherto excluded Florence Nightingale from this chapter. She certainly contributed a scathing denunciation of the damage wrought to women's health by a life spent on trivial pursuits, but I am persuaded by F. B. Smith, *Florence Nightingale: Reputation and Power* (London and Canberra: Croom Helm, 1982), that her accounts of devastating depression and family conflict are highly suspect.

115. Elaine Showalter, *The Female Malady: Women, Madness, and English Culture, 1830–1980* (New York: Pantheon, 1985), p. 120. I have selected these phrases from Showalter's book merely because they make a particularly clear assertion of the point, but the point is upheld, explicitly and implicitly, in numerous other sources as well.

116. Sydenham quoted in Ilza Veith, "On Hysterical and Hypochondriacal Afflictions," *Bull Hist Med* 30(May–June 1956):234.

117. Donkin, "Hysteria," p. 625. On Mrs. Seaton's pregnancy, see Zuzana Shonfield, *The Precariously Privileged: A Professional Family in Victorian London* (Oxford and New York: Oxford University Press, 1987), p. 224; Vera Wheatley, *The Life and Work of Harriet Martineau* (London: Secker & Warburg, 1957), pp. 215–16, and ch. 11.

118. Phyllis Grosskurth, *John Addington Symonds, A Biography* (London: Longmans, Green, 1964), pp. 109–10, 118, 136, 177.

119. "Postpartum Disorders," *Harvard Medical School Mental Health Letter* 5(May 1989):2.

120. Lotte Hamburger and Joseph Hamburger, *Troubled Lives: John and Sarah Austin* (Toronto: University of Toronto Press, 1985), pp. 77–91, superbly evoke this terrible period in Sarah Austin's life.

121. Crichton-Browne, Introduction to *New Letters and Memorials of Jane Welsh Carlyle,* pp. lvii–lx. Also see Phyllis Rose, *Parallel Lives: Five Victorian Marriages* (New York: Alfred A. Knopf, 1984), pp. 250–54, and Harriet Blodgett, *Centuries of Female Days: Englishwomen's Private Diaries* (New Brunswick, N.J.: Rutgers University Press, 1988), p. 168.

122. Jo Manton, *Mary Carpenter and the Children of the Streets* (London: Heinemann Educational Books, 1976), pp. 63–64; Rachel Grant-Smith, *The Experiences of an Asylum Patient* (London: George Allen & Unwin, 1922), pp. 50–59; Arthur H. Nethercot, *The First Five Lives of Annie Besant* (London: Rupert Hart-Davis, 1961), pp. 47–50.

123. Blodgett, *Centuries of Female Days,* p. 230. See pp. 157, 168–69, for the diarists' appreciation of marriage and motherhood.

124. For an excellent case study of a family of such women, see M. Jeanne Peterson, "No Angels in the House: The Victorian Myth and the Paget Women," *American Historical Review* 89(June 1984):677–708.

125. Thomas S. Dowse, *Lectures on Massage & Electricity in the Treatment of Disease* (London: Hamilton, Adams, and Bristol: John Wright, [1889]), p. 128; Playfair, "Systematic Treatment of Aggravated Hysteria," pp. 309–10.

126. Addison, *Observations on Disorders of Females,* pp. 35, 50; Ashwell, *Treatise on Diseases Peculiar to Women,* p. 247; Tilt, *Diseases of Women and Ovarian Inflammation,* p. 92; Dowse, *Brain and Nerves,* p. 123. For an excellent, balanced evaluation of the relationship between Victorian doctors and their female patients, see Regina Morantz, "The Lady and Her Physician," in Hartman and Banner, eds., *Clio's Consciousness Raised,"* pp. 38–53. G. J. Barker-Benfield, "The Spermatic Economy: A Nineteenth Century View of Sexuality," *Feminist Studies* 1(1973):45–74, represents the unbalanced perspective.

127. See the story recounted in Dyhouse, "Mothers and Daughters in the Middle-Class Home," p. 36.

128. Nethercot, *First Five Lives of Annie Besant,* pp. 50, 150; Grant-Smith, *Experiences of an Asylum Patient,* pp. 53–56 (Goodhart was the author of *On Common Neuroses,* 1892); T. Clifford Allbutt, "Nervous Diseases and Modern Life," *Contemporary Review* 67(1895):219.

129. MacKenzie, "Women and Psychiatric Professionalization," pp. 117–18.

130. Clouston, *Clinical Lectures on Mental Diseases,* p. 44.

Chapter 7

1. Leonard G. Guthrie, *Functional Nervous Disorders in Childhood* (London: Oxford University Press, Oxford Medical Publications, 1907), p. 22.

2. See James Walvin, *A Child's World: A Social History of English Childhood 1800–1914* (Harmondsworth: Penguin, 1982), pp. 12–13; and John Burnett, ed., *Destiny Obscure: Autobiographies of Childhood, Education and Family from the 1820s to the 1920s* (Harmondsworth: Penguin, 1984) pp. 62–63.

3. James Sully, *Studies of Childhood* (London: Longmans, Green, 1895).

4. Thomas T. Higgins, *"Great Ormond Street" 1852–1952* (London: Odhams Press, for the Hospital for Sick Children, [1952]); Charles Newman, "The Rise of Specialism and Postgraduate Education," in F. N. L. Poynter, ed., *The Evolution of Medical Education in Britain* (London: Pitman Medical Publishing Co., 1966), p. 172; Walvin, *Child's World,* pp. 18–19, 21; F. B. Smith, *The People's Health 1830–1910* (London: Croom Helm, 1979), pp. 152–55.

5. On infant and childhood mortality, to the breakthrough period of 1902–1907, see Smith, *People's Health,* pp. 113–28, 136–52; Ellen Ross, "Labour and Love: Rediscovering

London's Working-Class Mothers, 1870–1918,'' in Jane Lewis, ed., *Labour and Love: Women's Experience of Home and Family, 1850–1940* (Oxford: Basil Blackwell, 1986), pp. 80–82; Walvin, *Child's World*, pp. 21–24.

6. Stuart Sutherland, *Breakdown: A Personal Crisis and a Medical Dilemma*, rev. ed. (London: Weidenfeld & Nicolson, 1987), p. 106.

7. "Nervous, and Other Diseases, Caused by Novel Reading," *Family Oracle of Health* 1(1824):177 (on calomel); Robert Gooch, *An Account of Some of the Most Important Diseases Peculiar to Women* (London: John Murray, 1829), pp. 361–64.

8. Sully, *Studies of Childhood*, p. 219.

9. "Night Terrors," in D. Hack Tuke, ed., *A Dictionary of Psychological Medicine*, 2 vols. (London: Churchill, 1892), 2:857; J. A. Symonds, *The Memoirs of John Addington Symonds*, ed. Phyllis Grosskurth (Chicago: University of Chicago Press, 1986), pp. 38, 64, 77, 86; George Cheyne, *The English Malady: or, a Treatise of Nervous Diseases of all Kinds, as Spleen, Vapours, Lowness of Spirits, Hypochondriacal, and Hysterical Distempers* (1733; Delmar, N.Y.: Scholars' Facsimiles & Reprints, 1976), pp. 71–72; Francis Warner, "Recurrent Headaches in Children," *Brain* 3(1880–81):309.

10. Symonds, *Memoirs*, pp. 57–58; Henry Maudsley, *The Physiology and Pathology of Mind* (London: Macmillan, 1867), p. 271; James Crichton-Browne, "On Dreamy Mental States," *Stray Leaves from a Physician's Portfolio* (London: Hodder & Stoughton, [1927]), pp. 7–9, 12, 16–18, 27, 19, 39–40.

11. P. C. Smith, "The Meaning of the Term 'Neurasthenia' and the Etiology of the Disease," *BJM*, 4 April 1903, p. 782; Clifford Allbutt, "Neurasthenia," in Clifford Allbutt and Humphry Davy Rolleston, eds., *A System of Medicine*, 2d ed. rev., 9 vols. (London: Macmillan, 1905–11), 8:789; Beatrice Webb, *The Diary of Beatrice Webb*, vol. 1: *1873–1892, "Glitter Around and Darkness Within,"* ed. Norman MacKenzie and Jeanne MacKenzie (Cambridge, Mass.: Harvard University Press, 1982), pp. 11, 64 (3 Dec. 1882); James Sully, *My Life and Friends: A Psychologist's Memories* (London: T. Fisher Unwin, 1918), p. 44.

12. J. Crichton-Browne, "Psychical Diseases of Early Life," *JMS* 6 (April 1860):292, 299, 315; Maudsley, *Physiology and Pathology of Mind*, p. 279; T. S. Clouston, *The Hygiene of Mind* (London: Methuen, 1906), pp. 127–28.

13. Ilza Veith, "On Hysterical and Hypochondriacal Afflictions," *Bull Hist Med* 30(May–June 1956): 235 (on Sydenham); J. Conolly, "Hysteria," in John Forbes, Alexander Tweedie, and John Conolly, eds., *The Cyclopædia of Practical Medicine*, 4 vols. (London: Sherwood, Gilbert, Piper, Baldwin, & Cradock, 1833–35), 2:574; Alfred T. Schofield, *Functional Nerve Diseases* (London: Methuen, 1908), p. 260. Also see Harry Campbell, *Differences in the Nervous Organisation of Man and Woman: Physiological and Pathological* (London: H. K. Lewis, 1891), pp. 155, 157, 169; and Guthrie, *Functional Nervous Disorders in Childhood*, p. 13.

14. Francis Warner, *The Study of Children and Their School Training* (London and New York: Macmillan, 1897), pp. vii, 10–11, 56, and "Results of an Inquiry as to the Physical and Mental Condition of Fifty Thousand Children seen in One Hundred and Six Schools," *Journal of the Royal Statistical Society* 56(1893):71–72. Gillian Sutherland, *Ability, Merit and Measurement: Mental Testing and English Education 1880–1940* (Oxford: Clarendon, 1984), pp. 10, 15–16, 21, valuably discusses and criticizes Warner's survey.

15. Warner, "Results of an Inquiry," p. 100, and *Study of Children*, pp. 57, 160–61, 236.

16. See David Newsome, *Godliness and Good Learning: Four Studies on a Victorian Ideal* (London: John Murray, 1961), p. 8.

17. Crichton-Browne, "Psychical Diseases of Early Life," p. 299, and Introduction to *New Letters and Memorials of Jane Welsh Carlyle*, ed. Alexander Carlyle, 2 vols. (London:

John Lane, The Bodley Head, 1903), 1:lv; J. Milner Fothergill, *The Maintenance of Health: A Medical Work for Lay Readers* (London: Smith, Elder, 1874), p. 37.

18. Frederick MacCabe, "On Mental Strain and Overwork," *JMS* 21 (Oct. 1875):401; D. Hack Tuke, "Presidential Address, Delivered at the Annual Meeting of the Medico-Psychological Association," *JMS* 27(Oct. 1881):341.

19. Guthrie, *Functional Nervous Disorders in Childhood*, p. 134, and title of ch. 10; Charles Dickens, *Dombey and Son*, ch. 11.

20. On medical advice concerning Buckle as a child, see *DNB*, s.v. "Buckle, Henry Thomas"; James Johnson, *Change of Air, or the Pursuit of Health* (London: S. Highley, 1831), p. 4; John T. Conquest, *Letters to a Mother, on the Management of Herself and Her Children in Health and Disease*, rev. and enl. ed. (London: Longman, 1848), pp. 324–25.

21. Thomas Dixon Savill, *Clinical Lectures on Neurasthenia*, 3d ed., rev. and enl. (London: Henry Glaisher, 1906), pp. 131–33; Guthrie, *Functional Nervous Disorders in Childhood*, p. 139.

22. James Crichton-Browne, *What the Doctor Thought* (London: Ernest Benn, 1930), p. 56.

23. Sutherland, *Ability, Merit and Measurement*, p. 7; James Crichton-Browne, "Acute Dementia," *WRLAMR* 4(1874):269, 276–77, 279–80 (for concern over factory children).

24. Sutherland, *Ability, Merit and Measurement*, pp. 7–8. These issues are explored in greater detail in Gillian Sutherland, *Policy-Making in Elementary Education, 1870–1895* (Oxford: Oxford University Press, 1973).

25. Great Britain, *Parliamentary Debates* (Lords), 3d ser., 281 (16 July 1883):1465–73.

26. Quoted by Lord Stanley of Alderley, in Ibid., col. 1466. In referring to the "recent spread of education," Crichton-Browne was doubtless thinking of the Education Acts passed before 1880, in 1870 and 1876. Although the notion that intense study could produce brain disease was at least two centuries old, it had never before been applied to working-class children, as Olive Anderson observes, in *Suicide in Victorian and Edwardian England* (Oxford: Clarendon, 1987), p. 353 n32.

27. J. Crichton-Browne, "Education and the Nervous System," in Malcolm Morris, ed., *The Book of Health* (London: Cassell, 1883), pp. 294–95, 310, 349–50.

28. Sutherland, *Ability, Merit and Measurement*, p. 8; Great Britain, *Parliamentary Papers* (Commons) vol. 61 (1884) (*Accounts and Papers*, vol. 15), "Elementary Schools (Dr. Crichton-Browne's Report)," p. 3 [of the report].

29. *Parliamentary Papers*, Crichton-Browne Report, pp. 7–11.

30. Ibid., pp. 13, 15, 20–28, 50–53.

31. J. G. Fitch, "Memorandum Relating to Dr. Crichton-Browne's Report," printed together with the report, p. 55.

32. Crichton-Browne to Spencer, 21 Sept. 1884, Herbert Spencer Papers, MS 791/180, University of London Library, Senate House, London; Crichton-Browne to Norman Kerr, 18 Sept. 1884, Autograph Letter Collection, Wellcome Institute for the History of Medicine, London. Also see Herbert Spencer, *An Autobiography*, 2 vols. (London: Williams & Norgate, 1904), 2:20.

33. Fitch, "Memorandum," p. 79; Crichton-Browne Report, pp. 32, 27–28. Also see Sutherland, *Ability, Merit and Measurement*, p. 8, for Crichton-Browne's "loose modes of argument."

34. Mrs. S. Bryant, *Over-Work: From the Teacher's Point of View* (London: Francis Hodgson, 1885), p. 3; Anderson, *Suicide in Victorian and Edwardian England*, pp. 256, 353.

35. Sutherland, *Ability, Merit and Measurement*, pp. 8–9, 13.

36. James Crichton-Browne, Introduction to Niels T. A. Hertel, *Overpressure in High Schools in Denmark* (London: Macmillan, 1885), pp. xix–xx; "An Oration on Sex in

Education," *Lancet,* 7 May 1892, pp. 1011–18; "The First Maudsley Lecture," *JMS* 66(July 1920):210.

37. Fothergill, *Maintenance of Health,* pp. 44, 46, 48–49.

38. Frederic William Maitland, *The Life and Letters of Leslie Stephen* (New York: G. P. Putnam's; London: Duckworth, 1906), p. 39; Kitty Muggeridge and Ruth Adam, *Beatrice Webb, A Life 1858–1943* (London: Secker & Warburg, 1967), p. 29; William Allingham, *A Diary, 1824–1889,* ed. H. Allingham and D. Radford (1907; Harmondsworth: Penguin, 1985), p. 245 (6 March 1876, quoting J. A. Froude's account of a conversation with Ruskin); Thomas Hughes, *Tom Brown's Schooldays* (1857), pt. 2, chs, 2, 6.

39. Johnson, *Change of Air,* p. 16; Guthrie, *Functional Nervous Disorders in Childhood,* p. 139.

40. Robert Farquharson, "The Influence of Athletic Sports on Health," *Lancet,* 9 April 1870, p. 515.

41. My comments about Martin Benson are heavily indebted to Newsome's analysis of his life, in Chapter 3 of *Godliness and Good Learning.*

42. Arthur Christopher Benson, *Beside Still Waters* (New York and London: G. P. Putnam's, 1907), pp. 13–14.

43. E. F. Benson, *As We Were: A Victorian Peep-Show* (1930; London: Hogarth Press, 1985), p. 78; Arthur Christopher Benson, *The Life of Edward White Benson, Sometime Archbishop of Canterbury,* abr. ed. (London: Macmillan, 1901), p. 173; Newsome, *Godliness,* pp. 157–61.

44. Newsome, *Godliness,* p. 173 (also pp. 166–67, for more fatherly exhortations to the young Martin).

45. A. C. Benson, *Life of E. W. Benson,* p. 173; Newsome, *Godliness,* p. 192; A. C. Benson, *Ruskin, A Study in Personality* (London: Smith, Elder, 1911), p. 17; Audrey C. Peterson, "Brain Fever in Nineteenth-Century Literature: Fact and Fiction," *Victorian Studies* 19(June 1976):456.

46. John Springhall's study, *Coming of Age: Adolescence in Britain 1860–1960* (Dublin: Gill and Macmillan, 1986), is largely devoted to the subject of working-class adolescence. Also see Burnett, ed., *Destiny Obscure,* p. 252.

47. T. S. Clouston, "Puberty and Adolescence Medico-Psychologically Considered," *Edinburgh Medical Journal* 26(July 1880), pp. 12–13. The *OED* has entries for "adolescence" and "adolescent" from the fifteenth century, so the words were not of new coinage.

48. Walvin, *Child's World,* p. 167, discusses the different "legislative judgements" about the age of electoral responsibility, criminal responsibility, and sexual consent.

49. On Cabanis, see Jan Goldstein, *Console and Classify: The French Psychiatric Profession in the Nineteenth Century* (Cambridge and New York: Cambridge University Press, 1987), p. 52. John Demos and Virginia Demos, "Adolescence in Historical Perspective," *Journal of Marriage and the Family* 31(Nov. 1969):634–36, summarize nineteenth-century American literature on "youth" and G. Stanley Hall's contribution.

50. Charles Mercier, "Melancholia," in Tuke, ed., *Dictionary of Psychological Medicine,* 2:792.

51. Schofield, *Functional Nerve Diseases,* p. 261; Crichton-Browne, "Sex in Education," p. 1016.

52. David Skae, "A Rational and Practical Classification of Insanity," *JMS* 9(Oct. 1863):311, 314–15; Clouston, "Puberty and Adolescence," pp. 7, 11–12.

53. See the summary of E. H. Hare's theory in "Is Schizophrenia New in the World?" *Harvard Medical School Mental Health Letter* 6(Aug. 1989):7.

54. Clouston, *Hygiene of Mind,* pp. 169–70; also Clouston, "Puberty and Adolescence," pp. 11, 14.
55. "Woman in Her Psychological Relations," *J Psych Med* 4(Jan. 1851):22.
56. Clouston, "Puberty and Adolescence," p. 6; H. B. Donkin, "Hysteria," in Tuke, ed., *Dictionary of Psychological Medicine,* 1:619. Also see Deborah Gorham, *The Victorian Girl and the Feminine Ideal* (London and Canberra: Croom Helm, 1982), pp. 85–87, 91, 93.
57. Mary Scharlieb, "Adolescent Girlhood under Modern Conditions, with Special Reference to Motherhood," *Eugenics Review* 1(1909–10):174.
58. Edward John Tilt, *On the Preservation of the Health of Women at the Critical Periods of Life* (London: Churchill, 1851), pp. 19–20, 20n; also Gorham, *Victorian Girl,* pp. 86–88.
59. See, for example, Henry Maudsley, "Sex in Mind and in Education," *Fortnightly Review,* n.s., 15(1874):473; Crichton-Browne, "Education and the Nervous System," p. 363, and "Sex in Education," p. 1015; also Carol Dyhouse, "Social Darwinistic Ideas and the Development of Women's Education in England, 1880–1920," *History of Education* 5(Feb. 1976):43–46.
60. W. S. Playfair, "Some Observations Concerning What is Called Neurasthenia," *BMJ,* 6 Nov. 1886, p. 854; Crichton-Browne, "Education and the Nervous System," p. 380. Some adolescent girls contracted an anemic sickness that the Victorians labeled *chlorosis,* from the greenish pallor of complexion that its victims allegedly developed. Although not considered a functional nervous disorder itself, chlorosis—diagnosed only in female adolescents—was often linked with hysteria in medical texts. Like neurasthenia, it had passed out of medical parlance by the late 1920s, once other explanations were forthcoming for its variegated symptoms. Karl Figlio offers his heavily ideological interpretation of the disorder in "Chlorosis and Chronic Disease in Nineteenth-Century Britain: The Social Constitution of Somatic Illness in a Capitalist Society," *Social History* 3(May 1978):167–97, and Joan Jacobs Brumberg, *Fasting Girls: The Emergence of Anorexia Nervosa as a Modern Disease* (Cambridge, Mass.: Harvard University Press, 1988), pp. 172–74, points out how the diagnoses of chlorosis and anorexia nervosa overlapped.
61. W. S. Playfair, "Remarks on the Systematic Treatment of Aggravated Hysteria," *BMJ,* 19 Aug. 1882, p. 310; T. S. Clouston, *Clinical Lectures on Mental Diseases,* 2d ed. (London: Churchill, 1887), pp. 43–45, and *Hygiene of Mind,* p. 172.
62. Scharlieb, "Adolescent Girlhood," p. 177.
63. All the information in this paragraph is culled from the invaluable volume edited and introduced by Van Akin Burd, *John Ruskin and Rose La Touche: Her Unpublished Diaries of 1861 and 1867* (Oxford: Clarendon, 1979), pp. 28, 31, 63–64, 78–89, 163, 166–68.
64. Ibid., pp. 169–70 (italics in original).
65. Maria La Touche to George MacDonald, [15 Oct. 1863], George MacDonald Papers, The Beinecke Rare Book and Manuscript Library, Yale University, New Haven, Connecticut (italics in original). All further citations from Maria La Touche's correspondence refer to this collection. Also see Burd, ed., *Ruskin and Rose La Touche,* p. 89.
66. Burd, ed., *Ruskin and Rose La Touche,* pp. 171 (from Rose's autobiography of 1867), 92 (quoting Ruskin's letter to a friend about her).
67. Maria La Touche to George MacDonald, [19 Nov. 1863].
68. John Ruskin to Mrs. William Cowper, 6 Aug. 1866, in *The Letters of John Ruskin to Lord and Lady Mount-Temple,* ed. John Lewis Bradley (Columbus, Ohio: Ohio State University Press, 1964), p. 79.
69. Maria La Touche to Louisa Powell MacDonald, 25 Sept. [1865].

70. Burd, ed., *Ruskin and Rose La Touche,* pp. 112, 114–15, 122, 131.

71. The apt adjective is Lorna Duffin's: see "The Conspicuous Consumptive: Woman as an Invalid," in Sara Delamont and Lorna Duffin, eds., *The Nineteenth-Century Woman: Her Cultural and Physical World* (London: Croom Helm; New York: Barnes & Noble, 1978), p. 38.

72. "Woman in Her Psychological Relations," p. 37; Clouston, *Hygiene of Mind,* p. 245. In *Emile* (1762), Jean-Jacques Rousseau adumbrated the nineteenth-century medical view of sequential stages of growth, with appropriate experiences at each level, and also warned against premature sensuality. See R. P. Neuman, "Masturbation, Madness, and the Modern Concepts of Childhood and Adolescence," *Journal of Social History* 8(Spring 1975):5; and Claudia Nelson, "Sex and the Single Boy: Ideals of Manliness and Sexuality in Victorian Literature for Boys," *Victorian Studies* 32(Summer 1989):525–50.

73. Walvin, *Child's World,* p. 46; Burnett, ed., *Destiny Obscure,* pp. 50–52; Eric T. Carlson and Norman Dain, "The Meaning of Moral Insanity," *Bull Hist Med* 36(March–April 1962):137.

74. Maudsley quoted in Aubrey Lewis, "Henry Maudsley: His Work and Influence," *JMS* 97(April 1951):271; George H. Savage, "Moral Insanity," *JMS* 27(July 1881):150; Ch. Féré, "Nerve Troubles as Foreshadowed in the Child," *Brain* 8(1886):235–36. Also see F. Barry Smith, "Sexuality in Britain, 1800–1900: Some Suggested Revisions," in Martha Vicinus, ed., *A Widening Sphere: Changing Roles of Victorian Women* (Bloomington, Ind.: Indiana University Press, 1977), p. 196; and Peter Gay, *Freud: A Life for Our Time* (New York: Norton, 1988), p. 144 (on Maudsley and childhood sexuality).

75. Walvin, *Child's World,* pp. 143–47 (on child prostitution); Anthony S. Wohl, "Sex and the Single Room: Incest Among the Victorian Working Classes," in Anthony S. Wohl, ed., *The Victorian Family: Structure and Stresses* (New York: St. Martin's Press, 1978), pp. 199–203, 211–12.

76. For an extended discussion of sexuality in boys' boarding schools and the campaign against it in the late nineteenth century, see J. R. de S. Honey, *Tom Brown's Universe: The Development of the English Public School in the Nineteenth Century* (New York: Quadrangle / The New York Times Book Co., 1977), pp. 167–203; also John Chandos, *Boys Together: English Public Schools 1800–1864* (New Haven and London: Yale University Press, 1984), pp. 284–319.

77. See Arthur N. Gilbert, "Doctor, Patient, and Onanist Diseases in the Nineteenth Century," *Journal of the History of Medicine and Allied Sciences* 30(July 1975):231–32; Robert H. MacDonald, "The Frightful Consequences of Onanism: Notes on the History of a Delusion," *Journal of the History of Ideas* 28(1967):429.

78. Clouston, "Puberty and Adolescence," p. 17; Coventry Patmore quoted in Katharine Moore, *Victorian Wives* (London and New York: Allison and Busby, 1985), p. 12; Scharlieb, "Adolescent Girlhood," pp. 175–76.

79. Logie Barrow, *Independent Spirits: Spiritualism and English Plebeians, 1850–1910* (London and New York: Routledge & Kegan Paul, 1986), p. 259.

80. Tilt, *Preservation of the Health of Women,* p. 42. On manliness, asexuality, and eternal boyhood, see Jeffrey Richards, "'Passing the Love of Women': Manly Love and Victorian Society," in J. A. Mangan and James Walvin, eds., *Manliness and Morality: Middle-Class Masculinity in Britain and America 1800–1940* (Manchester: Manchester University Press; New York: St. Martin's Press, 1987), pp. 105–107; also Newsome, *Godliness,* p. 238.

81. See Walvin, *Child's World,* p. 138; Smith, "Sexuality in Britain," pp. 197–98; Sterling Fishman, "The History of Childhood Sexuality," *Journal of Contemporary History* 17(April 1982):270, 277.

82. See the list of statutes in Walvin, *Child's World*, pp. 200–202.
83. "The Study of Childhood," *BMJ,* 21 May 1904, p. 1205.
84. Among the numerous works on this topic, two recent books are particularly valuable: Deborah Dwork, *War is Good For Babies and Other Young Children: A History of the Infant and Child Welfare Movement in England 1898–1918* (London and New York: Tavistock Publications, 1987), and Jane Lewis, *The Politics of Motherhood: Child and Maternal Welfare in England, 1900–1939* (London: Croom Helm; Montreal: McGill-Queen's University Press, 1980). For two very different approaches to Edwardian interest in child welfare, see Bentley B. Gilbert, "Sir John Eldon Gorst and the Children of the Nation," *Bull Hist Med* 28(1954):243–51; and Anna Davin, "Imperialism and Motherhood," *History Workshop,* issue 5(Spring 1978):9–65. The second volume of Ivy Pinchbeck and Margaret Hewitt, *Children in English Society,* 2 vols. (London: Routledge & Kegan Paul, 1969–73), contains an extended discussion of changing British attitudes toward, and policies for, child welfare in the Victorian and Edwardian years.
85. On the Child Study Society, see Davin, "Imperialism and Motherhood," pp. 55, 65 n180; on the milk question, see Dwork, *War is Good for Babies,* p. 87; for an example of Crichton-Browne's sympathetic concern about the elderly, see Crichton-Browne, "The Prevention of Senility," *The Prevention of Senility and A Sanitary Outlook* (London: Macmillan, 1905), especially pp. 65–66.
86. Burnett, ed., *Destiny Obscure,* p. 50; also pp. 260–61.
87. Crichton-Browne, "Psychical Diseases of Early Life," p. 313, and "Education and the Nervous System," pp. 305, 322, 332, 349; Guthrie, *Functional Nervous Disorders in Childhood,* p. 9.
88. James Crichton-Browne, *Physical Efficiency in Children* (London: King, 1902).

Chapter 8

1. J. A. Mangan, "Social Darwinism and Upper-Class Education in Late Victorian and Edwardian England," in J. A. Mangan and James Walvin, eds., *Manliness and Morality: Middle-Class Masculinity in Britain and America 1800–1940* (Manchester: Manchester University Press; New York: St. Martin's Press, 1987), pp. 135–36.
2. James Crichton-Browne, *What the Doctor Thought* (London: Ernest Benn, 1930), pp. 254–55. The essential work on the Edwardian preoccupation with national efficiency is G. R. Searle, *The Quest for National Efficiency: A Study in British Politics and Political Thought, 1899–1914* (Berkeley and Los Angeles: University of California Press; Oxford: Blackwell, 1971). Also see Jonathan Rose, *The Edwardian Temperament 1895–1919* (Athens, Ohio: Ohio University Press, 1986), ch. 4.
3. An Inter-Departmental Committee on Physical Deterioration was established in the wake of these allegations. See Bentley B. Gilbert, "Health and Politics: The British Physical Deterioration Report of 1904," *Bull Hist Med* 39(March–April 1965):143–53; Richard Soloway, "Counting the Degenerates: The Statistics of Race Deterioration in Edwardian England," *Journal of Contemporary History* 17(Jan. 1982):142–51. Also see George F. Shee, "The Deterioration in the National Physique," *Nineteenth Century* 53(May 1903):797–805.
4. Grant Allen, "Plain Words on the Woman Question," *Fortnightly Review,* n.s., 46(Oct. 1889):450n. See Richard Allen Soloway, *Birth Control and the Population Question in England, 1877–1930* (Chapel Hill: University of North Carolina Press, 1982), pp. 3–24, for a detailed analysis of the declining British birthrate between 1876 and 1914, and pp. 25–48, for the relationship between class and fertility in the same period; also see

Soloway, "Counting the Degenerates," pp. 153–54. For the British response to Eastern European immigrants, see Bernard Gainer, *The Alien Invasion: The Origins of the Aliens Act of 1905* (London: Heinemann Educational Books, 1972). Several social surveys after the mid-1870s, in fact, found the health of Jewish immigrant children to be surprisingly good.

5. Among the growing literature on Victorian racist thought, the following are particularly valuable: Christine Bolt, *Victorian Attitudes to Race* (London: Routledge & Kegan Paul, 1971); Nancy Stepan, *The Idea of Race in Science: Great Britain 1800–1960* (London: Macmillan; Hamden, Conn.: Archon Books, 1982), and George W. Stocking, Jr., *Victorian Anthropology* (London: Collier Macmillan; New York: The Free Press, 1987). Throughout this chapter, I have used the word "race" in the free-wheeling Victorian manner, the better to convey a sense of the way it figured, often inappropriately, in nineteenth-century literature.

6. Olive Anderson, *Suicide in Victorian and Edwardian England* (Oxford: Clarendon, 1987), pp. 66–70, 172, 242–44, 265, 336.

7. T. S. Clouston, "Puberty and Adolescence Medico-Psychologically Considered," *Edinburgh Medical Journal* 26(July 1880):10 (for the "guardians"); Alfred T. Schofield, *Behind the Brass Plate: Life's Little Stories* (London: Sampson Low, Marston, [1928]), p. 235.

8. Thomas Trotter, *A View of the Nervous Temperament* (London: Longman, Hurst, Rees, & Orme, 1807), pp. x–xi (italics in original).

9. James Johnson, *Change of Air, or the Pursuit of Health* (London: S. Highley, and T. G. Underwood, 1831), p. 16; Edwin Lee, *A Treatise on Some Nervous Disorders*, 2d ed. rev. (London: Churchill, 1838), p. 21.

10. Daniel Noble, *Facts and Observations Relative to the Influence of Manufactures upon Health and Life* (London: Churchill, 1843), pp. 49, 80–81.

11. See Stepan, *Idea of Race in Science*, pp. 11–13.

12. Lionel John Beale, *The Laws of Health, in Relation to Mind and Body* (London: Churchill, 1851), p. 75, and *The Senses, The Brain, and the Mind; Their Connections and Relations* (London: Harrison, 1860), p. 9. Also see Forbes Winslow, *On the Preservation of the Health of Body and Mind* (London: Henry Renshaw, 1842), p. 147n.

13. Janet Browne, "Darwin and the Face of Madness," in W. F. Bynum, Roy Porter, and Michael Shepherd, eds., *The Anatomy of Madness: Essays in the History of Psychiatry*, 2 vols. (London and New York: Tavistock Publications, 1985), 1:151–52.

14. For an excellent discussion of Morel, Moreau, and the place of degeneration theory in French psychiatry, see Ian Dowbiggin, "Degeneration and Hereditarianism in French Mental Medicine 1840–90: Psychiatric Theory as Ideological Adaptation," in Bynum, Porter, and Shepherd, eds., *Anatomy of Madness*, 1:188–232 (p. 230 n170 on Adam); on Morel and original sin, see G. E. Berrios, "Obsessional Disorders during the Nineteenth Century: Terminological and Classificatory Issues," in the same volume, p. 183 n79; on Morel's causative explanations, also see Eric T. Carlson, "Medicine and Degeneration: Theory and Praxis," in J. Edward Chamberlin and Sander L. Gilman, eds., *Degeneration: The Dark Side of Progress* (New York: Columbia University Press, 1985), pp. 123–24. A now somewhat outdated survey of the international furor over degeneration, from 1857 to the 1920s, is found in Richard D. Walter, "What Became of the Degenerate? A Brief History of a Concept," *Journal of the History of Medicine and Allied Sciences* 11(Oct. 1956):422–29. Daniel Pick, *Faces of Degeneration: A European Disorder, c. 1848–c. 1918* (Cambridge and New York: Cambridge University Press, 1989) is the most recent study that places the degeneration uproar in an international perspective.

15. "On the Degeneracy of the Human Race," *J Psych Med* 10(April 1857):159–208 (words quoted on p. 208); W. H. O. Sankey, "On Melancholia," *JMS* 9(July 1863):175.

16. J. Crichton-Browne, "Psychical Diseases of Early Life," *JMS* 6 (April 1860):285, 290, and "The History and Progress of Psychological Medicine," *JMS* 7(April 1861):29; Henry Maudsley, *The Physiology and Pathology of Mind* (London: Macmillan, 1867), pp. 367–408. Also see Aubrey Lewis, "Henry Maudsley: His Work and Influence," *JMS* 97(April 1951):263, 265–67.

17. J. Crichton-Browne, "Cranial Injuries and Mental Diseases," *WRLAMR* 1(1871):5; G. F. Glandford's address, quoted in T. Clifford Allbutt, "Nervous Diseases and Modern Life," *Contemporary Review* 67 (1895):218.

18. J. Milner Fothergill, *The Maintenance of Health: A Medical Work for Lay Readers* (London: Smith, Elder, 1874), p. 250.

19. T. S. Clouston, *The Hygiene of Mind* (London: Methuen, 1906), p. 38, and *Female Education from a Medical Point of View* (Edinburgh: Macniven and Wallace, 1882), p. 19. Allbutt was among those who challenged the validity of the nervous system–machine analogy, as in "Nervous Diseases and Modern Life," pp. 218–19.

20. Thomas Stretch Dowse, *Lectures on Massage & Electricity in the Treatment of Disease* (London: Hamilton, Adams, [1889]), p. 181. Also see Charles E. Rosenberg, "George M. Beard and American Nervousness," in his collection of essays, *No Other Gods: On Science and American Social Thought* (Baltimore: Johns Hopkins University Press, paperback ed., 1978), p. 103.

21. Address to British Medical Association Annual Meeting, 1882, in John Hughlings Jackson, *Selected Writings of John Hughlings Jackson,* ed. James Taylor, 2 vols. (London: Hodder & Stoughton, 1931–32), 2:342. For a discussion of Jackson's concept of "nervous disease as a process of dissolution," see James Taylor's "Biographical Memoir," in John Hughlings Jackson, *Neurological Fragments,* ed. James Taylor (London: Humphrey Milford, Oxford University Press, 1925), pp. 10–11.

22. James Sully, *My Life and Friends: A Psychologist's Memories* (London: T. Fisher Unwin, 1918), p. 202. Also see D. Hack Tuke, "Presidential Address to the Medico-Psychological Association," *JMS* 27(Oct. 1881):323; Taylor, "Biographical Memoir," p. 10; Rosenberg, "George Beard," pp. 105–106, for illuminating connections between faculty psychology and the theories of Spencer, Beard, and Jackson.

23. Th. Ribot, "Will, Disorders of," in D. Hack Tuke, ed., *A Dictionary of Psychological Medicine,* 2 vols. (London: Churchill, 1892), 2:1367–68.

24. Henry Maudsley, "Remarks on Crime and Criminals," *JMS* (1888), quoted in Arthur N. Gilbert, "Masturbation and Insanity: Henry Maudsley and the Ideology of Sexual Repression," *Albion* 12(Fall 1980): 273–74; George H. Savage's contribution to "Discussion on Neurasthenia and its Treatment," *BMJ,* 8 Sept. 1894, p. 522, and Savage, "Moral Insanity," *JMS* 27(July 1881):147–48; Seymour J. Sharkey, "Hysteria and Neurasthenia," *Brain* 27(Spring 1904):3–4; James Shaw, "Obsessions," *JMS* 50(April 1904):248–49 (for "the first to be lost").

25. George Rennie, "A Clinical Lecture on Functional Nerve Diseases," *BMJ,* 4 May 1901, p. 1065; Sharkey, "Hysteria and Neurasthenia," p. 24. Also see J. E. Chamberlin, "An Anatomy of Cultural Melancholy," *Journal of the History of Ideas* 42(1981): 696–97.

26. Alfred A. Mumford, "Some Considerations on the Alleged Physical Degeneration of the British Race," *Fortnightly Review,* n.s., 76(August 1904):331–32. Also see Chamberlin, "Cultural Melancholy," pp. 693–94, 703–705; and Soloway, "Counting the Degenerates," pp. 144–45 (on Mumford). The international success of Max Nordau's *Degeneration* (first published in German in 1892–93 and translated into French and English in 1894

and 1895, respectively) makes it clear that the equation of fin-de siècle art and literature with cultural decay and national decline was not a uniquely British reaction.

27. Soloway, "Counting the Degenerates," p. 159.

28. William Allingham, *A Diary, 1824–1889,* ed. H. Allingham and D. Radford (1907; Harmondsworth: Penguin, 1985), p. 239 (5 Oct. 1875).

29. Francis Warner, "Results of an Inquiry as to the Physical and Mental Condition of Fifty Thousand Children seen in One Hundred and Six Schools," *Journal of the Royal Statistical Society* 56(1893):99.

30. Stephen Jay Gould, *The Panda's Thumb: More Reflections in Natural History* (New York: Norton, paperback ed., 1982), p. 163, and his book devoted to this subject, *Ontogeny and Phylogeny* (Cambridge, Mass.: Harvard University Press, 1977). Also see Chamberlin, "Cultural Melancholy," pp. 695, 698.

31. P. C. Smith, "Neurasthenia, Degeneracy, and Mobile Organs," *BMJ,* 3 March 1906, p. 494. Also see Stephen Kern, "Explosive Intimacy: Psychodynamics of the Victorian Family," *History of Childhood Quarterly* 1(1973–74):438–41.

32. Clouston, *Female Education,* p. 19.

33. Henry Maudsley, "Sex in Mind and in Education," *Fortnightly Review,* n.s., 15(1874):472; E. Lynn Linton, "The Higher Education of Woman," *Fortnightly Review,* n.s., 40(Oct. 1886):503, 508, 510; Clouston, "Puberty and Adolescence," p. 9.

34. Carol Dyhouse, "Social Darwinistic Ideas and the Development of Women's Education in England, 1880–1920," *History of Education* 5(Feb. 1976):47, 53–55.

35. Francis Galton, *Memories of My Life* (New York: E. P. Dutton, 1909), pp. 310–23 ("Race Improvement"); Daniel J. Kevles, *In the Name of Eugenics: Genetics and the Uses of Human Heredity* (Berkeley and Los Angeles: University of California Press, paperback ed., 1986), pp. ix, 3, 59–60, 114; G. R. Searle, "Eugenics and Class," in Charles Webster, ed., *Biology, Medicine and Society 1840–1940* (Cambridge and New York: Cambridge University Press, 1981), pp. 219–21; Soloway, "Counting the Degenerates," pp. 152, 157. As all of these sources make clear, the label *eugenist* implied no complete package of social, political, or medical policies. Different people were drawn to different aspects of eugenic thinking for different reasons. Richard A. Soloway's latest study, *Demography and Degeneration: Eugenics and the Declining Birthrate in Twentieth-Century Britain* (Chapel Hill and London: University of North Carolina Press, 1990) appeared too recently for me to be able to incorporate its insights into my own work.

36. Soloway, *Birth Control,* pp. 122–23; Searle, "Eugenics and Class," pp. 223–26.

37. Searle, "Eugenics and Class," p. 226.

38. Mary Scharlieb, "Adolescent Girlhood under Modern Conditions, with Special Reference to Motherhood," *Eugenics Review* 1(1909–10):183. Also see Frank Mort, *Dangerous Sexualities: Medico-Moral Politics in England since 1830* (London and New York: Routledge & Kegan Paul, 1987), p. 180.

39. Lewis, "Maudsley," p. 263. These concerns provided a major theme in Maudsley's book, *Responsibility in Mental Disease* (London: H. S. King, 1874). Also see James Crichton-Browne, "The First Maudsley Lecture," *JMS* 66(July 1920):208.

40. Clouston, *Hygiene of Mind,* p. 264. I am indebted to Professor Richard Soloway for his informative letter to me concerning Crichton-Browne's affiliation with the Eugenics Education Society. Also see Soloway, *Birth Control,* p. 31.

41. Soloway, *Birth Control,* pp. 22, 161; Searle, "Eugenics and Class," p. 233 (on the basic conservatism of Edwardian eugenists). While some late Victorian and Edwardian liberals, and even socialists, selectively endorsed certain aspects of eugenic thought, I am persuaded that they were elitists first, and social reformers second.

42. Crichton-Browne to Galton, 5 March 1905, Galton Papers 133/5A, The Library, Univer-

sity College London; James Crichton-Browne, *The Doctor's Second Thoughts* (London: Ernest Benn, 1931), pp. 154–55. British eugenists were by no means unanimous in advocating the compulsory "sterilization of the unfit" before World War I or after.

43. James Crichton-Browne, *Victorian Jottings from an Old Commonplace Book* (London: Etchells & MacDonald, 1926), p. 73.

44. Crichton-Browne to Galton, 5 March 1905, Galton Papers 133/5A, The Library, University College London; Crichton-Browne, *Victorian Jottings*, pp. 72–73 (on eugenics and phrenology); Presidential Address, London Conference of the Sanitary Inspectors Association, August 1905, in James Crichton-Browne, *The Prevention of Senility and A Sanitary Outlook* (London: Macmillan, 1905), pp. 95, 124–29.

45. See Stepan, *Idea of Race in Science*, p. xviii, on the "typological conception of race," and Chamberlin and Gilman, eds., *Degeneration*, for its subtitle: *The Dark Side of Progress*.

46. Sully, *My Life and Friends*, pp. 238–39.

47. Thomas Laycock, "On the Naming and Classification of Mental Diseases and Defects," *JMS* 9(July 1863):160–62; Gould, *Panda's Thumb*, pp. 160–68, for an incisive analysis of Down's work. Nancy Stepan, "Biological Degeneration: Races and Proper Places," in Chamberlin and Gilman, eds., *Degeneration*, pp. 97–120, summarizes the application of degeneration theory to racist thought.

48. See Chamberlin, "Cultural Melancholy," p. 699, and Mort, *Dangerous Sexualities*, p. 188.

49. See "Report of the Privy Council upon Physical Deterioration," *Lancet*, 6 Aug. 1904, pp. 391–92; "National Health and Military Service," *BMJ*, 25 July 1903, p. 208; "Physical Deterioration," *BMJ*, 2 Jan. 1904, p. 37; Soloway, "Counting the Degenerates," pp. 138, 140–43, 149, 159–60; Bentley B. Gilbert, "Sir John Eldon Gorst and the Children of the Nation," *Bull Hist Med* 28(1954):247, and Gilbert, "Health and Politics," p. 148. Dowbiggin, "Degeneration and Hereditarianism," pp. 197–99, points out how little substantial evidence supported French medical endorsement of degeneration theory.

50. Shuttleworth's views were summarized in "The Study of Childhood," *BMJ*, 21 May 1904, p. 1205. On Shuttleworth, see Gillian Sutherland, *Ability, Merit and Measurement: Mental Testing and English Education 1880–1940* (Oxford: Clarendon, 1984), pp. 13, 15–16; and *Who Was Who, 1916–1928*, s.v. "Shuttleworth, George Edward."

51. George Savage, *The Increase of Insanity* (London: Cassell, 1907), p. 6.

52. Soloway, "Counting the Degenerates," p. 143.

53. "Degeneracy of Human Race," pp. 186–87 (italics in original).

54. Ibid., p. 187.

55. Dowbiggin, "Degeneration and Hereditarianism," pp. 199–200, comments on the disjunction between degeneration theory and therapeutic practice in nineteenth-century French psychiatry. Andrew Scull, "Was Insanity Increasing? A Response to Edward Hare," *British Journal of Psychiatry* 144(1984):434, suggests that psychiatric pessimism turned into "a relentlessly self-fulfilling prophecy."

56. "Degeneracy of Human Race," p. 192; Smith, "Neurasthenia, Degeneracy, and Mobile Organs," p. 495; Shaw, "Obsessions," pp. 238, 244; Leonard G. Guthrie, *Functional Nervous Disorders in Childhood* (London: Oxford University Press, Oxford Medical Publications, 1907), pp. 4, 22–23. Also see Eric T. Carlson and Norman Dain, "The Meaning of Moral Insanity," *Bull Hist Med* 36(March–April 1962):138.

57. Dowbiggin, "Degeneration and Hereditarianism," p. 199.

58. As Professor M. Jeanne Peterson suggested to me.

59. Galton, *Memories of My Life*, pp. 259–61; Maudsley explored the characteristics of the hereditary criminal class in *Responsibility in Mental Disease*. Also see Soloway, "Counting the Degenerates," pp. 157, 160.

60. Gould, *Panda's Thumb*, p. 164.
61. Henry Maudsley, "Insanity and Its Treatment," *JMS* (1871), quoted in Gilbert, "Masturbation and Insanity," p. 277.
62. Galton, *Memories of My Life*, p. 296.
63. Charles Darwin, *The Autobiography of Charles Darwin 1809–1882*, ed. Nora Barlow (New York: Norton, paperback ed., 1969), p. 130. Also see Loren Eiseley, *Darwin's Century: Evolution and the Men who Discovered It* (Garden City, N.Y.: Doubleday, Anchor Books ed., 1961), pp. 216–18, and Kevles, *In the Name of Eugenics*, p. 18.
64. Eiseley, *Darwin's Century*, pp. 205–209, 218–20; Kevles, *In the Name of Eugenics*, pp. 41–43. Harry Campbell, *Differences in the Nervous Organisation of Man and Woman: Physiological and Pathological* (London: H. K. Lewis, 1891), pp. v–vi, provides an example of how quickly Weismann's influence began to be felt in British medical texts.
65. Stepan, *Idea of Race in Science*, p. 87; Soloway, "Counting the Degenerates," pp. 144, 152–53.
66. James Crichton-Browne, "An Oration on Sex in Education," *Lancet*, 7 May 1892, p. 1018; *Prevention of Senility and A Sanitary Outlook*, p. 106; on Pavlov's work, *The Story of the Brain* (Edinburgh and London: Oliver & Boyd, 1924), pp. 23–24, and *Doctor's Second Thoughts*, pp. 217–18.

Conclusion

1. Sydney Smith to Sarah Austin, 23 Jan. 1840, quoted in Lotte Hamburger and Joseph Hamburger, *Troubled Lives: John and Sarah Austin* (Toronto: University of Toronto Press, 1985), p. 131; James Crichton-Browne, "The First Maudsley Lecture," *JMS* 66(July 1920):224; also see Aubrey Lewis, "Henry Maudsley: His Work and Influence," *JMS* 97(April 1951):266–67.
2. James Crichton-Browne, *The Doctor's Second Thoughts* (London: Ernest Benn, 1931), pp. 49–50; Weir Mitchell quoted in Carroll Smith-Rosenberg, "The Hysterical Woman: Sex Roles and Role Conflict in 19th-Century America," *Social Research* 39(Winter 1972):670.
3. See Sandra M. Gilbert, "Soldier's Heart: Literary Men, Literary Women, and the Great War," *Signs* 8(Spring 1983):423.
4. For the *Times* (London) article, see Charlotte MacKenzie, "Social Factors in the Admission, Discharge, and Continuing Stay of Patients at Ticehurst Asylum, 1845–1917," in W. F. Bynum, Roy Porter, and Michael Shepherd, eds., *The Anatomy of Madness: Essays in the History of Psychiatry*, 2 vols. (London and New York: Tavistock Publications, 1985), 2:169; E. Mendel, "Diagnosis of Mental Disorders," and W. S. Playfair, "Neuroses, Functional, The Systematic Treatment of," in D. Hack Tuke, ed., *A Dictionary of Psychological Medicine*, 2 vols. (London: Churchill, 1892), 1:375, 2:851.
5. Alfred T. Schofield, *The Force of Mind or the Mental Factor in Medicine* (London: Churchill, 1902), pp. 228, 235; George H. Savage, *The Harveian Oration on Experimental Psychology and Hypnotism* (London: Henry Frowde, for Oxford University Press, 1909), pp. 20–21; Arthur Hurst, *A Twentieth Century Physician: Being the Reminiscences of Sir Arthur Hurst, D.M., F.R.C.P.* (London: Edward Arnold, 1949), p. 103.
6. C. Hubert Bond, "The Need for Schools of Psychiatry," *JMS* 66 (Jan. 1920):10–11; Crichton-Browne, "First Maudsley Lecture," p. 201.
7. J. Crichton-Browne, "A Plea for the Minute Study of Mania," *Brain* 3(1880–81):349; Charles Mercier, *The Nervous System and the Mind. A Treatise on the Dynamics of the Human Organism* (London: Macmillan, 1888), pp. 9–10.

8. W. F. Bynum, "The Nervous Patient in Eighteenth- and Nineteenth-Century Britain: The Psychiatric Origins of British Neurology," in Bynum, Porter, and Shepherd, eds., *Anatomy of Madness*, 1:90.

9. Edwin G. Boring, *A History of Experimental Psychology*, 2d ed. (New York: Appleton-Century Crofts, 1950), pp. 459–60, 463, 488–94.

10. David Drummond, "Neurasthenia: Its Nature and Treatment," *BMJ*, 7 July 1906, p. 14.

11. J. S. Mill, *Autobiography* (London: Longmans, Green, Reader, & Dyer, 1873), p. 169. See the discussion of this passage in Barbara T. Gates, *Victorian Suicide: Mad Crimes and Sad Histories* (Princeton: Princeton University Press, 1988), p. 32.

12. Drummond, "Neurasthenia," p. 11.

13. The best book on the place of mesmerism in late eighteenth-century French culture is Robert Darnton, *Mesmerism and the End of the Enlightenment in France* (Cambridge, Mass.: Harvard University Press, 1968).

14. John Conolly, "Hysteria," in John Forbes, Alexander Tweedie, and John Conolly, eds., *The Cyclopædia of Practical Medicine*, 4 vols. (London: Sherwood, Gilbert, Piper, Baldwin, & Cradock, 1833–35), 2:562.

15. A. T. Myers, "Hypnotism, History of," in Tuke, ed., *Dictionary of Psychological Medicine*, 1:603–604; Savage, *Harveian Oration*, pp. 25–26; D. Hack Tuke, "Hypnosis Redivivus," *JMS* 26(Jan. 1881):531.

16. As, for example, in D. Hack Tuke, "On the Mental Condition in Hypnotism, *JMS* 29(April 1883):55.

17. A full discussion of Braid's work appears in J. Milne Bramwell, "James Braid: His Work and Writings," *Proceedings of the Society for Psychical Research* 12(June 1896):127–66. Also see Michael J. Clark, "The Rejection of Psychological Approaches to Mental Disorder in Late Nineteenth-Century British Psychiatry," in Andrew Scull, ed., *Madhouses, Mad-Doctors, and Madmen: The Social History of Psychiatry in the Victorian Era* (London: Athlone Press; Philadelphia: University of Pennsylvania Press, 1981), pp. 278–80.

18. Peyton Blakiston, *Clinical Reminiscences* (London: Churchill, 1878), p. 32.

19. Savage, *Harveian Oration*, p. 26; Myers, "Hypnotism," pp. 605–606; Tuke, "Hypnosis Redivivus," p. 531, and "Mental Condition in Hypnotism," p. 80. On Gully, mesmerism, and medical unorthodoxy, see Elizabeth Jenkins, *Tennyson and Dr. Gully* (Lincoln: The Tennyson Society, Tennyson Research Centre, 1974), pp. 9–11, and Janet Oppenheim, *The Other World: Spiritualism and Psychical Research in England, 1850–1914* (Cambridge and New York: Cambridge University Press, 1985), pp. 217–36.

20. See Ruth Harris, "Murder under Hypnosis in the Case of Gabrielle Bompard: Psychiatry in the Courtroom in Belle Epoque Paris," in Bynum, Porter, and Shepherd, eds., *Anatomy of Madness*, 2:199, 203–10.

21. J. Milne Bramwell, *Hypnotism: Its History, Practice and Theory* (London: Grant Richards, 1903), p. 437. Among the other works of Bramwell and Tuckey, see Bramwell, "Hypnotism: and the Treatment of Insanity and Allied Disorders by Suggestion," in Clifford Allbutt and Humphry Davy Rolleston, eds., *A System of Medicine*, 2d ed. rev., 9 vols. (London: Macmillan, 1905–11), 8:1007–17; C. Lloyd Tuckey, *Psycho-Therapeutics; or, Treatment by Sleep and Suggestion* (London: Baillière, Tindall, & Cox, 1889), and *The Value of Hypnotism in Chronic Alcoholism* (London: Churchill, 1892). Also see Clark, "Rejection of Psychological Approaches," pp. 281–83, and the entry in the *OED* on "psycho-therapeutic."

22. Thomas Stretch Dowse, *On Brain and Nerve Exhaustion. 'Neurasthenia.' Its Nature and Curative Treatment* (London: Baillière, Tindall, & Cox, 1880), p. 53.

23. Harris, "Murder under Hypnosis," pp. 198, 217, 219–21, 224–32, explores with great verve the issues raised in this paragraph.

24. Among many such assertions in their work, see Henry Maudsley, *The Pathology of Mind* (London: Macmillan, 1879), pp. 56–57; and William B. Carpenter, *Principles of Mental Physiology, with Their Applications to the Training and Discipline of the Mind, and the Study of its Morbid Conditions* (London: H. S. King, 1874), p. 616.

25. H. B. Donkin, "Hysteria," in Tuke, ed., *Dictionary of Psychological Medicine*, 1:626; also see Harris, "Murder under Hypnosis," pp. 206–10.

26. Daniel Hack Tuke, *Illustrations of the Influence of the Mind upon the Body in Health and Disease Designed to Elucidate the Action of the Imagination* (London: Churchill, 1872), pp. ix, 407–17; "Mental Condition in Hypnotism," p. 78, and "Hypnosis Redivivus," pp. 537, 543. Also see Clark, "Rejection of Psychological Approaches," p. 289.

27. Maudsley, *Pathology of Mind*, pp. 59–60; William Thorburn, "The Traumatic Neuroses," *Proceedings of the Royal Society of Medicine* 7(1913–14), pt. 2(Neurological Section):10.

28. As Clark persuasively argues, in "Rejection of Psychological Approaches," pp. 288–92.

29. John Forrester, "Contracting the Disease of Love: Authority and Freedom in the Origins of Psychoanalysis," in Bynum, Porter, and Shepherd, eds., *Anatomy of Madness*, 1:259–62, suggests that doctors were wary of hypnotism because it gives the patient power to limit medical authority by refusing to be hypnotized or cured by hypnosis. The evidence strongly indicates, however, that British psychiatrists were far more worried about too little will in hypnotized patients than too much.

30. J. M. Charcot and Pierre Marie, "Hysteria, mainly Hystero-Epilepsy," in Tuke, ed., *Dictionary of Psychological Medicine*, 1:628, 640; Clifford Allbutt, "Neurasthenia," in Allbutt and Rolleston, eds., *System of Medicine*, 8:783, 786; Savage, *Harveian Oration*, pp. 35–40; Schofield, *Force of Mind*, p. 227, and *Nerves in Disorder. A Plea for Rational Treatment* (London: Hodder & Stoughton, 1903), pp. 163–64.

31. Benson's commentary on his hypnotic treatment is quoted in David Newsome, *On the Edge of Paradise. A.C. Benson: The Diarist* (London: John Murray, 1980), pp. 229, 234–35.

32. Tuke, "Hypnosis Redivivus," pp. 533–36 (for Carpenter's views, as well as his own), and "Mental Condition in Hypnotism," p. 79. Also see J. P. Williams, "Psychical Research and Psychiatry in Late Victorian Britain: Trance as Ecstasy or Trance as Insanity," in Bynum, Porter, and Shepherd, eds., *Anatomy of Madness*, 1:239–40.

33. Peter Gay, *Freud: A Life for Our Time* (New York: Norton, 1988), p. 103.

34. Ibid., p. 63n.

35. F. W. H. Myers, "The Mechanism of Hysteria," *Proceedings of the Society for Psychical Research* 9(1893–94):12–15; J. Michell Clarke, "Hysteria and Neurasthenia," *Brain* 17(1894):125.

36. Eder subsequently became a Jungian. Information in this paragraph is derived from Ernest Jones, *Free Associations: Memories of a Psycho-Analyst* (London: Hogarth Press; New York: Basic Books, 1959); J. B. Hobman, ed., *David Eder: Memoirs of a Modern Pioneer* (London: Gollancz, 1945); and Vincent Brome, *Ernest Jones: Freud's Alter Ego* (New York: Norton, 1983)—an unsatisfactory and frustrating book. Also see Gay, *Freud*, pp. 183–87; Martin Stone, "Shellshock and the Psychologists," in Bynum, Porter, and Shepherd, eds., *Anatomy of Madness*, 2:243; Samuel Hynes, *The Edwardian Turn of Mind* (Princeton: Princeton University Press, 1968), p. 164; Jonathan Rose, *The Edwardian Temperament 1895–1919* (Athens, Ohio: Ohio University Press, 1986), p. 180.

37. Ernest Jones, "The Treatment of the Neuroses, Including the Psychoneuroses," in William A. White and Smith Ely Jelliffe, eds., *The Modern Treatment of Nervous and Mental Diseases*, vol. 1 (London: Henry Kimpton; Glasgow: Alexander Stenhouse, 1913), pp. 339, 343.

38. Ibid., p. 334.
39. Daniel N. Robinson, *An Intellectual History of Psychology,* rev. ed. (New York: Macmillan, 1981), p. 386, insists that outraged Victorian proprieties cannot account for the initially frosty response to psychoanalysis from the international psychiatric community. Also see Gay, *Freud,* pp. 144–45 (on Freud's gradual acceptance of infantile sexuality) and 338 (on middle-class society's repressive role).
40. As Frank Mort observes in *Dangerous Sexualities: Medico-Moral Politics in England since 1830* (London and New York: Routledge & Kegan Paul, 1987), p. 189. Also see Jane Caplan, "Sexuality and Homosexuality," in Cambridge Women's Studies Group, *Women in Society: Interdisciplinary Essays* (London: Virago, 1981), pp. 157–59; Gay, *Freud,* pp. 146, 610; Phyllis Grosskurth, Introduction to J. A. Symonds, *The Memoirs of John Addington Symonds,* ed. Grosskurth (Chicago: University of Chicago Press, 1986), pp. 21–22.
41. Allbutt, "Neurasthenia," pp. 759–60, 788 (italics in original).
42. Mercier made his point in such works as *A Text-Book of Insanity and Other Mental Diseases,* first published in 1902, but entirely revised for the second edition in 1914, and in his essay on "Vice, Crime and Insanity," in vol. 8 of Allbutt and Rolleston, *System of Medicine.* For further comments on British psychiatric repudiation of psychoanalysis, see Clark, "Rejection of Psychological Approaches," pp. 298–300, and Stone, "Shellshock and the Psychologists," pp. 243, 255.
43. James Crichton-Browne, Foreword to G. Rutherford Jeffrey, *Common Symptoms of an Unsound Mind* (London: H. K. Lewis, 1923), p. xiv; Armstrong-Jones quoted in Stone, "Shellshock and the Psychologists," p. 247.
44. James Crichton-Browne, *Victorian Jottings from an Old Commonplace Book* (London: Etchells & MacDonald, 1926), pp. 64, 105–106.
45. James Crichton-Browne, *What the Doctor Thought* (London: Ernest Benn, 1930), pp. 227–28, 248–49.
46. James Crichton-Browne, *The Doctor's After Thoughts* (London: Ernest Benn, 1932), pp. 138–41. Also see *From the Doctor's Notebook* (London: Duckworth, 1937), p. 130.
47. Stone, "Shellshock and the Psychologists," pp. 246–47, 255.
48. See Jones, "Treatment of Neuroses," p. 342.
49. Robinson, *Intellectual History of Psychology,* pp. 385–86, compares the attitudes of Janet and Freud toward evidence; Donkin's introduction to Peter McBride, *Psycho-Analysts Analysed* (London: Heinemann Medical Books, 1924) as quoted in Ruth First and Ann Scott, *Olive Schreiner* (London: Andre Deutsch, 1980), p. 151n.
50. Charles S. Myers, *Present-Day Applications of Psychology, with Special Reference to Industry, Education and Nervous Breakdown* (London: Methuen, 1918), p. 44; T. S. Eliot to Julian Huxley, 26 Oct. 1921, as quoted in T. S. Eliot, *The Waste Land: A Facsimile and Transcript of the Original Drafts including the Annotations of Ezra Pound,* ed. Valerie Eliot (New York: Harcourt Brace Jovanovich; London: Faber & Faber, 1971), p. xxii.
51. D. Hack Tuke, "Presidential Address to the Medico-Psychological Association," *JMS* 27(Oct. 1881):333.
52. Janet's *Les Obsessions et la psychasthénie* was first published in 1903. See G. E. Berrios, "Obsessional Disorders during the Nineteenth Century: Terminological and Classificatory Issues," in Bynum, Porter, and Shepherd, eds. *Anatomy of Madness,* 1:173–74; and Barbara Sicherman, "The Uses of a Diagnosis: Doctors, Patients, and Neurasthenia," in Judith Walzer Leavitt and Ronald L. Numbers, eds., *Sickness and Health in America: Readings in the History of Medicine and Public Health* (Madison, Wisc.: University of Wisconsin Press, 1978), p. 26.
53. W. H. B. Stoddart, *Mind and Its Disorders. A Text-Book for Students and Practitioners* ·

(London: H. K. Lewis, 1908), pp. 354, 362. For his Freudian views, see W. H. B. Stoddart, *The New Psychiatry* (London: Baillière, Tindall, & Cox, 1915).

54. Alfred T. Schofield and R. Murray Leslie, "Psychasthenia," *BMJ*, 23 Nov. 1912, p. 1458.

55. Charles Mercier, *A Text-Book of Insanity and Other Mental Diseases*, 2d ed. rev. (London: George Allen & Unwin, 1914), p. xiii; T. S. Clouston, *Unsoundness of Mind* (London: Methuen, 1911), pp. 172–73. Stanley W. Jackson, *Melancholia and Depression: From Hippocratic Times to Modern Times* (New Haven and London: Yale University Press, 1986), pp. 270–73, summarizes the development of Kraepelin's concept of the manic-depressive family of disorders.

56. Richard Hunter, "Psychiatry and Neurology," *Proceedings of the Royal Society of Medicine* 66(April 1973):360.

57. Jones, "Treatment of the Neuroses," p. 332.

58. Lewis, "Maudsley," p. 271.

59. Myers, *Present-Day Applications of Psychology*, p. 41.

INDEX